GASTROENTEROLOGY NURSING
A Core Curriculum

Gastroenterology Nursing

A Core Curriculum

Coordinated by the

**Society of Gastroenterology
Nurses and Associates**
Core Curriculum Committee

illustrated

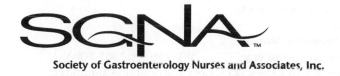

Society of Gastroenterology Nurses and Associates, Inc.

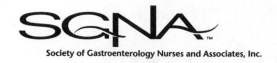

Society of Gastroenterology Nurses and Associates, Inc.

Publisher: The Society of Gastroenterology Nurses and Associates, Inc.
Editor: Vanessa Griffin
Project Manager: Cynthia Mangahis Friis, MEd BSN RN

THIRD EDITION

Printed in the United States of America

Library of Congress Cataloging in Publication Data
Gastroenterology nursing: a core curriculum / coordinated by the Society of Gastroenterology Nurses and Associates, Core Curriculum
Committee.—3rd ed.
     p.;   cm.
   Includes bibliographical references and index.
   ISBN 0-9702133-7-9 (hardcover)
   1. Gastrointestinal system—Diseases—Nursing.
   [DNLM: 1. Gastrointestinal Diseases—nursing.   WY 156.5 G2565 2003]
   I. Society of Gastroenterology Nurses and Associates. Core Curriculum Committee.
RC802.G363 2003
616.3'3'0231—DC22

                                                    2003018888
                                                    CIP

SGNA CORE
CURRICULUM COMMITTEE

Trina Van Guilder, RN, BSN, CGRN
University of Kentucky
Georgetown, Kentucky
Education Committee Program Chair

Cathleen Ferraro, RN, BA, CGRN
Dartmouth Hitchcock Medical Clinic
Rutland, Vermont
Education Committee Board Liaison

Linda Amick, RN, CGRN
Veterans' Administration Medical Center
Lexington, Kentucky

Linda Holmes, BSN, RN, CGRN
Bethesda Naval Hospital
Bethesda, Maryland

Jennifer Gleason, LPN, CGN
Tacoma Endoscopy Center
Puyallup, Washington

Betty McGinty, BS, RN, CGRN
Saint Josephs Hospital
Atlanta, Georgia

Nancy Robertson, RN, CGRN
The Methodist Hospital
Houston, Texas

Cynthia Mangahis Friis, RN, BSN, MEd
SGNA Headquarters
Chicago, Illinois
Staff Liaison

CONTRIBUTORS

The third edition of *Gastroenterology Nursing: A Core Curriculum* is made possible by the following contributors and reviewers who so generously shared their time, knowledge and expertise on this project.

Margaret Mays, RN, CGRN, BSN
Chapter 1
Dayton Veterans' Administration Medical Center
Dayton, Ohio

Randall V. Brinson, BSN, RN
Chapter 2
Dallas Southwest Medical Center
Dallas, Texas

Genia M. Spaulding, BS, MSN, CGRN
Chapter 3
Endoscopy Center North
Cincinnati, Ohio

Cynthia Gail Burton, RN, CGRN
Chapter 4
Baptist Physician's Surgery Center
Lexington, Kentucky

Jo E. Malham, RN
Chapter 5
Memorial Medical Center
Springfield, Illinois

Linda Amick, RN, CGRN
Chapter 6
Veterans' Administration Medical Center
Lexington, Kentucky

Marian Kerbleski, BSN, RN
Chapter 7
San Francisco Medical Center
San Francisco, California

Marianne Houlne, RN, CGRN
Chapters 8 & 9
Valley Internal Medicine
Renton, Washington

Colleen Kelley Keith, MSN, RN, CGRN
Chapters 10 & 11
The King's Daughters' Hospital
Madison, Indiana

Cathy S. Birn, MA, RN, CGRN, CNOR
Chapter 12
Memorial Sloan Kettering Cancer Center
New York, New York

Cynthia D. Schwab, RN, CGRN
Chapters 13 & 14
Saint Josephs Hospital
Atlanta, Georgia

Deborah Chandler, MS, BS, RN, CGRN
Chapters 15 & 16
Piedmont Hospital
Atlanta, Georgia

Donna Duncan, BSN, RN, CGRN
Chapters 17, 18 & 19
Saint Josephs Hospital
Atlanta, Georgia

Priscilla Ann Taylor, RN, CNS-FARNP
Chapters 20 and 21
UCLA Medical Center
Los Angeles, California

Diane Clain, MSA, RD
Chapter 22
Proctor, Vermont

Leslie Stewart, RN, CGRN
Chapter 23
Jersey Shore Medical Center
Neptune, New Jersey

Terri Herzog, BSN, RN, CGRN
Chapter 24
Rush University
Chicago, Illinois

Janet Hannah, RN, CGRN
Chapter 25
Loudoun Hospital
Leesburg, Virginia

Christine L. Smith, BSN, RN
Chapter 26
Johns Hopkins Hospital
Baltimore, Maryland

Julie A. Hanby, RN, CGRN
Chapter 27
Methodist Hospital
Houston, Texas

Mary B. McCoy, RN
Chapter 28
Methodist Hospital
Houston, Texas

Sandra L. Leveritt, RN
Chapter 29
Methodist Willowbrook Hospital
Houston, Texas

Gail E. Schlueck, MSN, CGRN
Chapter 30
San Francisco General Hospital
San Francisco, California

Deborah Walz, BSN, RN, CGRN
Chapter 31
Desert Samaritan Medical Center
Mesa, Arizona

Nancy Robertson, RN, CGRN
Chapter 32
The Methodist Hospital
Houston, Texas

REVIEWERS

Rosemary Becker, ADN, CGRN
Chapter 1
St. Francis Medical Center
Trenton, New Jersey

Judy Gugerty, MS, RN, CNOR
Chapter 2
Jewish Hospital
Louisville, Kentucky

Diane Fox, MS, RN, CGRN
Chapter 3
Private Consultant
Germantown, New York

Karen Laing, RN, CGRN
Chapter 4 & 28
Fairview Southdale Hospital
Minneapolis, Minnesota

Geraldine Simpson, ADN
Chapter 5
Mayo Clinic
Jacksonville, Florida

Rose Ann Freier, BSN, RN, CGRN
Chapter 6
Harris Methodist-Fort Worth
Fort Worth, Texas

Ann Hayes, BSN, RN, CGRN
Chapter 7
Veterans' Administration Medical Center
San Francisco, California

Joyce B. Packer, RN, BS, CGRN
Chapter 7
Veterans' Administration Medical Center
San Francisco, California

Marsha L. Ellett, DNS, RN, CGRN
Chapter 7 – Pediatric
Indiana University/Purdue University
Indianapolis, Indiana

Constance J. Saxton, RN, CGRN, BSN
Chapters 8 & 9
Mercy Hospital of Tiffin
Tiffin, Ohio

Debra Hoffman, BS, RN, CGRN
Chapters 10 & 11
University of Colorado Hospital
Denver, Colorado

Margaret G. Coffey, MSN, BSN, RN, CGRN
Chapter 12
Memorial Health University Medical Center
Savannah, Georgia

Cathy M. Dykes, MS, RN, CGRN, CCRC
Chapter 13
University of Texas at Southwestern Medical School
Dallas, Texas

Cheryl L. Calabro, RN, BSN
Chapter 13 – Pediatric
Children's Mercy Hospital
Kansas City, Missouri

Mary Anne Malone, RN, CGRN
Chapter 14
Samaritan Hospital
Troy, New York

Daphne Pierce-Smith, RN, MSN, CCRC
Chapters 14 & 17 – Pediatric
Emory University School of Medicine
Atlanta, Georgia

John Cavazos, RN, BSN, CGRN
Chapter 15
Northeast Methodist Hospital
San Antonio, Texas

Lynn E. Mattis, RN, MSN
Chapter 15 - Pediatric
Johns Hopkins Hospital
Baltimore, Maryland

Maureen Mehelic, BSN, RN, CGRN
Chapter 16
Saint Luke's Hospital
Chesterfield, Missouri

Rita Malfeo-Klein, RN, BSN
Chapter 16 - Pediatric
The University of Chicago Children's Hospital
Chicago, Illinois

Anne E. Streeter, BSN, RN, CGRN
Chapter 17
Saint Mary's Hospital
Grand Rapids, Michigan

Sandra A. Cialfi, MBA, BSN, RN, CGRN
Chapter 18
Brigham and Women's Hospital
Boston, Massachusetts

Susan N. Peck, MSN, CRNP
Chapter 18 - Pediatric
Children's Hospital of Philadelphia
Philadelphia, Pennsylvania

Kathryn South, BSN, RN, CGRN
Chapter 19
Integris Baptist Medical Center
Oklahoma City, Oklahoma

Cindy R. Brown, RN, BSN
Chapter 19 - Pediatric
University of Nebraska Medical Center
Omaha, Nebraska

Michael Lyons,
Chapters 20 & 21
Tacoma Digestive Disease Center
Tacoma, Washington

Rosemary Young, RN, MS
Chapters 20 & 22 - Pediatric
University of Nebraska
Omaha, Nebraska

Carrie Bartlett, RN, MPH
Chapter 21- Pediatric
Children's Hospital of New Orleans
New Orleans, Louisiana

Cathleen Ferraro, RN, BA, CGRN
Chapter 22
Dartmouth Hitchcock Medical Clinic
Lebanon, New Hampshire

Catherine DeAngelo, RN, AD, CGRN
Chapter 23
Jersey Shore Medical Center
Neptune, New Jersey

Adelina McDuffie, MS, RN, CPNP
Chapter 23 - Pediatric
Children's Specialty Group
Norfolk, Virginia

Eleonor Vergara, BSN, RN, CGRN
Chapter 24
Rush University
Chicago, Illinois

Cindy Crawford, RN
Chapter 24 - Pediatric
Baptist Medical Center
Jacksonville, Florida

Shari Huffman, MN, CPNP
Chapter 24 - Pediatric
Baptist Medical Center
Jacksonville, Florida

Linda Holmes, BSN, RN, CGRN
Chapter 25
Bethesda Naval Hospital
Bethesda, Maryland

James M. Gulizia, MD, PhD
Chapter 25 - Pediatric
University of Nebraska Medical Center
Omaha, Nebraska

Donna Beitler, RN
Chapter 26
Johns Hopkins Hospital
Baltimore, Maryland

Benita Riley, RN, MS
Chapters 26 & 31 - Pediatric
New York, New York

Robbie K. McAllister, RN, CGRN
Chapter 27
MD Anderson Cancer Center
Houston, Texas

Darlene Gassoway, BSN, RN, CGRN
Chapter 29
Saint Luke's Episcopal Hospital
Houston, Texas

Sandra J. Thomas, RN, CGRN
Chapter 30
Cape Coral Hospital
Cape Coral, Florida

Evon L. Dowd, RN, CGRN, BS
Chapter 31
Rockford Gastroenterology Associates
Rockford, Illinois

Carol Ponsolle, RN, CGRN
Chapter 32
Minnesota Gastroenterology
St. Paul, Minnesota

Theresa M. Shalaby, RN, BSN
Chapter 32 - Pediatric
Pediatric GI Children's Hospital
Pittsburgh, Pennsylvania

PREFACE

Diagnostic and Therapeutic Endoscopy continues to offer new advancements in technology each year. As Endoscopy techniques have advanced throughout the years, we have exceeded all previous expectations once thought possible through the use of an Endoscope.

As these Endoscopy technologies continue to advance so does the need to keep our nurses and associates informed of changes within the field. The need for current, evidence based practices, standards development and training become vital to the delivery of patient care within every Endoscopy department.

In response to this need, the Core Curriculum was originally published in 1993 and has since been reviewed and updated on a regularly scheduled basis. This current publication represents the third edition. It provides the most updated information on practices in Endoscopic procedure technologies, pharmacology, reprocessing of Endoscopy equipment, current SGNA role delineation statements, review of surgical interventions common to the gastrointestinal tract and much more.

This Core Curriculum serves as a reference designed to meet the needs of all members of the GI & Endoscopy team. It provides a knowledge base for GI & Endoscopy Nursing and hence, serves as a valuable study guide for certification in Gastroenterology.

This edition recognizes the variety of educational backgrounds of gastroenterology nurses and associates, as well as the many different settings in which they practice. As in the first edition, the word nurse is used throughout when describing tasks or situations shared by all disciplines. RN is used in instances where tasks or judgments are solely the responsibility of the registered nurse.

I wish to thank the authors, reviewers, and editors of the first edition, because this text was built on the solid foundation they laid. In addition, I would like to thank the 2002-2003 SGNA Education Committee who worked diligently to recruit expert SGNA members from across the nation as contributors and reviewers for this publication. This represents an enormous amount of effort and knowledge sharing on the part of the author's. The information provided in this Curriculum is supported by evidence based practice.

This edition is clearly an outstanding example of the SGNA Education Committee uniting together with SGNA's membership to provide an outstanding publication made available to Endoscopy departments across the nation.

Final acknowledgements and thanks to Cindy Friis, the SGNA Educational Staff Liaison, for her persistence and compassion in working with over 60 contributors, reviewers, and the Education Committee to gather, organize and edit revised content.

Trina VanGuilder, RN, BSN, CGRN
SGNA Education Committee Chair

CONTENTS

GASTROENTEROLOGY
NURSING
A Core Curriculum

GASTROENTEROLOGY NURSING PRACTICE

Chapter 1

THE GASTROENTEROLOGY NURSE AND ASSOCIATE

This chapter reviews the background leading to the development of specialized health care workers in the area of gastroenterology. The scope of practice in this setting is outlined, as are the competencies required to provide quality care for patients who are having endoscopic diagnostic and therapeutic treatments. Educational preparation and job qualifications are addressed. Practice settings and the types of positions needed and required responsibilities and functions are emphasized.

Learning objectives

After reviewing the content of this chapter, the gastroenterology nurse should be able to:

1. Trace the evolution of gastroenterology nursing as an area of specialization.
2. Discuss the scope of practice in the gastroenterology setting and the educational requirements needed to practice gastroenterology nursing.
3. Describe the general responsibilities and functions of the gastroenterology nurse and associate.
4. Delineate the roles of the gastroenterology nurse and associate, as specified by the Society of Gastroenterology Nurses and Associates, Inc. (SGNA).
5. Give examples of the job responsibilities of nurse managers, staff nurses, and associates in a typical gastroenterology unit.

BACKGROUND AND HISTORICAL PERSPECTIVE

As far back as records show, the care of the sick has constituted a role in everyday life. Witch doctors performed their rituals and departed, leaving someone else to follow through with the care. Nursing care was first differentiated from medicine in the fourth century by Hindu physician B.C. Charaka, who referred to the "aggregate of four," composed of the physician, the drug, the nurse, and the patient. Hippocrates referred to caregivers as assistants to the physi-

cian. There are accounts from the pre-Christian era of nurses involved in caring for the sick. Archaeological discoveries describe early nursing procedures as dressing wounds and feeding patients.

The Egyptians had a highly developed medical community wherein the members of the medical profession were organized so they could protect the secrets of their practice. The Egyptians were as progressive as today's physicians in that they had specialists dedicated to one disease, such as treatment of the eyes, head, or stomach. Accounts of the Egyptians, Greeks, and Romans all refer to the existence of midwives, whose art was the care of child-bearing women. When their civilizations declined, medical care of women deteriorated and was not brought back to its former stage of development until the seventeenth century.

During the Middle Ages, nursing was done primarily by women and was the function of many religious orders. Between 500 and 1300 A.D., nursing care consisted of only the most menial tasks, such as bathing, feeding, and bed-making. The nuns, who were chiefly responsible for this care, were assisted by women who were being punished for thievery or prostitution. It was not until the nineteenth century that education and dignity were brought to the nursing profession. Florence Nightingale emancipated upper-class women from idleness and encouraged them to serve humanity. As women became educated, the care of the sick began to improve.

Throughout the nineteenth century, prominent women became involved in promoting the cause of nursing. School nursing, industrial nursing, and other nursing specializations began to emerge. As technology increased and physicians needed more time to learn and implement new techniques and practices, the responsibilities of nurses also increased. During the 1940s, Frances Reiter first described the nurse with advanced education and clinical competence as a "nurse clinician." This was the precursor of the nursing specialties that we recognize today.

Development of gastroenterology

As early as the time of Hippocrates, specific mention was made of the GI tract in medicine. Hippocrates recorded use of a candle to inspect the rectum. In 1795, Bozzini documented the use of a rigid sigmoidoscope. Almost 100 years later, Kussmaul made the first attempt to visualize the stomach with a rigid tube. Rigid esophagoscopy developed slowly over the next 50 years, with progress being dependent primarily on the quality of the light source. The rigid instrument was able to survey only a small portion of the stomach, and it carried a significant hazard because of the possibility of perforation.

In 1932, a semiflexible instrument was designed by Rudolph Schindler. The Schindler gastroscope remained the model for development of gastroscopes for the next 30 years. The semiflexible gastroscope was based on the principle that a series of convex lenses could transmit light undistorted through a flexible tube if the distal tube was not bent beyond a certain angle. Risk of perforation was reduced by the placement of a rubber obturator at the tip.

In 1958, Hirschowitz, Curtiss, Peters, and Pollard published their report of a new gastroscope, the fiberscope, which revolutionized gastroenterology. The development of fiberoptic scopes was made possible by the earlier work of **Professor Harold Hopkins** of Reading University in the United Kingdom. Hopkins worked with John Logie Baird, the inventor of television, to design fiberoptic bundles that would transmit an image. The optical principles are dependent on the total internal reflection of light in each fiber. The fiber bundles are of two types: noncoherent bundles, which conduct light but not images, and coherent bundles, which produce high-quality images.

Modern, flexible fiberoptic instruments have the same basic features as those developed in the early fifties. The simplicity, ease of use, and safety of the earlier instruments caused the rapid adoption of this new technology.

Development of gastroenterology nursing

Gastroenterology nursing was first recognized as an area of specialization in 1941, when a group of physicians called the American Gastroscopic Club met at Dr. Rudolph Schindler's home in Chicago. This group was later named the Gastroscopic Society and was the forerunner of the American Society for Gastrointestinal Endoscopy. At that time, Dr. Schindler was the recognized master gastroscopist and his wife, Gabriele, was the first gastroenterology assistant. **Gabriele Schindler** was always at her husband's side, soothing the patient, helping with positioning, and assisting during the procedure. The memory of Gabriele personifies the spirit of professionalism and caring that has become the mark of excellence for today's gastroenterology nurses and associates. Beginning in 1985, SGNA has annually presented the Gabriele Schindler Award in recognition of high standards and outstanding achievement in gastroenterology nursing.

The next several decades brought about many changes in gastroenterology nursing practice and education. Fiberoptic instrumentation developed rapidly and the demand for skilled personnel to care for patients, instrumentation, and equipment increased, resulting in the need for dedicated personnel to work with patients who were undergoing endoscopic procedures. Physicians demanded a specialized unit within the hospital to perform GI procedures. A nurse or assistant was required to attend the patient and assist the physician with the procedure. Initially, the role of the gastroenterology nurse was to support the patient while the physician inserted the scope. It soon became evident that a successful unit called for someone who would not only care for the patient but also set standards and develop some order within the unit. There was a need for procurement and maintenance of instruments, checking patient consent forms, dispensing and documentation of medications, documentation of patient responses to treatment, and recording of information for hospital reports.

As the complexity of procedures increased, government and regulatory agencies added another aspect to the knowledge base required. The Centers for Disease Control and Prevention (CDC), Joint Commission on Accreditation of Healthcare Organizations (JCAHO), and other organizations all put forth guidelines, which required that gastroenterology personnel be informed of these new regulations and guidelines and integrate them into practice settings. Persons functioning in gastroenterology units felt a need for a support group or network of individuals to unite those associated with the practice of gastroenterology.

Society of Gastroenterology Nurses and Associates

The new guidelines and the subsequent need for support groups led to the formation of the Society of Gastrointestinal Assistants (SGA) in 1974. The first members of this group sought identification, respect, and national recognition of their activities. Their goals were to collect information, establish guidelines for future professionals, and expand specialized educational opportunities. SGA decided to hold annual meetings in May, concurrently with the annual educational meeting of gastroenterologists.

As the Society grew, the need to communicate information to the membership on an ongoing basis became evident. Therefore, in 1977 the first issue of the *SGA Journal* was published. Since 1989, the title of the journal has been *Gastroenterology Nursing*. Also in 1977, nine regional societies were established to give members the opportunity to meet during the year in geographically accessible areas. The number of regional societies has increased gradually to more than 65 and continues to increase.

In 1989, SGA changed its name to the **Society of Gastroenterology Nurses and Associates, Inc. (SGNA),** to better reflect the composition of its membership. According to a 2001 report, SGNA members include registered nurses (RNs, 80%); licensed practical nurses (LPNs, 8%); licensed medical technicians or technologists (LMTs or MTs), radiology technologists (RTs), equipment technicians, and associates (3%). The remainder comprised affiliate members such as vendors, managers, and consultants.

The American Nurses Association (ANA) and independent specialty groups believed there was merit in establishing a mechanism to measure the competency of nurses in the practice setting. Certification for gastroenterology nursing had its beginning in the early 1980s. A standing committee on certification was established by SGA to develop a certification program for gastroenterology clinicians. In 1985, the Certification Committee became the independent Certifying Council for Gastroenterology Clinicians, Inc.. In 1986, a total of 666 candidates took the first certifying examination. This voluntary certification program is aimed both at assuring the patient that the caregiver has acquired a proficient level of knowledge and at publicly recognizing the individual nurse/associate. The membership of SGNA continues to grow as the Society demonstrates its commitment to further education and practice for the member.

In 1990, to be consistent with the professional society, the name was changed again to the Certifying Board for Gastroenterology Nurses and Associates (CBGNA). Further refinement of the certifying process began that same year. Task analysis and role delineations serve to differentiate competency areas for the RN and the associate. Two distinctly different examinations are now administered. For information about the examination contents and requirements for certification, contact CBGNA directly.

SCOPE OF PRACTICE

Delineating a **scope of practice** is the responsibility of a professional society. The practice of nursing is further defined by state regulatory agencies and institutional policies and procedures.

As the professional society for nursing in the United States, ANA has assumed the responsibility of providing a current definition of nursing that reflects the dynamic, evolving role of professional nurses. In 1978, the Executive Committee of ANA's Division on Medical-Surgical Nursing Practice appointed an ad hoc committee to identify and describe the parameters of medical-surgical nursing. A statement on the scope of medical-surgical nursing practice was published in 1980. This statement defines the practice, delineates its dimensions, and outlines the functions of a professional nurse. This comprehensive definition served as a guide to emerging specialty organizations and societies.

SGNA has developed a scope of practice that is directly related to the development of a task analysis for certification. Gastroenterology nursing practice is defined as the nursing care of patients with known or suspected GI problems who are undergoing diagnostic or therapeutic endoscopic procedures. Nursing care includes the care and treatment necessary to provide comfort, assist individuals in the promotion and maintenance of health, provide for the physical and emotional needs of the patient, and provide safe and proficient care during endoscopy and other specialized procedures. It encompasses patient assessment, nursing diagnosis, outcome identification, planning, implementation,

and evaluation of patient care. The biological, psychological, and social components of the patient's response or adjustment to illness or disability are also taken into account. Gastroenterology nurses and associates use and adapt theories in microbiology, communication, ethics, and the behavioral sciences to form the basis of practice. That practice is continually influenced by the patient's physiological alteration, the patient's and family's needs for support and assistance, collaboration between medicine and nursing, and the level of professional autonomy in the practice setting.

EDUCATION AND TRAINING

SGNA continues to broaden its scope of practice and update standards for practice and the certification process. It is also essential to develop requirements for education and training of personnel who will be working in this practice setting, because those factors have direct effect on the quality of patient care provided.

Educational requirements for RNs include graduation from an accredited school of nursing and a license to practice nursing. SGNA recommends that RNs specializing in the field of gastroenterology have at least 1 year of general medical-surgical experience. This enables the **gastroenterology nurse** to practice acquired skills and be exposed to "first-line" management. In general, individuals should possess the following educational backgrounds:

1. Solid education and training in the biological sciences.
2. Pertinent experiences in the health care field.
3. Familiarity with hospital and other practice settings.

Specific content areas that might be incorporated into a specialty training program include the following:

1. Anatomy and physiology of the GI tract and relationships to pathophysiology and relevant diagnostic and therapeutic procedures.
2. Techniques of management and administration of a gastroenterology unit.
3. Skills in patient care, teaching, and staff development.
4. Care and maintenance of clinical instruments.
5. Pharmacology and IV therapy.
6. Emergency situations.
7. Research methods and application of published research to the practice setting.
8. Ethical, professional, and legal standards inherent in professional conduct.

Throughout this text and in documents published by SGNA, the term *gastroenterology nurse* includes both RNs and LPNs or licensed vocational nurses, because many aspects of their practice overlap. Material pertaining only to RNs is clearly identified. A **gastroenterology associate** is defined as a "health care professional with varied educational background engaged in the field of gastroenterology." This educational background may include certification, such as an RT or operating room technologist (ORT) has, or on-the-job training, such as a patient care technician receives. In a hospital setting, the associate is legally accountable to an RN (JCAHO, 1996). Unless otherwise specified, the term *nursing* is used to describe the spectrum of professional responsibilities and tasks undertaken by nurses and associates.

JOB RESPONSIBILITIES AND FUNCTIONS

Gastroenterology health care workers perform a variety of functions in various practice settings. SGNA members work in hospitals, clinics, free-standing endoscopy units, operating rooms, and physicians' offices. General areas of responsibility include patient care, care of instruments and equipment, management, teaching and research, and documentation. Gastroenterology nurses also perform some gastroenterologic procedures independently, including esophageal and anal manometry, gastric analysis, and rigid and flexible sigmoidoscopy.

Patient care

Gastroenterology team members are responsible for the care of patients undergoing diagnostic and therapeutic gastroenterologic procedures. Preparation before a procedure includes instruction on physical preparation of the patient, such as food or medication restrictions. It is also important to meet the patient's psychological needs by reassuring the patient, explaining the procedure, and instilling confidence. A brief history is taken to evaluate and assess any pertinent medical or surgical conditions. Baseline vital signs are recorded, and a brief physical assessment is done.

During the procedure, care is directed at ensuring the patient's physical safety and psychological well-being. Emphasis is placed on monitoring and assessing the patient, because the physician must concentrate his or her attention on the procedure. The nurse or associate must have a thorough understanding of the purpose of the procedure and how the procedure will be performed. He or she assists the physician with various technical aspects of the procedure, such as biopsy, polypectomy, or coagulation. The nurse or associate continues to offer reassurance to the patient throughout the procedure. The nurse continually assesses the patient's response to sedation and to the procedure, intervening when appropriate.

At the completion of the procedure, the nurse continues to monitor the patient's response to the procedure and to any medication administered. Patients who are sedated during the procedure will require time to recover. Assessment is also directed toward identification of potential and/or actual complications related to the procedure. The nurse must ascertain that the patient has met the institution's discharge criteria before the patient is released. At discharge, the patient receives a written explanation about follow-up care and how to contact health personnel if problems arise. A family member, if available, should be included in any discharge education to ensure a clear understanding of postprocedure instructions.

Management

The scope of nursing management and the responsibilities of the manager of the gastroenterology department vary depending on the types of procedures performed and the services provided. Management functions include developing the organizational structure of the department (e.g., lines of communication and authority), standards for practice, policies and procedures, position descriptions, and performance appraisals. Management also involves developing a budget, determining staffing patterns, coordinating services, projecting for new/replacement equipment needs as technology changes, and being fiscally accountable to the department.

Care of instruments and equipment

Gastroenterology nurses and associates must demonstrate technical competency in instrument and equipment care. Knowledge of the decontamination process is essential. Understanding the current facts about disinfection and sterilization ensures safe patient care. Nurses and associates must also know how to maintain the instruments and equipment and arrange for repair when required.

Teaching and research

Individuals working in the gastroenterology department have a responsibility to share knowledge. This may be done through staff development and orientation programs or through continuing education. Participation in professional organizations also offers an excellent opportunity to exchange information. The manager of the department has the responsibility to assess the level of expertise of the staff and encourage employees to plan for their own personal and professional growth. It remains the responsibility of individual nurses or associates to identify their own learning needs, acquire necessary knowledge, and stay abreast of current technologies.

Participating in and communicating clinical research are also vital parts of the gastroenterology nurse's or associate's role. Research may entail participation in drug trial studies, testing new instruments or procedures, or evaluating the effectiveness of treatment. Whatever the research, the nurse or associate must have some background in data collection, documentation, analysis, and interpretation. Publication offindings is essential for communicating results of research to the health care community. In addition, presentation of a paper or poster at a professional meeting is an excellent way for the nurse or associate to meet the responsibility of expanding current knowledge. Knowledge of research techniques also allows for critical evaluation of published materials.

Documentation

Documentation of patient care and maintenance of records and department reports are other responsibilities of the gastroenterology team member. Documentation requirements vary according to institutional policy and the particular endoscopy setting, but the JCAHO stipulates the following minimum documentation requirements:

- Documentation of a preprocedural patient assessment, including physical and psychosocial factors, current medications, treatment, and previous medical, anesthesia, and drug history; review of the patient's symptoms and general history of the current GI complaint.

- Documentation of the procedure performed; equipment used; staff involved; drugs, fluids, and anesthesia administered; unusual events and intervention; patient status at the conclusion of the procedure; type of specimen(s) obtained and disposition; and postprocedure diagnosis.
- Documentation of the postprocedural physical and mental status of the patient including but not limited to vital signs, level of consciousness, drugs and IV fluids, unusual events and intervention, discharge instructions, and disposition of patient.

SGNA has available a documentation guideline that details pertinent JCAHO documentation requirements and lists types of information that might be included on preprocedure, procedure, and postprocedure forms, and when providing discharge instructions to outpatients.

ROLE DELINEATION

The following role delineation statements have been issued by SGNA to outline the scope of practice of nurses and associates.

Role delineation of the registered nurse in a staff position in gastroenterology and/or endoscopy

The role of the RN has expanded with the changes in advancing technology and newly-defined patient needs. Recognizing that the role of the staff nurse in gastroenterology and/or endoscopy is still evolving, the following is a statement on the current activities common to this role.

Preface

The purpose of this role delineation is to broadly describe the responsibilities and functions of the RN in a staff role specializing in gastroenterology and/or endoscopy nursing. The roles the nurse assumes depend on his or her basic nursing preparation, specialized formal or informal education, and clinical experiences. Certification as a gastroenterology registered nurse (CGRN) validates the acquisition of such skills and knowledge. The RN practices in a variety of settings, such as hospitals, private offices, ambulatory surgery centers, and clinics. The RN functions within the scope of practice as defined by the state nurse practice act, job description of the employing facility, SGNA Standards of Practice, and ANA's Code of Ethics.

Role delineation statement

The RN is accountable for the quality of nursing care rendered to patients. The RN assumes responsibility for assessing, planning, implementing, directing, supervising, and evaluating direct and indirect nursing care for patients in the gastroenterology/endoscopy setting. The RN is responsible for determining the education and competency level of assistive personnel to whom he or she is delegating. The specific patient populations to whom direct care is provided include adults, adolescents, and children with GI disorders/diseases.

The role of the RN includes but is not limited to the following:

1. Establish nursing diagnoses.
2. Provide health education and procedural teaching to patients and significant others.
3. Administer and evaluate pharmacological and other therapeutic treatment regimens.
4. Establish priorities and make ethically sound decisions to ensure safe patient care.
5. Assist the physician during diagnostic and therapeutic procedures to promote optimal patient outcomes by team collaboration.
6. Respond to emergency situations to promote optimal patient outcomes by recognizing changes in the patient's health status.
7. Perform diagnostic studies as ordered by a physician.
8. Document patient data to ensure continuity in the provision and coordination of patient care.
9. Manage follow-up care.
10. Collaborate with other health care professionals.
11. Act as a resource for others.
12. Serve as a mentor for other nurses.
13. Participate in continuing education and achieving/maintaining certification.
14. Participate in data collection for research and using scientific findings to improve patient outcomes.
15. Monitor performance by developing and participating in quality management activities.
16. Participate as an active member in professional and consumer organizations, contributing to professional publications and presentations at professional meetings.

Role delineation of the licensed practical/vocational nurse in gastroenterology and/or endoscopy

The role of the licensed practical/vocational nurse (LP/VN) has expanded with the changes in advancing technology and newly defined patient needs. Recognizing that the role of the LP/VN in gastroenterology and/or endoscopy is still evolving, the following is a statement on the current activities common to this role.

Preface

The purpose of this role delineation is to describe the responsibilities and functions of the LP/VN specializing in gastroenterology and/or endoscopy nursing. The roles the LP/VN assumes depend on his or her basic nursing preparation, specialized formal or informal education, and clinical experiences. Certification as a gastroenterology nurse (CGN) validates the acquisition of such skills and knowledge. The LP/VN practices in various settings, such as hospitals, private offices, ambulatory surgery centers, and clinics. The LP/VN functions within the scope of practice as defined by the state nurse practice act, job description of the employing facility, SGNA Standards of Practice, and National Federation of Licensed Practical Nurses (NFLPN) Code for Licensed Practical/Vocational Nurses.

Role delineation statement

Under the supervision of a licensed RN or physician, the LP/VN is accountable for the quality of nursing care he or she provides to patients. Utilizing the nursing process, the LP/VN assumes responsibility for planning, implementing, directing, and evaluating nursing care for assigned patients in the gastroenterology/endoscopy setting. The specific patient populations to whom direct care is provided include adults, adolescents, and children with GI disorders/diseases.

The role of the LP/VN includes but is not limited to the following:

1. Observe, record, and report significant changes requiring intervention or changes in the patient's care plan.
2. Implement interventions within the limitations of licensure and institutional policy.
3. Provide health education and procedural teaching to patients and significant others.
4. Administer and evaluate pharmacological and other therapeutic treatment regimens within the limitations of licensure and institutional policy.
5. Contribute to the planning, implementation, and evaluation of patient care.
6. Establish priorities and make ethically sound decisions to ensure safe patient care.
7. Assist the physician and/or RN during diagnostic and therapeutic procedures to promote optimal patient outcomes by team collaboration.
8. Respond to emergency situations to promote optimal patient outcomes by recognizing changes in the patient's health status.
9. Perform diagnostic studies as ordered by a physician.
10. Document patient data to ensure continuity in the provision and coordination of patient care.
11. Assist with follow-up care.
12. Collaborate with other health care professionals.
13. Act as a resource for others.
14. Serve as a mentor for others.
15. Participate in continuing education and achieving/ maintaining certification.
16. Participate in data collection for research and using scientific findings to improve patient outcomes.
17. Monitor performance by developing and participating in quality management activities.
18. Participate as an active member in professional and consumer organizations, contributing to professional publications, and presentations at professional meetings.

Role delineation of assistive personnel

The changing health care environment has compelled the reassessment of the roles and tasks involved in providing patient care in endoscopy and gastroenterology practice settings. The following is a statement on the role of assistive personnel (unlicensed personnel; e.g., GI assistants, GI technicians, medical techs) who have direct patient care responsibility and are supervised by an RN.

Preface

Assistive personnel are accountable to and perform duties under the direct, on-site supervision of the RN when providing delegated patient care. As the person accountable for the outcomes of the patient care provided during the endoscopy experience, the RN is responsible for assessing patient care needs and determining the education and competency level of assistive personnel to whom he or she is delegating.

Role delineation statement

Assistive personnel contribute to optimal patient outcomes by providing delegated patient care activities after demonstrating competency, and within the following limits. Assistive personnel can:

1. Assist in collecting data for an objective assessment to identify the patient's needs, problems, concerns, or human responses (e.g., vital signs).
2. Assist, under the direction of the RN, in the implementation of the established plan of care.
3. Assist the physician and RN during diagnostic and therapeutic procedures. Respond to emergency situations as directed by the RN.

Assistive personnel will:

1. Provide and maintain a safe environment for the patient and staff by complying with regulatory agency requirements and standards set forth by professional organizations and employers.
2. Be responsible for personal continuing education.
3. Be knowledgeable about professional and practice issues related to the field of endoscopy/gastroenterology.
4. Comply with ethical, professional, and legal standards inherent in patient care and professional conduct (e.g., patient's bill of rights).
5. Participate in organizational performance improvement (PI) activities as directed.

Role delineation of the advanced practice nurse in Gastroenterology /Hepatology and Endoscopy

The changing health care environment has led to the development of expanded roles for nurses with graduate degrees in clinical specialties. Recognizing that the advanced practice nursing role in gastroenterology/hepatology and endoscopy is still evolving, the following is a statement on the current activities common to this role.

Preface

The purpose of this role delineation is to broadly describe the responsibilities and functions of the advanced practice nurse (APN) specializing in gastroenterology/hepatology and endoscopy nursing. The APN may be either a clinical nurse specialist or nurse practitioner who has completed an advanced degree in nursing (master's or doctorate) and who, through study and supervised clinical practice, has become an expert in a clinical area of nursing—in this instance, gastroenterology/hepatology and endoscopy. The scope of practice of the APN is distinguished by the level of complexity, responsibility, and autonomy of practice. The APN works in a variety of settings, such as hospitals, private offices, ambulatory surgery centers, and clinics. The APN functions within the scope of practice as defined by the state nurse practice act, job description of the employing facility, SGNA Standards of Practice, and ANA's Code of Ethics.

Role delineation statement

The APN provides service through direct care, consultation, research, education, and collaboration with other health care professionals. The specific patient populations to whom direct care is provided include adults, adolescents, and/or children with GI or hepatic disorders/diseases. The care provided may include, but is not limited to, advanced assessment, diagnosis, treatment/care planning, implementation, evaluation, and patient education. The following are general statements describing the major principles of the role.

The role of the APN includes but is not limited to the following:

1. Perform a comprehensive history and physical assessments.
2. Order and/or perform diagnostic studies.
3. Establish medical and nursing diagnoses.
4. Prescribe, administer and evaluate pharmacological and other therapeutic treatment regimens.
5. Manage follow-up care.
6. Collaborate with other health care professionals.
7. Act as a consultant for other providers regarding the medical and nursing care of clients.
8. Serve as a mentor for other nurses.
9. Identify and provide learning opportunities for other providers.
10. Document patient data to ensure continuity in the provision and coordination of patient care.
11. Establish priorities and making ethically sound decisions to ensure safe patient care.
12. Identify groups, families, and individuals at risk and developing a plan to address those risks, including, but not limited to, education programs, screening programs, and patient education materials.
13. Participate in continuing education and achieving/maintaining certification.
14. Participate in research and use of scientific findings to improve client outcomes.
15. Monitor performance by developing and participating in quality management activities.
16. Be a leader in professional and practice issues through active membership in professional and consumer organizations, publication of scholarly works, and presentations at professional meetings.

POSITION DESCRIPTIONS

The categories of individuals who perform functions in the gastroenterology department include:

- RNs, who may have titles such as supervisor, manager, head nurse, staff nurse, clinical nurse specialist, nurse clinician, nurse educator, nurse practitioner, nurse researcher, or patient care facilitator; and
- Associates, a group that may include LPNs, technicians, technologists, aides, or ancillary personnel.

The **position descriptions** for all of these individuals vary according to the practice setting and its organizational structure. The duties also vary depending on the size and number of procedures performed. In a hospital setting the location of the gastroenterology department in the organizational structure also has an effect on the types of responsibilities assigned to different personnel. Another variable is the method used throughout the hospital to formulate position descriptions and the subsequent evaluation mechanisms.

Position descriptions usually include a number of common elements, including: the title of the position; the department in which the position belongs; the person to whom the individual is responsible; a job summary; job qualifications such as level of education, experience required, and personal habits and characteristics; and specific duties or functions.

Nurse manager

Examples of the duties and responsibilities for the manager of the gastroenterology department include the following:

Planning and organization
1. Plan, coordinate, and direct the flow of patients through the gastroenterology department.
2. Allocate space and physical resources according to patient and physician need.
3. Develop and review department performance improvement standards.
4. Develop and update clinical competencies.

Management
1. Conduct performance reviews for assigned staff.
2. Monitor clinical performance for compliance with established standards and policies.

Staff allocation
1. Adjust staffing to meet workload volume.

Fiscal responsibility
1. Formulate and implement annual budget.

Education/orientation
1. Support staff orientation and cross-training through instruction, case selection, assignment of preceptors, and ongoing evaluation.
2. Assist staff in ongoing educational process.

Professional commitment
1. Actively participate in meetings or committees as assigned.
2. Actively pursue certification in the specialty.

Relationships, teamwork, delegation, and communication are other areas that might be included in the manager's position description.

Staff nurse (RN)

Selected examples of some of the duties and responsibilities that may be assigned to an RN staff nurse include the following:

Nursing process

1. Assessment
   a. Make initial observations of the patient on arrival at the gastroenterology unit.
   b. Formulate nursing diagnosis based on data collected.
   c. Provide assessment documentation that reflects the full range of patient needs, including physical, psychosocial, spiritual, and safety.
   d. Continue assessment of the patient throughout entire stay in the gastroenterology unit.
2. Nursing diagnosis
3. Outcome identification
4. Planning
   a. Individualize the plan of care, based on patient assessment.
   b. Prepare rooms, equipment, and supplies to accommodate the patient load.
5. Implementation
   a. Implement the plan of care.
   b. Assist physician with procedures.
   c. Monitor the patient before, during, and after the procedure.
   d. Provide patient education.
6. Evaluation
   a. Evaluate and document the patient's response to the nursing and medical plan of care.

Patient teaching

1. Assess patient's needs to include family or significant other when appropriate.
2. Provide patient with relevant information regarding diagnosis, medications, diet, and other therapy.

The above is only a sampling of the responsibilities that might appear. Other categories may include research and professional development.

Associate

Examples of duties and responsibilities that might be expected of associates include the following:

1. Assisting the physician with procedures
2. Implementing the plan of care under direction of an RN
3. Decontaminating instruments and equipment
   a. Receive and decontaminate instruments, equipment, and reusable supplies.
4. Sterilization and reprocessing
   a. Prepare items to be sterilized and maintain sterility through proper handling.
   b. Operate equipment used for cleaning and disinfecting endoscopic equipment.
5. Handling and storage
   a. Receive and place supplies in assigned storage area.

* * *

Examples of position descriptions, orientation programs,

and competency tools are available in a handbook published by SGNA (2002).

REVIEW TERMS

gastroenterology associate, gastroenterology nurse, Professor Harold Hopkins, position descriptions, role delineation, Gabriele Schindler, scope of practice, Society of Gastroenterology Nurses and Associates, Inc. (SGNA)

REVIEW QUESTIONS

1. The first recorded gastrointestinal assistant was:
   a. Florence Nightingale.
   b. Frances Reiter.
   c. Gabriele Schindler.
   d. B.C. Charaka.
2. During what period was medicine so far advanced that they had what is equivalent to today's subspecialties?
   a. Egyptians.
   b. Pre-Christian era.
   c. Middle Ages.
   d. Greeks and Romans.
3. The individual who first developed the fiberoptic telescope used for GI procedures was:
   a. Hippocrates.
   b. Hopkins.
   c. Schindler.
   d. Baird.
4. The rationale for the rapid adoption of fiberoptic instruments includes:
   a. Simplicity, ease of use, patient safety.
   b. Complex lens system, noncoherent bundles.
   c. Perfect imaging and ease of use.
   d. Combination of noncoherent bundles and coherent bundles to make a perfect image.
5. The first Society of Gastrointestinal Assistants (SGA) was formed in what year?
   a. 1968.
   b. 1976.
   c. 1972.
   d. 1974.
6. The practice of gastroenterology nursing requires application of the nursing process. The components include:
   a. Communicating, planning, evaluation, follow-up.
   b. Assessing, planning, implementing, evaluating.
   c. Interviewing, observing, communication, listening.
   d. Assessing, planning, evaluating, follow-up.
7. A gastroenterology associate is defined as:
   a. A nurse who is engaged in the field of gastroenterology.
   b. A non-RN health care professional with varied educational background engaged in the field of gastroenterology.
   c. An individual with advanced education who is engaged in gastroenterology.

d. An individual who is responsible for transporting patients and caring for instruments and equipment.

8. Initial assessment of patients on arrival to the gastroenterology unit is usually the responsibility of the:

   a. Physician.

   b. Nurse manager.

   c. Staff nurse (RN).

   d. Associate.

9. A general requirement for a recently graduated nurse who is interested in practicing gastroenterology nursing is:

   a. To work for 1 year on a medical-surgical unit to gain experience.

   b. To work for a private GI physician to gain knowledge of diagnosis and procedures.

   c. To work in a special procedures unit for 1 year.

   d. To work in an ambulatory care unit to practice skills for 1 year.

10. The gastroenterology nurse and associate roles are differentiated in that:

    a. The nurse's role is to formulate a nursing diagnosis and plan care accordingly.

    b. The associate's role is to formulate a nursing diagnosis and plan care accordingly.

    c. The associate is responsible for assisting only with the procedure.

    d. The nurse is primarily responsible for documenting care provided.

BIBLIOGRAPHY

Barnie, D. (1989). Evaluation of nursing specialties. *SGA J 11,* 214-216. Williams & Wilkins.

Hirschowitz, B. Curtiss, L. & Pollard, A. (1958). Demonstration of a new gastroscope, the "fiberscope." *Gastroenterology 35,* 50-53.

Joint Commission on Accreditation of Healthcare Organizations (1996). *Accreditation manual for hospitals. (vol 1,* rev. ed.) Oak Brook Terrace, Illinois.

Shields, N. (1987). The role of professional organizations in the practice of GI nursing, *SGA J 10,* 112-113. Williams & Wilkins.

Society of Gastroenterology Nurses and Associates, Inc. (2000). Guidelines for nursing care of the patient receiving sedation and analgesia in the gastrointestinal endoscopy setting [Monograph], *Gastroenterol Nurs 23(3),* 125-9. Lippincott, Williams & Wilkins.

Society of Gastroenterology Nurses and Associates, Inc. (2001). Role delineation of unlicensed assistive personnel in gastroenterology. *Gastroenterol Nurs 24(4),* 208-9. Lippincott, Williams & Wilkins

Society of Gastroenterology Nurses and Associates, Inc. (2001). Role delineation of the licensed practical/vocational nurse in gastroenterology. *Gastroenterol Nurs 24(4),* 204-5. Lippincott, Williams & Wilkins.

Society of Gastroenterology Nurses and Associates, Inc. (2001). Role delineation of the registered nurse in a staff position in gastroenterology. , *Gastroenterol Nurs 24(4),* 202-3. Lippincott, Williams & Wilkins.

Sugawa, C. & Schuman, B. (1981). *Primer of gastrointestinal fiberoptic endoscopy.* Boston: Little, Brown.

Chapter 2

MANAGING THE GASTROENTEROLOGY DEPARTMENT

This chapter reviews the principles and functions inherent in managing human and material resources in a gastroenterology unit. Five functions of management are addressed, including planning, organizing, directing, controlling, and staffing. Each function is further defined and the process outlined in an effort to provide the manager of the gastroenterology unit with fundamental managerial concepts.

Learning objectives

After reviewing the content of this chapter, the gastroenterology nurse should be able to:

1. Discuss the five functions of management and provide examples of activities included in each function.
2. Describe the organizational structure of the gastroenterology unit.
3. Outline methods for accomplishing department goals through efficient use of personnel.

FUNCTIONS OF MANAGEMENT

Management can be defined as a process of getting things completed with the help of others. This means that individuals must be directed toward common goals. There are two criteria used to determine whether an individual in an organization is a manager. First, does the individual perform management functions? Second, does he or she have authority? If either of these two components is lacking, the structure of the organization or the individual in the management position should be reexamined. These two criteria are presented here because they are important to the success of any gastroenterology unit and because the manager must demonstrate competency and accountability in the area of management.

The five functions a manager performs are planning, organizing, directing, controlling, and staffing.

1. **Planning** is the first function performed; it determines in advance what should be done.
2. **Organizing** comes after the planning process; it involves dissecting the work into parts so that it can be accomplished.
3. **Directing** is the third management function and includes guidance, coaching, motivating, and supervising subordinates.
4. **Controlling** involves activities that are used to measure attainment of the goals outlined in the planning phase.
5. **Staffing** is not always a separate management function, but when it concerns hospital departments such as the gastroenterology unit, it is important to set staffing apart. It can be a time-consuming process that entails recruiting, training, and promoting of staff.

These five functions are performed by managers at every level of the organization. The amount of time spent on the various functions by the hospital administrator in relation to that of the gastroenterology unit manager will be different. For instance, the administrator probably spends more time planning and organizing, whereas the unit manager spends more time staffing, directing, and controlling.

In addition to performing management functions, the second key criterion that a manager must possess is **authority,** which is the legal or rightful power to command and act. The manager must be given the power to command or enforce order; otherwise, there would be disorganization and chaos. In today's work environments the words *responsibility* or *task* are used rather than the word *authority.* Nevertheless, an effective manager must understand his or her authority. Regardless of how an individual manager applies that authority, it is important to have it. This issue will be further explored when the directing function of management is examined.

Coordination should be a by-product of the performance of the five functions of management described in the following sections. It is described as the ability of a manager to direct individuals to perform efficiently.

PLANNING

Planning is the first function performed by the gastroenterology unit nurse manager and entails outlining a course of action that is realistic for the unit. Planning involves development of a purpose or mission, philosophy, goals, and objectives for the organization and development of "work maps" showing how these goals and objectives are to be accomplished.

In the planning stage, the gastroenterology manager attempts to forecast how trends in patient treatment modalities and technologies will affect the unit. Gathering data on an ongoing basis from suppliers of equipment, reading current journals, attending professional meetings, benchmarking, and viewing exhibits provide a basis for forecasting.

The manager also has to project the qualifications of future employees based on the level of knowledge and skills needed to perform tasks in the gastroenterology unit. The political climate of the health care setting and the timing of any anticipated staffing or management changes are also critical in planning. The manager must choose the best strategy and know when to plan changes that will provide a positive result.

During the planning phase, the manager decides how to best use available resources. Staff input is important, because this decision requires review of equipment and supplies. Is there a need to purchase or replace medical devices? Are the supplies and materials used in the unit appropriate and the best for the types of procedures being performed? Another planning task is to look at work methods and processes. Are there ways of being more efficient? Are there activities being done that are not necessary and could be changed? Is there a need to do any space planning? The physical space of the unit and the placement of equipment and furniture should be conducive to a smooth work flow. It is easy to understand the importance of planning and how it affects the ability to perform other management functions.

Budgeting is a managerial task that takes place in both planning and controlling functions. During the planning function, budgeting involves setting goals or policies that guide the unit throughout the year.

A prerequisite to performing the above planning tasks is the manager's ability to make decisions. Identifying problems, exploring alternatives, choosing alternatives, implementing decisions, and evaluating results will help in clarifying the purpose of the unit. The gastroenterology unit nurse manager must be skilled in using decision-making tools to select the best course of action from all of the alternatives presented. Problem solving is a skill that can be learned. Decision making tools that assist the manager include the probability theory, which operates on the assumption that things occur in a predictable pattern; simulations, models and games that help describe, explain, and predict phenomena; decision trees, which are graphic tools that aid in visualizing alternatives; critical path method, which is useful when looking at costs; and queuing theory, which is used when problems arise around service that is being provided.

ORGANIZING

Organizing is the second function of management and is the means by which a manager develops order and fosters productivity. Organizing involves the integration of resources in a unit and the assignment of activities within that unit so they can be most effectively executed. This entails establishing lines of authority within activities and between departments and examining the contributions people make to the organization and determining to whom one will report. The organizing process comes from the need for cooperation; the goal is to build, develop, and maintain a structure of working relationships that brings about the objectives of the unit in a positive way.

Types of organizational structures

The **organizational structure** determines the process by which a specific group of people distributes responsibilities, establishes lines of communication, identifies relationships, and establishes authority.

Organizational structures can be formal or informal. An informal structure develops in all organizations. It is concerned primarily with the personal and social relationships that are not seen on the organizational chart. Formal organizational structures can be designed or rescinded, but informal structures cannot, because they have not been instituted by the manager. The manager needs to know that the informal structure exists, how it operates, and how to use it to advance the objectives of the unit. By knowing how the informal organization works, the manager can avoid activities that will unnecessarily threaten or disrupt it.

Formal organizational structures can be either bureaucratic or adaptive. Bureaucratic structures imply subdivision, specialization, technical qualifications, rules, and standards. The newer, adaptive organizational models are more freeform, open systems that are flexible and lend themselves to a more participative atmosphere.

There are no rules regarding which type of organizational structure is best for the gastroenterology unit; whatever works for the unit and institution is acceptable. Different types of formal organizational structures that may be appropriate for the gastroenterology unit include line authority, functional organization, staff authority, matrix organization, and project organization

1. **Line authority** is probably the most traditional and easiest organization structure to use, because each position has authority over a lower one in the organization. It is a chain of command, a leader-follower relationship. This type of structure works well when there are levels of expertise within the unit. For example, the manager would be in charge, with the RN, LPN, or gastroenterology associate reporting to him or her, and the LPN and associate reporting to the RN.
2. **Functional organization** authorizes a specialist from a given area to enforce recommendations within a clearly defined area. This type of structure might work well in a gastroenterology unit where there is an all-RN

staff. One RN would act as the specialist or spokesperson for communication to the institution's administration.

3. In a **staff authority** structure, staff members serve in an advisory capacity to the line structure but have no authority. The primary responsibility of the staff is to assist personnel who are in a line authority or chain of command. Unfortunately, this structure does not allow personnel to take the initiative to implement change. Staff personnel function primarily through influence and by offering suggestions to assist line personnel to be more effective.

4. A **matrix organization** looks at individual subsystems within a complex structure. Depending on the complex structure, these subsystems can be totally dependent or have total autonomy. This is demonstrated in many decentralized systems in which subsystems are given the authority to work independently of other groups but toward a common goal.

5. **Project organization** is usually used to accomplish a specific task; when the task is completed the group is disbanded. This type of structure is beneficial when a specific task, such as evaluating a new product and recommending whether to purchase it, must be accomplished.

Regardless of the type of organizational structure used, it must be clearly defined for the unit to deliver quality care. Each team member must know the process for distributing responsibilities and how to communicate through appropriate channels. The organizational structure should facilitate the communication of staff ideas and concerns and the integration of quality. If it does not accomplish this, it should be reevaluated and a different type of structure should be tried. However, individual departments such as the gastroenterology unit may not be able to exert much influence and many times structure is imposed without input from all involved departments. The emphasis should be on a team approach to delivery of quality care.

Organizational principles

Certain principles help maximize the efficiency of the organizational structure and help the manager and employees function more effectively within that structure. These principles include unity of command, requisite authority, and continuing responsibility:

1. **Unity of command** implies clear lines of authority. The employee knows to whom they report and who is the final authority. This means that each member of the organization has a single immediate supervisor.

2. **Requisite authority** implies that when a subordinate has been delegated a task, he or she is given the final authority to accomplish the task.

3. **Continuing responsibility** refers to the fact that when a manager delegates responsibility for a function to a subordinate, the manager is still responsible for that function.

Recognition of these few basic principles assists the manager by enhancing the efficiency of the organizational structure.

Organizational tools

Organizational tools that are helpful for the gastroenterology manager include organization charts and job descriptions.

The organization chart is a graphic representation of how the unit is organized. It depicts formal organizational relationships, areas of responsibility, persons to whom one is accountable, and channels of communication. It is used for planning, administrative control, and policy-making.

Job descriptions are important, because they assist the manager with organizing the administration of the various functions. Descriptions specify the title of the position, the qualifications necessary to complete the duties listed, and the person to whom the employee is responsible.

Span of control

The span of control is often referred to as the *span of management* and is used to identify the scope of management responsibility. Although the manager remains the final authority, he or she delegates authority to subordinates who, in turn, supervise a group of employees.

Factors that influence the manager's capability to supervise include the following:

(a) the amount of experience and management training he or she has acquired (An experienced and well-trained manager is able to supervise more employees.);

(b) the amount and the nature of work a manager has to do;

(c) the willingness to accept responsibility;

(d) the characteristics of the employees themselves (if they are self-directed and possess a high degree of knowledge and skill, they may not need as much direction.); and

(e) the design and complexity of procedures and activities that take place in the unit.

One caution regarding the span of control for a small unit is that overly prudent supervision discourages problem solving and independent thinking and may give subordinates the feeling of being smothered. Today we see the influence of the concept of continuous performance improvement permeating the hospital structure. This type of management philosophy results in many benefits, such as reduced waste, improved services, increased success, and decreased cost of health care services.

DIRECTING

After organizing, the next step in the process of management entails directing personnel and activities in such a way that goals of the unit are met. Managers must demonstrate the ability to lead, motivate, and mentor employees through the issuance of directives, instructions, assignments, and orders. The main objectives are to complete work, to teach employees, and to be a role model. The gastroenterology unit manager should build an effective workforce and motivate each member of the team. Regardless of the level of management, directing is always an important function. It requires that a manager possess leadership skills and the ability to integrate a participative management style into the daily coordination of the gastroenterology unit. Every manager should become familiar with his or her own leadership style, managerial philosophy, and sources of power and authority.

Leadership

The emphasis in management today is on human skills. Leadership is defined as the process of influencing the activities of an individual or group in efforts directed at goal achievement. In other words, leadership involves accomplishing goals with and by means of people. People have not always been the focus of leadership theory. Some of the more popular schools of thought in organizational theory include the following:

1. The theory of **scientific management,** in which the function of the manager is to set up and enforce performance criteria to meet organizational goals. The focus is on the organization rather than the needs of the people within the organization.
2. The **human relations** theory, which stresses concern for the needs of the people versus the task. Some have felt that a predominant concern for the task represents authoritarian leadership behavior, whereas concern for relationships represents democratic leadership. The human relations theory is based on the idea that the real power of the organization is the interpersonal relations that develop within the working unit. Mayo illustrated this concept in the famous Hawthorne experiment done with the Western Electric Company.
3. The **managerial grid,** which includes both task and relationship concepts. This model tends to be an attitudinal model, because it measures the values and feelings of the manager. This theory considers five different types of leadership, based on the manager's concern for tasks versus people within the organization.
4. The **contingency model** of leadership, which holds that a manager's leadership style can be effective or ineffective, depending on the situation. This model defines three aspects of a situation that structure the leader's role: leader-employee relations, task structure, and position power. Like the managerial grid model, this model is two-dimensional, in that it reverts back to the basic leader behavior styles: task-oriented and relationship-oriented.
5. The **authoritarian/democratic leader behavior model** is another theory of leadership style. In this theory, the authoritarian leader places more emphasis on tasks. On the other end of the continuum, the democratic leader is more concerned about relationships. This popular theory is still used today. It coincides with McGregor's X and Y theory. There are two basic leadership styles on a continuum: On one end, the leader directs employees by telling them what to do and how to do it; on the other the leader influences employees by sharing responsibilities with them and involving them in decision making. In some cases the continuum is extended beyond democratic behavior into a permissive style of leadership known as laissez-faire. In this style, employees do as they please. There are no policies and procedures, and there is no sign of any formal leadership.
6. The **transformational leadership style** is the most current model. A transformational leader is one who motivates followers to perform to their full potential by influencing a change in perceptions and providing a sense of direction. This leadership style emphasizes collective purpose and mutual growth. It involves being committed, having a vision, being a risk taker, and empowering others.

Regardless of which model is used, the manager must develop and implement the leadership style that works best in accomplishing the goals of the unit.

Motivating

To be successful at directing employees, the manager must understand human behavior and what motivates employee performance. Much has been written on the topic of motivation, and there are classic theories with which all managers should be familiar. In the 1950s, however, advocates of the behavioral sciences became concerned about the lack of scientific validation behind the management theories that had been applied in the past. The management theories in use today developed from this concern.

Maslow was one of the first to initiate the human behavior school with his hierarchy-of-needs theory. He classified human needs into five categories: physiological, safety, love, esteem, and self-actualization. Maslow's theory has been and still is very influential in management and continues to stimulate much research.

Another popular theory today is Herzberg's motivation-hygiene theory, wherein job factors are classified as either dissatisfiers or satisfiers. Satisfiers, or motivators, are achievement, recognition, work, responsibility, advancement, and growth. The idea is that as an employee receives positive feedback, his or her level of performance increases. The job dissatisfiers, or hygiene factors, are supervision, company policy, working conditions, interpersonal relations, job security, and salary. These are not motivators because for the most part, they do not cause any improvement in performance. They only prevent poor morale. Herzberg believes that if a person finds the job interesting, he or she can tolerate the dissatisfiers.

According to management theory, the manager's style affects the degree to which he or she can stimulate employee performance. McGregor's X and Y theory is a good example. Theory X assumes that most people prefer to be directed, are not interested in assuming responsibility, and have to be constantly supervised. Theory Y assumes that the employee is mature, independent, and self-motivated.

Managers who believe that people are inherently lazy tend to use fear and threats to motivate personnel, delegate little responsibility, and do not include personnel in planning. Managers who philosophically believe that people are self-motivated and enjoy work use praise and recognition and provide opportunities for growth. Theory Y complements Herzberg's theory in that positive incentives are used to stimulate personnel.

Personal management styles reflect managers' beliefs about motivation. Webster's dictionary defines motive as "that within the individual, rather than without, which incites him to action; any idea, need, emotion, or organic state that prompts to an action." If managers want to motivate employees, they have to provide the motive—in other words, incite action from the employee. If this is true, one of the roles of the manager is to understand what really motivates employees and what stimulates certain behaviors. This can be determined by identifying what employees want from their jobs. Different people have different needs. Today, the trend is toward recognition, flexibility in the work setting, and a sense of responsibility and accountability. Employees want to participate in decision making, particularly as it relates to them and to their own jobs.

Participative management

Current management philosophy holds that the better a manager treats an employee, the better the employee will perform. The trend in nursing is toward participative management, with emphasis on self-directed work teams. This philosophy is based on the belief that employees are self-directed and self-motivated and can be self-managed. Group problem solving and decision making give employees a sense of ownership. When they are empowered, the staff is motivated to implement the decisions members have helped develop. Professional employees have a need for autonomy and for some control over their own behavior. The challenge presented to managers is to integrate the needs of the organization with those of the employees. It is essential to have a balance.

Gastroenterology managers must possess well-developed human interaction skills. Instead of being autocratic, they need to be encouraging when interacting with employees. Managers must relinquish control in the traditional, autocratic sense to manage effectively.

The manager must hone his or her listening skills. The manager should spend time interacting with the staff to develop a trusting relationship with each of the employees within the department. The effective manager tries to be available to discuss issues, problems, and concerns that come up during the usual workday. He or she listens to employees' ideas and assists with problem solving. Communication is one of the biggest challenges for managers. It is important to share information, to keep employees informed of happenings, and to gain their cooperation.

Managers who deliver positive rewards in some form for productive behavior find that the behavior is repeated. Employees need to be told when they do something right.

Acknowledgement of good work performance is a strong motivating force. It lets employees know they are doing what is expected of them. The better employees feel about themselves, the more eager they are to work hard and be productive.

CONTROLLING

Controlling is the fourth step in the management process. It entails setting standards, measuring performance, reporting results, and taking corrective action. In controlling, the manager is concerned with making certain that the solution to a problem is properly implemented. This involves feedback of results and follow-up to determine the extent to which the predetermined goals have been accomplished. The success of the gastroenterology department depends on the degree of difference between what should be done and what is done. Having set the standards, the manager has a responsibility to stay informed of the actual performance and monitor outcomes. This can be achieved through observation, reports, and verbal feedback.

The controlling function of management should not be separated from the other management functions. In the managerial process of planning, the manager sets goals that become standards against which performance is continually checked and appraised. There is a direct connection between planning and controlling. Control is directly interwoven with other managerial functions, in that a manager cannot expect to have good control over the department without following sound managerial principles in pursuing his or her duties. Well-made plans, workable policies and procedures, continual training of employees, and appropriate supervision all play a significant role in control.

A gastroenterology department is part of a total system. For the system to be under control, the following requirements are essential:

(a) procedures through which control is maintained must be understandable;

(b) deviations from the controls or procedures must be identified quickly;

(c) controls or procedures must be appropriate and economical;

(d) there must be flexibility in the system; and

(e) corrective action must be taken when required.

Controlling entails three basic steps: setting and communicating standards or objectives, checking and appraising performance, and taking corrective action with appropriate documentation.

Setting standards

The overall objectives of the hospital are broken down into relative objectives for each department. These objectives are established by the department manager and include parameters such as quality, time standards, quotas, schedules, budgets, and patient procedures. Both internal and external types of standards affect the department, and both must be taken into consideration by the manager.

The manager should keep in mind that standards must be realistic. They must be achievable and must be considered fair by both the employees and the manager. It is essential that the employees be involved in identifying realistic and attainable standards.

Not all standards are tangible. Some types of intangible standards are important, particularly in the hospital setting. These might be the reputation of the hospital and even the individual department, high morale among employees in the department, and effective patient care, so recovery is quick and the patient's stay is pleasant.

Setting standards may seem overwhelming when considering the many types of activities in the department. Therefore, the manager might break down the task to a more manageable size by focusing on selecting strategic standards and looking for critical performance indicators.

Checking performance

The second step in the process of control is to check on the performance. Once the standards have been set, it is the manager's responsibility to compare actual performance with these standards. This is done by observing the work, by personally checking on employees, by studying various reports, and by data analysis.

Taking corrective action

The third part of controlling is taking corrective action. The manager is not really controlling if he or she does not consistently take corrective action when indicated. Ideally, there are no deviations from expected performance. Realistically, however, there will be discrepancies or variations that will need attention. When deviations do occur, the manager must analyze the situation and look at the total picture. He or she must then decide what remedial action is necessary and what modifications will secure improved results in the future.

Managing the budget

One of the most important control devices available to the manager is the budget. The budget is prepared during the planning process and provides direction for the manager. The budget is simply a statement of estimated expenses and revenues for a predetermined time period (fiscal year). The two types of budgets are the operating budget and the capital budget.

Operating budget. The operating budget consists of consumable items and resources used to provide direct patient care. Operating expenses vary depending on the volume of patients and the procedures performed in the gastroenterology unit. In most cases, the operating budget is further divided into direct or indirect expenses. Direct costs include items such as salaries, medical and surgical supplies, repairs, and charges from other departments. Indirect costs are expenses assigned for overhead and facility use. The box below provides examples of items that are considered direct and indirect expenses.

An important part of the operating budget is determination of staffing requirements. The goal is to secure enough budgeted positions to provide quality care in a cost-effective manner. Some health care providers use a patient classification system or acuity level to determine appropriate numbers. Others look at the total number of shifts per week required by category of staff. The staffing budget must take into account the number and type of patients that will be seen in the unit each day, the hours the unit will be staffed, coverage for after-hours emergency procedures, and coverage for staff vacations and absenteeism.

The supply part of the operating budget is usually based on the previous year's expenses and projection of costs for the next fiscal year. Other factors to consider include inflation rates, changes in workload by procedures or patients, any new or different supplies, and purchasing contracts.

Capital budget. The second type of budget is the capital budget. This budget includes large purchases, such as equipment, furniture, or construction projects that amount to more than $500 and are usually depreciated. Most hospitals expect the department manager to make a formal request in a proposal format that incorporates the following: data specific to the item requested; alternative solutions such as purchase, rent, or lease; priorities and recommendations; cost and benefit analysis; and an implementation plan.

Whatever budgetary goals are in place, the manager who is administering the budget should have a part in preparing it and be responsible for monitoring it throughout the fiscal year. The gastroenterology manager should remember that budgets are merely a tool for management rather than a substitute for good judgment.

Examples of direct and indirect expenses

Direct Expenses
Salaries and wages
Per diem staff
Overtime
On-call personnel
Disposable items
Instruments
Medical and surgical supplies
Repairs
Pharmacy

Indirect expenses
Equiment depreciation
Building depreciation
Malpractice insurance
Employee health benefits
Accounting
Purchasing
Utilities
Housekeeping

STAFFING

Staffing is the final managerial function. Once planning and organizing have been accomplished, the manager of the gastroenterology unit must assign staff to carry out the unit's goals. Staffing involves employee selection, placement, training, and compensation. The manager's function is to hire, place, develop, and train the employees for the unit. In addition, the manager evaluates and appraises the performance of employees and either rewards their efforts and abilities or disciplines and at times even discharges employees who are not performing at acceptable levels.

Staffing functions

The staffing function is not done only at the time the department or unit is established; it is ongoing. The manager has a responsibility to make certain that employees possess the necessary capabilities and are competent to perform the tasks required in the gastroenterology unit. To ensure that the right employees are hired for the necessary positions, the manager has to "determine the need." This step entails deciding on the number and type of employees needed. In a small unit, several functions may be combined. Staffing needs can be determined only after careful study of the entire unit. The manager must match jobs with people. Using job descriptions that fully delineate the requirements of the job facilitates this process.

The manager will determine the number of employees and the staffing budget requirements based on the volume of procedures. He or she generally hires individuals to replace those who voluntarily resign, are dismissed, or transfer. When an additional employee must be hired, the goal is to recruit and select a person who is qualified to perform the duties outlined in the job description.

Selection of employees

The human resources department may initially interview and screen job applicants; however, qualified individuals will ultimately be presented to the manager before being hired. A copy of the applicant's curriculum vitae or resume should always be obtained to review the applicant's experience and qualifications. An interview provides additional information about the applicant's job knowledge and personality. At this point, the interview should focus on the individual's competencies and qualifications to perform the required duties in the gastroenterology department. Questions asked in the interview must follow guidelines established by the Equal Employment Opportunity Commission (EEOC). The manager compares prospective employees' strengths and weaknesses to choose the one who best fits the needs of the department. It is also a good practice to follow up on references provided by prospective employees. Sometimes these can be invaluable. Following up may entail making telephone calls or requesting letters of recommendation. A record should be kept of all prospective employees and should include the position applied for and the basis for the decision to hire or not to hire.

Orientation and staff development

Once the manager has hired the desired employee, it is the manager's responsibility to coordinate the orientation of the new person to the hospital and the unit. Orientation should include introduction to policies and procedures; rules and regulations specific to the hospital; and a thorough review of the tasks, duties, and responsibilities outlined in the employee's job description. This is best accomplished by utilizing a preceptor and competency statements.

The purpose of staff development is to provide opportunities for the individual employee's professional growth and development; as such, it goes beyond orientation and should be available for all employees on an ongoing basis. Staff development opportunities might include hospital or department in-services, courses, seminars, and independent study or projects.

Staffing assignments

Providing for patient care on a daily basis is also a function of staffing. Schedules should provide staff with information as to where and when they should be on duty. There are a variety of staffing patterns that can be used. The delivery system may be point-of-service care, managed care, functional nursing, team nursing, or primary nursing. Any of these delivery systems will accommodate the various theoretical models of nursing.

Another consideration for the gastroenterology unit manager is whether centralized or decentralized staffing is in place. Computers are used for centralized staffing by many departments. This type of scheduling is cost-effective and reduces the hours allocated to developing and implementing staffing needs. Decentralized staffing is accomplished by a manager and staff at the unit level. The advantage of decentralized staffing is that employees get more personalized attention and input.

Beyond Fundamental Managerial Skills

The managerial thoughts and ideas presented are merely overviews and therefore are not discussed in depth. The gastroenterology nurse manager should be able to assess his or her own level of competency and seek out resources that will enhance his or her motivation skills. In addition to the fundamental managerial skills required for success, it is critical to stay abreast of new ideas and approaches to accomplishing the task.

Managing in today's environment is a challenging responsibility. Emphasis is being placed on increasing productivity and quality through team development while reducing costs. The role of the manager is to coach, facilitate, and develop the staff. Essential skills include the abilities to delegate power, encourage staff to expand their talents, and encourage risk taking.

Some people believe that the individual leaders, rather than the organization, create excellence. In other words, it does not just happen; an individual makes it happen. The challenge for managers is to integrate a set of skills that Hickman and Silva believe are essential for the "new-age" executive. The following leadership skills enable the gastroenterology unit manager to engage in laying a strong foundation of excellence:

1. **Creative Insight: Asking the Right Question.** Insight means being able to get to the root of the prob-

lem. The manager is able to readily see opportunities, advantages, and strengths that result in new strategies for success.

2. **Sensitivity: Doing Unto Others.** Because people are the organization's greatest asset, the manager must find a way to bind them together so they will achieve high goals. The manager may choose to unify employees through one-on-one communication, ongoing education programs, creative incentive programs, and job security.

3. **Vision: Creating the Future.** This skill enables the manager to have a clear vision of changes that may occur.

4. **Versatility: Anticipating Change.** The versatile manager is prepared and readily adapts to the ever-changing world. A manager must be able to anticipate change, accept it, and use it to predict the future.

5. **Focus: Implementing Change.** A successful manager gives undivided attention to the task at hand. By focusing on priorities, the manager increasingly controls the situation.

6. **Patience: Living in the Long Term.** Patience is a virtue. The manager who is able to integrate and orchestrate the other five skills will, through patience, know how and when to use them. If every manager would commit to acquiring the above skills, organizations would evolve into a high level of excellence.

Managers are being pressured to develop new skills and abilities that will improve the productivity and quality of services provided. Primary developmental functions of a manager/leader involve energetically and dynamically supporting and coaching all employees within his or her area. They must determinedly assist in removing barriers to successful performance and continually assist the group in developing a dedicated and positive team orientation. The definition often includes the expectation of leaders to nurture partners internally and outside the organization, including excellent physician relations. Leaders must act as mentors for the team, be open to change, and be available to identify and assist other employees in efforts to improve. They must be able to facilitate, mediate, and negotiate through excellent verbal and written communication skills. These skills cannot be mastered overnight, but hard work and commitment will result in success.

CASE SITUATION

Patsy Bartlett is the gastroenterology unit nurse manager at Piedmont Hospital. Her daily activities include managing the unit and being clinically competent to assist with scheduled procedures. This combination produces frustration, because she must also develop a marketing plan to keep her hospital competitive in the health care marketplace.

Points to think about

1. Patsy realizes that it is essential that she devise a plan for the new laparoscopic procedures that will be implemented in her unit. What kind of information must she put together?

2. Sometimes Patsy wonders if she is capable of managing the gastroenterology unit, because it gets rather hectic and time is precious. What types of activities would demonstrate management ability?

3. Patsy believes that a participative management style works best for her gastroenterology department. What are some examples of behaviors that would reinforce this management style?

4. Patsy had a situation in which an employee would call in at 5 am and request the day off. What type of plan might Patsy use to alter this employee's behavior?

5. Patsy has been asked to develop a marketing plan to increase the volume of procedures performed in the gastroenterology unit. How might she approach this challenge?

Suggested responses

1. To prepare for the introduction of new laparoscopic procedures, Patsy should:
   - Perform a financial forecast based on the projected number of laparoscopic procedures.
   - Determine capital equipment needs relative to this new procedure.
   - Design an orientation/training program for personnel.
   - Revise the existing budget to include income and expenses associated with this procedure.

2. Examples of management activities might include:
   - Making changes in staffing schedules based on requests of personnel.
   - Reviewing monthly financial statements and justifying variances.
   - Meeting with staff to discuss problems encountered with cleaning the new laparoscopes.
   - Conducting a performance appraisal of an associate.

3. Examples of behaviors that would reinforce the participative management style include:
   - Staff involvement in the decision of who would cover weekend call.
   - Staff meeting regarding general low morale throughout the institution.
   - Staff meeting to obtain input regarding the replacement of obsolescent equipment.
   - Staff involvement in developing a policy for monitoring sedated pediatric patients.

4. To improve this employee's behavior, Patsy might:
   - Set up a meeting with the employee and attempt to gather objective data about the reasons for his or her behavior.
   - Explain to the employee that the schedule has already been completed and only needed personnel are assigned.
   - Explain that the employee's request should be made in advance, in accordance with written leave policies.
   - Provide positive feedback on behaviors that should be recognized.
   - Set mutual goals relative to requesting time off.

- Schedule a follow-up meeting to review progress.
- Document the counseling session including anecdotal notes.

5. To develop a marketing plan, Patsy might:
   - Use creative insight to begin looking at what problems currently exist and possible solutions that would result in identification of opportunities.
   - Use these opportunities to create a vision of what she would like the department to do and to outline a plan for accomplishing the goals set forth.
   - Be open to accepting the changes that have taken place and use them to advance toward the anticipated goals.

REVIEW TERMS

authority, functional organization, line authority, matrix organization, organizational structure, project organization, quality, staff authority

REVIEW QUESTIONS

1. Management of the gastroenterology department entails:
   a. Coordination of the five functions of management.
   b. Getting things done through others.
   c. Doing tasks yourself to ensure they are done correctly.
   d. Ensuring that the employee knows to whom to report.
2. The management function that entails establishing authority relationships between activities and departments is:
   a. Staffing.
   b. Controlling.
   c. Organizing.
   d. Directing.
3. Managerial components of planning include:
   a. Developing goals and objectives.
   b. Maintaining a structure of working relationships.
   c. Assigning work activities.
   d. Hiring new personnel.
4. Activities that the gastroenterology nurse manager performs in the directing function of management include:
   a. Counseling employees.
   b. Leading and guiding employees.
   c. Developing position descriptions.
   d. Conducting performance appraisals.
5. The emphasis in management today should be on:
   a. Motivation.
   b. Pay increases.
   c. Flexible staffing.
   d. Human skills.
6. For the manager to determine the staffing budget, it will be necessary to calculate:
   a. Full-time equivalents and flexible staff.
   b. Volume of procedures and required staff.
   c. Qualifications of the required staff.
   d. Volume and cost of procedures.

7. A person who delegates authority to others is accountable for:
   a. The tasks allocated to other workers.
   b. The tasks unassigned to staff.
   c. The tasks delegated to staff.
   d. The tasks of other managers.
8. The process of measuring the degree to which predetermined goals of the gastroenterology unit are achieved is called:
   a. Planning.
   b. Controlling.
   c. Staffing.
   d. Directing.
9. In an operating budget, salaries, overtime, benefits, and medical-surgical supplies are usually considered:
   a. Indirect expenses.
   b. Fixed assets.
   c. Direct expenses.
   d. Capital budget items.
10. The management skill that focuses primarily on the assets of people in the organization would be:
    a. Focusing on being a change agent.
    b. Constructing the operating budget.
    c. Performing a financial forecast.
    d. Developing sensitivity.

BIBLIOGRAPHY

Avilo, R. (1999). *Full leadership development: building the vital forces in organizations.* Thousand Oaks, CA; Sage.

Blake, R. & Mouton, J. (1964). *The managerial grid.* Houston, TX: Gulf Publishing.

Cardiner, G. (2001). *21st century manager.* Princeton, NJ: Peterson's Pacesetter Guides.

Dunham-Taylor, J. (2000). *Nurse executive transformational leadership found in participative organizations.* Journal of Nursing Administration, 30(5), 241-250.

Fielder, F. (1967). *A theory of leadership effectiveness* (1st ed.). New York; McGraw-Hill.

Finkler, S. & Kovner, C. (2000). *Financial management for nurse managers and executives* (2nd ed.). Philadelphia: W.B. Saunders.

Fisher, K. (1999). *Leading self-directed work teams: a guide to developing new team leadership skills* (2nd ed.). New York: McGraw-Hill.

Huber, D. (2000). *Leadership and nursing care management* (2nd ed.), Philadelphia: W.B. Saunders.

Kelly-Heidenthal, P. (2003). *Nursing leadership and management.* Clifton Park, NY: Delmar Publishing.

Kiernan, M. (1996). *The 11 commandments of 21st century management.* Englewood Cliffs, NJ: Prentice Hall.

Kouzes, J.M. & Posner, B.Z. (1995). *The leadership challenge: how to get extraordinary things done in organizations.* San Francisco: Jossey-Bass.

Marquis, B.L. & Huston, C.J. (2000). *Leadership roles and management functions in nursing* (3rd ed). Philadelphia: Lippincott.

Mayo, E. (1949). *The social problems of an industrial civilization.* Boston: Routledge.

Merriam-Webster's collegiate dictionary (10th ed.) (1998). Springfield, MA. Merriam-Webster.

Moorehead, G., & Griffin, R.W. (2001). *Organizational behavior: managing people in organizations* (6th ed.). Boston: Houghton Mifflin.

Shortell, S. & Kaluzyny, A. (2000). *Health care management: organizational design and behavior* (4th ed.). Clifton Park, NY: Delmar Publishing.

Tappen, R. N. (2001). *Nursing leadership and management concepts and practice* (4th ed.). Philadelphia: F.A. Davis.

Taylor, F. (1998). *Scientific management.* New York: Dover Publisher.

Udall, S. & Hiltro, J. M. (1996). *The accidental manager*. New York: Prentice Hall.

Yurko, L.C., Coffee, T. L., Fusilero, J., Yowler, C. J., Brandt, C. & Fratienne, R. B. (2001). Management of an inpatient outpatient clinic: an eight year review. *Journal of Burn Care and Rehabilitation* (22), 250-254.

Chapter 3

INFECTION CONTROL

This chapter describes the precautions that must be taken in the gastroenterology/endoscopysetting to control the risk of infection for patients and healthcare personnel. Standards jointly adopted by the Society of Gastroenterology Nurses and Associates (SGNA), the American Society of Gastrointestinal Endoscopy (ASGE) and the Association for Professionals in Infection Control and Epidemiology , Inc. (APIC) are summarized. General infection control principles, including the Spaulding classification system, are reviewed. Guidelines for decontamination and high-level disinfection of GI endoscopes are provided. In addition, automated reprocessors are discussed, as are recommendations for reprocessing reusable and single-use devices and accessory equipment. Populations who should be considered for antibiotic prophylaxis are presented.

Learning Objectives

After reviewing the content of this chapter, the Gastroenterology nurse should be able to:

1. Identify elements of an educational and continuous quality improvement program as they relate to infection control.
2. Discuss the Spaulding classification system as it applies to GI endoscopes and accessories.
3. Explain appropriate steps of decontamination and high-level disinfection of endoscopes.
4. Identify the special requirements for reprocessing of endoscopic retrograde cholangiopancreatography (ERCP) elevator channels.

Discuss the reuse recommendations of reprocessing single-use endoscopy devices andaccessories.

INFECTION CONTROL PRINCIPLES

It is imperative that all healthcare personnel be educated regarding appropriate infection control measures. Infection Control education is a critical part of the orientation and continuing education process for all staff including physicians, nurses and assistive personnel, regardless of the setting in which gastrointestinal endoscopy is performed (hospital, clinic, or office). An infection results when **microorganisms** enter the human body, multiply, and produce a reaction. For an infection to develop, all three of the following interlinking components in the chain of infection must be present: an infectious organism, a means of transmission, and a susceptible host. The infectious organism may be in the form of bacteria, viruses, fungi, protozoa, or helminthes (worms). Bacteria are the most common infectious agents in the clinical setting. Both endogenous and exogenous microbes can cause infections related to endoscopic procedures.

1. **Endogenous infections** occur when the microflora colonizing the mucosal surfaces of the gastrointestinal or respiratory tract gain access to the bloodstream or normally sterile body sites as a consequence of the procedure. Examples of endogenous infections include cholangitis following the manipulation of an obstructed biliary duct or endocarditis in patients with mitral valve regurgitation who have sustained transient bacteremia during esophageal dilatation.

2. **Exogenous infections** are the result of microorganisms introduced from a source outside the body. Exogenous organisms most frequently associated with transmission during endoscopy have been gram-negative bacteria or Mycobacteria. Recent reports of endoscopic related transmission include hepatitis C virus (HCV), Pseudomonas aeruginosa, Mycobacterium tuberculosis (M. tuberculosis), and Mycobacterium intracellulare (Alvarado & Reichelderfer 2000).The most common factors associated with transmission involved inadequate manual cleaning, inadequate exposure of surfaces to disinfectant, inadequate rinsing and drying and improper use of automated endoscope reprocessors.

Direct and indirect contacts are the most common methods of transmission in the clinical setting. Other methods include airborne transmission; vehicle transmission, such as by endoscopes; and vector transmission via an animal or insect. A susceptible host can be anyone who has a lowered resistance. Factors that contribute to host susceptibility are age, immune status, or underlying disease. Because of their inefficient immune systems, patients infected with the human immunodeficiency virus (HIV), transplant patients and patients receiving immunosuppressant therapy are highly susceptible to infection.

Microbial reservoirs and mechanisms of transmission

The ability of bacteria to form biofilms is an important factor in the pathogenesis of endoscopy-related infections, particularly as biofilms interfere with disinfection. Biofilms consist of colonies of organisms forming structures to maximize growth potential. Development of a biofilm begins when free-swimming bacteria attach to a surface. Cell-to-cell communication then signals formation of a biofilm with pillar and mushroom-like structures around which water can circulate. This allows both maximum exposure of the bacteria to circulating nutrients and a decrease in the accumulation of waste products. Biofilms have been found to adhere to the internal channels of endoscopes. This finding emphasizes the importance of strategies aimed at decreasing biofilm formation through meticulous mechanical cleaning of the endoscope.

To break the chain of infection the gastroenterology nurse must recognize the need for appropriate decontamination, disinfection and, in some cases, sterilization of instruments and patient care items. Each endoscopy setting must develop policies to identify whether disinfection or sterilization is indicated based on the item's intended use. Classifications for levels of disinfection, and categorization of equipment and patient care items were devised in the 1960s by Earl H. Spaulding. Spaulding classified equipment and patient care items as critical, semicritical, and noncritical, based on the risk of infection involved in their use.

1. **Critical items** are those that present a high risk of infection if they are contaminated. These objects or instruments that break the mucosal barrier or that enter sterile tissue of the vascular system. Examples of critical items in the gastroenterology unit are sclorotherapy or injection needles, biopsy forceps, and intravenous catheters. Sterilization is recommended for critical items.

2. **Semicritical items** come in contact with intact skin and mucous membranes but usually do not penetrate body surfaces. Endoscopes are considered semicritical items. Semicritical items generally require high-level disinfection with a disinfectant such as glutaraldehyde or peracetic acid (Rutala, 1996).

3. **Noncritical items** come in contact with intact skin but not mucous membranes. There is relatively little risk of transmitting infection with these items. Some examples of noncritical items are stethoscopes, blood pressure cuffs, and pulse oximeters. These items require disinfection with an intermediate or low-level germicide or simple cleaning with detergent and water, depending on the nature of the device and the degree of contamination (Rutala, 1996).

Sterilization is the complete elimination or destruction of all forms of microbial life. Sterilization may be accomplished by steam under pressure (autoclaving), dry heat, low temperature sterilization such as ethylene oxide (ETO) gas or plasma technologies, and exposure to liquid sterilant/disinfectants. Sterilization should be regarded as a process rather than a single event. The only circumstance in which sterilization of an endoscope is required is when the endoscope is to be used in a sterile operative field. The Centers for Disease Control and Prevention (CDC) classify levels of disinfection as sterilization, high-level disinfection, intermediate-level disinfection, and low-level disinfection.

1. **High-level disinfection** destroys all mycobacteria, all viruses, all fungi, and all vegetative bacteria, but not necessarily all bacterial spores. The Food and Drug Administration (FDA) cleared products with a high-level disinfectant claim to kill 100% of the test organism M. tuberculosis. High-level disinfectants are referred to as sterilant/disinfectants, because they are capable of sterilization with extended soak times.

2. **Intermediate-level disinfection** inactivates M. tuberculosis, vegetative bacteria, most viruses, and most fungi; It does not necessarily kill bacterial spores.

3. **Low-level disinfectants** can kill most bacteria, some viruses and most fungi but are not effective against M. tuberculosis or bacterial spores.

STANDARDS FOR INFECTION CONTROL IN ENDOSCOPY SETTING

Standards for Infection Control and Reprocessing of Flexible Gastrointestinal Endoscopes (SGNA, 2000) outlines areas of importance in any GI endoscopy setting. As mentioned earlier, education on infection control issues is a vital component in the orientation and continuing education for all personnel, including physicians, nurses, and assistive personnel. Areas to be covered include standard precautions, Occupational Safety and Health Administration (OSHA) regulations, reprocessing protocols for endoscopes and accessory equipment, the mechanisms of transmission of infection, factors that promote a safe working environment, safe handling of liquid chemicals, and waste management procedures. OSHA has mandated standards which require exposure control plans and use of sharps with engineered sharps injury protection where feasible in an effort to reduce transmission of blood-borne pathogens (OSHA, 2001). Personal protective devices including gloves, masks, eye protection and moisture-resistant gowns should be used to protect personnel from blood or body fluid exposure. Eye wash stations should be readily available in case blood, body fluids, or chemicals splash into the eyes of caregivers, patients, or others. Annual reviews and updates on infection control issues in gastroenterology/endoscopy are highly recommended.

Personnel issues must be addressed, including limits on who may reprocess endoscopy equipment. Individuals who reprocess endoscopes and accessories require detailed knowledge of the instrument design and specific methods required to produce an instrument safe for use. Such individuals should be carefully selected, trained by a knowledgeable preceptor, and meet annual competency standards. Temporary personnel should never be given the responsibility of reprocessing instruments in either a manual or automated system.

An ongoing continuous quality improvement program should place special emphasis on strict adherence to published protocol for reprocessing flexible GI endoscopes. Supervisory personnel should be familiar with these standards and designate an individual in the setting to monitor compliance.

Preventive maintenance of reprocessing equipment and liquid chemical germicide monitoring should be incorporated in the quality assurance plan. Procedures should be in place for reporting any identified transmission of infection.

Procedure rooms and reprocessing rooms should be separate. Attention should be given to designating clean and dirty areas in each of these rooms. The correct storage, use, disposal, and containment of spills of liquid chemical germicides and other reagents should be addressed.

Reprocessing endoscopes

Reprocessing of flexible GI endoscopes is accomplished in two distinct phases: decontamination, and high-level disinfection.

The first phase is decontamination (pre-cleaning). In any endoscopy setting, the primary objective of decontamination is to prevent drying of secretions and to remove large numbers of organic material and microorganisms. Manual pre-cleaning allows for removal of a significant amount of organisms, feces and foreign material from the endoscope. Several studies have shown that pre-cleaning alone to be effective in reducing microbial contaminants by as much as 4 loggs or 99.99% (Rutala and Weber 1995). Reprocessing standards endorsed by SGNA, ASGE, the American Gastroenterology Association (AGA), the American College of Gastroenterology (ACG), and the APIC require that manual pre-cleaning of the endoscope, including all of its channels and removable parts, must precede either manual or automated disinfection (ACG, 1996). This manual decontamination (pre-cleaning) is always necessary before disinfection or sterilization, because any remaining organic material may harbor or form biofilms that prevent contact of the liquid chemical germicide with surfaces of the endoscope or accessory, resulting in ineffective disinfection/sterilization processes. Because it is impossible to sufficiently clean and disinfect endoscopes that cannot be completely immersed in liquid, the use of nonimmersible endoscopes in now unacceptable in gastroenterology (ACG, 1996).

The following steps are required to decontaminate flexible endoscopes:

1. Immediately after removing the endoscope from the patient, wipe the exterior of the scope with an enzymatic detergent solution. Suction enzymatic detergent solution and air until the effluent becomes clear. All channels should be irrigated with copious amounts of enzymatic detergent to soften, moisten and dilute the organic material. Purge air and water channels according to the manufacture's directions and attach water-resistant caps as needed to protect the endoscope.

2. Inspect the endoscope for damage and perform an underwater leak test according to the manufacture's directions. A leak test involves applying air pressure to the inside of the scope insertion tube and watching for air bubbles, identifying a leak in the scope covering or internally into one of the channels. Flex the distal portion of the scope in all directions to detect minute leaks. If damage is detected, proceed accordingly to the directions of the endoscope manufacturer and repair service. An endoscope sent for repair should be considered contaminated medical equipment and labeled as such for shipping according to OSHA guidelines. Consult Occupational Exposure to Bloodborne Pathogens: Final Rule (29CRF 1910.1030) for more information.

3. Detach all removable parts. Irregular surfaces must be thoroughly brushed to ensure complete removal of organic debris. With the endoscope submerged in a fresh enzymatic detergent solution and using an appropriate size cleaning brush, brush all channels giving particular attention to crevices that are most likely to harbor contaminated organic material. Gently wipe/brush the tip of the endoscope to remove any debris or tissue that may be lodged in or around the air and water nozzle. When pre-cleaning the duodenal (ERCP) scope, the distal tip must be brushed with the elevator both up and down to ensure that no matter is lodged in that movable part.

4. Attach all channel-cleaning adaptors specific to the endoscope. Irrigate all channels with enzymatic detergent solution, to remove any dislodged debris, followed by a clean water rinse and air drying. Also rinse and dry the exterior of the endoscope.

After thorough decontamination, the next step is high-level disinfection. Flexible GI scopes are classified as semicritical devices and require high-level disinfection using FDA-cleared solutions. High level of disinfection is the standard of care for the reprocessing of GI endoscopes by professionals associations (SGNA, 2000) and recognized as the appropriate standard of care by regulatory bodies (Kobs, 1996).

Glutaraldehyde

The most commonly used agent for high-level disinfection remains glutaraldehyde. In 1993, the FDA assumed jurisdiction over the regulation of clinical germicides, and at that time required manufacturers of 2.4% glutaraldehyde (as part of the 510(k) clearance process for medical devices) to label their product recommending 45 minutes of exposure to gluteraldehyde at 25 C. The recommendation was based upon the length of time and temperature needed for gluteraldehyde to kill 100% of M. tuberculosis without any manual pre-cleaning (Rutala, Clontz, Webser, & Hoffman, 1991). Recognizing the crucial role of manual pre-cleaning, subsequent guidelines have suggested that once the recommended pre-cleaning has been done, 20 minutes of a glutaraldehyde immersion at room temperature is sufficient to achieve high-level disinfection. Current SGNA/ASGE/AGA/ACG guidelines support this practice (DeMarino, Gage, Leung, Ravich, Wolf, Zuckerman, & Zuccaro, 1996). Glutaraldehyde is irritating to the skin and can cause contact dermatitis. Exposure to gluteraldehyde vapors can irritate the eye and nasal mucosal. The National Institute for Occupational Health and Safety has set ceiling limits of gluteraldehyde vapors at .05 part per million (ppm). Maintaining ceiling limits below .05ppm can be achieved by using one or more of the following methods: ducted exhaust hoods, air systems that provide 7 to 15 air exchanges per hour, ductless fume hoods with absorbents for the vapors, tightly fitting lids on immersion baths, and automated endoscope processors. Equipment is available to monitor vapor levels.

Hydrogen Peroxide

Hydrogen Peroxide is a rapid oxidizer, which facilitates the removal of organic debris and is relatively free of toxic fumes. Although hydrogen peroxide is a potent antimicrobial agent, it can damage rubber and plastics and corrodes copper, zinc and brass. A 7.5% hydrogen peroxide/0.85% phosphoric acid solution, classified as a high-level disinfectant is acceptable for endoscope reprocessing, unless incompatible with endoscopic equipment. Chemical dilution must be monitored by regularly testing the minimum effective concentration of 6%

Peracetic acid

Peracetic acid is a combination of acetic acid, hydrogen peroxide and water. A 1% solution has a broad-spectrum activity against bacteria, fungi, spores and enteroviruses. The use of an automated processor dilutes 35% paracetic acid to a final concentration of .2%, adds a buffer and anticorrosive agent. Unlike gluteraldehyde, paracetic acid is consumed with each reprocessing cycle; hence the overall reprocessing costs may be higher. Health hazards associated with paracetic acid include severe burns from direct contact with skin, irreversible damage or blindness from direct contact to the eyes. Also, inhalation of vapors or mist will irritate the nose, throat, and lungs. Currently there are no ceiling limits on permissible levels of paracetic acid in the air by the National Institute for Occupational Safety and Health.

Orthophalaldehyde

Orthophalaldehyde (OPA) is a relatively new product cleared by the FDA as a high-level disinfectant. It contains .55% 1,2-benzenedicarboxaldehyde. OPA has an excellent stability over wide PH ranges and is nonirritating to the eyes and nasal passages.

Guidelines for high-level disinfection of endoscopes (SGNA, 1997) include the following:

1. Manual cleaning is a prerequisite to manual or automated reprocessing with a chemical sterilant/disinfectant.
2. Reusable sterilant/disinfectants must be tested each day prior use, to determine if the solution is above the minimum effective concentration (MEC). The brand-specific strip should be used to test the MEC. The sterilant/disinfectant should be changed when the MEC fails or when the solution use-life expires, whichever comes first. Never exceed the use-life claim.
3. Make sure that the endoscope and all of its removable parts are completely submerged in the sterilant/disinfectant. Fill all channels with the chemical solution.
4. Cover the soaking basins with a tightly fitting lid to contain the chemical solution and its vapors.
5. After meticulous cleaning, high-level disinfection is achievable with a 20-minute soak at 20 degrees C (68 degrees F or room temperature) using a 2%glutaraldehyde solution that tests above its MEC.
6. Follow label directions as to time and temperature requirements for any chemical/steralant other than a non-surfactant 2% glutaraldehyde.
7. Surfactant-added glutaraldehydes are generally not recommended for flexible endoscopes.
8. Flush all channels with air before removing the endoscope from the sterilant/disinfectant.
9. Rinse the endoscope, all channels and removable parts with clean water following disinfection. To prevent toxic effects of residual chemicals after disinfection, adequate rinsing is vital. Chemical colitis mimicking pseudomembranous colitis can result if the endoscope and all of its parts are not thoroughly rinsed. Sterile water or water filtered through a 0.2-um filter is preferable for the final rinse. If sterile water is not used the next step is essential.
10. Purge all channels with air; rinse with 70% isopropyl alcohol, and purge all channels with air again to promote thorough drying. Also dry the exterior of the endoscope and all removable parts before storage.
11. Store the reprocessed endoscope by hanging it vertically in a well-ventilated cabinet. All removable parts should remain detached during storage.
12. Endoscope cases should never be used for storage.

Reports of transmission of infection by endoscopes are rare but can happen. Most of the transmission cases are attributed to a breach in the recommended reprocessing protocols (Spach, Silverstein & Stamm, 1993). Because endoscopes may be used on patients with both recognized and unrecognized infections such as HIV and the herpes B virus (HBV), it is important that they be reprocessed according to the Standards for Infection Control and Reprocessing of Flexible Gastrointestinal Endoscopes after each use (SGNA, 2000). It is unnecessary to reprocess an endoscope or accessory any differently depending on the diagnosis of a patient; to do so would be considered a double standard of care.

(Rutala, 1996). The only exception to this is Creutzfeldt-Jakob disease, for which a consult from an infection control professional is necessary.

Automated reprocessors

Automated reprocessors have become commonplace in the endoscopy settings for standardizing parts of the reprocessing protocol and decreasing personnel exposure to sterilant/disinfectants. The reprocessor does not replace mechanical cleaning or pre-cleaning of endoscopes. The endoscope should never be loaded into any automated reprocessor until pre-cleaning is completed. Although some automated reprocessors have cycles for circulating enzymatic detergent solutions, the physical action of wiping and brushing are not done. As mentioned earlier, manual cleaning will remove significant amount of organisms, feces and foreign material from the endoscope and is effective in reducing microbial contaminants by as much as 4 loggs or 99.99% (Rutala &Weber, 1995). If the automated reprocessor does not include a final alcohol/air rinse cycle, the step must be done manually.

Many types of reprocessors are available commercially. Recommended features for a reprocessor are as follows:
* circulation of fluids through all channels at equal pressure with out trapping air;
* rinse and forced-air cycles following both detergent and disinfectant cycles;
* disinfectant should not become diluted with any fluids;
* self-disinfection;
* no residual water should remain in hoses or reservoirs;
* self-contained water filtration system; and
* cycles for final alcohol rinse and air drying.

Although automated reprocessors have many benefits, one shortcoming is that they may not generate sufficient pounds per square inch to sufficiently access most ERCP or duodenal scope elevator channels Because the elevator channels of these scopes have small lumens, a force greater than that which is generated by the automated reprocessor may be needed to force fluid through them. Improper reprocessing of elevator channels has been associated with cases of patient morbidity and mortality (Spach, Silverstein, & Stamm, 1993). If the automated reprocessor is not capable of processing a channel, the device should be manually reprocessed, including all steps of cleaning, high-level disinfection, rinsing and drying, using a 2-5 ml syringe. It is important to investigate whether the elevator channel will need additional attention with both the scope manufacturer and the manufacturer of the automated reprocessor (FDA&CDC,1999).

Accessory equipment

Some endoscope accessories such as biopsy forceps are critical devices and, as such, require sterilization. Because of their tightly wound, spring-like configuration, they are extremely difficult to clean mechanically and sterilization steps may fail if organic debris is not removed. The recommended method for reusable biopsy forceps is to clean with an ultrasonic cleaner and steam sterilization.

Water bottles are another accessory device requiring special attention. The water bottle and its connecting tubing should be sterilized or receive high-level disinfection daily. If high-level disinfected, a thorough rinse using sterile water should be used to remove any chemical residue. Water bottles should be filled with sterile water for endoscopic irrigation (Martin & Reichelderfer, 1994).

Reprocessing of single–use accessory equipment

It is important for the gastroenterology nurse to be able to sort accessory devices according to Spaulding's classification system to determine how to reprocess each accessory. In some cases the use of single-use devices (SUDs) may be desirable, because it eliminates the need for reprocessing. Recent attention has been focused upon reprocessing SUDs. This approach remains controversial. The FDA finalized it policy on the reprocessing of SUDs for reuse through a guidance document issued on August 2, 2000. The document, entitled "Enforcement Priorities for Single-Use Devices Reprocessed by Third Parties and Hospitals," details a regulatory framework subjecting hospitals and third-party reprocessors to the same regulatory requirements applicable to the original equipment manufactures. According to this guidance document, the FDA requires registration of parties doing the reprocessing and listing of the reprocessed devices; premarket notification and approval requirements; adverse event reporting; and labeling and manufacturing requirements. In May 2002 SGNA maintained the position that "critical medical devices originally manufactured and labeled for single-use should not be reused. The original equipment manufacturers' recommendation regarding reuse of SUDs supersedes all other recommendations by any other entity."

Sanitation

Safe and effective sanitation methods are an essential component of infection control practices within the gastroenterology unit. Such methods are necessary to remove any sources of contamination, thereby minimizing the hazards of cross-contamination and lessening the risk of nosocomial infections.

An EPA-registered tuberculocidal hospital-grade disinfectant should be used for general wipe-down of noncritical items, such as procedure carts and stretchers. Environmental surfaces such as walls and floors should also be wiped down on a routine basis. Policies and procedures must be developed and adhered to for routine housekeeping.

Visable spills of blood or blood-contaminated body fluid should be decontaminated immediately with a 1:100 solution of household bleach or a hospital-grade disinfectant.

Endoscopy schedules should be planned so there is sufficient time for adequate processing of instruments and for the cleaning and set-up of the unit for the next patient.

Waste Management

Waste management policies and procedures should be developed by each healthcare facility using local, state, and federal waste management regulations. The policies and procedures should include proper methods of handling and disposing of waste and the designated parties responsible for compliance with the waste management regulations. Adherence to these specific procedures will help the health and safety of both staff and patients.

CASE SITUATION

Alice Holmes is a 28-year-old female who presents to the endoscopy unit for a colonoscopy. She has several tattoos and multiple body piercings. She has had diarrhea off and on for the past month. Recently she has experienced bloody bowel movements.

Points to consider

Keeping in mind that Ms. Holmes has increased risks factors of being HBV positive, what protection should be considered for personnel during the colonoscopy?

Upon completion of the procedure, how should the accessories be cleaned?

How would the environment be cleaned at the conclusion of the procedure?

At the completion of the procedure, what steps must the gastroenterology nurse take to properly decontaminate and disinfect the flexible colonoscope before use on subsequent patients?

Suggested responses

1. Regardless of the patient's suspected immune status, personnel should apply consistent infection control practices, including:
   (a) wearing gloves when touching blood or blood contaminated fluids or instruments;
   (b) wearing masks and eye protection;
   (c) wearing fluid-resistant gowns or aprons when assisting with the procedure, cleaning and reprocessing the colonoscope and when anticipated soiling of clothing with blood or body fluids is anticipated; and
   (d) washing hands thoroughly between endoscopy procedures and patient contacts.
2. Disposable accessories may be used. If non-disposable accessories are used, they must be meticulously cleaned and disinfected or sterilized according to the manufacture's instructions. If biopsy forceps are being reprocessed they should receive ultrasonic cleaning and steam sterilization.
3. At the conclusion of the colonoscopy, the environment should be cleaned by:
   (a) confining and removing organic material;
   (b) using moisture-proof disposable drapes as protective covering for procedure carts and equipment;
   (c) using an EPA-registered "tuberculocidal" hospital disinfectant for general wipe-down of all noncritical equipment;
   (d) using a 1:100 dilution of household bleach for visible blood or body fluids;

   (e) discarding moist, grossly contaminated waste in a disposable, leak-proof container; and
   (f) transporting grossly soiled linen with minimal handling in labeled, leak proof bags.
4. To properly decontaminate and disinfect the flexible colonoscope, the nurse should:
   (a) consider the flexible colonoscope as a semicritical item that has been in contact with mucous membranes;
   (b) wash hands, don gloves, mask, and eye protection, and protect skin and clothing with a fluid-resistant gown;
   (c) thoroughly inspect the colonoscope for damage, perform a leakage test; and
   (d) manually pre-clean, high-level disinfect, using appropriate sterilant/disinfectants, dry and store the endoscope in accordance with SGNA infection control guidelines and the manufacture's instructions.

Additional Considerations

Healthcare workers in all gastroenterology/endoscopy settings should be immunized with hepatitis B vaccine. Personnel should also be screened annually for tuberculosis by Mantoux skin testing.

Antibiotic prophylaxis for gastrointestinal endoscopic procedures should be decided on a case-by-case basis. General guidelines have been established by the ASGE for the prevention of endoscopically induced systemic or distant infections. It is recommended that high-risk patients receive antibiotics prior to stricture dilation, varix sclerosis and ERCP/obstructed billiary tree. High-risk patients include those with prosthetic valve, history of endocarditis, systemic pulmonary shunt, and synthetic vascular shunt less than one year old. It is also recommended that all patients with obstructed bile ducts and pancreatic pseudocyst receive prophylactic antibiotics prior to ERCP. In an effort to decrease risk of soft tissue infection, all patients undergoing endoscopic feeding tube placement should receive prophylaxis (ASGE, 1995).)

BIBLIOGRAPHY

Alvarado, C.J. & Reichelderfer, M. (2000). APIC Guideline for Infection Prevention and Control in Flexible Endoscopy. *American Journal of Infection Control 28, 139.*

American Society of Gastrointestinal Endoscopy (1995). Antibiotic Prophyalaxis for Gastrointestinal Endoscopy, Clinical Guideline. *Gastrointestinal Endoscopy 42,* 630-5.

Block SS. Peroxygen compounds. In: Block SS, editor. *Disinfection, sterilization and preservation.* 4th ed. Philadelphia:

DiMarino, A.J., Gage, T., Leung, J., Ravich, W., Wolf, D., Zuckerman, G. & Zuccaro, G. (1996). American Society of Gastrointestinal Endoscopy: Reprocessing of flexible gastrointestinal endoscopes. *Gastrointest Endosc 43,* 540-6.

Food & Drug Administration [FDA] and Center for Disease Control [CDC], (1999). *Public Health Advisory: Infections from Endoscopes Inadequately Reprocessed by an Automated Endoscope Reprocessing System.* [On-line.] Available: http://www.fda.gov/cdrh/safety/ endore-process.html

Liquid disinfecting and sterilizing reprocessors used for flexible endoscopes, Health Devices. 23:212-253,1994.

Occupational Safety & Health Administration (2001). *Compliance Directive: Bloodborne Pathogens Standard* [On-line]. Available: http://www.needle-stick-syringe-injury.com/pgs/needle-stick-osha.html.

Rutala, W. A. (1996). APIC guideline for selection and use of disinfectants. *American Journal of Infection Control 24,* 45-7.

Rutala, W. A., Clontz, E.P., Weber, D.J. & Hoffman, K. K. (1991). Disinfection practice for endoscopes and other semi-critical items. *Infection Control Hosp Epidemiol 12,* 282-8.

Semour, S. & Block, S. S. (Eds.) (2000). *Disinfection, sterilization and preservation* (5th ed.). Philadelphia: Lippincott Williams & Wilkins.

Society of Gastroenterology Nurses and Associates, Inc. (2002). *Reprocessing of endoscopic accessories and valves* (position statement). Chicago: Author.

Society of Gastroenterology Nurses and Associates, Inc. (2002). *Reuse of single-use critical medical devices* (position statement). Chicago: Author.

Chapter 4

ENVIRONMENTAL SAFETY

This chapter identifies the different types of environmental hazards that are present in gastroenterology settings and the precautions that the nurse and associate can take to protect both patients and healthcare personnel. These recommended practices are intended as achievable recommendations representing what is believed to be an optimal level of nursing practice. Policies and procedures will reflect variations in practice settings and or clinical situations that determine the degree to which the recommended practices can be implemented. The potential hazards may be associated with electrical equipment, chemical agents, ionizing radiation, latex sensitivity-allergen, accidental injury, electrosurgery, laser, workplace violence, and disaster planning.

Learning Objectives:

After reviewing the content of this chapter, the gastroenterology nurse and associate should be able to:

1. Identify potential hazards in the endoscopy unit that may have a potential to cause harm to patients or personnel, including electrical equipment, chemical agents, radiation, latex sensitivity, accidental injury, electrosurgery, laser, workplace violence, and disaster planning.
2. Describe steps that may be taken to minimize the dangers associated with these hazards.
3. Explain the responsibilities of gastroenterology personnel for ensuring a safe environment.

Basic safety regulations that govern institutional and healthcare facilities are found in the standards, guidelines, and codes of local, state, and federal agencies, such as Occupational Safety and Health Administration (OSHA), and voluntary standard-setting groups, such as the Joint Commission on Accreditation of Healthcare Organizations (JCAHO) and the National Fire Protection Association (NFPA).

It is the legal, ethical and moral responsibility of all gastroenterology personnel to be aware of these safety standards and how they affect patient care in the gastroenterology suite.

ELECTRICAL SAFETY

Electrical equipment and potential hazards associated with the use of electrical equipment should be identified and safe practices established. Light sources, cautery devices, laser, and video imaging equipment are all powered by electrical energy, as are lights, radiographic equipment, and many operating tables in surgery. The most common hazards relative to electricity are fire, burns, shock, or electrocution.

Staff members should demonstrate competence in using electrical equipment. All electrical equipment should be inspected before use. Inspection should include, but not be limited to, the following activities:

(a) check outlets and switch plates for damage;

(b) check power cords and plugs for fraying or other damage; and inspect (i.e., by a biomedical technician or electrical safety officer) new equipment before it s introduced into the practice setting.

Any direct contact with 110 or 220-volt wiring has the potential for **electrocution.** If the voltage is high enough; it can damage the brain and respiratory center, resulting in apnea.

Low-voltage currents frequently affect the heart, causing cardiac fibrillation or arrhythmias.

Complications of electrocution may include vascular injury, loss of consciousness, damage to the respiratory center, infection or eye damage.

To prevent fires and reduce the risks of burns and electrocution associated with electrically powered equipment, gastroenterology personnel can take the following measures:

(a) use appropriate precautions when using flammable gases or liquids;

(b) before use, check the integrity of all electrical equipment, including cords, switches, plugs, and wall receptacles;

(c) be sure that all electrical equipment is properly grounded;

(d) do not use multiple-outlet adapters or two-wire extension cords, and do not remove ground pins from three-pin plugs;

(e) avoid routing power cords through heavy traffic areas, and avoid rolling equipment over electrical cords;

(f) follow manufacturers' recommendations and standards for all electrical equipment;

(g) follow institutional policies and procedures regarding testing electrical equipment; never use an electrical device that has not been given a stamp of approval from the biomedical department;

(h) remove and report any questionable electrical equipment; and

(i) never place containers of liquid on electrical equipment.

Even when staff members take all reasonable precautions, it is still possible for a fire to occur in the endoscopy suite. To handle a fire quickly and effectively, gastroenterology personnel must participate in periodic fire drills in which they may practice using firefighting equipment. In addition, there should always be written policies and procedures for handling a fire emergency. Fire policies and procedures should be reviewed regularly and whenever a new type of equipment is installed.

If a fire occurs, it is important to proceed with the following steps:

(a) remove patients and staff from the immediate danger zone, if feasible;

(b) sound the alarm, and proceed according to institutional fire policy;

(c) close all doors to confine smoke and flame;

(d) smother or extinguish flames, if possible, using a **Halon** extinguisher for an electrical fire;

(e) never use water to extinguish an electrical fire;

(f) disconnect electrical equipment from its power source;

(g) activate circuit breakers and gas supply valves as directed by institutional policy;

(h) treat materials that are melting, dripping, or smoking as if they are actually burning to eliminate the possibility of their igniting or reigniting; and

(i) direct firefighters to the location of the fire.

When fire involves a patient directly, personnel should remove burning articles or smother the flame with a blanket. Smoldering, charred debris should be extinguished and removed from the patient immediately. Personnel should never use fire extinguishers directly on the patient because of the danger of cryogenic tissue damage or disposition of dangerous residue. After the fire has been extinguished, all burned material and equipment should be saved so the cause of the fire can be determined.

ENSOCOPIC IMAGING SYSTEMS

Like any other electrical device, endoscopes and their imaging systems must be checked for proper functioning before each use. Gastroenterology personnel should adhere to the following procedures:

(a) check the integrity of all electrical cables before use;

(b) do not handle equipment when hands, feet, body, or floor is wet;

(c) never use the light source as a supply table;

(d) ensure that all components of the imaging system are correctly connected;

(e) check the video image on the monitor(s) for clarity, and ensure additional equipment (e.g., image manager, printer, slide maker, computer) set-up is correct before use;

(f) turn on all system components and suction to make sure they are functioning properly; and

(g) turn the light source or processor off when not in use.

ELECTROSURGICAL AND CAUTERY DEVICES

Electrosurgical (ESU) and cautery units are among the most hazardous electrical devices in the endoscopy unit. Proper care and handling of electrosurgical equipment is essential to patient and personnel safety. It is used routinely to cut and coagulate body tissue with high-radio-frequency electrical current. These recommended practices do not endorse any specific product. Biomedical services personnel in practice settings should develop detailed routing safety and preventive maintenance inspections and maintain records.

Burns can result from: (a) poorly-applied patient **dispersive electrodes** (formerly called grounding pads), or (b) when electrical current seeks an alternate pathway out of the body, such as through ECG electrodes or metal objects like IV poles and x-ray tables. Bipolar units may be safer than monopolar modality, because the current returns through the electrode itself rather than the patient. It is important to follow the manufacturer's instructions for testing the equipment before the procedure. In the monopolar mode it is also important to place the dispersive electrode properly on the patient, and smaller size pads on the neonate or pediatric patient. It should not be placed near or on a bony prominence, skin over an implanted metal prosthesis, scar tissue, or places where circulation is likely to be impaired. The dispersive electrode should never direct current flow close to the site of a cardiac pacemaker. Any patient with an implantable cardiac defibrillating device should have the device inactivated before undergoing any procedure in the GI lab where there is a likelihood of an ESU or cautery device being used.

ESUs and cautery devices should be used on the lowest effective power setting for the endoscopic procedure. These settings should be confirmed orally to the operator/endoscopist before activation to ensure they are correct. An audio tone should be heard when the device is activated so that everyone knows when it is in use. The ESU or cautery unit should be turned off or placed in standby mode after each use.

If power settings above those expected are required to cut or coagulate, check the electrical pathway from the patient to the machine to rule out faulty or improper connections.

Most generators will sound an alarm if the electrical circuit is incomplete. If the problem is not obvious and easily correctable, the machine should be removed from service. Incomplete circuitry may lead to patient burns or shock to those touching the unit.

When caring for patients with pacemakers, personnel should take additional precautions that include, but are not limited to the following:

(a) checking with the manufacturer of the pacemaker and the patient's cardiologist regarding its function during use of the ESUs;

(b) ensuring that the distance between the active and dispersive electrodes is as short as possible;

(c) placing both electrodes as far from the pacemaker site as possible;

(d) keeping all ESU cords and cables away from the pacemaker and its leads;

(e) having a defibrillator immediately available for emergencies;

(f) using the lowest possible power setting on the ESU;

(g) evaluating the pacemaker continuously for proper function with continuous ECG monitoring; and

(h) having a magnet or a control unit available.

The patient's pacemaker may interpret electrocautery as cardiac activity and inhibit the pacemaker from initiating a heartbeat. These recommendations are available to reduce the potential for pacemaker inhibition.

When caring for a patient with an automatic implantable cardioverter/defibrillator (AICD) caregivers should take precautions that include, but are not limited to, the following:

(a) have the AICD device deactivated before the ESU is activated;

(b) have a defibrillator immediately available; and

(c) have continuous ECG monitoring during the procedure.

Argon enhanced coagulation (AEC) technology should be used according to the manufacturer's written instructions. As the AEC unit uses electrical current, the considerations and safety issues are the same as using any monopolar ESU. This will require personnel to take precautions, but not limited to:

(a) observe all safety measures for the ESU

(b) avoid placing the electrode in direct contact with tissue

(c) activate the argon gas flow and the ESU simultaneously

(d) limit the argon gas flow to the lowest level possible

(e) purge the argon gas line of air before each procedure and flush air out of the argon gas line by

(f) activating the system after moderate delays between activations.

MAINTENANCE

Every piece of electrical equipment must have an operation manual and receive routine preventive maintenance checks performed by the biomedical engineering department. Inservices should be held on a regular basis to update staff members on new equipment or changes in old equipment.

Health care facilities' policies and procedures for the use and maintenance of electrosurgery equipment must be in compliance with the Safe Medical Devices Act (SMDA) of 1990. If patient or personnel injuries or equipment failures occur, the ESU and the active and dispersive electrodes should be handled in accordance with the Safe Medical Devices Act of 1990. Device identification, preventative maintenance and service information, and adverse event information should be included in the report from the practice setting. Maintaining the ESU, the active and dispersive electrodes, and packaging allows for a complete systems check to determine the electrosurgical system integrity.

LASER SAFETY

The most dangerous aspects of laser are misdirection, scattering of the laser beam, smoke inhalation, and fire hazards. Whenever lasers are in use there is a potential for fire, damage to the skin or eyes, and respiratory tract irritation of patients and personnel. To prevent such injuries, personnel should follow these guidelines:

(a) place a warning sign of the door leading into the room where the laser is in use

(b) provide protective eyewear for all patients and personnel. The optical density of the eyewear should be equivalent to the wavelength of the laser used

(c) use instruments that are anodized or covered with non-reflective coating to prevent inadvertent beam reflection

(d) place the laser in the standby mode when it is not in use and allow the physician access to only one foot pedal when it is in use

(e) use lasers with a tamperproof audio tone that sounds when the beam is being activated

(f) use smoke evacuators and high-filtration masks to minimize the inhalation of the smoke produced in laser procedures

(g) flammable or combustible materials should not be used near the site; and

(h) follow all guidelines for electrical safety.

Policies and procedures should establish authority, responsibility, and accountability, and serve as operational guidelines. An introduction and review of laser safety policies and procedures should be included in the orientation and ongoing education of personnel to assist in the development of knowledge, skills, and attitudes that affect patient care.

All health care personnel working in laser treatment areas should attend a laser safety educational program that includes periodic updates to reinforce safe use of lasers. This program should provide participants a thorough understanding of all laser procedures and technology required for establishing and maintaining a safe environment during laser procedures.

RADIATION SAFETY

Certain waves of electromagnetic energy can penetrate matter by disrupting bonds between atoms and creating electrically charged ions. Such waves are termed **"ionizing radiation."** Radiation is a hazard because of its ability to modify molecules within body cells, thus causing cell dysfunction, alteration or halt in cell replication, or cell destruction. The effects of radiation may be somatic or genetic.

The primary source of ionizing radiation in the endoscopy unit is radiography equipment. Fluoroscopy allows the physician and staff to view and monitor the placement of catheters, stents, dilators, or endoscopes. In addition, portable x-ray machines may be used for diagnostic purposes.

The United States Nuclear Regulatory Commission (NRC) Title 10, Part 20, Code of Federal Regulations, "Standard for Protection Against Radiation," states an annual maximum permissible dose (MPD) for a whole body (trunk and head), active blood-forming organs, and gonads of 5 rem. The lens of the eye has an MPD of 15 rem per year, whereas the extremities and skin have an MPD of 50 rem per year. The 1994 revised regulations of the NRC created a new classification of radiation worker that they called "the declared pregnant woman." The NRC has limited the dose to the embryo/fetus to 0.5 rem (500m rem) over the entire pregnancy. Also, they recommend a uniform monthly exposure rate to the embryo/fetus of 50m rem/month.

There is no level of ionizing radiation that is not potentially harmful. Unnecessary exposure can be minimized in the following ways:
(a) decreasing the time of exposure;
(b) increasing the distance from the source;
(c) placing a shield between the radiation source and the body; and
(d) questioning all female patients of childbearing age about the possibility of pregnancy before radiographic procedures.

The following protective guidelines may help minimize the exposure of gastroenterology patients and personnel to ionizing radiation:
(a) wear lead-lined aprons, thyroid collars, gloves, and protective eyewear in accordance with institutional guidelines;
(b) use patient gonadal shielding as appropriate;
(c) wear film badges during procedures in which radiation exposure is encountered;
(d) analyze exposure levels monthly;
(e) alternate personnel for procedures that require radiation, and limit exposure time for personnel holding patients and/or films;
(f) when the fluoroscope is in use, instruct personnel not to turn their unshielded backs to the radiographic equipment and to maintain as great a distance from the x-ray beam as possible;
(g) allow only trained personnel to operate and maintain all radiographic equipment;
(h) be certain that the contrast medium selected is effective for the type of study being done;
(i) to help reduce unnecessary repeat procedures, be sure the patient is properly prepared and positioned (expose only the area of study to the film or fluoroscopy); and
(j) consult with a radiation safety office regarding equip-

ment inspection, analysis of radiation exposure badges, and educational in-services.

When handled properly and efficiently, ionizing radiation can be safe and effective during diagnostic and therapeutic procedures in the endoscopy unit.

LATEX SENSITIVITY/ALLERGEN

The incidence of latex allergies is on the rise. Complete avoidance in the endoscopy unit to latex is the only way to prevent increased sensitization and possible life threatening "anaphylactic" reaction. Identification of all patients' allergies, including **latex allergy,** is important before any endoscopic procedure is performed. A latex-free environment can make procedures safer for the latex-allergic patient. Gastroenterology nurses, associates and personnel have the responsibility to assess and educate the patients relative to latex allergy to promote positive patient outcomes in the endoscopy setting. The following individuals are at risk for developing latex allergy:
(a) workers with ongoing latex exposure, e.g. those in healthcare who frequently change latex gloves;
(b) individuals with a tendency to have multiple allergic conditions;
(c) persons with allergies to certain foods, especially avocado, potato, bananas, tomatoes, chestnuts, kiwi fruits, and papaya; and persons with spina bifida, asthma, or a history of multiple surgical procedures.

Our one intent is to provide guidance to the endosocopy staff practicing in facilities where powdered gloves are still in use. Collaboration with all healthcare providers including the physician will promote a safe environment for the latex allergic patients and healthcare workers.

Some of the following recommendations may be unnecessary if low-allergen and powder free gloves are utilized throughout the healthcare facility. Any specific requirements should be implemented based on the patient needs.
1. Notify the endoscopy unit 24-48 hours before the scheduled procedure regarding "latex alert."
2. Schedule the procedure as the first case of the day.
3. Remove all latex items from the patient area and procedure room; prepare a safe post-procedure recovery area for the patient.
4. Remove boxes of latex gloves from all areas and replace them with latex-free gloves, both sterile and nonsterile if applicable.
5. Educate the patient, family, or significant other(s) regarding the latex-safe plan and provide assurances regarding the involvement of all healthcare providers.
6. Double check all supplies and equipment for latex, including IV tubing and bags.
7. Use latex-free IV tubing or replace injection ports with three-way stopcocks.
8. Use medication in ampules or latex-free vials when available. Do not puncture rubber medication stoppers with a needle; instead, remove the rubber stoppers before withdrawing the medications.
9. Use glass or latex-free plastic syringes.

10. Use latex-free blood pressure cuffs. If they are not available, wrap the patient's arm to prevent blood pressure or tourniquet cuff tubing from coming into contact with the patient's skin.
11. Mark the patient's chart "Latex Allergy."
12. Provide latex-sensitive patients with a "Latex Allergy" identification band.
13. Remind all healthcare team members of the necessity for following latex avoidance procedures.
14. Prepare for a possible allergic response with IV fluids and drugs for treatment.

The above recommendations are designed to promote a safe healthcare environment for the latex-sensitive or latex-allergic patients and healthcare workers. The recommendations may not apply to every individual, and each facility should have in place latex-safe policies, procedures and protocols.

CHEMICAL SAFETY

Gastroenterology personnel come into daily contact with a large number of chemicals, some of which carry high exposure risks. There are certain common-sense rules for handling chemicals.

1. Always read and follow label directions.
2. Employees should have (a) easy access to, and (b) an understanding of the information provided on the material safety data sheet that accompanies all hazardous chemicals.
3. Employees should be familiar with a spill-containment plan specific for the liquid chemical germicide used. The information from the specific material safety data sheet should be incorporated into the plan.
4. Mix chemicals only in accordance with directions.
5. Use the rules of standard precautions as if the chemicals were body fluids: if it will come in contact with hands wearing gloves; if it might splash, wear a face shield and protective clothing; always wash hands after exposure to any chemical.
6. After the use of disinfectants, rinse instruments or surfaces thoroughly to remove any harmful residue.

One of the most frequently encountered hazardous chemicals in the endoscopy unit is glutaraldehyde. Because glutaraldehyde is water-soluble and vaporizes readily, its main effects are on the mucous membranes and the eyes. Short-term exposure can cause nose and throat irritation, burning of the eyes, and headaches.

When handling glutaraldehyde, gastroenterology personnel should wear rubber gloves such as nitrile or butyl gloves, goggles, a mask or a face shield, and an impervious gown. Glutaraldehyde should only be used in areas that have adequate ventilation. It should be stored in a tightly covered container in a cool, dry place. Sinks, showers, and eyewash stations should be available. If glutaraldehyde comes in contact with the eyes, the eyes should be flushed with water for a full 15 minutes. Skin should be washed thoroughly; clothing should be removed and washed before reuse. In case of excessive inhalation, the individual should be moved to fresh air and treated medically as symptoms warrant.

Another hazardous chemical that gastroenterology personnel are exposed to is formaldehyde, which is primarily as a tissue fixative. Like glutaraldehyde, formaldehyde is soluble in water and therefore mainly affects the mucous membranes and the eyes. To minimize exposure, workers should wear gloves, goggles, aprons, and masks. Formaldehyde should be stored in an airtight container. Personnel should be informed about possible adverse reactions. First-aid measures are the same as for glutaraldehyde.

Peracetic acid is another variety of **liquid chemical germicide.** In its reconstituted form, it is extremely irritating to the eyes, mucous membranes, skin, and to the respiratory tract. It should be stored in a dry area. Staff should be familiar with written procedures for disposing of partially or fully reconstituted peracetic acid. Supply of peracetic acid should be rotated and expiration dates routinely checked.

Isopropyl (rubbing) alcohol is also found in endoscopy suites. Gloves should be worn when using this chemical and care should be taken to avoid splashing, because it may cause corneal burns and eye damage. Isopropyl alcohol is highly flammable and therefore should be stored in tightly closed containers, away from heat, flames, or sparks. In case of excessive inhalation, the individual should be moved to fresh air and given medial support. In case of ingestion, the individual must receive immediate medical treatment.

Mercury-filled dilators, must be inspected on a regular basis to ensure that they are intact and to avoid leakage. Always follow the manufacturer recommendations and guidelines regarding replacement and expiration dates.

ACCIDENTAL INJURY

A few simple preventive measures go a long way toward helping gastroenterology personnel reduce the risk of accidental injury to themselves and/or their patients.

Human errors related to the operation of medical devices in the endoscopy unit can be minimized by utilizing built-in safety features such as the audible activation indicator on an ESU, providing adequate operator training/inservices, and preventative maintenance service of equipment regularly.

With the enactment of the new Safe Medical Devices Act, healthcare facilities are now required to report device-related injuries and illnesses to the Food and Drug Administration (FDA) and to the manufacturer. If problems develop, the FDA has the authority to recall certain devices.

Accidental falls are another potential source of injury. To avoid accidental falls in the endoscopy unit, the following steps should be taken:

(a) hallways and doorways should be free of equipment and carts;
(b) rooms should be kept neat and orderly; and
(c) electrical cords, cables, and accessories should be placed so that personnel do not trip or fall.

Mental or physical exhaustion can also contribute to the risk of accidents. Proper lifting techniques must be practiced. Devices are available to assist with heavy lifting and should be used whenever possible. Comfortable temperatures, noise control, ventilation, and adequate lighting are essential.

OSHA is the federal agency responsible for regulating workplace environments to ensure safety. It is important that the endoscopy unit comply with all applicable OSHA standards.

DISASTER PLANNING

Healthcare personnel must be prepared to respond quickly and effectively to internal or external disasters. Although rare, the occurrence of such events is a real possibility and must be anticipated. Personnel must be familiar with policies for fire, severe weather, and other disasters.

An internal disaster plan that includes procedures for moving patients out of the unit or evacuating them from the building should be devised and posted or accessible. Simulated disaster drills help personnel evaluate how they would function in a crisis.

WORKPLACE VIOLENCE

Workplace violence (WPV) is increasing across all clinical areas. The National Institute for Occupational Safety and Health (NIOSH) defines WPV as "any physical assault, threatening behavior, verbal abuse occurring in the workplace setting." The gastroenterology personnel are as vulnerable in the endoscopy unit as any other. By increasing individuals' sensitivity and awareness of potential violent incidents, this may help to identify a potentially violent situation before it escalates. Prevention is the best protection you can provide staff.

Policies and procedures for WPV should be established for all healthcare facilities. On the institutional level, OSHA makes the following recommendations for abatement of WPV:

(a) develop a crisis management plan;
(b) require mandatory training for all workers in prevention techniques, restraint and seclusion procedures, and multicultural diversity techniques;
(c) increase staff-to-patient-ratios when applicable; and
(d) identify patients with increased potential for violence.

We must work to keep our profession healthy, physically and mentally, by reporting workplace violence events and practicing what should be mandated to us in training. Learning to spot violence and defusing it before an event takes place is the key. Recognizing that WPV is not "part of the job" is the first step to change.

REVIEW TERMS

electrocution, Halon extinguisher, dispersive electrodes, Argon enhanced coagulation, laser, ionizing radiation, latex allergy, liquid chemical germicide

CASE SITUATION

Sam Little, age 68, was admitted to the endoscopy unit for a gastroscopy after radiographic x-rays were suggestive of a possible gastric mass. Mr. Little has a extensive medical history which include multiple surgeries, drug and food allergies.

Points to think about

1. The initial nursing assessment should include all surgeries, drug and food allergies.
   a. What particular foods are potentially significant for latex sensitization?
   b. Is there a significance if the patient has had multiple surgeries? If so, why?
2. Did the primary care physician relay any information regarding a potential latex alert?
3. Had the endoscopist seen the patient prior to their arrival for their appointment in endoscopy?
4. What immediate nursing responsibilities are implemented if a "latex allergy/sensitivity" is documented?

Suggested responses

1. During the initial interview it is determined that the patient has a latex allergy or sensitivity, the following must be completed:
   (a) immediately remove all latex items from the patient's area;
   (b) prepare the procedure room with removal of all latex gloves, IV accessories, etc and replace with non latex items;
   (c) coordinate with all healthcare team members including the physician;
   (d) be prepared to treat the patient with specific medications before the procedure is initiated; and
   (e) be sure all persons involved with this patient's care are aware of the latex allergy/alert and have a safe environment.
2. During the interview and implementation of care of the patient with latex allergy, be sure to include the patient, family, and/or significant other.

REVIEW QUESTIONS

1. An electrical fire that does not involve the patient directly should be handled by:
   a. Using a Halon extinguisher.
   b. Throwing water on it.
   c. Immediately removing the patient from the room.
   d. Suffocation with a fire blanket.
2. When out of use, an ESU device should:
   a. Be set down on a drape.
   b. Be placed in a safe location.
   c. Remain in the endoscopist's hand.
   d. Be handed to an assistant.
3. To avoid accidental injuries to patients and personnel when a laser is in use, it is important to:
   a. Use protective eyewear.
   b. Post "laser in use" signs.
   c. Use nonreflective instruments.
   d. All of the above.

4. For laser procedures, the optical density of the protective eyewear used is determined by:
    a. The physician's preference.
    b. The procedure that will be performed.
    c. Institutional policies and procedures.
    d. The wavelength of the laser being used.

5. When ionizing radiation is in use, pregnant healthcare worksers should:
    a. Wear a lead-lined apron, thyroid collar, and protective eyewear in accordance with institutional guidelines.
    b. Wear a film badge.
    c. Limit the dose to the embryo/fetus to 0.5rem (500m rem) over the entire pregnancy, with a uniform monthly exposure rate to the embryo/fetus of 50m rem/month.
    d. All of the above.

6. If a piece of electrical equipment malfunctions, it should be:
    a. Fixed by gastroenterology personnel.
    b. Removed from service and reported according to institutional policy.
    c. Used again to see if the problem recurs.
    d. Reported to the FDA.

7. The primary source of ionizing radiation in the endoscopy suite is:
    a. Portable radiographic equipment.
    b. Fluoroscopy.
    c. Radionuclides.
    d. CT scans.

8. If glutaraldehyde accidentally comes in contact with a healthcare worker's skin, he or she should:
    a. Wash the area thoroughly.
    b. Rinse the area with water only.
    c. Apply burn ointment.
    d. Cover the area with a bandage.

9. Under the new Safe Medical Devices Act, healthcare facilities are required to report device-related illness and accidents to:
    a. The manufacturer.
    b. OSHA.
    c. The FDA.
    d. The FDA and manufacturer.

10. Plans for evacuating patients in the event of an external or internal disaster should be:
    a. Posted in an obvious location.
    b. Recorded in institutional policies and procedures manuals.
    c. Practiced in simulated disaster drills.
    d. All of the above.

11. If a procedure is scheduled for a latex allergic patient, the following should be done:
    a. Schedule the procedure the first of the day.
    b. Complete a detailed medical history including medication allergies, surgeries, and food allergies.
    c. Refer the patient to the operating room.
    d. A & B.

BIBLIOGRAPHY

Anderson, C. (Ed.) (2001). Defining the Severity of Workplace Violent Events among medical and nonmedical samples, *Gastroenterology Nursing 24:5*, 225-230.

Association of periOperative Registered Nurses (2002). *Recommended Practices for Safe Care Through Identification of Potential Hazards in the Surgical Environment.* Denver, CO.

Association of periOperative Registered Nurses (2002). *Recommended Practices for Environmental Responsibility.* Denver, CO.

Association of periOperative Registered Nurses (2002). *Recommended Practices for Laser Safety in Practice Setting.* Denver, CO.

Association of periOperative Registered Nurses (2002). *Recommended Practices for Electrosurgery.* Denver, CO.

Association of periOperative Registered Nurses (2002). *Latex Guidelines.* Denver, CO.

Johnson & Johnson Medical, Inc. (1994). *Material Safety Data Sheet, Enzymatic Detergent.* New Brunswick, New Jersey.

Joint Commission on Accreditation of Healthcare Organizations (1997). *Accreditation manual for hospitals.* Oakbrook Terrace, IL.

Jordan, S. (1996). Using glutaraldehyde-based instrument sterilants safely. *Infection Control Steriliz- Technology 2:11,* 30-5.

Kneedler, J. & Dodge, G. (1987). *Perioperative patient care* (2nd ed.). Boston: Blackwell Scientific.

Marousky, R. (1991). The Material Safety Data Sheet (MSDS): A guide to chemical safety in the OR. *Today's OR Nurse 13,* 6-11.

Patterson, P. (1991). Advice for users on Compliances with Devices Act. *OR Manager 7,* 1.

Society of Gastroenterology Nurses and Associates, Inc. (2001, January). *Safe Operation of Radiographic Equipment during GI Endoscopic Procedures.* Chicago.

Society of Gastroenterology Nurses and Associates, Inc. (January, 2001). Radiation Safety in the Endoscopic Setting. *Gastroenterology Nursing 24:3,* 143-6.

Stephens Scientific, a Division of Richard-Allen Scientific (1996). *Material Safety Data Sheet (MSDS): Formaldehyde 4% Solution.* Kalamazoo, Michigan.

Ulrich Chemical, Inc. (1997). *Material Safety Data Sheet (MSDS): Isopropyl Alcohol 70%.* Indianapolis, Indiana.

Wai, D.M. (Ed.) (2001). A Guide to Caring for your Latex Allergic Patient. *Gastroenterology Nursing 22:6,* 262-5.

Walina, C. (1988). Occupational Hazards in the Endoscopy Suite. *SGA Journal 11,* 100-5.

Chapter 5

STANDARDS FOR PRACTICE

This chapter acquaints the gastroenterology nurse with the standards for practice that guide gastroenterology nursing. Standards for practice in the context of this chapter are viewed as any standards used by gastroenterology nurses and associates to define the professional practice. These include the Society of Gastroenterology Nurses and Associates (SGNA) Standards for Practice, the American Nurses Association (ANA) Standards of Clinical Nursing Practice, and the Joint Commission on Accreditation of Healthcare Organizations (JCAHO) hospital standards. The JCAHO statement of patients' rights and responsibilities and SGNA's infection control guidelines are summarized. Pertinent standards, regulations, and guidelines issued by governmental agencies are also reviewed.

LEARNING OBJECTIVES

After reviewing the content of this chapter, the gastroenterology nurse should be able to:

1. Outline the expected behavior of the gastroenterology nurse as set forth in the SGNA Standards for Practice.
2. Discuss the JCAHO standards the influence gastroenterology practice in the hospital setting and the JCAHO statement of patients' rights and responsibilities.
3. Explain how regulations and guidelines developed by specific government agencies guide practice in the endoscopy unit.

STANDARDS DEFINED

Standards are an acknowledged measure of comparison for quantitative or qualitative value, such as a model, criterion or rule of professional behavior. They can be used as guidelines in the workplace or with any legal issues.

Standards for practice are conceptual statements that can describe practice outcomes. They are not intended to specify how an outcome is to be achieved, but rather what is to be achieved. Standards of care can be defined as measurable statements that can be the means to accomplish practice outcomes. They define criteria against which the nurse's level of performance may be measured. As technology and knowledge advances, so must the approach to practiced outcomes. Standards should be continually updated and validated in the practice setting.

SOURCES OF STANDARDS AND GUIDELINES IN GASTROENTEROLOGY NURSING

Standards and guidelines that provide direction for gastroenterology nurses include standards of nursing practice, accreditation standards, community standards, standards of technical practice, and the regulations and guidelines issued by various governmental agencies.

Standards of nursing practice have been developed by the Society of Gastroenterology Nurses and Associates (SGNA), the American Nurses Association (ANA), the Association of Operating Room Nurses (AORN), and other nursing organizations.

Accreditation standards include those developed by the Joint Commission on Accreditation of Healthcare Organization (JCAHO).

Community standards are based on legal and ethical principles that affect standards of practice in the endoscopy unit, by way of statements for patients' rights and responsibilities.

Standards of technical practice may be developed in individual endoscopy units, with reference to guidelines issued by professional associations, such as SGNA's Recommended Guidelines for Infection Control. Technical standards must be congruent with other standards that apply to the gastroenterology nurse and associate.

A number of federal regulations and guidelines also affect the practice of gastroenterology nursing.

SGNA STANDARDS FOR PRACTICE

The Standards of Clinical Nursing Practice and Role Delineations were first published in 1991, revised in 1998, and adopted by the SGNA Practice Committee and the Board of Directors in 2001.

These standards for practice are qualitative, conceptual outcome statements, intended to specify the expected result of the care provided. They describe what is to be accomplished, not how those outcomes are to be achieved. The criteria necessary to meet these standards should be individualized for each work setting, based on the policies, procedures, and practices of the institution, and the education and professional licensure of its staff.

The SGNA Standards for Practice reflect a variety of personnel collaboration to ensure optimal patient outcomes for diagnostic and therapeutic procedures, and for purposes of health maintenance, restoration or palliation. They are broad enough to encompass the implementation of the Standards of Care relating to the roles of each gastroenterology staff member: advanced practice nurses, registered nurses, licensed practical/vocational nurses, and assistive personnel/technicians.

The standards are designed to be applicable across a continuum that covers independent, collaborative, and dependent aspects of practice. Gastroenterology nurses and associates perform some tasks independently, and some are dependent of the performance or judgment of other personnel. These will differ significantly depending upon the Nurse Practice Act in each individual state, professional or vocational licensure, educational background, and institutional nursing practice policy constraints. Similar policies may be devised for independent, collaborative, and dependent activities of an LPN/LVN or assistive personnel/technician.

The SGNA Standards for Practice are listed below, accompanied by some examples, criteria, or standards of care that may specify how each standard can be adapted to an individual practice setting.

STANDARD I: QUALITY OF CARE

Standard: The Gastroenterology Nurse continually and systematically evaluates the quality and effectiveness of nursing practice.

Measurement Criteria

1. The nurse participates in quality-of-care activities as appropriate to the individual's position, education, and practice environment.
2. The nurse uses the results of quality-of-care activities to initiate changes in nursing practices.
3. The nurse identifies and implements precepts of palliative care when indicated

Example: Nurse uses reversal agents to return to baseline status.

STANDARD II: PERFORMANCE APPRAISAL

Standard: The gastroenterology nurse evaluates his/her own nursing practice in relation to professional practice standards and relevant statutes and regulations.

Measurement Criteria:

1. The nurse engages in performance appraisal on a regular basis, identifying areas of strength as well as areas for professional practice development.
2. The nurse seeks constructive feedback regarding his/her own practice.
3. The nurse takes action to achieve goals identified during performance appraisal.
4. The nurse participates in peer review as appropriate.
5. The nurse is knowledgeable of and applies professional standards of care and guidelines for practice as a personal performance benchmark.

Example: Nurse participates in monthly staff meetings.

STANDARD III: EDUCATION

Standard: The gastroenterology nurse acquires and maintains current knowledge in nursing practice.

Measurement Criteria:

1. The nurse completes an orientation based on individual learning needs that have been identified for the performance description and practice setting in which the individual will perform.
2. The nurse identifies learning needs based on performance behaviors that include critical thinking, interpersonal, and technical skills. The nurse demonstrates accountability for maintaining competency and participates in educational activities relevant to professional issues and trends in gastroenterology nursing practice.

Example: Nurse attends continuing education courses.

STANDARD IV: COLLEGIALITY

Standard: The gastroenterology nurse contributes to the professional development of peers, colleagues, and others.

Measurement Criteria:

1. The nurse shares knowledge and skills with colleagues and others.
2. The nurse provides peers with constructive feedback regarding their practice.
3. The nurse contributes to an environment that is conducive to clinical education of nursing students as appropriate.
4. The nurse uses appropriate interpersonal communication techniques to avoid defensive responses and resistance to changing practice.
5. The nurse assists colleagues in building or maintaining the competencies necessary to provide safe, effective care to patients.

Example: Nurse acts as a mentor/preceptor in the endoscopy unit.

STANDARD V: ETHICS

Standard: The gastroenterology nurse's decisions and actions on behalf of patients are determined in an ethical manner.

Measurement Criteria:

1. The nurse's practice is guided by the Code for Nurses with Interpretive Statements (ANA, 1985).
2. The nurse maintains patient confidentiality.
3. The nurse acts as a patient advocate.
4. The nurse delivers care in a non-judgmental and nondiscriminatory manner that is sensitive to diversity, including culture, race, religion, age, gender, sexual preference, ethnicity, and personal preference.
5. The nurse delivers care in a manner which preserves/protects patient autonomy, dignity, and rights.
6. The nurse seeks available resources to help formulate ethical decisions.
   Example: Nurse ensures the patient's right for privacy.

STANDARD VI: COLLABORATION

Standard: The gastroenterology nurse collaborates with the patient, significant others, and healthcare providers in providing patient care.

Measurement Criteria:

1. The nurse communicates with the patient, significant others, and healthcare providers regarding patient care and the nurse's role in the provision of care.
2. The nurse consults with other members of the healthcare team for patient care as needed.
3. The nurse makes referrals, including provisions for continuity of care, as needed.
   Example: After procedure, the nurse provides patient report to the primary care nurse and the endoscopy unit nurse after a procedure.

STANDARD VII: RESEARCH

Standard: The gastroenterology nurse uses the findings of peer-reviewed, published scientific research in practice, and seeks opportunities to participate in research activities.

Measurement Criteria:

1. The nurse uses interventions substantiated by valid, scientific research as appropriate to the individual's position, education and practice environment.
2. The nurse participates in research activities as appropriate to the individual's position, education and practice environment.
   Example: Nurse collaborates with physicians on drug research project.

STANDARD VIII: RESOURCE UTILIZATION

Standard: The gastroenterology nurse considers factors related to safety, efficacy and cost in planning and delivering patient care.

Measurement Criteria:

1. The nurse evaluates factors related to safety, effectiveness and cost when two or more practice options would result in the same expected patient outcome.
2. The nurse assigns tasks or delegates care based on the needs of the patient and the knowledge and competence of the provider selected.
3. The nurse assists the patient and significant others in identifying and securing appropriate services available to address health-related needs.
   Example: Nurse refers patient and family newly diagnosed with Crohn's Disease to the Crohn's and Colitis Foundation of America, for support and additional education.

In addition to the Standards for Practice listed above, JCAHO accreditation standards demand that all gastroenterology nurses and associates adhere to JCAHO requirements in the hospital setting.

JCAHO STANDARDS

The Joint Commission on Accreditation of Healthcare Organizations (JCAHO) is an independent health care-standards-setting and accrediting agency. Their mission is to continuously improve the safety and quality of care provided to the public through the provision of health care accreditation and related services that support performance improvement in health care organizations. Standards developed by JCAHO reflect optimal achievable health care practices. They are reviewed and revised continually as warranted by technological developments, new knowledge, changes in government regulations, and consumer demands for accountability.

Accreditation by the JCAHO is recognized as a symbol of quality, and that an organization's ability can meet with certain performance standards. To earn accreditation, an organization must undergo an on-site evaluation and must demonstrate compliance within standard key areas, such as patient rights. The standards focus not simply on what the organization has, but what is actually does. Accreditation also considers performance expectations for activities that affect the quality of patient care and have the experience of a good outcome.

During a JCAHO accreditation survey, the health care organization's compliance with JCAHO standards, is judged on the following information:

   (a) Documentation of compliance provided by the hospital;
   (b) Verbal answers to questions concerning the implementation of a standard, or examples of its implementation, that will enable a judgment of compliance to be made;
   (c) Interviews with patients and staff members; and
   (d) On-site observations by JCAHO surveyors.

To meet JCAHO standards, in-hospital endoscopy/gastroenterology units must have certain specific characteristics. The Accreditation Manual for Hospitals, 1997 has 17 separate sections covering different aspects of hospital management and patient care. Of these, the section most pertinent to gastroenterology nurses and associates covers operative and other invasive procedures. Other relevant requirements deal with hospital-sponsored ambulatory care; infection control; nursing care; and plant, technology, and safety management.

Surgical and Anesthesia Services: JCAHO requires that surgical and anesthesia services are available to meet patients' needs; that patients with the same health status and condition receive comparable surgical and anesthesia care throughout the hospital; that there is effective collaboration among departments/services providing and supporting surgical and anesthesia services; and that surgical and anesthesia services participate in the hospital's performance improvement program.

Hospital-Sponsored Ambulatory Care Services: JCAHO requires that ambulatory care services are safe and effective and are integrated with other departments/services of the hospital; that staff participate in relevant educational programs or activities; that written policies and procedures address specific issues; that structures, systems, policies, and procedures are in place for safety management, life safety, equipment management, and utilities management; that comprehensive medical records are kept; that structures designed to improve the quality of patient care are in place; and that the ambulatory care unit participates in the hospital's performance improvement program.

Infection Control: JCAHO requires that there is an effective hospital-wide program for infection surveillance, prevention, and control; that a multidisciplinary committee is responsible for monitoring and correcting infection control practices; that a qualified individual(s) has responsibility for infection control activities; that there are written infection control policies and procedures; and that the infection control program is coordinated with support services, such as central services, housekeeping, and linen/laundry.

Nursing Care: JCAHO requires that patients receive nursing care (based on a documented assessment of their needs) conducted by an RN; that all members of the nursing staff are competent to fulfill assigned responsibilities; that patient care programs, policies, and procedures based on nursing standards of patient care and standards of nursing practice are developed; that the hospital's plan for providing nursing care is designed to support improvement, and innovation in nursing practice and is based on patient needs and the hospital's mission; that nursing leaders participate in the hospital's decision-making structures and processes; and that nursing care is monitored and evaluated as part of the hospital's performance improvement program.

Plant, Technology, and Safety Management: JCAHO requires the existence of a safety management program concerned with the physical environment and staff activities; a life safety management program, covering fire safety and the safe use of buildings and grounds; an equipment management program; and a utilities management program.

PATIENTS' RIGHTS AND RESPONSIBILITIES

The gastroenterology nurse has a responsibility to ensure that the rights of the patient are preserved. Patients have responsibilities that they and their significant other should consider if any hospitalization occurs. The JCAHO Accreditation Manual for Hospitals lists a number of basic patient rights and responsibilities as follows.

Patients' Rights:

- **Access to care.** All patients have a right to access treatment or accommodations that are available or medically indicated, including access to protective services (JCAHO RI 1.5).
- **Respect and dignity.** Patients have the right to considerate, respectful care at all times and under all circumstances, with recognition of their personal dignity.
- **Privacy and confidentiality.** Patients have the right to expect that any interviews, examinations, or consultations will be conducted with consideration for their privacy and that their hospital records will remain confidential.
- **Patient safety and security.** Patients have the right to expect reasonable safety and security insofar as hospital practices and environment are concerned (JCAHO RI 1 13).
- **Identity.** Patients have the right to know the identity and professional status of individuals providing services to them, to know which practitioners are primarily responsible for their care, and to know of any professional relationships among individuals or institutions involved in their care.
- **Information.** Patients or their legally authorized representatives have the right to obtain complete, current, and understandable information concerning their diagnosis, treatment, and any known prognosis.
- **Communication.** Patients have the right of access to people outside the hospital by means of visitors and by verbal and written communications; interpreters should be provided where language barriers are a problem. Any imposed restrictions of patient visitors, mail, telephone calls, or other forms of communication are to be evaluated for therapeutic effectiveness. If restrictions are necessary, the patient and/or family will receive a complete explanation to determine limitations(JCAHO RI 1.3 6.1).
- **Consent.** Patients and their families have the right to reasonable informed participation in decisions involving the care (JCAHO RI 1.2.2).
- **Consultation.** Patients have the right to consult with specialists at their own request and expense.
- **Refusal of treatment.** Patients have the right to refuse treatment to the extent permitted by law.
- **Transfer and continuity of care.** Patients have the right to receive a complete explanation of the need for and alternatives to any transfer to another facility or organization and the right to be informed of any continuing health care needs following discharge from the hospital.
- **Hospital charges.** Patients have the right to an itemized and detailed explanation of the total bill for services rendered in the hospital.
- **Hospital rules and regulations.** Patients should be informed of hospital rules and regulations applicable to their conduct and about the hospital's mechanisms for handling patient complaints.

- **Pastoral counseling.** Patients have the right to pastoral counseling on request. (JCAHO RI 1.3.5)
- **Advance directives.** Patients have the right to make their own decision about the care they receive or appoint a spokesperson on their behalf. Advance directives will include withholding resuscitative services, forgoing or withdrawal of life-sustaining treatments, and decisions involving care at the end of life (JCAHO RI.2.4).
- **Voice dissatisfactions.** The patient has a right to voice dissatisfactions about patient care-related issues (JCAHO R1.3.4).
- **Ethical issues.** The patient has the right to consideration of ethical issues during the development of the plan of care (JCAHO R1.I).
- **Research.** All patients participating in research projects are given the right to a description of benefits (JCAHO RI.2.1.5), a description of potential discomforts and risk (JCAHO RI 1 .2.1 .2), and a description of alternative services (JCAHO RI 1,2,1,3). In addition, research patients have the right to a full explanation of services, especially those which are experimental in nature. The research patient has the right to refuse participation without compromising services. Patients will receive informed consent addressing the following issues: name of person providing information, date forms are signed, verification of rights to privacy, confidentiality, and safety (JCAHO RI 1.2,1.4, RI 1.2.1.5, RI.3).
- **Organ donation.** Patients have the right to information concerning organ donation in accordance with institutional organ donation policy (JCAHO RI 2).
- **Written statement.** Each patient has the right to written statements concerning his or her patient rights (JCAHO RI 4).
- **Ethics.** Patients have the right to the adherence of institutional ethics established to include behaviors of marketing, admissions, transfers, discharge, billing, and relationships with other care providers and institutions.

PATIENT RESPONSIBILITIES

The JCAHO states that hospitals have the right to expect behavior on the part of patients and their significant others that is reasonable and responsible. Each patients' responsibilities are:

- **Providing information.** The patient is responsible for providing, to the best of his or her knowledge, accurate and complete information about present complaints, past illnesses, hospitalizations, medications, and other matters relating to his or her health. The patient and family are responsible for reporting perceived risks in their care and unexpected changes in the patient's condition. The patient and family help the hospital improve its understanding of the patient's environment by providing feedback about service needs and expectations.
- **Asking questions.** Patients are responsible for asking questions when they do not understand what they have been told about their care or what they are expected to do.

- **Following instructions.** The patient and family are responsible for following the care service, or treatment plan developed. They should express any concerns they have about their ability to follow and comply with the proposed care plan or course of treatment. Every effort is made to adapt the plan to the patient's specific needs and limitations. When such adaptations to the treatment plan are not recommended, the patient and family are responsible for understanding the consequences of the treatment alternatives and not following the proposed course.
- **Accepting consequences.** The patient and family are responsible for the outcomes if they do not follow the care, service, or treatment plan.
- **Following rules and regulations.** The patient and family are responsible for following the hospital's rules and regulations concerning patient care and conduct.
- **Showing respect and consideration.** Patients and families are responsible for being considerate of the hospital's personnel and property.
- **Meeting financial commitments.** The patient and family are responsible for promptly meeting any financial obligation agreed to with the hospital.

Gastroenterology nurses and associates should respect the rights of all patients and their families, regardless of race, religion, sex, disease status, national origin, or sources of payment of care. Gastroenterology patients and their families must be made aware of their responsibilities to caregivers, health care institutions, and other patients.

SGNA-RECOMMENDED GUIDELINES FOR INFECTION CONTROL

These standards were prepared, written and adopted by SGNA Practice Committee and the Board of Directors in 2000. They are to be recommended or adapted for all settings where gastrointestinal endoscopy is practiced. These guidelines were developed to complement SGNA's 2000 "Guidelines for the Use of High Level Disinfectants and Sterilants for Reprocessing of Flexible Gastrointestinal Endoscopes."

These guidelines minimizes the potential hazards in maintaining a safe environment, free from the possibility of spreading disease from patient to patient or patient to gastroenterology nurse or associate. They include recommendations for decontamination, disinfection, and sterilization of endoscopes and accessories; methods and practices to ensure a safe environment; and guidelines for the protection of personnel.

Infection control guidelines should be reviewed in depth by each gastroenterology nurse. They may also be adapted as appropriate for use in individual hospital-based and private practice settings.

FEDERAL REGULATIONS AND GUIDELINES

In addition to the infection control guidelines developed by SGNA, several governmental agencies, including the Centers for Disease Control and Prevention (CDC), Environmental Protection Agency (EPA), Food and Drug

Administration (FDA), and Occupational Safety and Health Administration (OSHA), have promulgated guidelines and regulations that have and impact on disinfection and sterilization practice within gastroenterology.

CENTERS FOR DISEASE CONTROL AND PREVENTION

The CDC is recognized as the lead federal agency for protecting health and safety of people, at home or abroad, providing credible information in health decisions, disease prevention and education. The CDC formulated general guidelines for the prevention and control of nosocomial (hospital acquired) infections. Most applicable to patient care in the endoscopy unit is the Guideline for Handwashing and Hospital Environmental Control, which covers hand washing; cleaning, disinfecting, and sterilizing patient care equipment; microbiological sampling; management of infective waste; housekeeping; and laundry.

CDC guidelines have no force of regulation or law and may be modified as appropriate in individual health care settings, they represent the best available compilation of practical, well-founded infection control practices. Some of the recommendations are based on well-documented epidemiological studies; in areas where little scientific evidence is available, the guidelines are based on reasonable theoretic rationales.

ENVIRONMENTAL PROTECTION AGENCY (EPA)

The EPA is the federal agency that approves products for disinfectant registration after review of labeling and supporting data submitted by manufacturers. The EPA classifies chemical germicides as sporicides, general disinfectants, hospital disinfectants, sanitizers, and "others."

The EPA is responsible to carry out certain laws enacted by Congress. One of its functions is to regulate solid waste, which includes hazardous waste, such as toxic, ignitable, corrosive, and reactive waste. In November 1988, this agency was commissioned to establish a demonstration program for tracking medical waste when federal regulations were signed into law.

The EPA developed specific guidelines for handling infectious waste from "the cradle to the grave." The guidelines cover designation of waste; handling, storage, packaging, and transporting waste; selection of appropriate treatment and disposal methods; monitoring of treatment methods; and compliance with state and local requirements.

FOOD AND DRUG ADMINISTRATION (FDA)

The FDA is the federal regulatory agency responsible for controlling the safety and effectiveness of drugs, devices, and instrumentation.

The complexity of medical devices and the increased number of new products resulted in Congress developing the comprehensive Medical Device Amendments of 1976 to the Federal Food, Drug, and Cosmetic Act. The primary reason for the amendments was to ensure that any new device was safe and effective before it was put on the market. Congress divided medical devices into two groups and three classes based on the potential hazards of the device. Devices were also categorized: pre-amendment, post-amendment, substantially equivalent, implant, custom, investigational, and transitional.

There are essentially two ways that a new device gets on the market. If the manufacturer can establish substantial equivalence, pre-market notification is all that is required. However, if the new device is not similar to a pre-amendment device, a Pre-market Approval Application (PMA) must be filed.

Therefore, most manufacturers file a "Pre-market Notification," which is referred to as a 510(K), before introducing a new product. This is a request by the manufacturer to the FDA to market a device. If the FDA does not approve, the only alternative is the lengthy process of submitting a PMA.

In some situations, the manufacturer may need to conduct clinical studies to support a PMA or 510(K) submission. If this is the case, the device may need to be distributed and used for investigational purposes. An Investigation Device Exemption (IDE) is obtained to ensure that the pre-clinical testing makes use of a predetermined protocol.

The FDA has also established a reporting system whereby the health care practitioner must report problems with medical devices. The Safe Medical Device Act of 1990 requires health care facilities to submit a report twice a year regarding device-related injuries and serious illnesses. Based on the user reports, the FDA has the authority to recall devices.

OCCUPATIONAL SAFETY AND HEALTH ADMINISTRATION (OSHA)

OSHA is the federal regulatory agency responsible for enforcing safety and health regulations in the workplace. The primary function of OSHA is to protect the health care worker by making sure that employers comply with health and safety provisions of the federal laws. OSHA can inspect the workplace at any time on request of the employees. OSHA issued a compliance directive, instruction CPL 2-2.-44A, "Enforcement Procedure for Occupational Exposure to Hepatitis B Virus (HBV)." These are guidelines used by enforcement officers who conduct inspections of practices required to implement CDC standard precautions. Other proposed rules for protecting employees in the work setting were published in OSHA 29 CFR Part 1910, "Occupational Exposure to Bloodborne Pathogens."

Health Insurance Portability and Accountability Act

The Health Insurance Portability and Accountability Act of 1996 (HIPAA) is federal regulation affecting the entire health care industry. Originally, this legislation was designed to provide health care coverage benefits for individuals who may have pre-existing conditions and were also in the process of changes places of employment. As the legislation developed, all areas of patient confidentiality was included to protect patients' personal health information. These regulations are considered the most significant changes to the health care industry since the advent of Medicare diagnosis related groups (DRGs).

HIPAA requires the health care industry to standardize around a single set of formats related to acquiring, claiming, and reimbursing for health benefits and services. Virtually everyone who provides health care is affected by the HIPAA law. There are serious economic and criminal penalties for not complying with the HIPAA standards.

This law focuses on privacy rules that allow patients more control over their health information and how it is disseminated. Protected health information is defined as individually identifiable health information that is oral or maintained in any form or medium. Written consent is by the patients before anything can be done with the patient personal health information.

Only health professionals with a "need to know" status should have access to a patient's personal health information. Oral communications must be safeguarded for privacy. Every person working in a health care facility is responsible for protecting patients' personal health information. Providers must be continually on the alert to eliminate areas where patient confidentiality may be breached and institute steps to prevent the inadvertent dissemination of private information. Health care providers must provide every means possible to protect patients' privacy including shutting doors, pulling curtains in semi-private areas, and taking patients to private areas where discussions can be done without the risk of other people obtaining the information.

Endoscopy units must have their overall operations reviewed on a regular basis to ensure all patient personal health information is protected. This includes where patient records are placed before, during, and after procedures and any other information that may be inadvertently viewed by people who do not "need to know."

CASE SITUATION

Jeannie Allan, a 56-year-old woman, has just been admitted to the endoscopy unit for a colonoscopy. She has had rectal bleeding for the past 2 months and is concerned about what the doctor will find when he performs the colonoscopy. She has a history of ulcerative colitis and has had problems with her bowels for 25 years. She is concerned that she may have cancer and does not want her husband to know until a diagnosis is defined. The nurse preparing Mrs. Allan for her procedure follows a set of pre-determined standards for practice. These standards are put forth by the SGNA and serve as a guide to gastroenterology staff members.

Points to think about:

1. What activities might a endoscopy nurse perform on behalf of Mrs. Allan to ensure her right to privacy and confidentiality in the endoscopy unit?
2. In preparing for Mrs. Allan's colonoscopy, what types of activities might be conducted to meet the standard of "preventing harm to the patient"?
3. What type of information about Mrs. Allan should the nurse document that would demonstrate nursing actions and the patient's responses to those actions?

Suggested responses:

1. To ensure Mrs. Allan's right to privacy and confidentiality, the endoscopy nurse might:
   a. Establish mutually with the patient what information she would liked discussed in front of her family.
   b. Make sure that any information discussed with other staff and the patient's physician is communicated discreetly and in a professional manner, so it is not overheard by the patient's family or by other patients and their families.
   c. When preparing for the colonoscopy, take care to keep the patient covered with an appropriate drape.
2. The types of activities that might be performed to protect the patient from harm would include:
   a. Decontaminating and disinfecting endoscopic instruments
   b. Ensuring the informed consent has been obtained before the procedure
   c. Performing safety check of electrical equipment that has the potential to burn the patient or cause fires.
3. Examples of a nursing action and patient response the nurse would document are as follows. Nursing action: administration of midazolam (Versed) Response: patient is calm

REVIEW TERMS

Standards of practice, Standards of care, ANA: American Nurses Association, CDC: Centers for Disease Control and Prevention, EPA: Environmental Protection Agency, FDA: Food and Drug Administration, OSHA: Occupational Safety and Health Administration, JCAHO: Joint Commission on Accreditation of Health care Organization

REVIEW QUESTIONS

1. Accreditation standards are developed by:
   a. SGNA.
   b. CDC.
   c. JCAHO.
   d. ANA.
2. Measurement of comparison for quantitative or qualitative value are called:
   a. Standards of care.
   b Guidelines.
   c. Standards of practice.
   d. Criteria.
3. Which of the following is not a source of standards of nursing practice:
   a. Professional consensus.
   b. Expert opinions and theories.
   c. Scientific research.
   d. State licensing authorities.

4. JCAHO standards apply to:
   a. In-hospital endoscopy units.
   b. Independent endoscopy units.
   c. Physician's offices.
   d. All of the above.

5. According to the JCAHO Accreditation Manual for Hospitals, patients are responsible for:
   a. Ensuring their own safety.
   b. Providing an accurate medical history.
   c. Providing an interpreter if they do not speak English.
   d. Participating in medical research.

6. Which of the following is not covered in the SGNA infection control guidelines:
   a. Decontamination, disinfection, and sterilization of endoscopes and accessories.
   b. Recommendations for a safe environment.
   c. Protection of personnel.
   d. Isolation practices.

7. The federal agency responsible for monitoring the safety of medical devices is:
   a. OSHA.
   b. EPA.
   c. FDA.
   d. CDC.

8. The CDC guidelines for the prevention and control or nosocomial infections:
   a. Have the force of law.
   b. Are an accepted compilation of practical recommendations.
   c. Are applicable only to hospital settings.
   d. Are all based on conclusive scientific research.

9. Before participation in a research program the patient will be given an explanation of all except:
   a. A description of benefits.
   b. Alternative services.
   c. Names of others enrolled in the research project.
   d. Potential risk and discomforts.

10. JCAHO considers endoscopy units to be in what category of services:
    a. Ambulatory care.
    b. Surgical and anesthesia services.
    c. Nursing care.
    d. Outpatient services.

BIBLIOGRAPHY

American Nurses Association (1996). *Quality assurance workbook*. Kansas City, MO: Author.

American Nurses Association (1991). *Standards of clinical nursing practice*. Kansas City, MO: Author.

Brent, N. (1997). *Nurses and the Law, A Guide to Principles and Applications*. Philadelphia, Pennsylvania: W.B. Saunders.

Boyce, J.M. & Pittet, D. (2002). Guideline for hand hygiene in health care settings. Atlanta, Georgia, Centers for Disease Control and Prevention.

Comprehensive accreditation manual for hospitals: the official handbook. (1997). Oakbrook Terrace, Illinois: Joint Commission on Accreditation of Healthcare Organizations.

Joint Commission on Accreditation of Healthcare Organizations (1990). *Accreditation manual for hospitals, 191, Vol. 1*. Oakbrook Terrace, IL: Author.

Kessler, D., Pape, S. & Sundwall, D. (1987). The federal regulation of medical devices. *New England Journal of Medicine 336,* 317-57.

Kneedler, J. (1976). A standard: what is it and how to use it. *AORNJ 23:55,* 1-554. AORN.

Patterson, P., (Ed.) (1991). Advice for users on compliance with devices act. *OR Manager 7:1.*

Smith, J.M. (2002). Alert! New revisions to HIPPA privacy rules. *Journal of the National Medical Association May: 94(5),* 285-6.

Society of Gastroenterology Nurses and Associates, Inc. (2001). *Standards for practice, SGNA Monograph Series,* Chicago, Illinois.

Society of Gastroenterology Nurses and Associates, Inc. (2000). Standards for infection control and reprocessing of flexible gastrointestinal endoscopes [Monograph]. *Gastroenterology Nursing : 23(4),* pp.172-179.

Chapter 6

PROCESS IMPROVEMENT

Transforming the commitment to quality care from an idea into a reality is one of the challenges health care professionals face. The emphasis on quality is being driven by customer demand for health care that is appropriate, timely, safe, efficient, and cost-effective. Customers also expect services to be provided in a caring and respectful manner. This chapter provides guidelines for integrating a process improvement plan in the gastroenterology unit.

Learning objectives

After reviewing the content of this chapter, the gastroenterology nurse should be able to:

1. Define the term *quality* as it pertains to patients undergoing gastroenterology procedures.
2. Outline the steps that must be taken to develop a process improvement plan.
3. Identify indicators for measuring process improvement for gastroenterology patients.
4. Formulate ideas for improving quality within the gastroenterology unit.

RATIONALE FOR A QUALITY PROGRAM

In the last decade industry and health care have moved from an environment of quality improvement to a continuous **process improvement** model. Quality improvement is a retrospective process; process improvement is prospective or concurrent. Process improvement is a methodology designed to allow for scientific analysis of the way we do our work. Although there are several models of process improvement utilized in health care institutions, they all have the same basic principles: (a) most problems are process rather than people issues, (b) the people closest to the process know it the best and have an interest in improving the process, and (c) decisions should be made based on measurable data.

Many individuals once believed quality was undefinable and therefore not measurable. In *Service Quality*

Improvement: The Customer Satisfaction Strategy for Health Care (1994), quality is defined as "consistent conformance to customer expectations and needs." These needs and expectations can be precisely measured with the correct indicators. Also, just as technology is rapidly changing, so are the needs of customers. Health care is not stagnant, nor should processes in health care become stagnant.

Process improvement includes more than patient care. Each department needs to identify all of its customers: physicians, patients, other hospital departments such as radiology and pathology, insurance providers and the staff within the department. It encompasses all the work that is done in and around the gastroenterology department or office setting.

The Joint Commission on Accreditation of Healthcare Organizations (JCAHO) in 1996 defined process improvement as "a systematic, hospital-wide approach to process design and performance measurement, assessment, and improvement." This process is collaborative and interdisciplinary. A process is defined by JCAHO as "a goal-directed, interrelated series of actions, events, mechanisms or steps."

INTEGRATING QUALITY INTO THE GASTROENTEROLOGY DEPARTMENT

To implement any process improvement plan, the management team must have a commitment to the process, and training in the principles of the process. Staff must also be trained in the principles of continuous process improvement and be empowered to make changes in how they do their work. This does not happen overnight, but the successful manager will assist the staff in using the process to make decisions. Staff must not become satisfied with the "status quo." Some units may have many effective processes in place. However, that doesn't mean that they can't become great processes. Over time, some processes even break down and customer satisfaction drops.

Before a process improvement plan can be developed, the unit's vision and mission statement must be formulated. If the unit is hospital-based, it is important that the vision and mission statement reflect the global vision and mission statement of the institution. From the vision and mission statement, quality finds focus.

According to Christopher (1994), vision sets direction, and mission provides the roadmap. The tools of continuous quality improvement are then utilized to produce the necessary results to provide efficient, cost-effective, quality processes for patients, physicians, and other customers.

A vision statement for a gastroenterology unit might be:

The gastroenterology unit will provide quality diagnostic and interventional therapeutic care to all individuals utilizing the unit.

The mission statement might be:

The gastroenterology unit will provide a cost-effective, efficient, state-of-the-art environment for all persons utilizing the unit.

MEASURING QUALITY

The foundation for a comprehensive process improvement plan is a working knowledge of the process and the tools necessary to achieve the goal. These include flowcharting the process, establishing work teams with defined roles, and expertise in the collection and interpretation of data. When developing the plan for process improvement, there are several criteria to consider when selecting the initial process. Choose one which does not involve multiple departments, improving chances of success because the unit has control of the outcome. The vision and mission statement act as the base or foundation of the unit. The challenge is to translate those broad statements into measurable indicators. In addition, choose a process that is fairly simple. For instance, if getting lunch is a problem for the unit, gather a representative group of the staff and establish who will be the leader of the group, who will keep the minutes (usually done on a flip chart so all participants can see them), who will be the timekeeper, and who will keep the group on track. Once the roles have been assigned, make a list of the reasons it is difficult to get lunch. After the list is made, group similar reasons together. The participants can then decide how they would like to address the issue. Because the staff addressed the issue and came up with an improvement to the process of getting lunch, there is compliance with the solution. The next step is to decide when and how the issue will be evaluated.

Quality indicators and thresholds

A clinical **indicator** is a measurable variable used to assess the degree to which outcomes or expectations are being met. The identification of indicators for the gastroenterology unit is a complex process that requires a high level of clinical expertise. Those responsible must develop suitable indicators so the important aspects of care may be measured or evaluated effectively.

The following are criteria for developing effective quality indicators:
  (a) objectivity;
  (b) specificity;
  (c) measurability;
  (d) comprehensiveness;
  (e) clinical validity;
  (f) relevancy; and
  (g) efficiency.

There are three types of standards: structure, process, and outcome. Because indicators are used to measure standards, there are three types of indicators. The following are some examples of indicators that might be appropriate for the gastroenterology unit:

1. Proper cleaning and disinfection of equipment (structure).
2. Emergency equipment available and functional for all procedures (structure).
3. Number of incomplete procedures because of poor bowel prep (process).
4. Number of patients who do not have necessary lab work pre-procedure (process).
5. Patient/family who rate satisfaction with nursing care as 80% or above (outcome).
6. Patients having sclerotherapy who have blood pressure and pulse within ±5% of their baseline value (if available) before discharge (outcome).
7. To facilitate the data collection, indicators must be stated in a concise manner. For example, it would be easy to check the chart for pre-procedural and post-procedural vital signs to see if the last outcome standard was met properly. Keep in mind that indicators must be easy to use or they will probably not be used at all.

Once indicators are developed, it is important to establish thresholds or acceptable rates of activity that determine when to evaluate care. Indicators can be designated as either rate-based or sentinel events indicators.

1. **Rate-based indicators.** These are established on the premise that there are usually exceptions to standards of care. When establishing a threshold, acceptable rates for clinical events are established based on the literature, on expert opinion, or on hospital experience.
2. **Sentinel event indicators.** These represent standards of care that, if not followed, may result in serious outcomes. A sentinel event is a negative outcome that is serious enough to merit investigation of every instance. An example might be a transfusion reaction or a perforation of the bowel during a procedure. Nurses in the gastroenterology department probably will not establish sentinel event indicators, because these are usually monitored by the medical staff quality committee.

Monitoring quality

The JCAHO *Accreditation Manual for Hospitals,* in Performance Improvement Standard I, requires that the hospital has a planned, systematic, hospital-wide approach to process design and performance measurement, assessment, and improvement. These activities are collaborative and interdisciplinary. New processes are designed well. Data are systematically collected. The hospital collects data on important processes or outcomes related to patient care and organization functions.

The manual also requires that there is a written plan for the process improvement program that describes the program's objectives, organization, scope, and mechanisms for overseeing the effectiveness of monitoring, evaluation, and problem-solving activities.

In determining quality, the gastroenterology nurse must rely on facts rather than opinions. It is not enough to have all the goals, objectives, standards, and indicators in written form. There must be a formal process for monitoring process improvement. It is helpful to involve the entire staff in this process, because it gives each person an inside look at measuring quality. In "Achieving Impressive Customer Service", Leebov and Scott (1994) emphasize the benefit of customer satisfaction surveys and the part nurses play in these. In one process improvement plan, nurses were assigned to ask satisfaction questions to three patients/family members a week. This way, each nurse got feedback on the unit's work but the results were then added together with all of the other nurses' reports, to get an overall picture of units processes.

If the gastroenterology unit is hospital-based, there is usually a quality improvement program in place and a coordinator to help facilitate this process. It is imperative that someone assume the responsibility for monitoring and evaluating the quality of care delivered in the freestanding gastroenterology unit as guided by the Comprehensive Accreditation Manual for Ambulatory Care (CAMAC).

Monitoring the quality of care involves data collection, tabulation, evaluation, and reporting. It begins with the task of data collection. Data collection specifications must detail exactly what indicators to use, how much data to collect, and how often. It may not be necessary to create new forms for data collection. Existing forms, such as the patient's record, incident reports, patient satisfaction questionnaires, infection rates, and the observations of the staff providing care, may be appropriate.

The frequency with which information is collected should be based on the volume of patients and recurrence of problems. It is recommended that data be gathered, reviewed, and reported regularly, based on a calendar developed for that purpose. Processes may be looked at monthly, quarterly, semi-annually, or annually, depending on its importance to satisfaction with the unit. Any indicators exceeding the established threshold require investigation of the quality and appropriateness of care.

Once the information has been collected, it must be tabulated so it can be evaluated and compared to acceptable variance levels. It is important to determine in advance what percentage of variance will be acceptable for a specific standard. If one of the indicators in the gastroenterology unit states that all patients' allergies are verified before the delivery of any medication, there would be no variance. The expectation is that this standard is met 100% of the time.

Evaluation involves determining the degree to which the key quality elements were met, as well as taking a look at whether or not the care delivered is still considered state-of-the-art.

The next step is to report the findings. This may require developing a form to serve as a tracking mechanism. It may be helpful to use control charts that depict trends or patterns of performance.

In conclusion, to measure the quality of care provided, it is necessary to establish the following components:

(a) written indicators and thresholds;
(b) tools for data collection and tabulation;
(c) predetermined acceptable levels of variance for evaluating each indicator; and
(d) a means for reporting the findings.

Taking the above steps will provide a means of measuring and documenting the process improvement plan that is recommended by JCAHO.

IMPROVING QUALITY

Once the data have been collected and evaluated, the next step is to identify the area(s) that need improvement. It is important that staff receive frequent updates on current process improvement activities. The emphasis should be on developing strategies that will improve the process.

Effective methods for improving quality start with a commitment to making changes. The following is a brief list of strategies for implementing change and improvement.

1. **Education and training.** Education is essential when implementing any new change. Without adequate knowledge, people cannot be expected to understand the need for change. Training in process improvement should start at orientation and be a part of annual review.

2. **Team approach.** Involve the entire unit. A basic tenet of process improvement is that those closest to the issue are the ones who understand it best and need to be involved in the solution. The Joint Commission on Accreditation of Healthcare Organizations (JCAHO) in 1994 advises that when a process involves more than one department, the group improving the process must reflect that cross-departmental activity.

3. **Start with an easily attainable,** timely process improvement.

Once the strategies for process improvement have been established, they must be written, communicated, and monitored. Process improvement effectiveness relies on a clearly written plan of action. The written plan is so important that JCAHO has made it a required part of the process improvement plan. If the gastroenterology unit is hospital-based, the written plan should include the overall hospital-wide process improvement plan.

Once the written plan is developed, it must be evaluated on a regular basis to ensure that the changing needs, expectations, and outcomes of customers are being met in a timely, effective manner.

CASE SITUATION

Josie Smith presents in the emergency room at 8 p.m. with a food bolus lodged in her esophagus. The gastroenterologist is finally called at midnight after a barium swallow has been attempted, leaving the esophagus full of barium. The endoscopy call person is called shortly after midnight by the gastroenterologist, and they finish the procedure at 2:30 a.m. The endoscopy call person is then responsible for cleaning the endoscope and cart before going home.

Points to think about

1. How often does this happen?
2. What is the process in the emergency room before calling the gastroenterologist?
3. Why is a barium swallow done before calling the gastroenterologist?
4. Does the barium put the patient at increased risk?

Suggested responses

To address the above questions, apply process improvement principles such as the following:

1. Keep track of call procedures after a specified time (e.g., 2200).
2. What kinds of procedures are being done after that time?
3. Flowchart the process from the time the patient presents in the emergency room until the gastroenterologist is called. Possibilities include:
   a. Length of time patient spends before seeing a physician
   b. Actions taken by emergency room physicians before calling the gastroenterologist.
4. Form a team, including representatives from the emergency room (physicians and nurses) and the gastroenterology unit (physicians and nurses).
5. Mutually develop a protocol for patients presenting with a food bolus lodged in the esophagus.
6. Monitor results.
7. Evaluate findings.
8. Initiate improvements, if needed, and continue to monitor and evaluate the process until objectives are consistently met.

REVIEW TERMS

indicator, process improvement

REVIEW QUESTIONS

1. Leaders in health care have defined quality as:
   a. Undefinable and not measurable.
   b. A continuous conformance to meet the needs and expectations of the customers.
   c. The degree to which actions taken or not taken maximize the probability of beneficial outcomes.
   d. A distinguishable attribute.

2. Models of process improvement must be based on which of the following principles?
   a. Most problems are related to process rather than people.
   b. The people closest to the process should be involved in improving it.
   c. Decisions should be made on measurable data.
   d. All of the above.

3. Improvement process for a gastroenterology unit is defined by guidelines developed by:
   a. JCAHO and CAMAC.
   b. SGNA and CBGNA.
   c. CIA and FBI.
   d. OSHA and APIC.

4. An objective:
   a. Is an observable activity.
   b. Is more specific than a goal.
   c. Should be realistic.
   d. All of the above.

5. True or false: a goal is a desired outcome, should reflect the mission statement, and should be realistic.

6. For indicators to be effective, they must:
   a. Be subjective.
   b. Evaluate outcomes.
   c. Be complex.
   d. Be measurable.

7. Improving quality in the patient care setting should be based on:
   a. Correcting the problem.
   b. Finding the person at the bottom of the problem.
   c. Regulatory rules alone.
   d. Improving the process.

8. A quality improvement program should include:
   a. Written, measurable indicators and thresholds.
   b. Tools for data collection and tabulation.
   c. Means of evaluating the plan.
   d. All of the above.

9. True or false: Once an improvement plan is in place, it does not need to be reevaluated unless a problem occurs.

10. One effective strategy for improving the quality of care is to:
    a. Provide education and training.
    b. Assign the manager total responsibility for making changes.
    c. Discipline those who are responsible for failure to meet objectives.
    d. Change the goals and objectives.

11. The mission statement of the unit should be:
    a. Independent of the institution's statement.
    b. Formulated before a process improvement plan can be developed.
    c. Reflective of the overall philosophy of the unit, based on the beliefs of the team members.
    d. Written as the final step in developing a process improvement plan.

BIBLIOGRAPHY

Christopher, W.F. (1994). *Vision, mission, total quality.* Portland, OR: Productivity Press.

Joint Commission on Accreditation of Healthcare Organizations (1994). *Framework for Improving Performance.* Oakbrook Terrace, IL: JCAHO.

Joint Commission on Accreditation of Healthcare Organizations (1996). *Accreditation manual for hospitals*, 1996 edition, Oakbrook Terrace, IL: JCAHO.

Joint Commission on Accreditation of Healthcare Organizations (2002). *Primer on indicator development and application.* Oakbrook Terrace, IL: JCAHO.

Leebov, W. & Scott, G. (1994). *Service Quality Improvement: The Customer Satisfaction Strategy for Health Care.* Chicago: American Hospital Publishing, Inc.

Leebov, W., Scott, G. & Olson, L. (1998). *Achieving Impressive Customer Service-7 Strategies for the Health Care Manager.* New York: Jossey Bass, Inc, A Wiley Company.

Maradieque, A. (1989). Quality assurance as reflected in documentation. *SGNA Journal 12,* 135-7.

Walton, M. (1986). *The Deming management method.* New York: Pergee Books.

Chapter 7

THE RESEARCH PROCESS

This chapter provides an overview of the steps involved in the nursing research process and reviews some of the statistical methods used to analyze data derived from descriptive research. In addition, the measures of central tendency and ethical considerations in nursing research are reviewed. The chapter ends with a case situation in which nursing research is conducted in a clinical setting and applied to clinical practice.

Learning objectives

After reviewing the content of this chapter, the gastro-enterology nurse should be able to:

1. Define basic terms used in research design.
2. Outline the seven steps performed in a research study.
3. Identify indexes of central tendency used to describe typicality and variability in study samples.

Research in nursing has occurred only over the past 30 to 40 years. Nursing research originated with Florence Nightingale during the Crimean War in the 1850s. She published her notes on nursing in 1859. The United States established the National Center for Nursing Research (NCNR) within the National Institute of Health (NIH) in 1986. This provided needed financial support for nursing research.

NCNR was promoted to full institute status within NIH in 1993. National Institute of Nursing (NINR) elevates nursing research on the same level as other health disciplines.

Nurses are well prepared for research—research is a form of rigorous problem solving, as is nursing. The requisite skills for competent practice are also essential in research; careful observation, strict documentation, and systematic assessment. Clinical nurses contribute greatly to nursing science by identifying research problems, collecting data, and subscribing to evidence-based practice.

Whether a research study is straightforward or complex, no investigation is productive without thoughtful planning. Careful contemplation and planning culminate in valuable research.

THE GOALS OF RESEARCH

Nursing research provides a scientific foundation for knowledge of nursing practice. This knowledge is essential for description, exploration, explanation, prediction, and control of nursing phenomena (Polit, Beck &Hungler, 2001).

Description

Description is the primary aim in many nursing studies. When controlled, systematic, empirical observations are made, descriptive accounts of the phenomenon under study may become significant contributions. For example, a recent study described enema techniques used by experienced nurses.

Exploration

Unlike descriptive research, the aim of exploratory studies is to expose factors that influence, relate to, cause, or affect a phenomenon. Coexisting variables are observed, and the frequency with which they coexist is analyzed in this type of research. For instance in gastroenterology nursing, the incidence of colon polyps in rural, urban, and suburban populations might be explored as part of a larger effort to link environmental/genetic factors to colon polyp formation.

Explanation

Research aimed at explanation is related to theory building. Theories represent a method of deriving, organizing, and integrating ideas about the manner in which phenomena are related. A study based on the effects of pre-procedural teaching on the level of anxiety experienced by patients who have undergone a colonoscopy might use the information theory to explain the role of nursing in stress reduction. In nursing, there has been particular emphasis on the need for developing theories of nursing.

Prediction and control

A **variable** is defined as a characteristic or attribute that takes on different values within a given population. Many research studies attempt to demonstrate a relationship between variables by manipulating one, the **independent variable,** and observing for a predicted change in another, the **dependent variable.** In such studies, a researcher must be able to predict the influence of the independent variable and control the influence of extraneous variables. For example, Hayes and Buffum (2001) studied the relationship intervention to enhance patient recall about postprocedural instructions. Subjects were randomized into a control group (without a wristband) or an intervention group (with a wristband). Although the researchers predicted it would make a difference, results showed no significant difference in the average memory score between both groups.

Nursing research may also be classified as either basic or applied.

1. **Basic research** is concerned with adding to the body of knowledge. It links the study in question to accepted models or theories.
2. **Applied research** focuses on an immediate solution to a practical problem. Most nursing research has been applied research.

The next section describes the seven steps performed in the research process.

STEPS IN THE RESEARCH PROCESS

The scientific research process is reiterative. Investigation at one stage of the study often casts light on an earlier stage, causing the researcher to return to the earlier step to refine a research problem or to revise study methods. Rarely does discovery proceed in a linear, sequential manner. Seldom does a researcher start at the first step in the process and proceed in orderly fashion through the remaining sequence of steps. Nonetheless, all research includes the following seven steps.

1. Identify the problem.
2. Review the literature.
3. State the aims of the study and formulate a hypothesis.
4. Design the study.
5. Carry out the study plan.
6. Analyze the data.
7. Share the results.

Step 1. Identify the problem.

Research often begins with a problem in everyday practice. The act of stating a research question or problem initially gives the project direction. In the beginning, problem statements are often too broad and vague and must often be refined and limited to make the project manageable.

By examining the level of interest in the topic and exploring the feasibility of the investigation, the researcher may be able to narrow the focus of the study and arrive at a research problem or question that is practical. In fact, the feasibility of a study is sometimes a study in itself. When a study appears feasible, it is important to consider the level of outside interest and the researcher's own motivation before pursuing a research idea. Is there interest among the professional community in the findings to come out of the proposed research? Is the researcher sufficiently interested in the topic to sustain motivation to study the problem until the work is completed?

Interest level and motivation are only two of the factors that influence the feasibility of a project. The following are several others:

(a) Time. Is the scope of the problem such that it can be studied within the time allotted for the study?
(b) Availability of subjects. Can the researcher obtain a sufficient number of subjects to investigate the problem?
(c) Cooperation of others. Researchers rarely conduct investigations independently. Are the necessary resources available? Will it be a problem to get the necessary permissions from subjects, guardians, institutional administrators, and so on?
(d) Facilities and equipment. What facilities and equipment will be needed, and will they be available to complete the study?
(e) Money. Will funding be needed? If so, how much? Does the anticipated cost outweigh the value of the expected findings?
(f) Experience of the researcher. Is the problem from a field in which the researcher has some experience? If not, is there another, more experienced investigator who has substantive knowledge of existing concepts, findings, and theories who can guide the researcher in developing methods of study, and who can help avoid research problems requiring sophisticated measuring instruments and/or complex statistical analyses?
(g) Ethical considerations. Could the study impose unfair or unethical demands on the participants?

Step 2. Review the literature.

Before beginning research it is wise to review existing literature related to the topic, including previous research on the same or a similar topic. Several objectives are met in doing so. The researcher may learn that:

(a) the proposed problem has already been solved;
(b) it is necessary to investigate a different question en route to the problem;
(c) the problem has been studied, but not sufficiently to rule out further investigation, in which case it may be feasible to replicate the study according to methods outlined in the literature;
(d) certain research designs are appropriate for the proposed topic, whereas others are not;
(e) certain important variables must be examined; or
(f) other researchers have made mistakes that must be avoided.

In short, searching existing literature will help to clarify and refine the focus of the research, thus enabling the researcher to define the scope of the study so it becomes more feasible.

What to look for in research reports. When reviewing previous research, various types of information may be uncovered.

1. **Facts, statistics, or findings.** This is probably the most important category of information, because it represents the results of other research efforts. It includes progress other investigators have made when examining the topic.

2. **Theory or interpretation.** This type of information is also significant, because it concerns the relationship between the idea or topic of interest and an existing body of knowledge surrounding that topic.

3. **Methods and procedures.** Literature focused on research instruments and procedures is useful, because it saves the researcher from redeveloping and revalidating measurement tools that already exist.

4. **Opinions, speculation, anecdotes, clinical impressions, or narrations of incidents and situations.** These categories of information are value-laden and subjective. They serve to broaden the researcher's understanding of the problem and help deal with snags that may occur. Because it is important to remain as objective as possible, the researcher should avoid the temptation to rely heavily on such sources.

Where to find research reports. Individual books, journals, and other periodicals are rich with information. However, browsing through these sources to find pertinent information may be a bit overwhelming. Fortunately, there are tools that allow for more efficient retrieval of relevant data, including the following:.

1. **Abstracts.** Abstracts contain summaries of journal articles. Although not detailed, they are useful in determining whether or not an article will be relevant to the topic at hand.

2. **Indexes.** Printed indexes, such as *Index Medicus,* can unlock vast stores of literature on every subject imaginable. If the topic requires information from disciplines other than nursing (e.g., chemistry, genetics, psychology), a librarian can identify relevant indexes on these subjects.

3. **Computer databases.** Relevant information can be identified quickly by searching computerized databases such as MEDLINE plus at **http://www.medlineplus. gov/,** PubMed at **http://www.ncbi.nlm.nih.gov/ entrez/query.fcgi?db=PubMed,** or the United States Library of Medicine at **http://www.nlm.nih.gov/ databases/databases.html.** These sites are free and easily accessible. Librarians can usually help with a search strategy if needed. Resources are readily accessible, usually free, in large medical institutions. A librarian can help develop an efficient search strategy.

4. **Bibliographies.** Bibliographies provide compilations of references to books, periodicals, and reports on a particular topic. Annotated bibliographies provide additional comments about the purposes or findings of studies and sometimes include information about the quality of the work. Bibliographies

can also identify other investigators with experience in the area of interest.

5. **Personal contact.** Contacting other investigators can help clarify information they have published and help the researcher refine his or her own purpose and methods. Any or all of these tools may be a fruitful means of retrieving pertinent literature on the topic of interest.

How to evaluate and screen research reports. The researcher should critically consider all sources of information. When written by the person or persons who performed the study, a research report is considered a primary source of information. A secondary source describes research performed by other investigators. Reviews of the literature, for example, are secondary sources. Primary information sources should be used as much as possible. In addition, when reviewing a study, the researcher should examine its relevance, the validity and reliability of the instruments used (as discussed in the section on study design), control of extraneous variables, the sample size, and the statistical and clinical significance of the results. Finally, negative findings should be considered. It is not uncommon to encounter conflicting reports, an indication that more research is necessary.

Step 3. State the purpose of the study and formulate hypotheses or research questions.

The review of the literature concludes with the purpose, aims, or objectives. These are general statements that delineate what the researcher hopes to accomplish or learn from a particular research study.

Research questions and **hypotheses** are more specific than the aim or purpose; they address the relationship between variables to be tested during the study. A particular study may have several research questions or several research hypotheses, and the same study could have both hypotheses and research questions.

Research questions are written in the present tense and ask general questions about the relationship between variables, as in the following example: "What is the relationship between the amount of dietary fiber ingested and the frequency of bowel movements?"

Research hypotheses are more specific, are written as declarative sentences, and state the direction of the relationship between two or more variables: "Adult subjects who eat a high-fiber diet will have more stools than those who do not."

The statistical or **null hypothesis** is used for statistical testing. It is always stated in the opposite direction from the research hypothesis, and it indicates that there is no relationship between the variables: "Adult subjects who have a high-fiber diet will have the same number of stools as those who do not." In other words, the independent variable, dietary fiber, has no effect on the dependent variable, frequency of stools. If the statistical test demonstrates no relationship between the variables, the null hypothesis is accepted. If a relationship is supported by statistical testing, the null hypothesis is rejected. Most researchers only write the research hypothesis, because the null hypothesis is its opposite and is therefore understood.

Step 4. Design the study.

Steps in actual study design are as follows:

1. Determine how to sample the study population (e.g., a random sample, a convenience sample).
2. Decide on a setting in which to carry out the study (e.g., a hospital, an office endoscopy setting, a specific geographical location).
3. Select measures for collecting data (e.g., develop a new survey instrument, use a previously validated instrument).
4. Specify procedures to collect the data (e.g., informed consent, assignment to group, collection of data).
5. Decide which statistical procedures should be used (e.g., mean, median, standard deviation).

In nursing research, three study designs are predominantly used. They are the survey, the experiment, and the case study. While all surveys are partially descriptive in nature, the primary intent of the experiment and the case study is to prove or disprove a hypothesis.

To conduct a survey, interviews or self-completion questionnaires are used.

An experiment generally involves **quantitative** measurement before and after some treatment or intervention is rendered.

A case study is almost exclusively **qualitative.** In this design, data are collected through observation. Sampling methods and measures for data collection are essential steps in study design.

Sampling the population. Sampling refers to the process of selecting a study group to represent the entire population. The overriding concern in assessing a sample is its representativeness. Sampling plans are essentially one of two types: probability sampling and nonprobability sampling.

Random sampling is the simplest of the probability sampling designs. It involves selection from the population (or a subpopulation) at large, and it is performed in such a way that each member of the population has equal probability of being included in the sample. Probability sampling is the more respected of the two types, because greater confidence can be placed in the representativeness of the sample.

Accidental sampling is a nonprobability sampling technique that entails using the most readily available persons or objects as participants in the study (Polit et al., 2001). Researchers must be careful about generalizing results to the population at large when sampling by this nonprobability technique since it may not be representative.

In many experimental designs, an **experimental group** and either a control group or a comparison group are selected. The experimental group is made up of subjects who receive an experimental treatment or intervention. The **control group** is made up of subjects who do not receive an experimental treatment or intervention. Their performance provides a baseline against which the effects of the treatment can be measured. A **comparison group** is a selection of subjects whose scores on a dependent variable are used as the basis for evaluating the scores of group of primary interest. The phrase *comparison group* is used rather than the phrase *control group* when the investigation does not use a true experimental design (Polit et al., 2001).

The terms **double-blind** and **placebo effect** refer to design features of research studies. A double-blind experiment is one in which neither subjects nor investigators are aware of which subjects are in the experimental group and which subjects are in the control group. In an investigation of the effects of a drug, for example, neither the drug administrator nor the subjects are aware of whether the drug administered is the experimental drug or placebo. A placebo is a material whose appearance is identical to the drug under investigation. Using a placebo allows researchers to separate psychological effects induced by drug administration (the placebo effect) from the real effects of the drug.

Measurement for collecting data. Measurement is the assignment of numbers to objects according to specific rules (Polit et.al., 2001). These rules allow researchers to assign values consistently from one subject or event to another. Nurses taking measurements for research studies follow the same kinds of rules they follow when performing measurements in nursing practice. For example, patients are weighed at the same time each morning, in exactly the same way, with exactly the same amount of clothes every time. These rules of measurement are used in research to ensure the accuracy of the results.

There are four levels of measurement: nominal, ordinal, interval, and ratio. Nominal data are the weakest form of measurement and are used to organize data into categories such as gender, race, religion, and marital status. Ordinal data are data that can be arranged according to rank, such as pain intensity, anxiety, and coping ability. When measuring pain, we might ask the subject to rate his or her pain on a scale from 0 to 10. A rating of 10 would be greater than a rating of 7, which would be greater than a rating of 3; however, the measurement method is too crude to consider these ratings as exact distances apart. Another example of a rank order scale is: strongly disagree, disagree, neutral, agree, and strongly agree.

The next level of measurement, interval level, is characterized by rank order data that occur at specific intervals. An example is temperature. Because the intervals on the thermometer have equal gradations, you can say that a measurement of 101° is 4° higher than a measurement of 97°. However, because interval level data do not have a genuine zero point, you cannot say that 40° is twice as warm as 20°or that 0° means that there is no temperature.

The highest level of measurement, ratio, has all the characteristics of interval-level data plus a genuine zero point. Weight and height are ratio levels of measurement; therefore we can say that 40 pounds is twice as much as 20 pounds. Although there is a difference between interval and ratio-level measurements, they are treated the same way statistically.

The level of measurement is the major concern when selecting the appropriate statistic to test a particular hypothesis. Nonparametric statistics are used to test the relationship between variables measured at the nominal or ordinal level. Examples of nonparametric statistics include the chi-square (for nominal level data) and the Mann-Whitney U test (for ordinal level data). Parametric statistics such as the t-test and analysis of variance are used to test hypotheses whose variables are measured at the interval or ratio level.

Before initiating the research study, researchers must ensure the validity and reliability of all instruments used to measure the variables. A valid instrument is one that measures what it is supposed to measure. For example, you would use a sphygmomanometer to measure blood pressure; you would not measure blood pressure with a questionnaire. Reliability refers to the reproducibility or consistency of the measurement. For example, you would expect a particular person to weigh the same if he or she stepped on and off the scale several times in succession. You would expect two people to obtain the same heart rate if they were auscultating the same person's heart at the same time.

Questionnaires and surveys are valuable measurement instruments, but establishing their validity and reliability is often complicated. New researchers should try to find data collection instruments that have already undergone extensive validity and reliability testing.

Step 5. Carry out the study plan.

There is little to be said about this step in the research process, except to emphasize that this phase requires careful observation, strict documentation, and systematic assessment. This phase of research is labor-intensive, and it is the most important in terms of the outcome and reliability of the results.

Step 6. Analyze the data.

When planning a research study, some beginning researchers give inadequate attention to plans for data analysis. Failure to consider how the data will be analyzed almost inevitably results in collecting useless data. A second concern is that researchers who are unfamiliar with statistical methods might think that if they just plug the numbers into the computer, they will receive accurate statistical analyses. Although computer packages makes statistical analysis quick and easy, researchers must ensure that data are accurate, that appropriate statistics were chosen, and that the research design met the assumptions of the statistics chosen. For example, researchers who want to use a t-test must meet certain assumptions of the test (e.g., ensure that data are measured at the interval or ratio level, randomly assign subjects to treatment and control groups, and select an adequate sample size) to have confidence in the statistical findings.

Once the data analysis is complete, but before conclusions can be drawn, it is wise to pause and consider the nature of the scientific approach as it pertains to nursing research. Respect for the powers of the scientific approach must be tempered by a familiarity with its limitations and flaws. Because many of the persistent and intriguing questions in nursing concern morality and ethics, and because no scientific method can be used to answer these questions, it is inevitable that the nursing process will never rely solely on

scientific information. Moreover, the problem of measurement is a substantial one in nursing. Although there are reasonably accurate measures of physiological phenomena, comparable measures for psychological phenomena, such as pain and anxiety, are still being refined.

Finally, every study, no matter how sophisticated, has some flaws. Investigators are inevitably faced with compromises and constraints that must be acknowledged when conclusions are drawn. Consumers of research need to understand these limitations to evaluate the usefulness of the information provided.

Step 7. Share the results.

Disseminating results of a study is absolutely essential, whether the findings were those that were hypothesized or not. Both expected and unexpected findings add to our knowledge and our understanding of the world of nursing and health care.

The results of a research study may be reported in the following ways:

(a) Writing and publishing an article that describes the study and the results obtained;

(b) Giving an oral presentation of the study findings at a local or national meeting;

(c) Presenting the findings with a poster at a local or national meeting; or

(d) Presenting the findings within the local area at informal group meetings, in-services, or work.

ELEMENTARY DESCRIPTIVE STATISTICS: A REVIEW OF CENTRAL TENDENCY

When conducting a study, nurse researchers are frequently interested in the typical member of a group. They may care to know, for example, how much information typical colostomy patients have about diet or how much postprocedure pain the typical endoscopy patient experiences.

The layperson tends to think of typicality in terms of a group *average*. However, this term is ambiguous because there are three commonly used kinds of averages, or measures of **central tendency:** the mode, the median, and the mean. Furthermore, an average alone sometimes gives inadequate information about the typicality of a characteristic, as is true when there is considerable variability in the group. Variability refers to the spread or dispersion of data values around the mean and may be quite different between two groups, whereas the mean value in either group is the same. Consequently, it becomes necessary to talk about typicality not only in terms of averages (the mode, the median, or the mean) but also in terms of variability.

In this section, measures of central tendency are reviewed. In addition, two indexes of variability are described: the range and the standard deviation.

Mode

The **mode** is the numerical value that occurs most frequently in a set of values. It is not necessary to calculate to derive the mode; rather, the researcher simply inspects the set of values. For example, in the following set of values the mode is 14.

14 10 12 14 14 14 22 16 14 8 12 12 14

Median

The median is an index of average *position* in a set of values. It does not take into account the quantitative values of individual scores. Specifically, the median is that point in a set of values above which and below which 50% of the values lie. Notice that to find the median, it is necessary first to order the values. In this first set of values, there are five elements:

2 8 6 0 5

Once they are ordered, it is easy to see that 5 is the median value:

0 2 5 6 8

Also notice that in a set of values containing an even number of elements, finding the median requires computing a midpoint between two values. Examine the set of values below. The median of this set of values is 6.

0 2 5 7 8 9

Because the median is insensitive to extreme values, it is often preferred as the index of central tendency when the distribution of values is skewed, as in this example:

0 2 5 7 8 99

Despite the extreme value of one element in the set (99), the median remains 6. In this instance, the median gives a truer picture of what is *typical* of the set.

Mean

The **mean** is the index of central tendency that is usually referred to as the average. The mean is simply the sum of the values in a set, divided by the number of elements in a set. So, for the following set of values:

4 2 6 15 8

The mean is calculated in this way:

$$\frac{4 + 2 + 6 + 15 + 8}{5} = \frac{35}{5} = 7$$

Of the three indexes of central tendency, the mean is the most stable. If repeated samples are drawn from a population and some characteristic is measured, the means for these samples would fluctuate less than the modes or the medians. When researchers work with interval or ratio level measurement, the mean, rather than the mode or median, is almost always the statistic reported. However, as in the instance above in which 99 was an extreme value, there are some circumstances in which the mean would give a distorted picture of what is typical for a group.

The concept of **variability** is concerned with the degree to which subjects in a sample vary from one another with respect to some critical attribute. Sampling strategies can have a dramatic effect on variability. If, for instance, the aim of a study is to determine the variability of systolic pressure in any given sample of the population, and the sample studied is an accidental sample of patients seen in one emergency room, the variability of systolic pressures is likely to be greater than if the sample were selected from the junior class of a local high school. Because emergency room patients are more likely to present with extremes of pressure, the range of pressures may be greater than those among a young, healthy population. Consequently, it is necessary to describe variability in ways that account for situations like this one. Indexes like the range and standard deviation are used to give meaning to the concept.

Range

The **range** is simply the highest score (or value) minus the lowest score in a given set of values. Examine the range of systolic pressures in an accidental sample of emergency room patients:

110 138 88 246 122 116

The range of systolic pressures in this sample is 246 minus 88, or 158. Now examine the range of systolic pressures in a random sample of high school juniors:

110 118 122 116 112 118 116

The range in this sample is 118 minus 110, or 8. The systolic pressures among the first group sampled are widely dispersed, whereas pressures in the second group are more narrowly dispersed.

Standard deviation

A more complicated measure of variability is the standard deviation. The standard deviation measures the spread among values in a set around the average value in the set, or simply how far away the numbers in a list are from their average. The standard deviation is considered more reliable than the range as a measure of variability because, like the mean, it takes into account every value in the set of values. To calculate the standard deviation, examine systolic pressures from the high school juniors sample:

110 118 122 116 112 118 116

The formula for finding the standard deviation is as follows:

$$SD = \sqrt{\frac{\sum(\text{deviation scores}^2)}{n-1}}$$

where $\sum$ indicates "the sum of," and n = the number of subjects in the sample.

The first step in finding the standard deviation is to compute the mean pressure. After adding the seven pressures and dividing by 7, it can be seen that the mean pressure is 116. The next step is to find the spread or deviation score for each pressure in this group. A deviation score is equal to the sample score minus the mean score. For this group, the deviation scores are, respectively:

-6 2 6 0 -4 2 0

Because the standard deviation is a type of average deviation, it might seem logical to find the standard deviation by totaling the deviation scores and then dividing by the number of subjects. The difficulty in this approach is that the sum of a set of deviation scores is always 0. The standard deviation overcomes this problem by squaring each deviation score before summing. So the third step in computing the standard deviation is to square the deviation scores:

36 4 36 0 16 4 0

Where n = 7 subjects in the sample, the equation looks like this:

$$SD = \sqrt{\frac{(36+4 +36 +0+16+4+0)}{}}$$
(7-1)

Finishing the computation, the standard deviation is calculated as follows:

$$SD = \sqrt{\frac{96}{6}} = \sqrt{16} = 4$$

What does the standard deviation indicate about variability? In general, the greater the standard deviation, the more variable the data. Conversely, the smaller the standard deviation, the less variable the data. If the mean blood pressure of two populations is equal, yet the standard deviation in one sample is 17, while the standard deviation in the second sample is 3, it is obvious that the blood pressures of the first sample are more variable than the blood pressures of the second sample. The standard deviation provides a picture of the distribution of the data base. In a normal distribution, 67% of the sample will be within one standard deviation of the mean, 95% within two standard deviations of the mean, and 99% within three standard deviations of the mean.

The standard deviation can also illustrate the relative value of using the mean to describe typicality of an entire data set. The larger the standard deviation, the less reliable the mean is as an indicator of typicality. Conversely, the smaller the standard deviation, the more reliable the mean is as an indicator of typicality.

MORAL AND ETHICAL ISSUES IN NURSING RESEARCH

The fundamental principles that are discussed in this section should guide nurse researchers when they study human problems. First, subjects should be protected from harm and discomfort. The phrase "harm and discomfort" is not limited to physical injury. Nurse researchers also need to address emotional concerns.

The second principle is that participation in research must always be voluntary.

The participant in a research study also has the following rights:

(a) self-determination;
(b) privacy;
(c) confidentiality;
(d) the right to maintain self-respect;
(e) the right to withdraw without penalty; and
(f) the right to services.

The right to self-determination requires further explanation. To voluntarily participate in a research study the participant needs to give informed consent. The subject should have access to the following information:

(a) the purpose of the project and its general value;
(b) all procedures used in the study and why;
(c) the subject's part in the study and how much time and energy will be required;
(d) any possible pain, discomfort, stress, or loss of autonomy or dignity; and
(e) how privacy, confidentiality, and anonymity will be

guarded and the process whereby data will be used.

Before a human subjects study can begin, it must be reviewed by an approving body, usually an Institutional Review Board (Polit et. al., 2001).

The moral and ethical edicts discussed must be strenuously applied in protecting the rights of vulnerable participants who may be incapable of giving informed consent or are at high risk for unintended side effects. These include children, disabled (emotionally, mentally or physically), institutionalized, or pregnant subjects.

CASE SITUATION

Denise Heckel is a gastroenterology nurse in a metropolitan hospital. For over a month the staff will cooperate with Denise by helping her study the effects of preprocedural visits on the anxiety level of endoscopy patients. The subjects Denise selects for the study must be adults (18 years or older) who are scheduled for upper and lower endoscopies and who are English-speaking, oriented to their surroundings, and able to hear and give accurate information. Denise is also measuring the amount of midazolam used for patient sedation before and during the endoscopic procedure.

Points to think about

1. What steps should Denise follow to study her target population?
2. What purpose or purposes (e.g., description, exploration, explanation, prediction and control) might Denise fulfill in performing her study?
3. What factors should Denise have explored to determine whether or not her study will be feasible?
4. What hypothesis might Denise test in a study of this nature?
5. What variables might influence her results? Which variables has she controlled? Which variables may she yet need to control?

Suggested responses

1. Denise should take seven steps when conducting her study:
   Step 1: Identify the research problem.
   Step 2: Review the literature.
   Step 3: State the aims and expected outcome of research.
   Step 4: Design the study.
      a. Sample the population to be studied.
      b. Decide on a setting in which to do the study.
      c. Select measures for collecting data.
      d. Specify data collection procedures.
      e. Decide how the data will be analyzed.
   Step 5: Collect the data.
   Step 6: Analyze data and draw conclusions.
   Step 7: Share research results.
2. Denise might fulfill any of the following predominant aims of research, depending on the nature of her study:

(a) **Description**. Describe the clinical manifestations of stress before endoscopy by using Selye's model of stress.

(b) **Exploration**. Explore factors that influence anxiety, such as content of preprocedural information (sensory versus procedural information); age; sex; contact with nurse versus admission clerk; and patient's past experiences.

(c) **Explanation**. Explain the nursing role in preprocedure visits as reduction of uncertainty, using information theory.

(d) **Prediction**. Predict that some action will reduce patient anxiety before endoscopy.

3. To determine whether or not her study will be feasible, Denise should explore the following factors:

(a) The time allotted;

(b) Availability of a sufficient number of subjects;

(c) Cooperation of others and availability of the necessary permissions;

(d) Availability of facilities and equipment;

(e) The amount of funding needed, if any, to perform the study and whether the anticipated cost outweighs the value of the expected findings;

(f) The availability of an experienced investigator who can provide guidance in developing methods of study and can help avoid research problems requiring sophisticated measuring instruments and/or complex statistical analyses; and

(g) Whether the study could impose unfair or unethical demands on the participants; whether she can obtain informed consent; and, if not, whether she can justify not obtaining informed consent in terms of the benefits to patients versus the harm done.

4. Some hypotheses that Denise might test in a study of this nature include the following:

(a) That sensory information and procedural information, rather than procedural information alone, reduce patient anxiety.

(b) That patients who receive information the evening before their procedure experience less anxiety than patients who receive information immediately before endoscopy.

(c) That preprocedure information is more effective in reducing both anxiety and the need for sedation during endoscopy when patients have had positive experiences or no experience with outpatient surgery than when patients have had negative experiences; that is, negative prior experience influences preprocedural anxiety.

(d) That midazolam premedication offers no benefit over no premedication in reducing anxiety when preprocedure visits have been performed.

5. Variables that might influence Denise's results include patient age and sex; timing of preprocedure visits; con-

tent of information provided; predisposition toward anxiety; length of visit; format of visit; past experiences; present emotional circumstances; reason for procedure; and many others.

Variables that Denise has controlled are age, type of procedure, and ability to communicate with an English-speaking investigator. She has yet to control all other variables.

REVIEW TERMS

central tendency, comparison group, control group, dependent variable, double-blind, experimental group, hypotheses, independent variable, mean, median, mode, null hypothesis, placebo effect, population, qualitative, quantitative, random sampling, range, sampling, standard deviation, variability, variable

REVIEW QUESTIONS

1. If a research study examines the effects of preprocedural visits on the anxiety level of patients undergoing upper and lower endoscopies and controls the amount of sedative used, what is the dependent variable?
   a. Anxiety level.
   b. Preprocedure visits by an endoscopy nurse.
   c. The amount of sedation required.
   d. Type of endoscopic procedure scheduled.

2. In the case situation described in this chapter, "adults (18 years or older) who are scheduled for upper and lower endoscopies and who are English-speaking, oriented, and able to hear and give accurate information" describes:
   a. All patients seen in the endoscopy clinic.
   b. The population selected for the study.
   c. A random sample from the population at large.
   d. All of the variables in Denise's study.

3. Patients who are participating in a study of the effects of preprocedure visits (by an endoscopy nurse) on patient anxiety are assigned to one of two groups using a table of random numbers. Group 1 receives routine preprocedure care, including an instructional pamphlet. Group 2 receives the same care and pamphlet but also receives a visit from an endoscopy nurse. Which statement best describes Groups 1 and 2?
   a. Group 1 is a random sample, whereas Group 2 is not.
   b. Group 2 is the experimental group, whereas Group 1 is the control group.
   c. Group 2 is the comparison group, whereas Group 1 is the control group.
   d. Group 1 is the experimental group, whereas Group 2 is the control group.

4. When doing a literature review on the topic of interest, a researcher reads a review article that mentions another study that contradicts her hypothesis. How should the researcher evaluate this information?
   a. She should consider it irrelevant information.
   b. She should consider it a primary source of information and rely on it heavily.

   c. She should disregard it, because it conflicts with other information.
   d. She should view this conclusion skeptically until she has had a chance to read the contradictory study herself.
5. To calculate how long it will take her to complete her study, a researcher must compute the average number of patients treated each day in her clinic. How might she find this average?
   a. She could read it in a review of the literature.
   b. She could scan clinic records and see that, on most days, there are 20 patients treated.
   c. She could sum the total number of patients treated last year and divide it by the number of days the clinic operated.
   d. She could compute the difference between the highest number of patients treated and the lowest number of patients treated per day over the last year.
6. If the most sedation required by a member of a study group was 1.7 mg/kg, and the least amount required was 0.8 mg/kg, the range of sedation required for this group would be:
   a. The least and the greatest amount required to produce sedation.
   b. The average of the greatest and least amounts required to produce sedation.
   c. 1.7 mg/kg minus 0.8 mg/kg.
   d. 2.5 mg/kg.
7. Which statement best describes a null hypothesis?
   a. A conclusion statement saying that the study results are inconclusive.
   b. A hypothesis that states there is no relationship between the variables under study.
   c. A hypothesis to be ignored.
   d. A hypothesis that was never pursued, because the idea is too preposterous.
8. A placebo is a:
   a. Treatment.
   b. Measure of central tendency.
   c. Theory.
   d. Sample.
9. $SD = \sqrt{\dfrac{\Sigma(\text{deviation scores}^2)}{n-1}}$
   is the formula for:
   a. The mean of a sample.
   b. The mode of a sample.
   c. The standard deviation.
   d. The deviation scores.
10. During a study of the effects of preprocedural visits on the anxiety level of patients undergoing endoscopies, the researcher measures the level of anxiety by asking subjects to rate their anxiety on a scale from 0 to 10. What level of measurement is this?
   a. Interval.
   b. Nominal.
   c. Ordinal.
   d. Ratio.

BIBLIOGRAPHY

Barrish, J.O. & Gilger, M.A. (1993). Colon cleanout preparations in children and adolescents. *Gastroenterol Nurs 16*, 106.

Bums, N. & Grove, S.K. (1997). *The practice of nursing research: conduct, critique, and utilization* (3rd ed.). Philadelphia: W.B. Saunders.

Ellett, M. & Beausang, C. (2002). Introduction to qualitative research. *Gastroenterol Nurs 25*, 10.

Fullhart, J.W. (1993). Generating ideas for research. *Gastroenterol Nurs 15*, 244.

Gilger, M.A. (1993). Conscious sedation for endoscopy in the pediatric patient. *Gastroenterol Nurs 16*, 75.

Gruber, M. (1995). Understanding published research reports, or how to "study" a study. *Gastroenterol Nurs 18*, 33.

Hayes, A. & Buffum, M. (2001). Educating patients after conscious sedation for gastrointestinal procedures. *Gastroenterol Nurs 24*, 54.

Nightingale, F. (1859). *Notes on Nursing: What it is and what it is not.* Philadelphia: J.B. Lippincott.

Polit, D.F., Beck, C.T. & Hungler, B.P. (2001). *Essentials of nursing research: methods, appraisal, and utilization.* Philadelphia: J.B. Lippincott.

Schmelzer, M. (2001). Understanding the research methodology: should we trust the researchers' conclusions? *Gastroenterol Nurs 23*, 269.

Schmelzer, M. & Wright, K.B. (1996). Enema administration techniques used by experienced registered nurses. *Gastroenterol Nurs 19*, 171.

Tealey, A.R. (1994). Percutaneous endoscopic gastrostomy in the elderly. *Gastroenterol Nurs 16*, 151.

Thome, S.E., Radford, M.J. & Armstrong, E. (1997). Long-term gastrostomy in children: caregiver coping. *Gastroenterol Nurs 20*, 46.

Tinstman, C. (1995). Understanding the role of the Institutional Review Board. *Gastroenterol Nurs 18*, 153.

Waltz, C., Strickland, O. & Lenz, E. (1991). *Measurement in nursing research* (2nd ed.). Philadelphia: I.A. Davis.

Young, R.J. (1996). Pediatric constipation. *Gastroenterol Nurs 19*, 88.

NURSING PROCESS

Chapter 8

ASSESSMENT

This chapter explores the nursing process, defined as a systematic, interactive approach to nursing care using problem-solving techniques. The nurse's experience and education provide a foundation of knowledge that can be used to assist patients to meet identified outcomes logically and progressively. Although our experiences and education may vary considerably the nursing process provides a shared vision of practice that brings continuity to the nursing care of a patient. The nursing process is composed of five interrelated steps: assessment, diagnosis, planning, implementation, and evaluation (Alfaro-Lefevre, 2002).

1. **Assessment:** Continuously collecting data about health status to monitor for evidence of health problems and risk factors that may contribute to health problems. Assessment is the primary focus of this chapter, is considered the most crucial step.
2. **Diagnosis:** Analyzing data to clearly identify actual and potential health problems and strengths.
3. **Planning:** Determining desired outcomes (specific goals) and identifying interventions to achieve the outcomes.
4. **Implementation:** Putting the plan into action and observing initial responses.
5. **Evaluation:** Determining how well the outcomes have been achieved and deciding whether changes need to be made.

Learning objectives

After reviewing the content of this chapter, the gastroenterology nurse should be able to:

1. Delineate the essential elements that constitute the basis of the nursing process.
2. Discuss the nursing process as a part of collaborative practice.
3. Identify the steps of a nursing assessment and specifically as it applies to the assessment of the gastrointestinal patient.
4. Identify the types of data collection and the types of data specific to the gastrointestinal patient.
5. Discuss the nursing assessment of the patient receiving sedation and analgesia in the gastrointestinal endoscopy setting.

ASSESSMENT PROCESS

The first step in the nursing process is **assessment,** a continuous activity performed throughout contact with a patient. It entails systematically gathering data about a patient that is then analyzed to form a nursing diagnosis. To obtain valid data, the nurse must be able to use well-developed communication, interviewing, and physical assessment techniques. The initial assessment begins a process of updating that will continually evaluate the effectiveness of therapy and determine the course of clinical care. Reassessment must occur at regular intervals to evaluate the patient's response to care and to insure that care is appropriate. **Collaborative problems** are patient conditions best managed by a multidisciplinary team approach. Some agencies require documentation of multidisciplinary team efforts in planning, giving care, and in planning for discharge. The concept of collaborative care can be expanded to include the overall care of a patient that may involve several hospital and office visits to treat an existing condition. The nurse makes independent decisions for both collaborative problems and nursing diagnoses. The difference is that for nursing diagnosis, nursing prescribes the definitive treatment to achieve the desired outcome; in contrast, for collaborative problems, prescription for definitive treatment comes from both nursing and medicine"(Carpenito, 2002; Alfaro-LeFevre, 2002).

"Over time, patients may receive a range of care in multiple settings from multiple providers. Health care providers need to offer a continuum of care. Services should flow continuously from assessment through treatment and reassessment. A patient's care should be coordinated among practitioners"

(Joint Commission on Accreditation of Healthcare Organizations [JCAHO], 2000).

A nursing assessment differs in purpose from a medical assessment. The aim of a medical assessment is to define the existence of medical problems and identify underlying pathology. The purpose of a nursing assessment, on the other hand, is to identify human responses to medical conditions, treatments and changes in activities of daily life. In addition to the identification of adverse patient responses, the classification system for nursing diagnoses has expanded to include assessment of patient strengths and a nursing focus on patient health maintenance and health promotion behaviors. Lynda Juall Carpenito lists four types of nursing diagnosis: actual, risk, possible, wellness, or syndrome. These concepts will be discussed in Chapter 9.

The American Nurses Association has designated the North American Nursing Diagnosis Association (NANDA) as the official organization to develop the classification system for nursing diagnosis. "This evolving classification system increasingly reflects both the art and science of nursing" (Carpenito, 2002).

Types of nursing assessments

The appropriate type of assessment is determined by the clinical situation, client status, time available, and purpose of the data collection. Assessments can be divided into four general categories: initial assessment, focus assessment, time-lapsed assessment, and emergency assessment (Craven & Hirnle, 2003).

1. **Initial assessment.** This type of assessment involves initial identification of normal functional status and collection of data concerning actual or potential dysfunction. This is the baseline for reference and future comparison. This can also be described as a comprehensive assessment of patient health.
2. **Focus assessment.** This type is a status determination of a specific problem identified during previous assessment.
3. **Time-lapsed reassessment.** In this type of assessment, the nurse compares client's current status to the baseline obtained previously; detects changes in all functional health patterns after extended period of time has passed.
4. **Emergency assessment.** This is the identification of a life-threatening situation.

Steps of a nursing assessment

A patient's entire plan of care is based on the assessments made by attending health care providers. The nursing assessment is used to determine a need for nursing service and to assist other professionals (e.g. physicians, pharmacists, nutritionists, social workers,) in determining their activities. Rosalinda Alfaro-LeFevre has identified five key phases of assessment (2003):

1. collecting data;
2. validating (Verifying) data;
3. organizing data;
4. identifying patterns/ testing first impressions; and
5. reporting and recording data; reporting significant data. (Alfaro LeFevre, 2002)

COLLECTING DATA

Systematic guidelines for collecting data ensure that comprehensive, holistic data will be collected. If data collection is well planned, nursing diagnoses follow easily. Problems in data collection arise when the data are inappropriately organized, when pertinent data are omitted, irrelevant or duplicate data are collected, erroneous or misinterpreted data are collected, too little information is acquired, interpretation of data (rather than observed behavior) is recorded, and/or when failure to update the database occurs.

The nurse uses the interview, the physical examination, and observation, review of records and diagnostic reports, and collaboration with colleagues to establish the database (Carpenito, 2002; JCAHO, 2000).

INTERVIEW

The intent of the **nursing interview** is to record a patient's unique qualities. When this goal is met, the planning of individualized care becomes possible. The nursing interview will be a reflection of the type of assessment needed at that time. A patient that comes to the primary care setting will most likely require a more complete and comprehensive assessment than the patient with an acute problem that is being seen in an emergency setting. Data collection focuses on identification of a client's present and past health status. This includes coping patterns (strengths and limitations), functional status, response to therapy (nursing, medical), risk for potential problems, and desire for higher level of wellness (Carpenito, 2002).

All nurse-client interactions are based on communication. "Your ability to establish rapport, ask questions, listen and observe is the key to a positive nurse-patient relationship and essential to getting the facts. People who seek health care, whether they're well or acutely ill, are in an extremely vulnerable position; they need to know that they are in good hands and that their main concerns will be addressed" (Alfaro-Lefevre, 2002). The term **therapeutic communication** describes techniques that encourage the client or family to share views and feelings openly (Carpenito, 2002). A skilled interviewer uses interpersonal skills to convey a sense of warmth and concern that will make the patient more at ease and willing to share necessary personal information.

The nursing interview gives the client/patient an opportunity to provide a personal account of their present health status. **Subjective data** collection compiles information from the patient's perspective as it relates to their clinical presentation. Subjective data usually include feelings of anxiety, discomfort, or mental stress. The presence of pain is a subjective finding. Only the patient can provide information about the frequency, location, duration, or intensity of pain (Elkin, Perry & Potter, 2000).

Interviewing techniques should be responsive to the individual qualities of the patient that may affect the ability of the nurse to collect pertinent data. Educational level, level of consciousness, and language barriers are examples of possible limiting factors for an effective interview. As stated by the JCAHO "The nursing assessment should consider religious and cultural practices, emotional barriers, desire and motivation to learn, physical and cognitive limitations, language barriers and the financial implications of care choices" (JCAHO, 2000).

Assessment of the **spiritual domain** is another important aspect of competent nursing care. Spirituality involves a person's inner resources and values that guide and give meaning to life. All areas of nursing assessment provide important data for developing nursing diagnoses that address the patient's spiritual needs. Assessment findings that indicate anger, doubt, loss of hope or purpose in life, questions about moral and ethical implications of a therapeutic regimen, or display of self-blame are manifestations of spiritual distress in the patient. Accurate assessment of the patient's spiritual well-being contributes to the development of a holistic plan of care for the patient.

PHYSICAL EXAMINATION

The **nursing physical examination** verifies information uncovered in the nursing history interview and contributes new objective data. A physician's physical assessment focuses on pathology and etiology (cause of disease). The nursing exam is used to verify and expand on the data that has been gathered during the nursing interview.

The nursing physical exam and observation of the patient contribute much of the **objective data** to the nursing evaluation of the patient. In comparison to the subjective data surrounding a patient's perception of their situation, the objective data compiles information that can be measured and validated by others. Some nurses in expanded roles perform comprehensive physical examinations. All nurses conduct selected aspects of physical assessment for nursing purposes (Elkin, Perry & Potter, 2000).

Physical measurements of any patient must include vital signs. Height and weight may also be included. In addition, the patient's heart, lungs, and abdomen should be assessed. Assessment of other systems may be appropriate, depending on the patient's condition and health problems.

Physical assessment of a patient is performed in four phases: **inspection, palpation, percussion,** and **auscultation.** The steps of a general assessment will be covered briefly at this time with a more detailed explanation later in this chapter as it relates to the gastrointestinal patient (Craven & Hirnle, 2003).

1. **Inspection.** Inspection is concentrated watching. It is close, careful scrutiny, first of the individual as a whole and then each body system. During inspection, the patient's anatomic structures are considered and any abnormalities present are noted.
2. **Palpation.** Palpation follows and often confirms points you noted during inspection. Palpation applies your sense of touch to assess these factors: texture, temperature, moisture, organ location and size, as well as any swelling.
3. **Percussion.** Percussion is tapping the person's skin with short, sharp strokes to assess the underlying structures. The strokes yield a palpable vibration and a characteristic sound that depicts the location, size, and density of the underlying organ.
4. **Auscultation.** Auscultation is listening to sounds produced by the body, such as the heart and blood vessels and the lungs and abdomen. Certain sounds, such as congested breathing or bowel tones, can be heard without a special device but most body sounds are very soft and must be channeled through a stethoscope.

OBSERVATION

"The observation of a patient begins the moment the nurse meets the patient. It can provide important information about a patient's status. Observation includes looking, watching, examining, scrutinizing, surveying, scanning, and appraising. Using knowledge of nursing care, physical assessment, basic sciences, social sciences, and pathophysiology, nurses observe clients in a sophisticated manner" (Craven & Hirnle, 2003).

The skill of observation involves the sense of vision, smell, hearing and touch to observe aspects of a patient that can provide additional information to the collection of data. How does the patient look? Visual clues can give insight to a patient's level of comfort or discomfort. The patient's body size, hydration, and nutritional status can be seen. A patient's manner and interactions with others are also important components to an assessment. A keen sense of smell is used when assessing a patient. Any body or breath odors may indicate an underlying physical condition. For example, foul smelling breath may signify an oral or pulmonary infection or may indicate gastrointestinal bleeding. Patients with esophageal or gastric cancer often present with foul smelling breath as well. A fruity breath odor may indicate a metabolic disorder such as ketoacidosis in diabetes mellitus. Alcohol on a patient's breath may be a one explanation for physical findings. Hearing is important to listen to any physical abnormalities that may need further investigation as in an abdominal assessment. Listening to what the patient says is not only important in terms of subjective data collection, but can also give insight as to the patient's level of mental capability, consciousness, education. These are especially aspects to consider when planning teaching strategies for the patient and family. Touch is used as a part of physical assessment, but also to provide warmth and reassurance.

Review of records and diagnostic reports: A nurse's role often involves more than the review and interpretation of data. A nurse generally supervises patient teaching and appropriate preparation for diagnostic tests. Diagnostic work is an interdisciplinary function that involves coordination and communication among nurses, physicians, laboratory personnel, radiology department and diagnostic specialty units. The nurse's role is often pivotal in the organization of services and the acquisition of patient diagnostic data. During more complex or invasive procedures nurses often assist to provide patient care and monitoring.

Lab values and diagnostic reports provide vital information to use to formulate a medical diagnosis. This information is also very useful to develop the nursing diagnosis. It is extremely important to be aware of the significance of the test and lab results as you gather data to formulate a plan of care for each patient. For this text we will be concentrating more on lab values and diagnostic tests that are of special interest to the gastrointestinal nurse. A discussion will follow in the section entitled "Care of the gastrointestinal patient".

COLLABORATION WITH COLLEAGUES TO ESTABLISH THE DATABASE

A team of health professionals working together can provide continuity to their service and improve patient outcomes. Communication with other team members is ongoing as the patient is evaluated and re-evaluated to ensure effective therapy. Nurses often consult and collaborate with many specialty team members such as physicians, pharmacists, physical therapists, counselors, spiritual advisors as well as members of the primary care team such as technicians and patient care assistants. All information gathered from other team members is important to data collection and validation.

Validating data. To keep data free from error, bias, and misinterpretation, it must be confirmed or verified periodically. The act of verifying or confirming data is also known as validation. To verify data return to the five steps of data collection and review the data from the various sources used to establish the database. Does information strengthen your initial impression or do inconsistencies exist? Review records and test results to compare information with acquired data. Do the sources of information appear reliable? Any discrepancies will require further investigation and re-evaluation.

Validation becomes particularly necessary when data discrepancies exist. For example, a nurse who receives verbal communication of no known allergies, yet notes a recorded allergy to penicillin, should validate the patient's drug allergies. Validation is also critical when the source of the assessment data may not be reliable or when serious harm to the patient could occur as a result of inaccurate data.

Organizing data. Cluster the data into groups of information that help you to identify patterns of health or illness. A variety of frameworks exist for the orderly collection and recording of assessment data. To approach a nursing diagnosis cluster data about a patient's strengths and talents and functional health patterns as well as information derived from the physical assessment of the patient. Physical examination is extremely valuable to the assessment of the patient and is separated from functional assessment for organizational purposes only. Data should also be organized to focus on levels of priority in patient care (Carpenito, 2002).

Identifying patterns/testing first impressions. After clustering data into groups of related information, initial impressions of patterns of human functioning will become apparent. These impressions should be tested to decide if the patterns are as they appear. Testing first impressions involves deciding what's relevant, making tentative deci-

---

Potential Diagnostic Data in Gastroenterology

Laboratory Tests

CBC: Hb, HCT, differential leukocyte count
PT, PTT, INR
Electrolytes
Ketones and protein
Amylase
Lipase
Creatinine
Serum cholesterol
LDH, AST, ALT, ALP
Glucose
Bilirubin
Serum albumin
CPK

Imaging Studies

Type 1: Simple radiographic pictures in which structures are enhanced either by natural differences in radio density or by differences enhanced through instillation of a contrast agent.
- Chest radiograph
- Flat plate of abdomen
- Upper GI series, may include esophagogram
- Lower GI series/ Barium enema
- Oral cholecystogram
- Contrast radiographs

Type 2: A cross-sectional look at internal organs by sound waves, x-ray beams, or measurement of magnetic resonance signals
- Computed Tomography-CT scan
- Ultrasonography
- Magnetic Resonance Imaging- MRI

Type 3: Pictures of internal organs detected by radio-active tracers and gamma cameras after the intravenous injection of a radioisotope
- Nuclear imaging scan
- Endoscopic Exams
- Esophagogastroduodenoscopy
- Colonoscopy
- Proctosigmoidoscopy
- Anoscopy
- Endoscopic Retrograde Cholangiopancreatography
- Laparoscopy
- Tests of Gastrointestinal motor activity
- Manometry
- Microscopic examination of tissue
- Liver Biopsy
- Cytology
- Mucosal biopsy
- Tests of digestive function
- Gastric Analysis
- Fecal Analysis
- Misc. Tests
- PH studies
- Bernstein test
- Virtual Colonoscopy
- Video Capsule

sions about what the data may suggest, and focusing assessment to gain more information to fully understand the situations at hand" (Alfaro-Lefevre, 2002). Combine subjective and objective information from health care assessments, the patient and family to confirm or invalidate initial data. Decide what is relevant or irrelevant and continue the process to relay appropriate information to other members of the team verbally and through a process of written documentation.

Reporting and recording data; reporting significant data. Data collected in an assessment should be documented in the medical record and /or verbally reported to other members of the health care team. Data is of little benefit unless it is effectively communicated in a timely manner. Acceptable timeframes for communication will depend on the patient's condition. Critical information must be recognized and communicated immediately to ensure timely intervention.

Documentation of patient data fulfills the standard of care that requires the communication of a patient's health status. Data should be recorded legibly, good grammar should be used, and only standard medical abbreviations should be included. To speed data retrieval, the data should be formatted under headings and organized categorically whenever possible. Some information is more appropriately recorded in narrative form, whereas other information should be charted on a flow sheet.

Documentation of patient data must comply with certain legal requirements. Written records are the most readily acceptable as evidence in a trial. Specifically, the nurse must chart everything observed, carried out, changed, taught, evaluated, or initiated. The database should contain descriptive, subjective, and objective information as supported by documented facts.

To avoid ambiguity when documenting data derived from a conversation or interview, the patient should be quoted verbatim or the entry should be noted as a paraphrase. Similarly, clarifying errors avoids miscommunication of data. A nurse can correct a written error by striking the notation with a single line, enclosing it in parentheses, writing "error" above it and initialing it (Craven & Hirnle, 2003).

Data Collection: The Gastroenterology Assessment

Because of the vague nature of symptoms of GI disorders, digestive diseases are among the most difficult to assess. Patients with illnesses unrelated to the gastrointestinal tract may present with gastrointestial symptoms such as nausea, vomiting, abdominal pain, altered appetite, and/or bowel changes. On the other hand, certain GI disorders may produce symptoms that are extraintestinal. For example, one of the most common extraintestinal manifestations of inflammatory bowel disease is arthritis. To complicate matters further, some digestive symptoms may not be disease-related at all but may be a side effect of medication. For this reason, all complaints are potentially meaningful and therefore merit attention.

The nursing assessment of the gastrointestinal patient follows the same guidelines as the general assessment with a focus on gastrointestinal data collection. The steps for a focused gastrointestinal assessment include the interview, physical exam, observation, and review of records and diagnostic reports.

Interview

The first objective is to arrive at a clear statement of the patient's health problem or chief complaint. The nurse must be alert to manifestations of pain, noting the location, intensity, and whether or not the pain radiates. Associated symptoms may also be significant. For example, testicular atrophy, gynecomastia, and alopecia may be associated with hepatic cirrhosis. Commonly experienced symptoms to inquire about include nausea, vomiting, diarrhca, constipation, appetite, significant weight loss or gain, dysphasia, odynophagia (painful swallowing), chest or abdominal pain, jaundice, and the passage of blood in vomitus or stool. The timing of symptoms in relation to the ingestion of food is also important. Ingestion of food constitutes physiologic stress to the gut much the same as exercise can apply stress to the heart to illicit symptoms in an ailing heart.

Equally important is the pattern with which symptoms occur. Relevant history of GI symptoms, including the duration of the diagnosed GI problem (if it has been diagnosed) and any evidence of complications stemming from GI disease should be documented. The nurse should establish the patient's normal GI status, clarify how the patient's status has changed, and note any stratcgics the patient may have used to manage the problem. Possible familial tendency toward the problem as manifested in relatives, as well as the presence of risk factors for GI disease should be explored and documented.

Nutritional assessment is an important aspect of a gastrointestinal comprehensive assessment. The provision of adequate nutrition and its ability to be metabolized is vital to the maintenance and repair of the body. Alteration in nutritional status is manifested by recent significant weight loss or gain, overweight or obese appearance, underweight or malnourished appearance, decreased energy levels, altered bowel patterns, and altered appearance of the skin, hair, teeth, and mucus membranes. Documentation should include patterns of consumption and elimination and relationships between diet and symptoms, diet and medications, diet and lifestyle, diet and emotional states (Craven & Hirnle, 2003; JCAHO, 2000).

Nutritional problems can be the result of the inability of the body to use ingested nutrients. Diseases such as inflammatory bowel disease can cause poor nutrient absorption. The inability to tolerate certain foods can cause malabsorption syndromes. Celiac disease, which is characterized by anintolerance to the gluten found in wheat, rye, oats, and barley, can cause small bowel mucosal villi to atrophy, decreasing their absorptive abilities. Lactose intolerance occurs when there is a deficiency of lactase, the digestive enzyme that breaks down the sugar found in milk. Any obstruction of the intestinal tract caused by scar tissue, benign or cancerous growths, or structural abnormalities will alter nutritional status. Surgical removal of absorptive sections of the intestine will interfere with the ability to maintain a balance of the associated nutrients. Decreased bile salts, the absence of normal digestive secretions from disease (e.g. secondary to pancreatic insuffiency), or from medication regimes may also result in decreased utilization of nutrients. Increased excretion or protein loss characterizes many GI disorders including abscesses, fistulas, Crohns, or ulcerative colitis (Craven Hirnle, 2003).

Care should be taken to evaluate and address the nutritional needs of each patient. Periods of stress can alter nutritional needs and leave the patient at risk for nutritional deficiencies. Increased metabolic demands can be a response to the emotional stresses that accompany hospitalization or physical stresses such as infection or wound healing. In addition, they frequently accompany conditions marked by increased tissue destruction including cancer, ulceration and necrosis. Psychological states can affect a person's desire to eat. Anorexia nervosa is an eating disorder in which the person refuses to eat due to fear of becoming overweight.

Nutritional problems can also include conditions of weight gain. Overweight status and conditions of obesity can be a physiologic stress to the body. Obesity can impose physical limitations on a patient that can limit mobility as well as putting one at increased risk for certain conditions such as heart disease.

Medications are frequently the cause of GI distress and can disrupt the normal uptake of certain medications. A medication profile should be obtained. The patient's profile should include medication or food allergies. The patient's past and present use of medications taken for GI problems should be explored. If the patient has experienced or is presently experiencing side effects from these medications, this fact should also be recorded. Likewise, it is important to evaluate whether or not the patient is experiencing or has experienced the desired effects of the medication. Finally, current use of other prescription and nonprescription medications should be described.

Individuals identified at nutritional risk during the initial interview should undergo a comprehensive nutritional assessment. This includes a dietary history and intake information, physical examination for clinical signs, anthropometric measures, and laboratory tests. Nutritional assessment skills are specialized but identification of a patient at risk can begin a process of communication to other health team members that will ensure an appropriate evaluation.

Routine laboratory tests are of particular value in nutritional assessment because they are objective, can detect preclinical nutritional deficiencies, and can be used to confirm subjective findings. "The best routinely performed laboratory indicators of nutritional status are hemoglobin, hematocrit, cholesterol, triglycerides, total lymphocyte count, and serum albumin. Glucose low- and high-density lipoproteins, prealbumin, transferring, and total protein levels also provide meaningful information" (Jarvis, 2000).

Physical Examination

This section describes techniques used in inspection, auscultation, palpation, and percussion of the abdomen. Inspection and auscultation should always precede percussion and palpation. This order is different than the suggested sequence for the general physical assessment of a patient but particularly important when assessing the abdomen. Stimulation of the abdomen caused by percussion and palpation affect normal bowel activity.

Inspection

The examiner should note the patient's breathing pattern (chest versus abdominal breathing) and be alert for scars, distended veins, and signs of abdominal trauma that may be relevant to the present illness. In addition, striae, which may evidence significant weight loss, should be noted. Upon inspection of the contour, the examiner should observe symmetry of the abdomen (above and below the umbilicus). Distention will present as a rounded contour. The umbilicus is useful as an aid when distinguishing causes of distention. It may be everted in ascites, whereas it remains unchanged in gaseous distention. Peristaltic waves can sometimes be observed, particularly if the patient is thin. This observation becomes significant when an obstruction is present.

Auscultation

Bowel sounds originate from the movement of air and fluid through the small intestine. The nurse should observe the frequency and rhythm of intestinal peristaltic sounds, by listening with the diaphragm of a stethoscope. Bowel sounds vary considerably in normal individuals. Normal bowel sounds do not rule out bleeding or other pathology. Normal bowel sounds are soft, high-pitched sounds. Bowel sounds are normally intermittent. Before declaring that no bowel sounds are present, it is important to listen in each quadrant for a total of 4 to 5 minutes. Findings significant on auscultation include the following:

(a) bruits, which may indicate cardiovascular abnormality rather than GI pathology;

(b) high-pitched tinkles and peristaltic rushes, which are audible when intestinal obstruction occurs; and

(c) decreased or absent bowel sounds, which can suggest paralytic ileus, gangrene, peritonitis, or inflammation.

Palpation

Touch is most useful in identifying tenderness, temperature changes, and masses. Both shallow and deep palpation should be performed during assessment. Findings significant to digestive diseases include fluid waves, abnormal organ size, rebound tenderness, masses, and hernias. Examination of the size, shape, position, consistency, mobility, and tension of the major organs concludes physical assessment of the abdomen. Abdominal tenderness should be assessed and characterized.

Percussion

Based on much the same concept as ultrasound, percussion is performed with two hands. Sound waves produced by striking one object against another allow an examiner to note the presence of air, fluid, and solid matter in the abdomen.

To perform percussion, the examiner should place the distal phalanx of the middle finger of the nondominant hand flat against the area to be percussed. This finger is the only part of the examiner's hand that should be in contact with the abdomen. With the tip of the flexed middle finger of the dominant hand, the examiner should sharply strike the distal joint of the phalanx on the abdomen. Sounds generated by this action reflect the size, density, and characteristics of the underlying abdominal structures and can be described as flat, dull, resonant, hyperresonant, and tympanic. Tympany generally denotes large amounts of gas in the stomach and intestines, whereas dullness is normally noted over a full bladder, mass, or organs such as the liver or spleen. The presence of fluid is not always easy to differentiate from other conditions but is suspected when there is abdominal distention with bulging flanks, a fluid wave, and shifting dullness when the patient is turned on one side.

Nursing care of the patient in the endoscopy setting

"The delivery of health care in the field of gastroenterology and endoscopy is expanding, thus modifying the traditional role of the registered nurse (RN). Care of the patient undergoing an endoscopic procedure continues to be more critical in nature, more complex in technology, and more comprehensive in scope. Nursing care of the patient has changed to include a continuous comprehensive nursing assessment, administration and maintenance of conscious sedation under the direction of a physician, administration of reversal agents, use of state of the art equipment during diagnostic and complex therapeutic procedures and documentation of all of the above" (Society of Gastroenterological Nurses & Associates, Inc. [SGNA], 2000).

Specific guidelines for the documentation of care provided for the patient in the gastrointestinal endoscopy setting have been developed by the SGNA as well as guidelines for the nursing care of the above. These modules serve as guidelines for nursing care and responsibilities in the endoscopic procedural setting.

CASE SITUATION

Eleanor Russell, age 73, arrives in the gastroenterology department holding area. She originally went to the emergency room (ER) complaining of nausea and vomiting, severe right upper quadrant abdominal pain, and sternal pain with pressure radiating to her back. The ER nurse communicates to you that Mrs. Russell described a family history of gallbladder disease and was diagnosed with cholecystitis several months ago. In addition, he reports that Mrs. Russell's symptoms became worse after eating a peanut butter and Swiss cheese sandwich and a milkshake yesterday for lunch. Her ECG is normal, and she is currently on Coumadin for thrombophlebitis in her right leg. The ER nurse tells you that Mrs. Russell's stool is negative for occult blood but that her prothrombin time (PT) partial thromboplastin time (PTT) is abnormal. He also adds that the patient is febrile.

Her physician has diagnosed Mrs. Russell with cholecystitis and cholelithiasis. He now awaits the results of further laboratory studies and an abdominal ultrasound examination to confirm or rule out gallstone obstruction of the common bile duct. The physician asks you to prepare for endoscopic retrograde cholangiopancreatography (ERCP).

As you greet Mrs. Russell, you notice that her face is rigid and pale. She is scanning her environment nervously, and her eyes are open wide. Her hands are cool, moist, and trembling; you observe a large bruise near her left wrist. Her respirations are rapid and shallow as she tells you, "I've never had anything like this before. My daughter was supposed to have talked to my doctor about my diet..."

Points to think about

1. What steps should a nurse carry out in assessing Mrs. Russell before diagnostic ERCP?
2. What subjective data are evident thus far? What objective data?
3. Which data might need validation?
4. Which data would require documentation in Mrs. Russell's records?
5. What additional preprocedure assessment should the nurse undertake before preparing for the ERCP procedure?

Suggested responses

1. In assessing Mrs. Russell before diagnostic ERCP the nurse should take the following steps.
   a. Collect Data;
   b. Validate Data;
   c. Organize Data;
   d. Identify patterns/test first impressions; and
   e. Report and Record Data.
2. The following subjective and objective data are evident.
   a. **Subjective data:** Nausea, sternal pain with pressure radiating to her back, symptoms became worse after eating a peanut butter and Swiss cheese sandwich and a milkshake.
   a. **Objective data:** Mrs. Russell's ECG is normal; her face is rigid and pale; she is scanning her environment nervously with eyes open wide; her hands are cool, moist, and trembling; she has a large bruise near her left wrist; respirations are rapid and shallow; a reported history of gallbladder disease in the family, a personal history of cholecystitis and a nursing report of fever, occult negative stool, and an abnormal PT and PTT.

3. Because the ER nurse communicates that Mrs. Russell was diagnosed with cholecystitis several months ago, her symptoms became worse after lunch yesterday, that her stool is negative for occult blood, her PT/PTT is abnormal and she presents with fever, the nurse might need to validate these data in the record and with the patient.

4. The nurse must document everything observed, carried, out, changed, taught, evaluated, or initiated.

5. During a preprocedure phase the nurse should perform and document a nursing assessment. The assessment factors should include physical, psychosocial, current medications, treatment, and previous medical, anesthetic and drug history. Review of patient's symptoms and history will supply any pertinent information to be documented

REVIEW TERMS

assessment, data, database, nursing examination, nursing history, nursing interview, nursing process, objective data, observation, subjective data, validation, collaborative practice, cholecystitis, cholelithiasis

REVIEW QUESTIONS

1. A nursing assessment:
   a. Is a systematic approach to nursing care.
   b. Is always comprehensive.
   c. Is a process of identifying a patient problem.
   d. Should precede a nursing history.

2. Which statement is true of physical assessment of the abdomen?
   a. The order in which inspection, palpation, percussion, and auscultation are performed is only important if the patient is in pain.
   b. Percussion and palpation should be performed before auscultation and inspection.
   c. Bowel sounds are normal if none are heard in four abdominal quadrants over a period of 4 to 5 minutes.
   d. Bowel sounds characterized by high-pitched tinkles and peristaltic rushes are abnormal.

3. A preprocedural assessment includes:
   a. Determination of baseline vital signs.
   b. Verification of current medications in use.
   c. Verification of NPO status.
   d. All of the above.

4. Validation is the act of:
   a. Clarification.
   b. Verification.
   c. Repeating a patient's responses twice.
   d. Checking to be sure a nursing history was taken.

5. Which of the following might the gastroenterology nurse record as objective nursing assessment data concerning a patient who presents in the ER with apparent biliary colic:
   a. A medical diagnosis of choledocholithiasis.
   b. "Patient is anxious."
   c. "Patient ate a peanut butter and cheese sandwich yesterday at lunch."
   d. "Patient is scanning her surroundings with wide open eyes."

6. By which method(s) could a patient's medication history be validated:
   a. By asking the patient what medications he or she takes.
   b. By reading the prescription labels on the bottles of medicines the patient provides.
   c. Both a and b.
   d. Neither a nor b.

7. A nurse's sense of vision, hearing, smell and touch are important features of:
   a. The observation of a patient.
   b. Collection of subjective data
   c. A patient diagnostic review.
   d. Patient interview and data analysis

8. The purpose of nursing assessment is to:
   a. Identify underlying pathology.
   b. Identify teaching needs.
   c. Monitor for evidence of patient health care needs.
   d. Analyze data to identify actual or potential health problems.

9. A multidisciplinary team approach to patient care is characterized by:
   a. A coordination of care among practitioners.
   b. A continuous flow of patient care service.
   c. A collaborative approach to manage health problems.
   d. All of the above.

10. A patient returns to the clinic after 2 weeks of taking a new prescription for reflux. The most appropriate assessment for a follow-up visit is:
    a. A comprehensive assessment
    b. A focused assessment
    c. A time-lapsed reassessment
    d. A limited assessment

BIBLIOGRAPHY

Alfaro-LeFevre, R. (2002). *Applying nursing process: Promoting Collaborative Care* (5th ed.). Philadelphia: Lippincott, Williams and Wilkins.

Carpenito, L.J. (2002). *Nursing Diagnosis: application to clinical practice* (9th ed.). Philadelphia: Lippincott, Williams and Wilkins.

Craven, R. & Hirnle, C. (2003). *Fundamentals of Nursing: Human Health and Function* (4th ed.). Philadelphia: Lippincott, Williams, and Wilkins.

Elkin, M., Perry, A. & Potter, P. (2000). *Nursing Interventions and Clinical Skills*, (2nd ed.). St. Louis, MO: Mosby.

Jarvis, C. (2000). *Physical Examination and Health Assessment* (3rd ed.). Philadelphia, PA: W.B. Saunders.

Joint Commission on Accreditation of Healthcare Organizations (2000). *Comprehensive Accreditation Manual for Hospitals.* Chicago: JCAHO.

Lewis, S., Heitkemper, M. & Dirksen, S. (2000). *Medical Surgical Nursing, Assessment and Management of Clinical Problems.* St. Louis, MO: Mosby.

Society of Gastroenterology Nurses and Associates Inc. (2000). *SGNA Guidlelines for the Nursing Care of the Patient Receiving Sedation and Analgesia in the Gastrointestinal Endoscopy Setting.* Chicago, IL: SGNA.

Society of Gastroenterology Nurses and Associates Inc. (1998). *Standards of Clinical Nursing Practice and Role Delineation Statements.* Chicago, IL: SGNA.

ORGANIZATIONS:

North American Nursing Diagnosis Association (NANDA)
1211 Locust Street
Philadelphia, PA 19107
800-647-9002
E Mail-www.virtualer.com

American Nurses Association
600 Maryland Avenue SW
Suite 100 West
Washington, DC 20024
202-651-7012
E-Mail-http://www.ana.org/

Chapter 9

NURSING DIAGNOSIS

This chapter discusses the nurse's role in diagnosing actual or potential health problems specific to patients with GI disorders. Nursing diagnosis is defined and differentiated from medical diagnosis. Examples of functional health patterns and the subsequent nursing diagnoses for gastroenterology patients are presented.

Learning objectives

After reviewing the content of this chapter, the gastroenterology nurse should be able to:
1. Define nursing diagnosis.
2. Differentiate between nursing diagnosis, medical diagnosis, and collaborative diagnosis.
3. Formulate a nursing diagnosis using an approved classification system.
4. Discuss actual, potential, and possible nursing diagnoses applicable to gastroenterology patients.

The term *nursing diagnosis* first appeared in the literature during the 1950s. Because of the implications associated with diagnosis and the idea that only physicians made diagnoses, nurses were reluctant to use the term. They were more comfortable using the word *problems* to refer to a patient's need requiring nursing intervention. Periodically through the 1960s and 1970s, the literature proposed descriptions of nursing diagnoses. Finally, an article by Lester King, M.D., in the *Journal of the American Medical Association* refuted the idea that only physicians could diagnose, thereby clearing the way for more exploration of the concept of nursing diagnosis (McFarland & McFarlane, 1996). King outlined three criteria that must be present to make a diagnosis:

1. A preexisting series of categories or classes that provide a reference for the diagnosis.
2. An entity to be diagnosed.
3. A judgment that the assessed response or phenomenon belongs to a particular class or category.

At that point, nurses began to develop a classification system for nursing diagnosis. This work was started through conferences on classification of nursing diagnoses and is still in progress today through the North American Nursing Diagnosis Association (NANDA). Other individuals and groups have played a role in identifying and testing human response patterns that result in a diagnostic label. The nursing field is now attempting to use the concept of nursing diagnosis as the linchpin in establishing autonomy and bringing unity to the profession. Only the future holds the results of these efforts.

NURSING DIAGNOSIS DEFINED

Nursing diagnosis is a clinical judgment about individual, family, or community responses to actual or potential health problems/life processes. Nursing diagnosis provides the basis for selection of nursing interventions to achieve outcomes for which the nurse is accountable (NANDA, 1990).

Nursing diagnosis provides a useful and practical method for organizing nursing knowledge so that the expertise of nursing can be defined, clarified, and developed.

Nursing diagnoses are based on the data obtained from the patient in the course of the nursing assessment. Assessment is the initial component of the nursing process; it should always be done when the patient is admitted to the preprocedural area. The plan of care is initiated when the nurse interprets assessment findings and determines pertinent nursing diagnoses.

A nursing diagnosis provides a concise statement of the interpretation of data collected. This concise statement describes the nature, source, and manifestations of health changes that the nurse is licensed to identify and treat through independent and interdependent nursing intervention.

Nursing diagnosis has become a critical link in the application of the nursing process. The same problem-solving skills are required to analyze the data obtained during an assessment and to make judgments and decisions about the problems that prevent patients and families from responding in a normal, healthy fashion. The process of determining a nursing diagnosis entails the use of clinical reasoning and judgment, which result in labeling the patient's health problem. This labeling is the product of collecting data, interpreting the information collected, grouping and clustering related facts, and assigning a name to the groupings.

Carpenito (2000) has described nursing diagnosis as both process and structure. Nursing diagnosis as process refers to the second step of the nursing process, when the nurses analyze the data collected during the assessment step and evaluates the health status. Often the diagnostic statement that results from the process of nursing diagnosis is also referred to as a nursing diagnosis. Nursing diagnosis as structure refers to specific labels or titles assigned to diagnostic categories that describe the health states that nurses can legally diagnose and treat.

The structure of a nursing diagnosis depends on its type. Carpenito has identified five types of diagnoses: actual, risk, possible, wellness, or syndrome. An **actual** diagnosis exists when the clinical state has been validated by the presence of major defining characteristics. **Risk** diagnoses represent the nursing judgment that an individual, family, or community is vulnerable to a potential problem. A **possible** nursing diagnosis describes a problem that is suspected by the nurse but needs more supporting data. **Wellness** diagnoses describe the individual, group, or family's transition from one level of wellness to a higher level of wellness and focus on patterns of wellness, healthy responses, and/or client strengths. **Syndrome** nursing diagnoses, a relatively new concept, describe a cluster of signs and symptoms. For instance, disuse syndrome is associated with a cluster of nursing diagnoses such as risk for constipation, risk for infection, risk for thrombosis, risk for activity intolerance, and risk for powerlessness (Carpenito, 2000).

From either perspective, process or structure, the value of the nursing diagnosis is that it provides a scientific basis for nursing practice so that desired patient outcomes and planned interventions are consistent with the patient's health problems.

NURSING DIAGNOSIS VERSUS MEDICAL DIAGNOSIS

The process used to identify a diagnosis or a patient problem is the same for nursing and medicine. Both nursing and medical diagnoses are concerned with gathering, sorting, interpreting, and analyzing data. However, **medical diagnosis** focuses on identification of a disease based on pathology and etiology, whereas **nursing diagnosis** focuses on the patient's present **health problems,** strengths and limitations, and methods of adapting to health problems. Table 9-1 provides examples of how nursing diagnoses and medical diagnoses differ.

Table 9-1. Nursing diagnosis versus medical diagnosis

Nursing diagnosis	Medical diagnosis
Directs nursing acts to be performed	Diagnoses medical condition
Identifies patient problems that the nurse is licensed to treat	Indicates a course of treatment
Made with the intention that nurses will perform interventions to alleviate, diminish, modify, or prevent a state of unwellness and maintain an optimum health state	Made with the intention of prescribing specific treatments to cure the disease or reduce injury
May change from day to day as the patient's response to therapy, health, and illness change	Remains the same as long as the disease persists

COLLABORATIVE DIAGNOSIS

Recently a distinction has been drawn between nursing diagnosis and collaborative diagnosis. A **collaborative diagnosis** is a statement of an actual or potential health problem that may occur from complications of disease, diagnostic studies, therapeutic procedures, or other treatment regimens. These are problems for which the nurse identifies a need to work with other members of the health care team toward resolution. Collaborative diagnoses require both nursing and medical intervention to diagnose, prevent, or treat. Carpenito (2000) defines collaborative problems as "certain physiological complications that nurses monitor to detect onset or changes in status." Nurses monitor patients to detect their onset/status and collaborate with physicians for definitive treatment.

It is important to remember that medical diagnoses, medical pathologies, diagnostic tests, treatments, and/or equipment names are not nursing diagnoses. Although the following data are considered when identifying health problems, they are not nursing diagnoses: therapeutic patient needs, therapeutic patient goals, a single sign or symptom, or invalidated nursing inferences.

FORMULATING A NURSING DIAGNOSIS

Chapter 8 discusses collection of data. It is essential that nurses understand what data are significant and how to obtain that important information. Knowledge of nursing science and other related biopsychosocial sciences is important to interpret the data and to accurately formulate the nursing diagnosis. Interpretation means sorting information and making a hypothesis for the occurrence of related events, conditions, or behavior. Nurses use clinical inferences in inductive reasoning when looking at functional patterns and observing patient responses. They then ask the questions: "What does this mean?" or "Why is he saying this?"

Cues are explored, data are collected, and the cues are *clustered*. Clustering involves making a judgment as to whether cues are consistent or inconsistent. The conclusion might be that the evidence does not support the existence of an actual problem, but that the patient is at risk for the problem to occur (a potential problem). Inconsistencies might be caused by conflicting reports from other members of the health care team, the patient, or the family or by unrealistic expectations on the part of the nurse because of inexperience or lack of knowledge.

The diagnosis statement states the health problem as related to the etiology and manifested by the signs and symptoms. For instance, constipation *(problem)* related to a diet high in dairy products *(etiology)* as evidenced by complaints of fullness, abdominal pain, and irregular bowel movement *(signs and symptoms)*. To identify these three factors, the nurse performs the following activities:

1. Clusters groups of subjective and objective cues to support the existence of a health problem.
2. Compares the collection of cues against established standards to identify any of the following:
   (a) changes in a patient's usual health pattern that are unexplained by expected norms for growth and development;
   (b) deviation from an appropriate population norm (e.g., lab values);
   (c) behavior that is nonproductive in the whole-person context; and
   (d) behavior indicating a developmental lag or evolving dysfunctional pattern.
3. Identifies the patient's strengths and problem areas and anticipates problems the patient is likely to experience. Several conclusions are possible:
   (a) There is no problem, and intervention is unnecessary.
   (b) There is an actual or potential problem.
   (c) There is a possible problem, which suggests the need to collect more data.
   (d) There is a clinical problem other than a nursing problem (a collaborative problem) that requires the nurse to consult with and sometimes cooperate with appropriate health care professionals.

Identifying specific nursing problems and prioritizing them helps to focus gastroenterology nursing practice and improve the quality of nursing care. Table 9.2 contains a partial list of approved nursing diagnoses classified by functional health problems. The classification system reflects areas in which assessment takes place.

Table 9.2 Potential nursing diagnoses for gastroenterology patients

Functional health problem	Nursing diagnosis
Health Perception Health Management Pattern	Health maintenance, impaired Noncompliance Self abuse, risk for Self care deficit Therapeutic regimen Management, ineffective
Nutritional metabolic pattern	Body temperature, altered Dentition, altered Fluid volume deficit Growth and development delayed Infection, risk for Nutrition, altered: less than body requirements Nutrition, altered: more than body requirements Nutrition, altered: potential for more than body requirements Oral mucous membrane, altered Skin integrity, impaired Swallowing, impaired
Elimination pattern	Bowel incontinence Constipation Diarrhea
Activity-exercise pattern	Activity intolerance Mobility, impaired physical Tissue perfusion, altered
Cognitive-perceptual pattern	Knowledge deficit Sensory-perceptual alteration
Sleep-rest pattern	Sleep pattern disturbance
Self-perception/self-concept pattern	Anxiety Body image disturbance Fatigue Fear Hopelessness Powerlessness Self-concept disturbance
Role relationship pattern	Communication, impaired Family process, altered Grieving Loneliness, risk for Role performance, altered Social isolation Social interaction, impaired
Sexuality pattern	Sexual dysfunction Sexuality patterns, altered
Coping-stress tolerance pattern	Adjustment, impaired Coping, ineffective Personal identity disturbed Powerlessness Self concept, disturbed Self esteem, disturbed
Life Principles	Spiritual distress Spiritual well-being, potential for enhanced
Safety/Protection	Protection, ineffective Self harm, risk for
Comfort	Comfort, impaired
Growth/Development	Development, risk for delayed

CASE SITUATION

In Chapter 8, Mrs. Russell, who has been medically diagnosed as having cholecystitis and cholelithiasis, was scheduled for a diagnostic endoscopic retrograde cholangiopancreatography (ERCP). During the preprocedural assessment, certain subjective data were identified, including:

- Nausea

- Sternal pain with pressure radiating to her back

- Symptoms becoming worse after eating peanut butter, Swiss cheese, and a milkshake

Objective data were also gathered, including:

- Normal ECG

- Febrile

- Face rigid and pale

- Scanning environment nervously with eyes open wide

- Hands cool, moist, and trembling

- Large bruise near left wrist

- Respirations rapid and shallow

Points to think about

1. Based on observations thus far, what are at least three functional health problems for Mrs. Russell?
2. According to Table 9-2, what are specific nursing diagnoses for Mrs. Russell's health problems?
3. What type(s) of nursing diagnoses were formulated?
4. Is there a collaborative diagnosis for Mrs. Russell? If interdependent nursing and medical interventions are necessary, what would the difference be in the nursing focus versus medical focus?

Suggested responses

1. Functional health problems the gastroenterology nurse might identify are:
   (a) Health perception-health management pattern
   (b) Coping-stress tolerance pattern
   (c) Nutritional metabolic pattern
   (d) Cognitive-perceptual pattern approved
2. Specific nursing diagnoses that correspond to these health problems might be:

Functional health problem	Nursing diagnosis
Health perception-health management pattern	Noncompliant with prescribed regimen
Self-perception/self-concept pattern	Anxiety
Nutritional metabolic pattern	Injury, potential for bruising, hemorrhage
Cognitive-perceptual pattern	Knowledge deficit related to disease and therapy

3. Nursing diagnoses might include the following types:
   (a) Actual problems: noncompliance with prescribed regimen, anxiety, and knowledge deficit.
   (b) Potential problem: injury, potential for bruising, hemorrhage.
   (c) Possible problem: nutrition, altered: possible less than body requirement because of pain when eating.
4. In Mrs. Russell's case the diagnosis of cholecystitis with cholelithiasis is a medical diagnosis. The nursing focus is on collecting data related to functional needs, with the outcome being care of the patient. The medical focus is on the medical history and a physical examination, with the desired outcome being care of the disease.

REVIEW TERMS

collaborative diagnoses, health problems, medical diagnosis, nursing diagnosis

REVIEW QUESTIONS

1. Which of the following was not one of King's criteria for making a diagnosis?
   a. A preexisting series of categories to provide a reference.
   b. An entity to be diagnosed.
   c. The existence of a medical pathology.
   d. A judgment that the assessed phenomenon belongs to a particular category.
2. The organization responsible for classification of nursing diagnoses is the:
   a. American Nurses Association.
   b. North American Nursing Diagnosis Association.
   c. Society of Gastroenterology Nurses and Associates.
   d. American Medical Association.
3. "Cholecystitis with cholelithiasis" is an example of a:
   a. Collaborative diagnosis.
   b. Nursing diagnosis.
   c. Medical diagnosis.
   d. Medical history.
4. A health problem is a:
   a. Problem attended to by all health care professionals.
   b. Deficit in knowledge about nutrition, exercise, and rest.
   c. Behavior.
   d. Condition related to health.
5. A collaborative diagnosis:
   a. Calls for multidisciplinary intervention.
   b. Requires cooperation between nurses responsible for pre-, intra-, and postprocedure patient care.
   c. Involves the nurse in identification, but not treatment.
   d. Is identified by more than one member of the health care team.
6. Formulating a nursing diagnosis provides:
   a. Important assessment data.
   b. An interpretation of the data collected.
   c. Interdependent nursing interventions.
   d. Outcome criteria for evaluation.
7. Nursing diagnosis focuses on the patient's:

    a. Pathology and etiology.

    b. Pathophysiology.

    c. Present health state.

    d. Health perceptions.

8. An example of an actual problem would be:

    a. Potential burn resulting from electrosurgery.

    b. Knowledge deficit related to disease and therapy.

    c. Fluid volume deficit, possible, caused by nausea and pain.

    d. Skin integrity, potential for impairment.

9. A nursing diagnosis for a patient admitted to the endoscopy unit for a diagnostic esophagogastroduodenoscopy who is not responding to treatment for a gastric ulcer might be:

    a. Knowledge deficit related to new experience.

    b. Sensory perception, altered.

    c. Bowel elimination, altered.

    d. Airway clearance, ineffective.

BIBLIOGRAPHY

Carpenito, L. (2000). *Nursing diagnosis: application to clinical practice* (9th ed.). Philadelphia: Lippincott, Williams and Wilkins.

Elkin, M., Perry, A. & Potter, P. (2000). *Nursing Interventions and Clinical Skills* (2nd ed.). St. Louis, MO: Mosby.

McFarland, G,. & McFarlane, E. (1996). *Nursing Diagnosis and Intervention* (3rd ed.). St. Louis, MO: Mosby.

North American Nursing Diagnosis Association (2000). *Taxonomy of nursing diagnoses.* St. Louis MO: NANDA International.

Chapter 10

PLANNING

This chapter will acquaint learners with the planning component of the nursing process. **Planning** entails determining what nursing activities will help the patient achieve the goals set forth in the outcome identification process. Trends in care planning are discussed, followed by an elaboration of the purposes of planning, responsibility for planning, and the activities involved in initial, ongoing, and discharge planning. The identification of treatment options, documentation of nursing orders, and outlining of care plans are also covered. Finally, considerations in planning care for gastroenterology patients are summarized.

Learning objectives

After reviewing the content of this chapter, the gastroenterology nurse should be able to:

1. List the advantages of planning patient care based on accepted nursing diagnoses.
2. Compare nursing and medical plans of patient care.
3. Describe three basic types of planning, including who performs each type.
4. Describe four means by which nurses can expand their existing repertoire of treatment options.

TRENDS IN PATIENT CARE PLANNING

Whenever nurses respond to an actual or potential health problem by determining expected patient outcomes and by identifying nursing activities for preventing, reducing, or resolving health problems, they are planning patient care. A plan of care may be a formal, documented plan or it may be implied by a documented set of nursing interventions. The Joint Commission for Accreditation of Healthcare Organizations (JCAHO) no longer requires that a formal nursing care plan be documented in a patient's hospital records. However, planning and documentation of care based on accepted nursing diagnoses, etiology, and scientifically sound intervention remain the hallmark of professional nursing practice. Furthermore, The Society of Gastroenterology Nurses and Associates (SGNA) has delineated its own position statement, *Role Delineation of the Registered Nurse in a Staff Position in Gastroenterology*, to accomplish the following:

(a) establish nursing diagnoses;
(b) establish priorities;
(c) document patient data to ensure continuity in care; manage follow-up care; and
(d) collaborate with other health care professionals.

Rationale for care planning

Although formal written care plans are no longer required, the planning of patient care is essential. Once assessment data are obtained, a nursing diagnosis is made, and desired outcomes are identified, a plan of action must be developed. Planning is the deliberate, systematic process of identifying nursing actions directed toward achieving desirable outcomes and preventing, reducing, or resolving patient health problems. This process involves **setting priorities** for care, determining patient goals and expected outcomes, selecting nursing actions and strategies, and documenting the plan of care. This is done so that the problem that is causing the greatest danger, discomfort, or pain to the patient be addressed first (Gardner, 2003). For example, if a patient is anxious about an impending procedure, the gastroenterology nurse assesses the patient's fear and considers the types of interventions that will alleviate the patient's anxiety. The patient will no doubt have less anxiety if the nurse explains the procedure in detail. The desired outcome in this situation is decreased anxiety. The planned intervention is to explain the procedure to the patient.

There are a number of important reasons listed for developing a plan of care:

1. A plan of care can identify patient problems that may be prevented, reduced, or resolved by nursing activities.

Once again, it must be recognized that the nurse cannot solve all patient problems. The patient may have problems that the family or significant other should assist in solving. There may be problems that should be referred to other members of the healthcare team for action.

2. A plan of action helps the gastroenterology nurse assign priorities for care and select nursing interventions or actions that meet the unique needs of the individual patient.

3. A documented plan provides a means of communicating information that will help other members of the healthcare team provide continuity of care.

4. The planning of care based on nursing diagnoses uses a universal language with which nurses can communicate about health problems, thus helping to build on the existing knowledge base of nursing science.

5. The planning of care based on nursing diagnoses gives a professional quality and character, rather than merely vocational assistance, to the act of nursing. It serves to separate nursing and medicine, bringing the two professions into a collegial relationship in which nurses can acknowledge and demonstrate their own unique knowledge base and contributions to their patients' health.

The planning of patient care has also taken on economic importance. Since the inception in 1983 of Medicare's system of prospective payment based on diagnosis-related groups, providers have been under increasing pressure to render quality care while accepting decreasing compensation for increasing costs. More than ever, it has become important for the nursing profession to delineate its product and to demonstrate that this product is cost-effective.

Nursing and medical plans of care

In some ways, nursing and medical plans of care are similar. Nursing and medical diagnoses share certain characteristics; both are abstractions derived from assessment and inferences based on scientific knowledge that summarize a cluster of signs and symptoms. Therefore, both nursing and medical plans of care prescribe monitoring of signs and symptoms, both are instituted and refined following initial and ongoing assessments, and both prescribe measures based on bodies of scientific knowledge. But because nursing and medical diagnoses differ (see Chapter 9), there are differences between nursing and medical plans of care. For example, nursing and medical diagnoses differ in causality. Nursing plans of care address psychological, environmental, and sociological factors contributing to disturbances in health, as well as biological factors. Moreover, because the act of diagnosis carries legal implications regarding the right to initiate treatment, nursing care plans based on nursing diagnoses focus on patient *responses* to medical treatment or on health problems nurses can independently treat. Thus interventions prescribed in nursing care plans include only actions that nurses can lawfully perform.

Clinical pathways

The evolution of healthcare delivery during the 1980s and 1990s has demanded quality patient care with controlled cost. Inpatient hospital stays have become shorter as insurance providers have reduced payment. Planned, efficient outcome-focused care has become crucial, not only for nursing, but also for all healthcare team members.

Clinical pathways (also referred to as clinical paths, care maps, critical pathways, collaborative plans of care, anticipated recovery paths, and multidisciplinary action plans) have been developed as "interdisciplinary plans of care that outline the optimal sequencing and timing of interventions for patients with a particular diagnosis, procedure, or symptom" (Ignatavicius and Hausman, 1995). These pathways are not designed to replace the nursing plan of care but rather to supplement it, prompting nursing diagnoses and interventions specific to the patient (Beyea, 1996).

In many respects, the clinical pathway is very similar to the nursing care plan. Specific patient outcomes are listed for achievement as daily outcomes and discharge outcomes. Sequenced interventions are planned along specific time lines. Unlike nursing care plans, the pathways are developed by multiple professionals, reflect interdisciplinary interventions, and track various aspects of care (Ignatavicius and Hausman, 1995). A care coordinator, frequently a nurse, may be assigned to oversee the patient's care. Variances or deviations from the pathway are documented. The variances may be a system variance, provider variance, or client variance (Beyea, 1996). Documentation of variances provides a basis for pathway revision, patient care evaluation, and continuous process improvement.

There are multiple benefits of clinical pathways. Pathways serve as teaching tools for patients and families, encouraging patient involvement in goal setting. Communication between healthcare team members, particularly during pathway development and revision, is improved. Education of new healthcare providers is enhanced. Pathways can also help demonstrate quality care to managed care companies, licensing bodies, and accrediting agencies such as JCAHO (Ignatavicius and Hausman, 1995).

Table 10-1 is an example of a clinical pathway for GI bleeding. The gastroenterology nurse plays an important role, particularly in teaching regarding the endoscopic examination and discharge care.

COMPREHENSIVE PLANNING

There are three basic types of planning that take place in the course of comprehensive care planning: initial planning; ongoing, problem-oriented planning; and discharge planning.

Initial planning

Initial planning is usually performed by the nurse who admits the patient and performs a nursing history and physical examination. Standardized care plans, including computerized care plans, agency-developed plans, care/clinical maps, and textbook plans, should be tailored to the patient's needs and may be initiated at this time.

To illustrate initial planning, the nurse's role in endoscopic variceal ligation (EVL) is reviewed. When the nurse is notified that a patient is going to undergo EVL, he or she completes initial planning, which includes assessment of the supplies and equipment needed to perform the procedure. Items to consider might include the following checklist:

(a) flexible gastroscope;

(b) overtube with bite block;

(c) suction apparatus including suction tip;

(d) ligation kit;

(e) topical anesthetic;

(f) sedative, depending on patient's hemodynamic stability; and

(g) devices for intraprocedure monitoring of vital signs.

The policies and procedures of the institution guide the initial planning phase. Ensuring the accessibility of an emergency cart, typing and crossmatching blood for patients with potential bleeding problems, and providing the staff with protective attire are all integral components of comprehensive planning.

The gastroenterology nurse uses assessment data obtained at admission to outline the plan of care. This includes any current medications, allergies that might cause complications, history of bleeding problems, and any procedures the patient has already undergone that are related to the reason for admission. In addition, the nurse reviews laboratory reports to identify any abnormal values that should be communicated to other members of the healthcare team.

To ensure that the patient will understand the purpose and expected outcomes of an endoscopic procedure, planned nursing interventions might include the following:

1. Allow the patient to ask questions and verbalize any concerns.

2. Support the patient by listening, showing concern, and encouraging questions.

3. Be prompt when performing procedures to avoid delays or postponement of procedures.

4. Involve family and significant others in discussions and questions about the procedure and care needed.

Ongoing planning

Ongoing problem-oriented planning is carried out by any nurse who has contact with the patient. This type of planning involves updating and individualizing nursing interventions. Typically, ongoing planning encompasses the following activities:

(a) clarifying nursing diagnoses;

(b) revising expected outcomes to make them more realistic and patient centered;

(c) developing new outcome statements and/or new diagnoses, as indicated by analyses of new data;

(d) identifying nursing actions that promote achievement of identified outcomes; and

(e) documenting patient responses to nursing interventions.

Actual or potential changes in the patient's health status that might occur before, during, or after the procedure should be documented. During the procedure, monitoring of physiological and hemodynamic parameters should continue. Changes may affect the nursing diagnosis, identified outcomes, and/or original plan of care. When changes occur, modification is essential to better accomplish the desired end results of care. Again, documentation is needed to ensure continuity of care and to facilitate measurement of outcomes.

Discharge planning

Discharge planning should be multidisciplinary, involving nurses, doctors, and dietitians; it may also involve social workers and/or case managers. Discharge planning begins on admission.

When a patient is admitted for an endoscopic procedure, an informed consent form is usually signed. Thus, the patient is agreeing to prescribed care. However, informed consent does not affect the patient's right to participate in or refuse treatment. Patient participation in the plan of care should begin when the patient is first seen by the gastroenterology nurse and should continue to discharge. Patients and their families may or may not take an active role in therapeutically managing the patient's illness. When taking the nursing history, the nurse should assess the role the patient wants to assume.

The establishment of a nurse-patient relationship with a participative patient will result in the patient actively assuming a role as a member of the healthcare team. This means that before, during, and after endoscopic diagnosis and treatment, the participative patient will want to stay informed about his or her health status, methods available to alter it, and ways to assist health professionals. If desired, the patient can be involved in all decisions, beginning at admission and ending at discharge. The patient should also be involved in establishing the outcomes expected from prescribed treatment.

The nurse must also anticipate and plan for the patient's needs after discharge. In discharge planning, the nurse working with the patient assists the patient and family in identifying appropriate community resources or options, such as home healthcare, respiratory therapy, or other appropriate agencies. In some institutions, a discharge planner or care manager may be available to assist the gastroenterology nurse in planning for care after discharge from the hospital or for care following procedures or treatments performed in a physician's office or outpatient setting. Discharge planning is crucial with the advent of shorter hospital stays.

There are certain factors the gastroenterology nurse must be aware of that influence patients' ability to participate in planning their own care. First are the basic beliefs about health to which the patient subscribes. A patient who does not believe in his or her susceptibility to illness may not want to take preventive measures. A typical example is the patient who consumes large amounts of alcohol and has cirrhosis of the liver. In many cases, family superstitions or folklore affect behavior toward healthcare. Other barriers to patient participation include distrust, lack of knowledge, pride, modesty, fear, impatience, religious beliefs, and cultural diversity.

Table 10-1. GI hemorrhage DRG 174 6-Day LOS

Consults for Consideration: (Date & Initial when completed) GI Medicine _____ Surgery _____ Dietary Dept. _____
Social Services _____ Home Care _____

	Day 1	Day 2	Day 3
Assessment Neuro/Psych:	Mental Status • LOC • restlessness • subjective statement of fatigue & weakness • explore anxiety/coping skills • begin assessment of knowledge of health care problem & potential modifiable risk factors (smoking, diet, alcohol, stress & exercise) • identify available & need family /human/ economic resources to resume independent self-care activities.	Mental Status • LOC • restlessness • subjective statement of fatigue & weakness • explore anxiety/coping skills • continue assessment of knowledge of health care problem & potential modifiable risk factors (alcohol, smoking, diet, stress, exercise) • collaborate w/ social services re: available & needed family /human/ economic resources to resume independent self-care activities.	Mental status • restlessness • subjective statement of fatigue & weakness.
Pulmonary:	RR & pattern.	RR & pattern.	RR & pattern.
Cardiovascular:	HR & BP for hypovolemia & tachycardia • rhythm for dysrhythmias • narrow pulse pressure • pulses & capillary refill.	HR & BP for hypovolemia & tachycardia • rhythm for dysrhythmias • narrow pulse pressure • pulses & capillary refill.	HR & BP for hypovolemia & tachycardia • rhythm for dysrhythmias • narrow pulse pressure • pulses & capillary refill.
GI:	Mucous membranes for dryness • bowel sounds • abdominal pain (location, stage, level, & duration), cramps, distention • nausea • vomiting • stool for frequency, color, & form • daily wgt.	Mucous membranes for dryness • bowel sounds • abdominal pain (location, stage, level, & duration), cramps, distention • nausea • vomiting • stool for frequency, color, & form • daily wgt.	Mucous membranes for dryness • bowel sounds • abdominal pain (location, stage, level, & duration), cramps, distention • nausea • vomiting • stool for frequency, color, & form • daily wgt.
GU:	I & O • uo >30 ml/h.	I & O • uo >30 ml/h.	I & O • uo >30 ml/h.
Integumentary:	Skin turgor, temp, color, & integrity • presence of diaphoresis, petechiae, or spider angiomata.	Skin turgor, temperature, color, & integrity • presence of diaphoresis, petechiae, or spider angiomata.	Skin turgor, temperature, color, & integrity • presence of diaphoresis, petechiae, or spider angiomata.
Focus	Fluid resuscitation/volume replacement • identify source of bleeding.	Fluid resuscitation/volume replacement • initiate PO fluid intake.	Increase in PO fluid • progressive increase in activity • teaching.
Diagnostic Plan	Chemistries • monitor HCT & hemoglobin q2-4h until stable • hemolytic profile w/ platelets • coagulation studies • liver function tests • blood grouping & crossmatch • stool for occult blood • specific gravity qs. *Consider:* urgent anoscopy, sigmoidoscopy, colonoscopy; or endoscopy (esophageal, stomach, duodenal) w/ cautery/injection &/or biopsy • gastric secretion pH & occult blood q4h • SaO2 pulse oximeter • cardiac monitor.	CBC w/ differential • continue monitoring HCT, hemoglobin, & electrolytes q6-8h until stable • repeat abnormal lab tests. *Consider:* visceral (mesenteric) angiography • nuclear bleeding scan w/ labeled red blood cells • gastric secretion analysis.	Repeat any abnormal lab tests(s). *Consider:* Contrast xray to rule out underlying pathology • further coagulation studies.

Therapeutic Interventions	Large - bore IV access • give 2 L IV NS/RL in 1-2 h then 150-200 ml/h (as tolerated) to keep uo >30 ml/h until stable • irrigate NGT q2h w/ 30 ml NS • NPO w/ frequent oral care • bedrest • cardiac monitor • O2 p.r.n. *Consider:* antacids • histamine H2 receptor blocker • sucralfate • antibiotics (if ulcers suspected) • IV vasopressin • packed red blood cells (if HCT <25%).	Clamp NGT for 12hrs • give sips of H2O PO • discontinue NGT if clamping tolerated • continue IV fluid hydration • start on clear fluids once NGT removed & no nausea • BRP w/ assistance • assist w/ hygiene.	Discontinue NGT • decrease IV fluids as PO fluid intake increased to maintain uo > 30 ml/h • progress diet from fluids to soft • change to PO meds • get OOB to chair t.i.d. • walk in hall w/ help b.i.d. • continue cardiac monitor & special gravity. *Consider:* oral iron, stool softener, & fiber supplement.
Patient/Family	Explain initial treatment/meds/fluids • instruct to call nurse for chest pain, SOB, dizziness, fast HR, diaphoresis, vomiting, diarrhea • explore potential precipitating factors (ASA, NSAID, smoking, alcohol, corticosteroids, family history, anticoagulants, prolonged retching) & document same • identify available & needed family/ human/ economic resources to resume independent self-care activities • identify Pt/family coping mechanisms • initiate discharge plan • discuss plan for daily review of plan care w/ Pt/family.	Explain need for adequate hydration • explain disease process • identify learning needs related to disease process & document same • discuss potential lifestyle changes p.r.n. (alcohol, smoking cessation, diet, stress management, wgt reduction, exercise program) • reassure that responses (anxiety, subjective feelings of emotional liability or inability to concentrate, etc.) are a normal reaction • encourage verbalization of anxiety/ fear • review, clarify, & confirm information given to date.	Collaborate w/ dietician & initiate diet teaching • teach to get up slowly from lying position • teach signs of intestinal bleeding (hematemesis, melena, hematochezia) • review meds & food/drug interactions.
Expected Outcomes	W/ volume replacement, hemodynamic stability is restored • active bleeding stopped • uo >30 ml/h • verbalizes treatment plan.	Tolerating PO fluids • plan for encouraging PO fluids documented • fluid & potassium in balance as evidenced by uo >30 ml/h, stable VS & stable HCT & hemoglobin • decrease in anxiety.	No parenteral therapy • increased tolerance of PO fluids & diet • nutritional assessment documented & calorie/protein needs identified • well hydrated • no bleeding • no abdominal distress • formed stools • independent ADL • verbalizes disease process & potential lifestyle changes.
Trigger(s)*	S & S of new bleeding w/ hypotension, tachycardia, & uo <ml/h. **Variance Management** Identification Analysis Action	Persistent hypotension, tachycardia, or uo <30ml/h • nausea/vomiting/abdominal pain. **Variance Management** Identification Analysis Action	Persistent hypotension, tachycardia, or uo <30ml/h • nausea/vomiting/abdominal pain. **Variance Management** Identification Analysis Action

Continued

From Birdsall C, Sperry S: *Clinical pathways in medical surgical practice*, St. Louis, 1997, Mosby.
*The presence of a trigger results in a variance to the path. Evaluation & intervention must be initiated and documented.

Table 10-1. GI hemorrhage DRG 174 6-Day LOS—cont'd

	Day 4	Day 5	Day 6
Assessment Neuro/Psych:	Mental status • restlessness • subjective statement of fatigue & weakness	Mental status.	Mental status.
Pulmonary:	RR & pattern.	RR.	RR.
Cardiovascular:	HR & BP for hypovolemia & tachycardia • BP for orthostatic changes • pulses & capillary refill.	BP for orthostatic changes • pulses	BP for orthostatic changes • pulses.
GI:	Appetite & food tolerance • stool for frequency, color, & form • daily wgt.	Appetite & food tolerance • stool for frequency, color, & form • daily wgt.	Appetite & food tolerance • stool for frequency, color, & form • daily wgt.
GU:	I & O • uo >30 ml/h.	Us qs.	Uo qa.
Integumentary:	Skin turgor, temp, color & integrity • presence of diaphoresis, petechiae, or spider angiomata.	Skin turgor & integrity.	Skin turgor & integrity.
Focus	Teaching • increased independence in ADL • increased activity & diet tolerance.	Discharge plan & teaching.	Self-care & discharge.
Diagnostic Plan	CBC w/ differential • repeat abnormal lab tests.	Repeat HCT & any lab study w/ abnormal value.	None.
Therapeutic Interventions	Discontinue IV • increased walking in hall • soft diet.	Encourage activity & independence in ADL.	Discharge • encourage lifestyle modifications.
Patient/Family Teaching/ Discharge Planning	Teach S & S of bleeding (thirst, frequent lip licking, light-headedness, dizziness, weakness/fatigue, impaired mental status, irritability, pallor, tremors, decrease in uo, dry skin & mucous membranes) • review meds, food/drug interactions, appropriate health-seeking behaviors, & when to seek medical care.	Review discharge plan, disease process, exercise plan, meds, & drug/food interactions • value of relaxation techniques & health-seeking behaviors by modifying lifestyle p.r.n. (smoking, stress, alcohol, diet, aspirin, other meds, etc.).	Review appointment dates for physician visit and discharge plan.

Expected Outcomes	Ambulates without assistance & independent in ADL • verbalizes meds information • demonstrates improved appetite • states signs of intestinal bleeding (hematemesis, melena, hematochezia) & to report same (red or brown-tinged vomitus & maroon, red, bloody, or tarry stools).	Verbalizes diet restrictions (avoid foods that previously caused discomfort, high-acid foods, hot pepper, caffeine, highly spiced food, & alcohol) & need to prevent constipation while on oral iron • denies subjective feelings of anxiety • verbalizes appropriate concerns & fears • states S & S of bleeding (thirst, frequent lip licking, light-headedness, dizziness, weakness/fatigue, impaired mental status, irritability, pallor, tremors, decrease in urine output, dry skin & mucous membranes) & when to seek medical care.	Verbalizes risk factors & health-seeking behaviors • states appointment date w/ physician.
Trigger(s)*	Pain, new bleeding, anorexia, decreased output • inability to maintain fluid & food intake needed for hydration & to meet caloric needs.	Inadequate fluid or dietary intake.	Inadequate fluid or dietary intake • unable to be independent in ADL.
	Variance Management Identification Analysis Action	**Variance Management** Identification Analysis Action	**Variance Management** Identification Analysis Action

From Birdsall C, Sperry S: *Clinical pathways in medical surgical practice*, St. Louis, 1997, Mosby.

*The presence of a trigger results in a variance to the path. Evaluation & intervention must be initiated and documented.

It is important to remember that a patient's level of involvement in his or her care can vary depending on the ability to overcome many of the above-mentioned barriers. However, nurses can influence their patients by providing them with support and encouraging them to be self-directed consumers of healthcare.

DETERMINING NURSING ACTIVITIES

Care planning involves determining age-specific nursing activities that will help the patient achieve predetermined health outcomes. Although patient outcomes are related to nursing diagnoses, nursing interventions stem from the etiology of the health problem. Consequently, whenever they are known, measures that address the etiology of the problem must be prescribed. Thus, for example, if the problem identified is "ineffective individual coping related to fear of hospitalization," then a nurse might prescribe information on coping strategies. Similarly, the nurse might write the orders "apply warming blanket to procedure table" and "increase room temperature to 75°F" in response to the diagnosis "body temperature, altered; potential" for an infant who is scheduled to undergo an endoscopic procedure.

Identifying treatment options

There are no substitutes for knowledge, experience, and resourcefulness when it comes to prescribing care. Furthermore, the nurse who responds to every patient problem with a procedure limits the effectiveness of the patient. The array of treatment options documented in research and in the empirical literature ranges from skilled nursing procedures to teaching and counseling, and simple acts of humanity, such as silence, humor, and touch. Strategies that may help nurses broaden their repertoire of nursing actions include the following:

1. Consult with successful colleagues, observe them, and talk with them about what they do.
2. Research the nursing literature for suggestions to improve care.
3. Talk with patients and family members about measures they have found most helpful in addressing their problems.
4. Consult standards of care, including those of the ANA and SGNA, institutional standards, standards of accrediting agencies such as JCAHO, and so on.

Selected treatment strategies should be tailored to the patient and compatible with the total plan of care. They must be consistent with the patient's values, beliefs, culture, and psychosocial background and must be realistic in terms of the abilities, time, and resources available.

Writing nursing orders

The following requirements pertain when writing **nursing orders:**

1. Using directive verbs, describe clearly and concisely the action to be taken (i.e., what, where, who, when, and how).
2. Date and sign the order; make a note when the plan is reviewed.

3. Use only accepted abbreviations.
4. For lengthy procedures, refer to policy manuals or other agency guidelines for steps in the routine.
5. Below are examples of nursing orders written in regard to endoscopy care:
   - "Assess patient's breath sounds immediately after procedure and with each set of postprocedural vital signs."
   - "Instruct parent not to lift the child up by the arms or sides for a period of 24 hours after the procedure."
   - "Explain to caregiver signs and symptoms of bleeding or hematoma and what to do if bleeding occurs."

Documenting the plan of care

The final phase of care planning is to document the plan. The plan documents nursing diagnoses, desired outcomes, and nursing orders. A well-documented plan directs nursing efforts and advances the four goals of nursing: to promote wellness, to prevent disease/illness, to promote coping, and to prevent injury. It is tailored to the individual patient and is based on scientific principles and incorporates findings of nursing research. A plan of care also addresses dependent and interdependent nursing functions and thus is compatible with the medical plan of care and other interdisciplinary efforts. It includes nursing responsibilities for fulfilling the medical plan of care, yet it guides nursing assessment priorities, teaching and counseling activities, and advocacy behaviors. It is designed to meet the patient's psychological, environmental, sociological, and physiological needs.

PLANNING CARE IN GASTROENTEROLOGY

Resources have been identified in this chapter to aid in gastroenterology care planning. In addition, Table 10-2 contains nursing care plans based on nursing diagnoses relevant to patients who undergo endoscopic procedures. Diagnoses in the first column represent health problems that gastroenterology nurses frequently treat. The patient outcomes listed are realistic and achievable within the short duration of the patient's stay in the endoscopy unit. Notice that all patient outcomes are behaviors or states that nurses can readily and objectively observe. The far right column lists the actions that nurses caring for these patients would take to treat each problem. These actions are based on scientific principles and incorporate the most recent findings of nursing research. Finally, notice that each intervention has a time frame. Time frames become important in evaluating patient care. When caring for patients in the endoscopy unit, these time frames may be short or long, which suggests that follow-up is required beyond the expected length of stay.

Barnie (1990a, 1990b, 1990c) has identified short-term goals applicable before, during, and after endoscopic procedures, as well as plans of care for the gastroenterology patient undergoing endoscopy. Although these plans incorporate medical diagnoses, they are based in part on nursing diagnosis and suggest useful interventions. Additional worthwhile guides to care planning are offered in the reference list.

Table 10-2. Sample endoscopy care plan

Nursing diagnosis	Patient outcome	Nursing activity
Anxiety/fear	Patient demonstrates effective coping mechanisms. Patient exhibits reduced physiological manifestations of anxiety/fear.	Instruct in relaxation techniques (e.g., deep breathing and imagery) preprocedure. Refer patient concerns to physician when appropriate, all phases of endoscopy experience. Allow time for questions preprocedure. Involve family/significant other for support preprocedure and post procedure. Minimize noxious stimuli; keep environment calm and unhurried, all phases. Use therapeutic communication and touch, all phases. Monitor patient for subjective and objective signs of anxiety, (i.e., shakiness, perspiration, increased heart rate, extraneous movement, hesitation, poor eye contact), all phases.
Alteration in comfort, actual or potential	Patient tolerates procedure, asking for medication as needed.	Teach patient system of ranking pain preprocedure. Support patient through discomfort by coaching patient in relaxation techniques (e.g., deep breathing, visualization) intraprocedure. Assess positioning for maximum comfort preprocedure and intraprocedure.
Knowledge deficit related to unfamiliar environment and procedure	Patient describes expected physiological and psychological responses to endoscopy.	Provide information about impending procedure using visual aids or appropriate literature preprocedure. Provide sensory information about procedure and sedation preprocedure.
Injury related to change in vital signs related to sedation; potential	Patient remains stable while sedated.	Obtain baseline vital signs on admission. Monitor BP, temperature, respirations, and pulse intraprocedure and postprocedure.
Injury related to instrumentation trauma (perforation and/or hemorrhage); potential	Patient experiences minimal trauma from endoscope.	Check lab work (CBC, PT/PTT, platelets) preprocedure. Insert bite block to protect teeth and pharynx intraprocedure. Verify that emergency equipment is in working order preprocedure. Monitor intake and output intraprocedure.
Aspiration, potential for	Patient's airway remains clear and unobstructed.	Position patient on left side preprocedure. Suction secretions prn preprocedure and intraprocedure.

The concept of causality concerns how a profession views cause-and-effect relationships between health problems and the factors that produce them. Medicine recognizes and seeks to treat biological causes of health problems. Nursing recognizes multiple causes or contributors to a problem, including psychological, environmental, and sociological factors, as well as biological causes.

The modes of therapy physicians and nurses may undertake independent of one another are defined by medical and nurse practice acts. Thus, because the nursing profession has defined its role as having independent, interdependent, and dependent aspects, nursing diagnosis focuses on the independent aspects of nursing practice.

CASE SITUATION

Two-year-old Nathan Mitchell has experienced persistent diarrhea for more than 10 days before admission and is severely dehydrated. The gastroenterology unit nurse reviews Nathan's nursing history and visits Nathan, who is combative and uncooperative despite the fact that his parents are doing all they can to comfort him. The nurse who admitted Nathan initiated a standard care plan used in the department for pediatric patients. He diagnosed Nathan by selecting the following from a list of health problems:

• impaired verbal communication;

- potential for injury, secondary to development (and combativeness);
- defensive coping;
- noncompliance, secondary to development;
- powerlessness; and
- anxiety, secondary to hospitalization.

he also added the following health problems:

- actual fluid volume deficit;
- impaired skin integrity (rectal excoriation);
- altered health maintenance; and
- ineffective family coping, disabling.

On examination, the gastroenterology nurse notices that the IV in Nathan's forearm has infiltrated, leaving it quite swollen and sore. The nurse discontinues Nathan's IV and elevates it on his teddy bear.

Nathan's parents accuse the doctors of giving Nathan medicine that he does not need, saying that rice cereal and milk have always been good for diarrhea. They believe the medicine is responsible for their child's poor appetite and vomiting. They also are grumbling about the day care center where they take Nathan, reporting that Nathan is the eighth child from the center to come down with severe diarrhea. While listening to their account of the day care center, another nurse takes the gastroenterology nurse aside to show the result of Nathan's stool culture: Nathan is infected with *Giardia lamblia*.

Points to think about

1. Which basic types of planning have occurred in this scenario? Which type of planning might be initiated at this time?
2. In choosing three priority health problems, what factors would be taken into consideration?
3. The nursing diagnosis "altered health maintenance," which was selected by the admitting nurse, is unfamiliar to the gastroenterology nurse. How would its meaning be determined?
4. In what ways will the nursing plan of care differ from the medical plan of care?
5. The gastroenterology nurse in this case usually cares for adults and therefore feels somewhat limited in her existing repertoire of pediatric treatment options. How might she expand her repertoire?

Suggested responses

1. The basic types of planning that have occurred in this scenario include:
   - initial planning, which was instituted by the admitting nurse;
   - ongoing, problem-oriented planning, which occurred when the gastroenterology nurse responded to a health problem (i.e., impaired skin integrity, secondary to IV infiltration) by setting a patient-centered outcome (to reduce pain and swelling caused by fluid extravasation) and identifying means of reducing or

resolving the problem (i.e., discontinuing the IV, applying the warm compress, elevating the arm); and
   - discharge planning with the parents (this planning may include contacting the public health department to investigate the day care center for the presence of *G. lamblia*).
2. Factors the nurse may take into consideration in choosing three priority health problems include:
   - the actual or potential threat of each problem to Nathan's well-being;
   - the parents' preferences and values, which will determine their participation in Nathan's therapy; and
   - potential problems; that is, risks peculiar to Nathan's age, health status, medical management, etc.
3. To determine the meaning of the nursing diagnosis "altered health maintenance" the gastroenterology nurse should refer to the North American Nursing Diagnosis Association (NANDA) taxonomy of nursing diagnoses. This reference not only defines health problems associated with each nursing diagnosis but also provides defining characteristics of health problems that differentiate them from other problems.
4. The nursing plan of care would differ from the medical plan of care in the following ways:
   - it addresses psychological, environmental, and sociological factors contributing to disturbances in health, as well as biological causes; and
   - it focuses on patient responses to medical treatment or health problems that nurses can independently treat. Interventions prescribed in it include only those actions that nurses can lawfully perform.
5. The gastroenterology nurse might expand her repertoire of treatment options by:
   - consulting with successful colleagues, observing them, and talking with them about what they do;
   - researching the nursing literature for suggestions to improve care;
   - talking with patients and family about measures they have found most helpful in addressing their problem; and
   - consulting standards of care, including ANA and SGNA standards, institutional standards, standards of accrediting agencies, etc.

REVIEW TERMS

nursing orders, planning, setting priorities

REVIEW QUESTIONS

1. Which of the following is not a valid reason for planning patient care based on nursing diagnoses?
   a. It is required by managed care companies.
   b. It enhances continuity of patient care.
   c. It improves the clarity of communication among nurses.
   d. It emphasizes the collegial relationship between nursing and medicine.

2. The nursing care plan:
   a. Is based on scientific principles and incorporates findings of nursing research.
   b. Advances nursing's four aims and is tailored to the individual patient.
   c. Is designed to meet developmental, psychological, and sociological needs of patients, as well as their physiological needs.
   d. All of the above.

3. A nursing plan of care addresses:
   a. Only the biological causes of the patient's health problems.
   b. Only those health problems that nurses can treat independently.
   c. Only nursing diagnoses.
   d. Independent, dependent, and interdependent aspects of nursing practice.

4. Assessment of the supplies and equipment needed to perform an endoscopic procedure is an example of:
   a. Initial planning.
   b. Admission planning.
   c. Ongoing planning.
   d. Discharge planning.

5. Intraprocedural changes in the patient's health status may affect:
   a. The nursing diagnosis.
   b. The expected outcomes.
   c. The plan of care
   d. All of the above.

6. Discharge planning is the responsibility of:
   a. The physician.
   b. The home health nurse.
   c. The nurse who has had the most consistent contact with the patient.
   d. Family members and significant others.

7. To help broaden the array of treatment options available to them, nurses should consult successful colleagues, the literature, standards of care, and:
   a. The taxonomy of nursing diagnoses.
   b. The plan of care.
   c. Patients and their families.
   d. Physicians.

8. In response to a patient's fluid deficit secondary to persistent diarrhea, which of the following nursing orders would be appropriate for the gastroenterology nurse to write?
   a. "Increase the IV rate following bouts of diarrhea."
   b. "Prepare patient for electrosurgery."
   c. "Monitor vital signs every 2 hours until diarrhea stops. Observe for signs of hypotension with widening pulse pressure."
   d. "Stools for culture in am and pm."

9. The final product of the planning phase of the nursing process is:
   a. A well-documented plan of care.
   b. The clinical pathway.
   c. A series of outcome statements.
   d. Nursing intervention.

10. The activity concerned with ranking nursing diagnoses in order of actual or potential threat to the patient's well-being is known as:
    a. Planning.
    b. Outcome identification.
    c. Establishing problem priorities.
    d. Cost containment.

BIBLIOGRAPHY

Barnie, D. (1990a). Care planning in the endoscopy unit: master care plan for the intraprocedure patient. *Journal Reprints II*, Rochester, NY: Society of Gastroenterology Nurses and Associates.

Barnie, D. (1990b). Care planning in the endoscopy unit: master care plan for the postprocedure patient. *Journal Reprints II*, Rochester, NY: Society of Gastroenterology Nurses and Associates.

Barnie, D. (1990c). Care planning in the endoscopy unit: master care plan for the pre-endoscopy patient. *Journal Reprints II*, Rochester, NY: Society of Gastroenterology Nurses and Associates.

Beare, P. & Myers, J. (1990). *Principles and practice of adult health nursing*. St. Louis, MO: Mosby.

Beyea, S. (1996). *Critical pathways for collaborative nursing care*. Menlo Park, CA: Addison-Wesley.

Birdsall, C. & Sperry, S. (1997). *Clinical pathways in medical surgical practice*. St. Louis MO: Mosby.

Carpenito, L. (2002). *Nursing diagnosis: application to clinical practice* (9th ed.). Philadelphia: Lippincott Williams & Wilkins.

Claussen, D.W. (1995). A clinical pathway for endoscopy. *Gastroenterol Nurs* 18(5), 182-5.

Edel, E., Johnson, P. & Tiller, S. (1989). Perioperative documentation: incorporating nursing diagnoses into the intraoperative record. *AORN J* 50, 596-600. Association of Operating Room Nurses.

Flaherty, G. & Fitzpatrick, J. (1978). Relaxation techniques to increase comfort of postoperative patients. *Nurs Res* 27, 3525.

Gardner, P. (2003). *Nursing Process in Action*. Independence, KY: Delmar Learning.

Gordon, M. (1984). *Manual of nursing diagnosis 1984-1985*. New York: McGraw-Hill.

Griffith, H., Thomas, N. & Griffith, L. (1991). MDs bill for these routine nursing tasks. *American Journal of Nursing* 91, 22-27.

Ignatavicius, D. & Hausman, K. (1995). *Clinical pathways for collaborative practice*. Philadelphia: W.B. Saunders.

Iyer, P., Taptich, B. & Bernocchi-Losey, D. (1995). *Nursing process and nursing diagnosis* (3rd ed.). Philadelphia: W.B. Saunders.

Kleinbeck, S. (1989). Developing nursing diagnoses for a perioperative care plan: a classroom research project. *AORN J* 49, 1613-25. Association of Operating Room Nurses.

Kneedler, J. & Dodge, G. (Eds.) (1989). *Perioperative patient care* (2nd ed.). Palo Alto, CA: Blackwell Scientific.

Kozier, B., Berman, A.J., & Erb, G.(1999). *Fundamentals of nursing: concepts, process, and practice* (6th ed.).Upper Saddle River, New Jersey: Prentice-Hall.

Labar, C. (1986). Filling in the blanks on prescription writing. *American Journal of Nursing 86*, 31-3.

MacKenzie, P.S. & Beresford, L. (1988). Planning and documentation: addressing patient needs in a day surgery setting. *AORN J* 47, 526-37. Association of Operating Room Nurses.

Malen, A. (1986). Perioperative nursing diagnoses: what, why, and how. *AORN J* 44, 829-39.

North American Nursing Diagnosis Association (1989). *Taxonomy I with official diagnostic categories*. St Louis, MO: Author.

Shaffer, F. (1988). Nursing care plan for fiberoptic procedures. *SGA J* 11, 124-5.

Society of Gastroenterology Nurses and Associates, Inc. (2003). *Manual of gastrointestinal procedures* (5th ed.). Chicago: IL: SGNA.

Society of Gastroenterology Nurses and Associates, Inc. (2001, February). *Role Delineation of the Registered Nurse in a Staff Position in Gastroenterology*. Chicago, IL: SGNA.

Taylor, C., Lillis, C. & LeMone, P. (1989). The nursing process. In Cleary, P., Faven, E. & Intenzo, D. (Eds.), *Fundamentals of nursing, the art and science of nursing care*. Philadelphia: J.B. Lippincott.

Winchester, C. (1991). A new approach to esophageal varices: endoscopic variceal ligation. *Gastroenterol Nurs 14*, 5-8.

Chapter 11

IMPLEMENTATION

This chapter will familiarize gastroenterology nurses with the implementation phase of the nursing process. General information about a variety of issues that arise during implementation of planned care is provided, followed by a discussion of variables that influence the way care is implemented and a list of specific guidelines for nursing intervention. The role of the gastroenterology nurse in communicating the care provided in the gastroenterology unit is explored. The last part of the chapter examines nursing activities that surround teaching, counseling, and advocacy of patient rights in gastroenterology nursing.

Learning objectives

After reviewing the content of this chapter, the gastroenterology nurse should be able to:

1. Describe the three broad areas of nursing activity that occur in the implementation phase of the nursing process.
2. Distinguish between independent, interdependent, and dependent nursing functions when implementing a plan of care.
3. Discuss six variables that influence the way a plan of care is implemented.
4. Define general guidelines for implementing care of the gastroenterology patient.
5. Describe four means of communicating nursing actions performed during the implementation phase of the nursing process.
6. List documentation requirements when implementing care of the gastroenterology patient undergoing endoscopy.
7. Discuss the nurse's role as teacher/counselor when implementing care of the gastroenterology patient.
8. Discuss the nurse's advocacy role as it applies to informed consent and ethical decision making.

FROM PLANNING TO IMPLEMENTATION

During the planning phase a patient's health problems are identified. Risks peculiar to the patient's age, health status, and medical management are considered to anticipate and prevent potential problems. During the planning phase these health problems are ranked or prioritized in order of actual or potential threat to the patient's well-being. Nursing interventions that will assist the patient toward achievement of identified outcomes are identified and prioritized.

Once documented, the plan outlines a set of nursing actions in a logical sequence that is designed to promote wellness, prevent disease and illness, promote recovery, and facilitate coping with altered functioning. It specifies *what* will be done, as well as *how, when, where,* and *by whom* (i.e., nurse, patient, or significant other). Each plan of care is tailored to the patient's individual needs, and each incorporates criteria for evaluating the effectiveness of nursing actions in assisting the patient toward achievement of desired outcomes.

In the implementation phase the plan becomes a blueprint that guides nursing care. Each nursing action performed is based on scientific principles and reflects the rights and desires of the patient and significant others. All actions are carried out safely, skillfully, and efficiently in a manner that provides continuity of care during each phase of recovery.

During the implementation phase, the following three broad areas of nursing activity occur:

1. the plan is put in motion;
2. the database is updated as data collection continues; and
3. nursing care and patient progress are documented and communicated

This chapter examines these three activities and the role of the gastroenterology nurse as teacher, counselor, and patient advocate.

PUTTING THE PLAN IN MOTION

During implementation, all of the steps outlined in the plan of care should be carried out efficiently and effectively. Whether or not all steps are executed by a nurse depends on the particular practice setting. The amount of time an institution and its nursing professionals allocate for teaching, counseling, and advocacy depends on the value and benefits they associate with each activity.

Carrying out the plan of care requires cognitive ability, interpersonal skill, and technical skill:

1. **Cognitive ability** is necessary not only to think critically about a patient's health problem but also to apply nursing theories to solve problems.

2. **Interpersonal skill** is a component of overall professional skills. Such skills, particularly the ability to communicate clearly, competently, and with caring, help elicit patients' trust and cooperation. A nurse's well-developed intellectual and interpersonal skills not only maximize the chance that healthy outcomes will be achieved but also ensure efficient implementation of care.

3. **Technical skill** is often necessary when implementing care. Required technical ability ranges from minimal to extensive, depending on the nature of equipment used to execute procedures and the complexity of the procedure. Examples of implementation measures that require technical skill are noninvasive measurement of arterial hemoglobin oxygen saturation during GI procedures using a pulse oximeter, insertion of a duodenal or nasogastric tube, performance of esophageal manometry studies, and monitoring of cardiac status using an ECG monitor.

Independent, dependent, and interdependent nursing functions are addressed in the plan of care and carried out during the implementation phase. These functions are explained as follows:

1. **Independent intervention** is action initiated without direction or supervision of other health care professionals and is instituted as the result of a nursing assessment. Actions taken in the course of independent intervention are those for which a nurse is legally accountable. Teaching, counseling, and advocacy of patient rights are examples of activities nurses can initiate freely.

2. **Interdependent intervention or collaborative intervention** is action performed in concert with the efforts of other health care professionals. For example, case study conferences organized by nurses and attended by related health professionals for the purpose of discussing patient care frequently result in action requiring cooperation and coordination between nurses and other professionals. These cooperative activities reflect nurses' interdependent function in providing care.

3. **Dependent intervention** is action performed under the supervision or direction of a physician and is most often directly related to the patient's disease. Dependent interventions include IV therapy, diet, and activity—the bulk of nursing activity in traditional practice settings.

Nurse practice acts in all states clearly indicate that nurses are to fulfill orders written or otherwise given by physicians. Yet it is important for nurses to understand their responsibility in dependent intervention; that is, although physicians are ultimately responsible for actions performed at their direction or under their supervision, nurses are required to clarify any doubts concerning the activities prescribed. The nurse who fails to do so risks a liability suit for the action.

Safety is the focus of many nursing activities carried out during implementation. Adhering to disinfection guidelines during processing of contaminated equipment, monitoring the environment for safety, and positioning according to physiological principles during or after operative procedures to avoid neurovascular damage and skin breakdown are typical nursing activities performed to safeguard patient safety. Verification of identification and informed consent, validation of reports of essential laboratory findings and diagnostic procedures, and routine inspection of hospital equipment to ensure proper function are other safety measures a nurse may carry out.

Managing time constraints

Huey (1988) has suggested three ways to free available time for implementing comprehensive nursing care:

(a) delegating technical and nonnursing tasks;

(b) revising policies to delete obsolete and/or unnecessary practices; and

(c) preventing complications.

Delegating tasks

Making high-quality nursing care possible is a matter of understanding nursing objectives and adhering to them. This frequently requires delegation of nonnursing tasks. Many practice settings have instituted professional practice models to allow nurses to use their time more efficiently and effectively. For example, Jakobsen (1990) suggests the following practical alternatives that reserve professional nurses for independent nursing functions.

1. The **Professionally Advanced Care Team (ProACT) model** instituted at the Robert Wood Johnson Hospital in New Brunswick, New Jersey, has restructured nursing services based on two nursing roles—the primary nurse, whose role is to remain with the patient throughout his or her hospital stay, and a clinical care manager, an RN whose role is to manage that stay. Added support is provided by pharmaceutical services, who manage everything related to medication and IV therapy (except administration), and "support service hosts," who provide housekeeping, dietary trays, and supplies.

2. In Miami, the **Partners in Practice (PIP) model** allows a nurse to team with a "practice partner." The nurse acts as mentor to a partner (usually an LPN or technician) who has been screened for interest in a nursing career. Once teamed, the RN's practice partner attends to tasks that do not have to be performed by an RN, as well as any other tasks the RN chooses to teach the partner (e.g., urine testing). Nurses acting as mentors find that

they have more time to teach and counsel patients and to consult with other members of the care team.

Another trend in nursing practice has the dual effect of allowing nurses to carry out planned care more efficiently and involving patients in self-care. Many professionals believe that alert, oriented, and reasonably intelligent hospitalized patients are quite capable of taking their own medications. Successful medication self-administration programs have been implemented with physician permission in clinical areas, including postpartum, cardiac, geriatrics, and oncology units.

Revising practice policies

To make high-quality nursing care possible through increased efficiency, nurses must cast off unnecessary rituals and adapt old techniques to accommodate new information. Protective isolation, for example, is a time-consuming ritual that has been found ineffective in preventing infection. In 1983 the Centers for Disease Control and Prevention (CDC) deleted protective isolation from their isolation guidelines, because it was shown that individuals at risk of infection are infected with their own organisms. Other related studies demonstrated that outcomes of patients treated in isolation versus in rooms with other patients do not differ significantly. Clearly, discarding policies surrounding protective isolation augments nursing care by increasing efficiency without diminishing the overall effectiveness of nursing intervention.

Preventing complications

Adapting procedures to incorporate new research findings can also free available time by minimizing the risk of complications. For example, nursing research suggests that using shorter, smaller catheters minimizes irritation to local veins while still allowing blood transfusion. If the catheter must be retained and thrombophlebitis occurs, a short catheter minimizes the extent of involvement. Thus, taking this measure minimizes the risk and severity of a complication of IV therapy, potentially increasing time available for important nursing functions.

Variables that affect the way care is implemented

Variables that influence how a plan of care is implemented fall into the following six categories:
1. Patient variables
2. Nurse variables
3. Standards of care
4. Research findings
5. Resources
6. Ethical and legal guides to practice

Patient variables

Every plan of care must be tailored to individual needs, a requirement that frequently calls for creative solutions to health problems. For example, a patient's previous response to nursing measures may affect his or her receptiveness to further intervention. Obviously, the patient whose past experiences with nursing care were unpleasant or unrewarding is less likely to be receptive. Diminished ability to participate in self-care also influences the way a plan of care is implemented. For example, a geriatric patient with arthritis may require assistance with ostomy care, whereas the otherwise healthy young ostomate will not. Sometimes a patient's willingness to participate in care becomes a factor when the nurse implements planned care. Psychological perceptions, religious beliefs, or socioeconomic factors may prompt a patient to reject all or some nursing intervention. For instance, an otherwise receptive patient who lacks the means to purchase meat may not comply with a high-protein diet regimen for weight loss that includes meat. In this case, interim measures to attain the outcome "Patient will select three servings of protein daily from a menu" may include teaching the patient how to identify complete proteins in combinations of vegetable proteins (e.g., grains, legumes) and dairy products.

Developmental differences can substantially influence planned care, especially among pediatric patients. Not only do actual and potential health problems (and therefore desired outcomes) differ within developmental age-groups (Table 11-1), but means of achieving outcomes also vary according to the child's unique developmental task for his or her age-group. Thus, when taking action (e.g., to reduce the fear and anxiety every child or adolescent experiences during endoscopy), it is necessary to identify the developmental task for the child's age-group and select age-specific treatment options. Similarly, it is necessary to consider whether outcomes and treatment options are realistic, given the patient's developmental circumstances.

Nursing variables

A nurse's cultivated level of expertise determines the number and kind of treatment options implemented. Moreover, nurses vary in the degree to which they like patient contact. The nurse who enjoys patient contact clearly has greater willingness and motivation to provide comprehensive care during implementation. How well or poorly a nurse manages time affects his or her efficiency and therefore the available time for carrying out all measures planned. On the other hand, many nurses continually struggle to provide time to implement total patient care yet remain frustrated by unpredictable and uncontrollable events.

Standards of care

Current standards of care determine nursing responsibilities and suggest liability limits. (**Liability** refers to the legal responsibility for nursing acts or failure to act, including the responsibility for financial restitution in the event of demonstrable damages resulting from negligent acts.) For example, among the Society for Gastroenterology Nurses and Associates (SGNA) standards, Standard II requires that nurses "initiate actions to ensure the continuity of effective nursing care before, during and/or after endoscopic procedures in the GI unit." Associated with this standard are seven criteria, including "instructs patient(s)/family(ies) in the proper

Table 11-1. Health problems specific to four pediatric age-groups.

Age	Developmental stage	Actual or potential health problems
Birth to 1 year	Trust versus mistrust	Sleep pattern disturbance Swallowing, impaired Hypothermia/hyperthermia, potential Fluid volume, altered: deficit or increase Impaired skin integrity Aspiration, potential: related to existing or coexisting conditions Infection, potential: related to existing or coexisting conditions Impaired gas exchange Ineffective thermoregulation Ineffective airway clearance Self-concept disturbance: maturational, related to deprivation Health Maintenance, altered: maturational, related to inadequate health practice Self-care deficit, inability to feed, toilet, or dress self
1 to 3 years	Autonomy versus shame and doubt	Impaired verbal communication Sleep pattern disturbance Impaired skin integrity Infection, potential: related to existing or coexisting conditions Self-concept disturbance: maturational, related to deprivation Health maintenance, altered: maturational, related to inadequate health practice Injury, potential for: related to development (e.g. poisoning, falls) Impaired social interaction Powerlessness, maturational or situational Coping, ineffective: situational or maturational Anxiety, situational Fear, situational Self-care deficit, inability to feed or toilet self
3-6 years	Initiative versus guilt	Coping, ineffective: situational or maturational Powerlessness, maturational or situational Anxiety, situational Fear, situational Sleep pattern disturbance, related to nightmares or fears Injury, potential for: related to developmental (e.g., poisoning, falls) Infection, potential: related to existing or coexisting conditions Self-care deficit, inability to dress self Self-concept disturbance: maturational, related to deprivation
7 to 11 years	Industry versus inferiority	Self-concept disturbance: maturational, related to peer pressure Noncompliance, situational Anxiety, situational Fear, situational Self-care deficit, inability to bathe self completely Impaired social interaction Violence, potential for: situational, related to inability to control behavior Health maintenance, altered: maturational, related to inadequate health practice

Modified from Carpenito L, 1983; North American Nursing Diagnosis Association: *Taxonomy I with official diagnostic categories*, St. Louis, 1989, NANDA; developed with assistance from Zelasny B, BSN, CCRN, Denver Children's Hospital, Denver.

preparation for diagnostic studies" and "provides written postendoscopy instructions to outpatients undergoing endoscopy and reviews those directions with the family/significant other, as appropriate." Gastroenterology nurses must therefore involve family and significant others in preendoscopy teaching.

Research findings

New information emerges continually, thereby giving rise to new treatment strategies. The nurse who is aware of research findings implements a more creative, varied, and comprehensive set of actions when solving health problems.

Resources

The best-laid plans are doomed to fail without adequate resources to enable implementation of the plan. Inadequate staffing, equipment, supplies, and other resources may reduce or alter the type of care rendered.

Ethical and legal guides to practice

Within the past decade, laws governing delivery and ethical dimensions of health care have become more complex. In many settings, hospital risk managers and ethical committees counsel hospital policy makers whose policies, in turn, influence modern nursing practice.

Guidelines for nursing intervention

The following guidelines for implementation of nursing care have been offered:

1. Before instituting any measure to treat a health problem, the patient must be assessed to be sure action is still necessary.
2. The nurse should be fully prepared to perform the planned action when he or she approaches the patient. All equipment should be ready, and the nurse should either know how to perform the nursing action or come with a nurse associate who does. The nurse should tell the patient why the action is being taken. Also, patients should be informed of any potential adverse responses to the procedure.
3. The nurse should approach the patient with a caring attitude, using language the patient understands. By communicating genuine concern for what the patient is experiencing, the nurse conveys regard for the patient's well-being.
4. The nurse should develop a large repertoire of skilled nursing interventions. The larger an array of options he or she has to choose from when treating health problems, the greater the likelihood of success.
5. The nursing actions chosen must comply with standards of care and be within ethical and legal institutional guidelines to practice.
6. The nurse should think critically about the plan of care, always questioning whether routines are really the best method of treatment. He or she should consult immediate colleagues, colleagues in related nursing fields, and relevant literature to discover more effective ways of managing health problems. The effectiveness of each action in terms of its positive and negative effects on the outcome should be evaluated.
7. The nurse should modify the prescribed interventions to accommodate patients' developmental and psychosocial circumstances, ability and willingness to participate in achieving desired outcomes, previous responses to nursing measures, and progress toward expected outcomes.

DATABASE UPDATING

Data collection continues throughout the implementation phase, and the database is continually updated. These activities serve three important functions during implementation in the following ways:

1. Comparing new data against the baseline database enables nurses to identify patterns and trends;
2. Collecting data following nursing intervention allows nurses to evaluate the effectiveness of nursing actions according to evaluation criteria listed in the care plan; and
3. As the database is updated, the plan of care can be revised.

Just as during the assessment phase, nurses collect both subjective and objective data. During implementation, however, subjective data are derived from confirmation or validation of responses to therapy and perceived progress as noted by the patient or significant others. Objective data are obtained by monitoring both the patient's response to nursing activity and the medical plan of care.

COMMUNICATING ABOUT CARE

Communicating about care with patient and family, colleagues, and other health professionals is vitally important for several reasons. It not only sparks involvement of patients and significant others but also ensures continuity of care as the responsibility for the patient's care shifts from one provider to the next. Communication is essential to the coordination and continuity of care, and it also promotes efficiency among members of the health care team. Informing colleagues of action enables nurses to supplement and complement each other's efforts, avoiding duplication and omission of effort. Communication about care should focus not only on nursing care provided and patient progress toward specified outcomes but also on the total plan of care rendered by physicians and all health professionals. Communication takes many forms, including documentation, discussion and verbal reports, conferences or consultation, and referrals.

Documentation

Documentation of care in written records is the most visible and permanent medium of communication with regard to implementation of nursing care. Documentation can refer either to an action or to a written record. As a process, documentation refers to the act of collecting, abstracting, and coding of client data and therapeutic processes for the purposes of communicating about patient care, supplying a supporting reference concerning the status or progress of a patient, and archiving evidence of care rendered.

Documentation, the most formal of all methods of communication, constitutes written, legal evidence of all pertinent intervention involving a patient. Documentation of care that has been rendered serves purposes beyond communication between colleagues, including the following:

1. **Planning.** Because patient records document not only baseline and ongoing data but also how a patient is responding to therapies, they are useful as resources for planning and modification of planned care.
2. **Process improvement audit.** Records provide a medium for studying the quality of care provided and the competence of nurses rendering care. Charts selected at random are audited against standards of care to determine if standards are being met. If discrepancies between practice and standards are found, action involving in-services, policy changes, counseling, and so on may be initiated to remedy substandard practices.

3. **Research.** The nursing record serves as a valuable source of data in nursing research. Each record represents a unique case study from which researchers hope to learn how to improve recognition and treatment of patient health problems.
4. **Education.** By reading a patient's chart, one can learn a great deal about clinical manifestations of disease, effective or less-effective treatment modalities, and factors that affect patients' abilities to achieve health outcomes.
5. **Legal evidence.** The nursing record serves an important function in implicating or absolving nurses when entered into court proceedings as evidence.
6. **Historical document.** Finally, because records are dated and retained for many years, they are sometimes useful as an indicator of a patient's past health.

Documentation requirements in the endoscopy unit

The following are examples of the types of documentation required for endoscopic procedures:

(a) procedure performed;
(b) date and time of the procedure;
(c) equipment used;
(d) staff present;
(e) anesthesia/sedation administered and patient's response;
(f) medications and response;
(g) vital signs and monitoring methods;
(h) oxygen therapy;
(i) use of cautery, electrocoagulation, or laser;
(j) dilators used;
(k) solution injected;
(l) specimens taken;
(m) photographs and/or x-rays taken;
(n) postprocedural diagnosis; and
(o) nursing notes and procedure nurse signature.

In addition to these procedural notes, SGNA's documentation guidelines also list the information required for preprocedural, postprocedural, and discharge documentation.

Discussion and verbal reporting

Communication of care takes several forms. Discussion between two or more individuals to identify problems and work toward their solution constitutes informal communication of care. More formal communication of care is accomplished by oral or written reporting. Formal reports convey new patient data and information about the patient's status and progress toward desired outcomes.

Conferences or consultation

Two types of conferences, which are listed as follows, are held in many practice settings for the purpose of communicating about care:

1. **Care conferences,** during which a specific case situation or situations are reviewed. Impressions are shared, treatment options are explored, and care is planned.
2. **Nursing rounds,** which are on-site conferences from which patient and family input is sometimes elicited and

from which direct observation can be made. At the same time, nursing care and patient progress can be evaluated.

Consultations with other health care professionals to seek advice, instruction, or information or to exchange ideas concerning patient care may be considered another form of conference communication. For example, gastroenterology nurses consult with clinical nurse specialists in their area concerning mutual patients.

Referrals

More and more, nursing has been recognized for its role in screening and referring patients who require or would benefit from adjunct services or existing community resources. The process of sending a patient to another source for aid or to another professional for appropriate action is known as **referral.** Both internal referrals to departments elsewhere within a facility and external referrals to other hospital facilities or outside agencies are useful in providing comprehensive holistic care. Most agencies have policies governing referrals that require submitting special forms. In addition, these policies specify who can make the referral, how it is to be done, and so on. When it is appropriate to make a referral, the nurse must give information to the receiving agency or department that will ensure continuity of patient care. Answering the question, "What would I need to know if I were to continue care of this patient?" will help to accomplish this end.

INDEPENDENT INTERVENTION: TEACHING, COUNSELING, AND ADVOCACY

During implementation, nurses actively determine their patients' needs for assistance and ability to meet basic human needs. The promotion of self-care through teaching, counseling, and advocacy frequently becomes important when assisting patients to meet desired outcomes.

Patient teaching

Whether teaching patients about an upcoming endoscopic examination or about self-care during or after their hospital stay, a nurse's role in teaching remains the same. Nurses implement patient education through the following four broad areas of activity:

(a) diagnosing a patient's knowledge deficit;
(b) planning learning activity;
(c) providing learning opportunities; and
(d) evaluating learning.

Diagnosing knowledge deficits

When identifying a knowledge deficit as a health problem, nurses base this diagnosis on an assessment of the patient's learning needs. This assessment must include not only evidence that the patient is unaware of information that might improve health behaviors but also that the patient is ready to learn and knowledge is a priority. Before nurses can effectively implement a teaching plan, they must also assess their own knowledge on the subject and become informed. It is often necessary to contact appropriate resource persons or obtain additional information to provide accurate, up-to-date facts to substantiate the lessons.

Planning the learning activity

Setting goals for the learning activity is an action very similar to that of identifying health outcomes. (See Chapter 10.) Learning goals must be realistic, and they may be short-term or long-term. McGregor (1988) advises that gastroenterology nurses and their patients agree in writing or via verbal contract concerning respective roles of both nurse and patient in the learning activity. In this way, nurses and patients identify measurable behaviors to help each other monitor progress toward the learning goals. For example, a contract might contain the following terms:

(a) "Nursing staff will provide written home bowel prep instructions by 5/12."

(b) "Mr. Franklin will review these instructions and verbally describe home bowel prep procedure at next office visit on 5/15."

Providing learning opportunity

In providing an environment conducive to learning, it is important for gastroenterology nurses to convey an attitude of support rather than condescension. Finding a room or space where distractions can be kept at a minimum also augments the patient learning opportunity. Adequate preparation for learning activities ensures that the learning content can be delivered in a logical and comprehensive manner. Involving the patient and family members and the patient's significant others also facilitates learning, encourages reinforcement, and ensures that proper follow-up is arranged by the patient and family. Finally, the nurse/teacher who exercises accomplished communication skills ensures not only that information is imparted in a clear, concise, and comprehensive manner but also that comprehension occurs. The learning opportunity may be facilitated by continually reminding the patient about the learning contract.

Evaluating learning

Methods for evaluating learning correspond to the type of skill learned. Cognitive skills are best evaluated by oral questioning or written questionnaire. Affective skills are better evaluated through observation of behavioral response. Psychomotor skills may be evaluated by return demonstration. Short-term goals (i.e., those that may be attained within 1 week) may often be evaluated during the period of hospitalization, but long-term goal evaluation must be referred to home health nurses, office nurses, or long-term care nurses.

Counseling

Counseling may be one of the most important gastroenterology nursing activities. Anxiety about hospitalization, the gastroenterology procedure, an outcome of surgery, or the results of laboratory studies can manifest itself in insidious ways that impede learning and healing. Fear, when suppressed, may precipitate a crisis marked by a total breakdown in a patient's coping mechanisms. To reduce fear and anxiety, gastroenterology nurses counsel patients throughout the course of therapy.

Counseling is the act of rendering guidance to a patient and/or significant other, an act that sometimes entails assisting the patient in problem solving. Counseling may be short-term, long-term, or motivational.

1. **Short-term counseling** is given when ineffective coping patterns surface that require immediate attention. The severity of the underlying emotional issue may cause disturbance ranging from a minor dilemma to a major crisis.

2. **Long-term counseling** is rendered consistently over a period of weeks or months and involves repeated contact with a nurse via telephone or personal visit.

3. **Motivational counseling** is performed either to stimulate a patient's inner drive to get well or to enhance motivation to cooperate in performing or learning to perform self-care. Motivational counseling generally requires an exploration of attitudes, values, and feelings underlying the disinterest in or indifference to recovery. To implement motivational counsel, nurses typically design incentives to stimulate drive and ambition.

In the gastroenterology unit, short-term counseling to enable patients to overcome anxiety and fear is an important function. Several factors influence the patient's vulnerability to crisis in the gastroenterology laboratory, including personality, cultural factors, and availability of support systems.

1. Anxiety-prone personalities are more vulnerable to crisis when faced with a physical threat than are persons not identified as anxious personalities.

2. Misperceptions related to religious belief or ethnic experiences and misunderstandings because of language barriers predispose patients to psychological stress.

3. Actual lack of supportive family and friends or perceived lack of professional support from a competent, knowledgeable, and willing staff may precipitate crisis.

Wheeler (1988) offers six signs of impending crisis that gastroenterology nurses should be alert for to prevent breakdown of existing coping mechanisms:

1. Debilitating fear of impending procedure, what physician will find, pain and anesthesia, lack of control.

2. Disorganized thought and behavior caused by an inability to use cognitive, judgment, or decision-making abilities.

3. Regressive dependency marked by helplessness and reduced ability to cope.

4. Inability to limit emotional reactions in a customary manner in the midst of loss of privacy, control, or both.

5. Inappropriate response to hospital personnel or family, manifested as withdrawal or isolation.

6. Maladaptive behavior as the result of intense and uncontrollable feelings: magical thinking, excessive fantasies, regressive behavior (frequently anger), or somatic delusion.

Wheeler (1988) suggests a counseling outcome and three criteria, listed as follows, for evaluating nursing intervention when implementing measures to assist a patient in emotional crisis:

Outcome	Criteria
Patient will exhibit adaptive behaviors.	1. Patient accepts tasks. 2. Patient talks openly about impressions and feelings during the experience. 3. Patient makes predictions and plans concerning recovery.

Wheeler also offers the following suggestions for short-term and long-term counseling intervention in crisis situations:

Short-term

1. Acknowledge the crisis: The event is stressful, yet competent personnel are standing by to help (this supports the patient's right to dignity.)
2. Encourage the patient to express feelings while listening empathetically.
3. Give information in nontechnical terms.
4. Explore coping alternatives.

Long-term

1. Explore the patient's past in an attempt to identify his or her strengths and similar situations in which the patient coped successfully. Avoid discussion focused on chronic past problems.
2. Reframe the situation by restating it in a more meaningful and positive way; for example, "You are angry because you care."
3. Consider a referral to a social worker, psychiatrist, or psychologist.

Advocacy

In nursing, the act of supporting patient rights is receiving greater emphasis by both consumers and nursing professionals. Consumer expectations and demands have evolved with changes in health care delivery. At the same time, nursing professionals have come to value the promotion of individual well-being and to respect the individual's right to self-determination.

Advocacy behaviors in nursing exhibit two components: informing patients and supporting them in their decisions. Informing patients enables them to make educated decisions. Information gastroenterology nurses can impart to help patients make educated decisions should include not only information about patient rights but also information concerning options.

This section elaborates on two areas in which the gastroenterology nurse can act to safeguard patient rights in gastroenterology: informed consent and assisting patients to make informed decisions when confronted by ethical dilemmas.

Informed consent

Endoscopic procedures are becoming more varied and technical, and the role of the gastroenterology nurse as an educator and advocate is becoming more important. When gastroenterologists and nurses work together to educate patients, there is no reason why any physically and mentally competent patient should not be totally informed about impending GI procedures. Yet nurses in the endoscopy unit frequently encounter circumstances in which they question a patient's comprehension of a proposed procedure or the risks involved. They also witness situations in which a patient's ability to freely consent to treatment is altered. The effects of anxiety, pain, medication, depression, or temporary or permanent disorientation are among the factors that can influence an individual's normal ability to judge and make decisions about his or her health care.

Although it is common to think of informed consent as a thing (i.e., a legal document), it is actually a process. **Informed consent** is an interaction between physician and patient, in which a meaningful exchange of information concerning an impending health care administration occurs. Only the patient or a legally authorized guardian may give consent, and a legal guardian may give consent only in the event that the patient is incompetent by reason of age (i.e., the patient is a minor and neither married nor self-supporting), physical inability, or legal incompetence (see below).

Informed consent is required on three occasions: on admission, before any diagnostic procedure or medical or surgical treatment is performed, and/or before any human experimentation is enacted. Furthermore, the conditions under which consent can be waived are very specific, as listed in the following explanations:

1. Consent is not needed in an emergency if there is immediate threat to life or health; if experts agree that an emergency exists; and/or if the patient is unable to consent and a legally authorized person cannot be reached.
2. Consent is not required for an action necessary to treat an unanticipated complication incurred during surgery when a legally authorized person cannot be reached.

A patient's refusal of treatment constitutes a slightly different circumstance. Refusal to consent must be documented and, when appropriate, accompanied by an explanation of consequences that the patient may incur by refusing. A release form should be signed and witnessed, relieving nurses, doctors, and the hospital of all liability for outcome of the treatment refusal.

Failure to obtain consent may result in charges of battery against the nurse, doctor, and hospital caring for the patient. Even when given, consent is legally valid only when the following conditions are met:

1. The physician and hospital make full disclosure concerning the proposed treatment or experiment.
2. The patient possesses competent judgment and decision-making ability.
3. The patient claims to comprehend the procedure and attending risks and aftereffects.
4. The patient gives consent voluntarily of his or her own free will.

Responsibility for obtaining consent rests with the person(s) who are to perform the therapeutic or diagnostic procedure or who are conducting the research study. Gastroenterology nurses may play a role in evaluating comprehension, assessing impediments to comprehension (including deficits in reasoning or judgment processes), or detecting deleterious influences on patient decision making (i.e., force, coercion, and/or manipulation).

Advocacy in ethical dilemmas

Reeder (1989) has proposed the following model of nursing ethics that upholds four ethical values, including fidelity, accountability, virtues, and caring:

1. **Fidelity** refers to the commitment, covenant, or contract nurses have with patients. It is fostered by accountability, virtues, and caring, and it implies a promise of advocacy and alliance in fulfilling patient needs.
2. **Accountability** requires responsibility and being answerable for breach of responsibility.
3. The relevant **virtues** are courage, honesty, and justice (i.e., treating all with equality and openness in the midst of certain risks and possible harms).
4. **Caring** is "a commitment to protecting and enhancing the dignity of patients.... It is attending to the 'objectness' of persons without reducing them to the moral status of objects."

There are three circumstances when nurses may experience moral conflict when implementing a plan of care:

(a)   moral uncertainty, which is an inability to recognize the nature of an ethical problem;

(b)   moral dilemmas, as when a conflict arises between two or more ethical principles with no obvious solution; and

(c)   moral distress, which is a conflict between an individual's knowledge of ethically appropriate action and institutional constraints preventing action.

One dilemma frequently encountered in the gastroenterology unit concerns whether or not to maintain nutrition of severely debilitated or vegetative patients through percutaneous endoscopic gastrostomy tubes.

McDonald (1986) notes that a nurse's role in facilitating ethical decision-making varies between institutions. Nonetheless, he suggests that nurses can be active in professional health care dilemmas via decision-making teams. He suggests that the current lack of nursing participation in ethical decision making is to some extent a function of traditional views of the nurse's role as held by physicians. Moreover, MacDonald suggests that the lack of preparation in nursing education systems surrounding ethical decision making causes nurses to shy away from participation. Finally, he suggests that avoidance of ethical decision making is also motivated by fear. Fear of superiors, of co-workers, of emotions, or even fear of greater responsibility can lead to complacency and passivity.

It may help to understand and accept the fact that in ethical dilemmas all participants are "morally equal." McDonald suggests the following ways nursing leaders can implement involvement:

1. Leaders must temporarily defer some leadership roles to others.
2. Each team member must assume equal responsibility and obligation for his or her own views.
3. A decision-making mechanism in which each team member's opinion is respected must be enacted to handle treatment dilemmas.

In addition, Barnie (1990) offers some basic guidelines to gastroenterology nurses who participate in ethical decision-making.

1. Teach, clarify, and reinforce medical information.
2. Remain as objective as possible, segregating personal opinions from the medical and legal options of the patient and family. Give insight without influence.
3. Provide a willing ear and a cautious mouth: listen empathetically; avoid hasty, emotional, and irrational accusations at all cost.
4. Approach patients respectfully and provide support for existing coping mechanisms.
5. Accept and support the family's legal decisions without imposing personal principles, morality, or religious beliefs.
6. Observe and communicate appropriately.
7. Work through appropriate channels, providing referrals to such resources as support groups or financial aid advisors when appropriate.

CASE SITUATION

Bennett Brandish is a 48-year-old executive with rectal polyps who is undergoing a colonoscopic polypectomy. He sought medical attention when he began to notice occasional blood in his stool. He reports having confidence in his physician, Dr. MacElroy, but has also heard "a few horror stories" about hospital care. Mr. Brandish is somewhat edgy, but he cooperates in his care. In fact, Mr. Brandish responded favorably to preprocedural teaching, listening carefully to the information given him and asking many questions. He claimed to feel "more in control of the situation."

He is now under conscious sedation for the colonoscopic polypectomy. Dr. MacElroy began to report difficulty maintaining light in the operative field just after the procedure began. The gastroenterology nurse has been attempting to troubleshoot the equipment difficulty when Dr. MacElroy notices that the patient has begun to hemorrhage.

Points to think about

1. In removing the rectal polyps, Dr. MacElroy has encountered one of the possible complications (hemorrhage) of the procedure and must now treat it. What intervention must the gastroenterology nurse take to help Dr. MacElroy correct the immediate problem?
2. Of the actions identified, which might the gastroenterology nurse be able to delegate?

3. Which of the actions identified are activities the nurse may initiate independently? Which must occur under Dr. MacElroy's direction and supervision?
4. What variables may influence how the nurse implements the actions identified?

Suggested responses

1. The gastroenterology nurse might identify the following actions to help Dr. MacElroy correct the problem.
   (a) Call for additional help.
   (b) Increase the IV flow rate.
   (c) Place the patient in the Trendelenburg position.
   (d) Insert a large-bore IV line.
   (e) Set up cautery equipment.
   (f) Continue to troubleshoot equipment failure.
   (g) Type and cross and send for blood (stat).
   (h) Change the suction canister.
   (i) Increase frequency of vital sign monitoring.
   (j) Administer oxygen through nasal cannula.
   (k) Plan to take further action; for example, to reverse narcotic.
   (l) Comfort Mr. Brandish as appropriate.
   (m) Document all actions, observations, and patient responses.
2. The following list includes actions the gastroenterology nurse might delegate.
   (a) Sending for blood.
   (b) Changing the suction canister.
   (c) Setting up the cautery.
   (d) Continuing to troubleshoot equipment failure.
3. Actions the gastroenterology nurse might take independently include the following.
   (a) Increasing the frequency of vital sign monitoring.
   (b) Planning further actions.
   (c) Counseling Mr. Brandish when appropriate.
   (d) Documenting actions, observations, and patient responses.

   Actions the nurse might implement, depending on Dr. MacElroy's directions and under his supervision, include the following:
   (a) Increasing the IV flow rate.
   (b) Placing the patient in the Trendelenburg position.

   In this circumstance, the nurse may need to prompt Dr. MacElroy to elicit direction, because he may be preoccupied with the hemorrhaging vessel.
4. Variables that may affect the way the nurse treats this situation may include the following:
   (a) Mr. Brandish's level of awareness of the problem;
   (b) The patient's coping style;
   (c) Rapidity of change in the patient's metabolic condition;
   (d) Whether or not the nurse has available support personnel;
   (e) Whether or not the nurse has backup equipment; and
   (f) The nurse's experience in similar situations.

REVIEW TERMS

advocacy, care conferences, consultations, counseling, dependent intervention, documentation, independent intervention, informed consent, interdependent intervention, liability, nursing rounds, referral

REVIEW QUESTIONS

1. The implementation phase of the nursing process is characterized by all of the following, *except that:*
   a. Evaluation criteria are developed, against which the effectiveness of nursing intervention can be measured.
   b. The nursing plan of care is put in motion.
   c. The database is updated as data collection continues.
   d. Nursing care and patient progress are documented and communicated.
2. The act of rendering guidance or assisting a patient with problem solving is:
   a. Referring.
   b. Consulting.
   c. Counseling.
   d. Teaching.
3. Whether or not a nurse allocates time for teaching, counseling, or advocacy behaviors is a function of all of the following, *except:*
   a. The nurse's ability to manage time.
   b. Whether or not the institution values these activities.
   c. Whether or not the nurse likes patient contact.
   d. Whether or not a doctor has ordered it.
4. A gastroenterology nurse might vary the way he or she comforts an anxious 10-year-old boy based on:
   a. The developmental task of children in the 7- to 11-year-old age-group.
   b. His willingness to participate in counseling.
   c. Recent findings concerning the impact of certain words in calming/provoking anxiety.
   d. All of the above.
5. Administering medication is:
   a. An independent nursing activity.
   b. An interdependent task.
   c. A dependent nursing obligation.
   d. A nonnursing chore.
6. Nurses accomplish patient teaching in four phases, including planning the learning activity, providing learning opportunity, evaluating learning, and:
   a. Correcting mistakes.
   b. Developing learning objectives.
   c. Explaining the patient's privacy needs to significant others.
   d. Helping patients make informed decisions.
7. The objective of the Partners in Practice model of professional nursing is to:
   a. Expand the types of actions nurses can take independently.

b. Involve the patient in self-care.

c. Increase cooperation between nurses and support services.

d. Allow RNs to use their time more efficiently and effectively.

8. A research nurse wants a gastroenterology nurse's patient to participate in a research study. Whose responsibility is it to obtain the patient's consent?

a. The research nurse.

b. The physician.

c. The legal department.

d. The gastroenterology nurse.

9. Before implementing any nursing action, the gastroenterology nurse should follow all of these guidelines, *except:*

a. Think critically about the plan of care, always questioning whether routines are really the best method of treatment.

b. Consult immediate colleagues, colleagues in related nursing fields, and relevant literature to discover more effective ways of managing health problems.

c. Before instituting any measure to treat a health problem, assess the patient to be sure that the action is still necessary.

d. Document his or her action.

10. Nurses participating in ethical decision making are "morally equal" and therefore need not:

a. Give insight without influence.

b. Fear the advice and opinions of physicians, hospital risk managers, and ethics committees.

c. Accept and support the family's legal decisions.

d. Work through appropriate channels, providing referrals to such resources as support groups or financial aid advisors when appropriate.

BIBLIOGRAPHY

Barnie, D. (1990). Percutaneous endoscopic gastrostomy tubes: the nurse's role in a moral, ethical, and legal dilemma. *Gastroenterol Nurs 12*, 250-4.

Black, M. (1988). Documentation in the GI lab. In Trivits, S. (Ed), *SGA Journal Reprints.* Rochester, NY: Society of Gastrointestinal Assistants.

Bodinsky, G. (1989). Documentation: charting to standardize. SGNA Monograph Series. Rochester, NY: Society of Gastroenterology Nurses and Associates.

Carpenito, L. (2002). *Nursing diagnosis: application to clinical practice* (9th ed.). Philadelphia: Lippincott Williams & Wilkins.

Huey, F. (1988). Working smart. *Am J Nurs 86*, 679-84.

Iyer, P., Taptich, B. & Bernocchi-Losey, D. (1995). *Nursing process and nursing diagnosis* (3rd ed.). Philadelphia: W.B. Saunders.

Jakobsen, E. (1990). Three new ways to deliver care. *Am J Nurs 90*, 24-6.

LaFontaine, P. (1989). Alleviating patients' apprehensions and anxieties. *Gastroenterol Nurs 11*, 256-7.

McAloose, B. & Gruber, M. (1990). SGNA standards of practice for gastroenterology nurses and associates. *Gastroenterol Nurs 12*, 229-31.

McDonald, D. (1986). Nurses on ethical teams—expanding their decision-making role. *AORN J 44*, 83-5. Association of Operating Room Nurses.

McGregor, P. (1988). Your patient's escort: teaching the significant other. *SGA J 10*, 234-5.

McGregor, P. (1987). Developing a patient questionnaire. *SGA J 10*, 50-1. Society of Gastrointestinal Assistants.

Mikels, C. (1989). Patient education for enhancement of compliance. *Gastroenterol Nurs 12*, 60-2.

Mikels, C. (1988). Patient education guidelines. *SGA J 11*, 43-4. Society of Gastrointestinal Assistants.

Monroe, D. (1990). Patient teaching for x-ray and other diagnostics. *RN 53*, 52-6.

North American Nursing Diagnosis Association (1989). *Taxonomy I with official diagnostic categories.* St. Louis, MO: Author.

Ord, B. (1990). Communication: care plan sharing. *Nurs Times 86*, 40-1.

Plumeri, P.A. (1990). Informed consent for endoscopy. In Trivits, S. (Ed.), *Journal Reprints II,* Rochester, NY: Society of Gastroenterology Nurses and Associates.

Reeder, J. (1989). Secure the future: a model for an international nursing ethic. *AORN J 50*, 1298-1307.

Taylor, C., Lillis, C. & LeMone, P. (2001). Implementing/documenting. In Cleary, P., Faven, E. & Intenzo, D. (Eds.), *Fundamentals of nursing: the art and science of nursing care* (4th ed.). Philadelphia: J.B. Lippincott.

Thurlow, J. (1989). Informed consent: every patient's right. *Gastroenterol Nurs 12*, 132-4.

Wheeler, B. (1988). Crisis intervention *AORN J 47*, 1242-8. Association of Operating Room Nurses.

Chapter 12

EVALUATION

The fourth and final component of the nursing process is evaluation. It is a dynamic, continuous indicator of the effectiveness of nursing interventions. It is a reflection of continuous reassessment of the plan of care, as priorities are modified to meet changing needs and goals.

Learning Objectives

After reviewing the contents of this chapter, the gastroenterology nurse should be able to:

1. Understand and explain the tasks involved in the evaluation process.
2. Understand and explain the purpose of the evaluation process.
3. Understand and explain the function of evaluation as it coordinates with the progressive steps of the nursing process.
4. Explain the continuous, cyclic evolution of the nursing process.
5. Identify therapeutic nursing interventions derived from each level of the nursing process appropriate to the plan of care that is developed to meet each individual patient's physical and behavioral needs.

THE NURSING PROCESS

The nursing process is an accepted framework of nursing practice, the components of which include Assessment, Planning, Intervention and Evaluation (APIE).

The Assessment Phase of the nursing process consists of a collection of data, both real and potential. Common words associated with this phase of the nursing process include: observe, gather, collect, differentiate, assess, recognize, detect, distinguish, identify, display, indicate, and describe. (Liese,2003).

The **planning phase** of the nursing process consists of utilizing the data collected to formulate patient goals and outcomes. It must be measurable, prioritized, and include not only the patient, but significant others, as well as all members of the health care team. Common words associated with this phase of the nursing process include: rearrange, reconstruct, determine, outcomes, formulate, include, expected, designate, plan, generate, short/long term goal, develop (Liese,2003).

The implementation phase of the nursing process is the action phase of the process. During this phase of the process, the plan of care is initialized. It involves direct care of the patient, and includes all treatments, procedures, and activities involving the patient. This phase of the process involves documentation of patient response to interventions. Common words associated with this phase of the nursing process include: document, explain, give, inform, administer, implement, encourage, advise, provide, and perform (Liese,2003).

The final phase of the nursing process and the portion we will deal with in greater detail in this chapter is **evaluation**. The evaluation phase of the nursing process is an analytical portion. During this phase it is determined if the interventions delivered were effective, and if goals previously determined require reassessment. It is a time for reassessment of the plan of care, with necessary modifications initiated relative to the objective response of the patient to the plan of care, and the extent to which goals were realized. Some common words associated with this phase of the nursing process include: monitor, expand, evaluate, synthesize, determine, consider, question, repeat, outcomes, demonstrate, reestablish.

The scientific basis upon which the practice of professional nursing is based has been delineated in guidelines set forth by the American Nurses Association (ANA). In *ANA Standard VI*, the evaluation portion of the nursing process is addressed. The process of evaluation is described as the analysis of the patient's progress toward the attainment of preset outcomes (goals). More specifically, it states that:

1. Evaluation is systematic, ongoing, and criterion-based.
2. The patient, family, and other health care providers are involved in the evaluation process as appropriate.
3. Ongoing assessment data are used to revise diagnoses, outcomes, and the plan of care as needed.
4. Revision in diagnoses, outcomes, and the plan of care are documented.
5. The effectiveness of interventions is evaluated in relation to outcomes. Documentation of the patient's progress toward achievable outcomes is retrievable (Fowler, 2002).
6. The patient's responses to interventions are documented (Fowler, 2002).

The nursing roles implicit within the framework of the nursing process are multidimensional, and include provision of care and coordination of care. It is inherent in professional accountability, and includes the appropriateness of nursing actions, the need to rearrange priorities, and an analysis of all aspects of the delivery of care.

Evaluation itself is a multidimensional process, and has multiple facets. Patient care is evaluated through direct observation, patient interviews, and review of the patient's documented records. Interventions (expected outcomes) are either met, not met, or ongoing. They are consistent with the established plan of care, and reflect the rights and desire of the patient, the patient's significant others, and other members of the health care team that are involved with the patient's care. As a health care provider, the nursing focus is on the patient and direct delivery of care. As a coordinator of patient care, the nursing role is largely predetermined by the profession's scope of practice. As a member of a professional discipline, we accept accountability for our actions, and thereby become advocates for our patients and our profession.

Nursing practice is based upon a scientific framework that is the foundation the profession's practice. These involve **critical thinking**, **communication** with patients and peers, and adherence to a **standard of care**, which can be measured. **Criteria** are measurable qualities, attributes, or characteristics that specify skills, knowledge, or health states (Taylor, Lillis, and LeMone, 1989). When analyzed within the framework of standards of care, they delineate nursing behaviors. Every standard of nursing care is accompanied by one or more measurable criteria that are required to be met, to qualify as having met the pre-established standard of care.

Direct and indirect nursing care are interventions derived through critical thinking, and documented as real and potential patient outcomes, set into motion by the implementation of predetermined tasks which address the patient's physical and emotional needs and requirements. The effectiveness of these interventions is the framework upon which the evaluation phase of the nursing process is built. It is a collaborative process that involves a continuous and ongoing interaction between the patient, the nurse, and the environment, on a verbal and nonverbal level. It is continually reassessed as patient priorities change, and preset goals are satisfactorily met.

Important points to remember when reassessing a patient for satisfactory goal resolution are the ability of the patient to achieve the goals set - are they realistic? Can the patient realistically manage the totality of the activities of daily living upon discharge, or does his physical or emotional state make this an unattainable goal? Was the patient involved when the goals to be attained were decided upon? More than the patient's disease process must be taken into account in the predetermination of patient goals and outcomes. These include, among many others, the patient's past and present coping mechanisms, his spiritual beliefs, the support systems available to the patient at the current time and in the future, the impact of the patient's cultural influences, the patient's current level of activity and its future status, and the effect of the patient's disease process and treatments on his self-image, his comfort level, and his ability to function independently.

STANDARDS OF CARE

Standards of Care serve as a blueprint for quality nursing care. They ensure that data collection is systematic and well documented, reflecting the patient's actual or potential health problem. They are individual to each patient, and are based upon current knowledge, reflective of both the patient's and the caregivers priorities in the pursuit of health restoration and maintenance. It is assessed jointly by the nurse, the patient, and his significant others, and is reassessed and revised as tasks are completed and goals are met.

Standards of care also provide a foundation for the development of performance evaluation tools, which provide the base for the development of sound quality assurance programs. They allow for peer review, provide a measurable body of knowledge that can be utilized for research purposes, and promote interdisciplinary collaboration and cooperation. Most importantly, it assures that quality of care remains consistent with existing standards.

Endoscopy nurses apply standards of care in their professional practice on a daily and ongoing basis. The endoscopy nurse evaluates the quality of care given to patients undergoing endoscopic procedures to determine the quality of care and the effectiveness of intervention. Professional practice is evaluated within the scope of professional practice standards and relevant regulatory agencies. Patient safety and effectiveness of patient intervention and care is an ongoing process.

The endoscopy nurse follows a specified plan of care to achieve desired patient outcomes in a safe efficient and cost-effective manner. Criteria assessed include patient comfort and stability, and the maintenance of equipment at the optimum level. Examples of the application of these standards and criteria in professional practice are delineated below.

Standard: The gastroenterology nurse will maintain all equipment appropriately to ensure safe, quality care of the patient undergoing an endoscopic procedure.

Criteria: All endoscopes will be cleaned and disinfected per the manufacturer's written guidelines and institutional policy.

Standard: The gastroenterology nurse correctly and thoroughly completes the documentation required for patients undergoing endoscopic procedures.

> **Criteria:** 1. Vital signs are recorded pre- and post-procedure.
> 2. Procedure start and completion times are accurately and appropriately documented.
> 3. The patient's tolerance to sedation is recorded.
> 4. The patient's post procedure discharge criteria are satisfactorily achieved.

In the plan of care, expected patient outcomes represent the heart of the evaluation process, since they reflect the desired outcomes as an actual task completed, and goal achieved.

Potential patient outcomes are assessed relevant to the patient's health status at the time of assessment, and environmental factors impacting upon the patient's ability to complete the tasks required in order to achieve the desired outcome (goal). Examples of actual and potential outcome influences are airway clearance and knowledge deficit.

Outcome: Ineffective airway clearance; potential.

Criteria: The patient is free from respiratory injury relative to sedation.

Outcome: Knowledge deficit relative to endoscopic procedure; actual.

Criteria: The patient will verbalize understanding of endoscopic procedure and preparation requirements necessary for it.

Evaluation of patient care is performed jointly by the nurse, the patient, and the balance of the health care team involved with the patient's care. It involves evaluating the extent to which the desired outcome was achieved, evaluating the effectiveness of nursing interventions, and evaluating the effectiveness of the overall plan of care.

The evaluation of an implemented plan of care is performed continually and systematically. It encompasses a series of tasks that quantify the effectiveness of our nursing planning and interventions. It includes Standards of Professional Performance, and has become the guideline for patient and institution specific plans of care, a framework for quality assurance programs, a scientific basis for professional and patient education. It also identifies areas of possible research exploration.

The ANA's's 1996 statement on the scope and standards of nursing practice presents the theoretical guideline from which the tasks utilized in the evaluation of the goals achieved are derived. (American Nurses Association, 2003) This theoretical guideline contains eight standards of practice.

Standard I.   Quality of Care

The systematic evaluation of the quality of care and the effectiveness of nursing practice.

Standard II.   Performance Appraisal

The evaluation of practice as measured by the standards of professional practice.

Standard III.   Education

The professional practitioner is obligated to participate in ongoing continuing education activities for the purpose of maintaining currency of professional expertise.

Standard IV.   Collegiality

The nurse contributes, to the best of his or her ability, to the professional development of others.

Standard V.   Ethics

The nurse is obligated to intervene on the behalf of patients in an ethical manner.

Standard VI.   Collaboration

The nurse collaborates with the patient's significant others and the multidisciplinary care team in the provision of quality care.

Standard VII.   Research

The nurse contributes to the scientific and theoretical basis of nursing by reviewing and applying current research in the professional practice.

Standard VIII.   Resource Utilization

The nurse includes in her plan of care interventions based upon the requirements for patient safety, effectiveness of care, cost of care, and the efficiency of the delivery of care.

The analysis of measurable outcomes are reviewed as concisely and systematically as they were assessed, planned, and implemented. The steps involved form the body of knowledge we know as the Evaluation Process.

STEP 1. Collecting evaluative data

The goal of the first analytical tool inherent in the evaluation of patient task accomplishment and goal achievement answers the question, "To what degree were predetermined patient outcomes achieved?" The answer can be found by employing several varying methods of analysis. The evaluative technique utilized will be determined upon whether the outcome evaluated is cognitive, psychomotor, or affective.

1. Cognitive outcomes define increases in knowledge. Data are collected by asking the patient to repeat or apply information to familiar situations.
2. Psychomotor outcomes address the achievement of new, learned skills. The patient demonstrating the new skill is an effective way of measuring goal achievement.
3. Affective outcomes are more difficult to evaluate, since they define less measurable behavioral differences. These outcomes relate to changes in the patient's values, beliefs, and attitudes. Behavior and social interactions are observed to evaluate the achievement of these outcomes.

When all evaluative data has been collected, it is compared with the standards of nursing care, expected outcomes, and professional regulations and policies.

Federal requirements for discharge planning process

Hospitals must identify at an early stage of hospitalization all meidicare clients who are likely to suffer adverse health consequences upon discharge if there is no planning.

The hospital must provide a discharge planning evaluation.

A registered nurse, social worker, or other qualified person must develop or supervise development of the evaluation.

Discharge planning must include an evaluation of the likelihood of needing posthospital services and of the availability of the services.

The evaluation must include the client's capacity for self-care or the possibility of the client being cared for in the environment from which the client entered the hospital.

The evaluation must be completed on a timely basis so that appropriate arrangements for posthospital care are made before discharge.

The discharge planning evaluation must be in the client's medical record.

From Perry AG, Potter PA: *Clinical nursing skills and techniques*, St Louis, 1994, Mosby. Originally from *Federal Register*, 53:116, June 16, 1988.

STEP 2. Analyzing outcome achievements and effectiveness of nursing interventions

Once the determination has been made as to whether identified patient outcomes have been achieved, an analysis of the variables that contributed to their success or failure becomes a valuable evaluative tool. The value of this step becomes apparent when the actual influences promoting outcome achievement, or the lack of it, are identified and reassessed.

STEP 3. Reassessment of the plan of care

The final task performed in the evaluation phase of the nursing process is reassessment. This is the time when data has been collected and documented, and is reassessed to determine the patient's progress toward the achievement of expected outcomes. The relevant data has been collected. Actual outcomes and potential outcomes are compared, and reassessment made accordingly. It is during the reassessment step of the evaluation phase that the nursing outcomes, goals and plans of care are reviewed and revised as necessary.

QUALITY IMPROVEMENT AS A FUNCTION OF THE NURSING PROCESS

Monitoring the quality of care is the responsibility of all health care workers, and is an important function of the evaluation phase of the nursing process. Documentation of patient intervention measures, and the utilization of measurable outcome criteria, provides the methodology by which standards of care can be monitored and evaluated, providing important information for use in quality improvement programs.

Effective quality improvement programs are consistent with scope of practice and regulatory and institutional policies. As performed on a smaller scale when evaluating patient care outcomes, it should be systematic, facility-wide, and provide data that can be utilized to improve delivery of care. Time and past experience has shown that although quality of care cannot be assured, but it can be monitored continuously, and thereby improved substantially. Historically, they are designed to evaluate which nursing interventions are the most optimal. These include patient satisfaction with the services provided, the quality of the technical aspects of the services provided (and the risk of injury or illness that are associated with them), the efficiency and cost management of the resources utilized, and the evaluation of the efficient utilization of the resources available (including cost containment of physical resources, and the time and type of utilization of medical personnel). Quality improvement, as an extension of the nursing process, is a bridge between direct patient care, and the balance of the members of the health care team. The ultimate goal for all is the achievement of a standard of excellence in an objective and straightforward manner. The ultimate goal–the improvement of patient care.

EXAMPLES OF EVALUATION OF CARE IN THE ENDOSCOPY SUITE

Example 1

Standard

Patients receiving conscious sedation are to be monitored continually for the development of adverse reactions.

Criteria

1. Personnel monitoring the sedated patient are fully conversant with their adverse reactions and the therapeutic interventions for each. These include appropriate dosage indications and medication contraindications, interactions with other medications, and the onset and duration of action of each medication that has been used.
2. All patients receiving conscious sedation are to have adequate and continually intravenous access.
3. Emergency equipment, including appropriate reversal agents and equipment, such as oxygen administration equipment and defibrillators, should be readily available whenever conscious sedation is administered.

Evaluation

1. Continuous intravenous access is adequately maintained throughout the duration of the patient's procedure and recovery.
2. Discharge criteria reflect that the patient has achieved a baseline level of functioning. These include, but are not limited to, the patient's return to a physiological level inclusive of adequate respiratory levels, a preprocedural level of consciousness, pink and intact skin color and condition, fully functional protective reflexes, and stability of vital signs.

Example 2

Goal

The endoscopy nurse will provide patient education that is commensurate with the patient's procedure, level of understanding, and cultural, religious and personal beliefs.

Criteria

1. The nurse will assess the patient's ability and readiness to learn by assessing learning needs and readiness to learn.
2. In collaboration with the patient and /or his significant others, the nurse will deliver patient teaching based on identified need.
3. The nurse will teach the patient/significant others in an environment that is conducive to their assessed learning needs.

Evaluation

1. The nurse will evaluate the patient's ability to meet the learning criteria through verbalization and discussion.
2. Teaching interventions will be modified according to the patient's assessed ability to meet the goal criteria.

CASE SITUATION

Leadville Community Hospital is continually reviewing and revising its standards of care, as its staff ceaselessly strives to deliver the safest and most cost-efficient patient care in Colorado. Delivery of care is continually reviewed and upgraded, as it is redesigned to meet the challenges of an ever more technologically and medically complex hospital environment.

Leadville Community Hospital is currently re-evaluating the patient discharge criteria to be used for their post-endoscopy outpatient population. Currently the endoscopy physician must evaluate the patient before he can be discharged from the hospital setting. The hospital is planning to implement a discharge program based upon a nursing evaluation of pertinent criteria. Hospital personnel members feel that this will help the endoscopy unit flow more efficiently. It allows the physician to continue with procedures uninterrupted, while at the same time, the postprocedure nursing staff ensures that patients have adequately met all the criteria for a safe discharge from the hospital.

The preset criteria upon which the nursing staff would evaluate a patient's ability to be safely discharged from the hospital would include:

(a) Return of vital signs to preprocedural levels;
(b) Return of LOC to preprocedural levels;
(c) Determination that oxygen saturation is within pre-determined parameters;
(d) An evaluation of the patient's ability to safely ambulate;
(e) An evaluation of the patient's skin color, warmth and dryness; and
(f) An evaluation of the patient's perception of pain on a scale of 1 - 10.

Gastroenterology nurse Sally Caulfield is monitoring Winston MacBride as he awaits discharge from the endoscopy unit following a colonoscopy with polypectomy of a large cecal polyp. Winston had been medicated with Meperidine (Demerol) and Midazolam (Versed) before the start of the procedure, and two times during the course of the procedure. His physician, Dr. Elkins, has written orders to discharge his patient when he is stable, and to have him follow-up with him in his office in one week.

Points to think about

1. How might the gastroenterology nurse evaluate her patient's readiness for discharge within the discharge criteria currently set forth by Leadville Community Hospital?
2. Sally noted that preprocedural teaching was completed and documented by the nurse who had admitted Winston 'to the endoscopy unit. This teaching was inclusive of potential and actual postprocedure changes in bowel movements, dietary restrictions, if necessary, medication restrictions, if necessary, and possible reasons he may need to contact his physician before his scheduled post-procedure appointment. These reasons might include rectal bleeding in large amounts, an elevated temperature over 100 degrees Fahrenheit, severe abdominal pain, and a rigid and distended abdominal area. When should evaluation of teaching take place and how might an evaluation be performed?
3. Assuming that Winston achieved all expected outcome criteria (met all necessary criteria set forth for patient discharge from the endoscopy unit), what evaluative statements would Sally document on the patient's chart? These evaluative statements should be pertinent to goals met and specific outcome criteria achieved, thereby adequately meeting the standards of the hospital for discharge.
4. When Sally evaluates Winston's progress one hour postprocedure, his vital signs are stable (within 20% of his preprocedural vital signs), he is alert and oriented to person, place and time, he is denying abdominal pain, and his abdomen is soft and non-distended. He is, however, complaining of nausea, and is declining oral intake of fluids. What actions might Sally implement, as she reassesses Winston's requirements, as based upon these new actual outcomes?
5. Sally is a member of her unit's Quality Improvement Committee. The committee is currently redesigning their postprocedure discharge policy to meet the needs of a growing and evolving patient population. What type of suggestions could she suggest to the rest of the committee that would accumulate measurable data for evaluation of the efficacy of the endoscopy unit's newly implemented, nurse-driven postprocedure discharge policy?

Suggested responses

1. Evaluation of a patient's progress toward a preset goal is a measurable process, with preset outcomes evaluated against preset criteria. The preset criteria, in this instance, are the parameters for discharge that the patient must achieve before he can be safely discharged from the hospital. The actual outcomes are based upon the patient's ability to achieve these preset criteria. As the nurse proceeds through each individual criterion for discharge, she will evaluate the patient's actual outcomes against these preset criteria. By carefully evaluating Winston's progress in achieving these predetermined outcome criteria (stable vital signs, LOC return to preprocedural levels, oxygen saturation level, ambulation ability, skin color warmth, dryness and turgor, and pain perception), Sally can make a determination of his readiness for discharge.

2. Patient teaching is the responsibility of every health care worker who comes into contact with the patient. Multiple staff members care for the patient as the plan of care progresses. It is the function of every person treating the patient to be able to assess the patient's level of understanding, and speak to any questions or concerns the patient might express as he proceeds with the plan of care. Patient perceptions of both physical and emotional experiences are altered on an ongoing basis as new information and experiences are processed. This is why the evaluation process is an ongoing process, which must be continually reassessed. Methodologies for evaluating patient teaching are directly proportional to the desired patient outcomes, and the type of learning need required of each. A cognitive outcome, such as a patient's understanding of potential changes in bowel function immediate post-colonoscopy, might be best assessed by asking the patient to repeat the information and verbalize understanding. At the very minimum, all patients should be evaluated for understanding of the plan of care at the implementation of the plan, during the patient's pre-assessment telephone interaction with the nurse, through to the pre-discharge level of understanding. Encouraging patients to verbalize their learning needs both before and after the procedure, and then evaluating the extent to which these individual needs were met, would facilitate an evaluation of their effectiveness. A new postprocedure plan could then be designed and implemented, based upon actual educational deficits assessed during this evaluative process.

3. At the time of Winston's discharge from the hospital, after the successful completion of his procedure, Sally's evaluation of her patient's readiness for discharge is based upon his having achieved the predetermined outcome criteria as set forth in the hospital's discharge policy. It is also dependent upon her evaluation and documentation of his understanding of any possible contraindications to activities of daily living, possible complications to take note of in the immediate postprocedure period, and his responsibility to follow-up with his doctor within a specified time frame. At the time of discharge, Sally would document Winston's discharge status, along with the degree each outcome criteria was met, partially met, or not met. All predetermined discharge criteria would be addressed, along with any discharge teaching and/or instructions, and Winston's level of understanding of each. Sally's discharge note might read as follows:

Patient is alert and oriented to person, place and time, and describes minimal discomfort. Vital signs are stable and within 20% of their preprocedural levels. Oxygen saturation is 100%. Ambulating without assistance and with a steady gait. Skin is pink, warm, and dry to the touch, with normal turgor. Oral intake tolerated well, with no nausea or vomiting noted. Patient describes post-discharge care measures, self-evaluation criteria, and verbalizes understanding of all teaching. Discharged to home in stable condition, in the care of his brother, Mike. He will follow-up with his physician, in his office, in one week, as per MD instructions.

4. The evaluation process is dynamic and continually altered by the patient's response to interventions. After each patient interaction, the degree to which expected outcomes have been achieved is reassessed. It is at this point that the plan of care can either be terminated (the patient is discharged to home), modified (new interventions are determined as necessary for the patient to achieve the outcome objectives desired), and/or continued. Planned care may be terminated if each outcome has been achieved; i.e. the patient may be discharged to home when all discharge criteria have been successfully met. If the patient is continually having difficulty achieving the desired outcome, the plan of care may require reassessment and modification. In the instance described here, Winston is refusing oral intake. Sally must now reassess Winston to determine how best to help him meet the outcome criteria; she must decide whether to give him ice chips and begin oral intake slowly, or to first administer an anti-emetic, and then offer oral intake again. If the patient just requires more time to achieve the desired outcome, the plan of care is continued unaltered. In this instance, Sally has decided to continue monitoring her patient until the cause of his nausea is determined, or the nausea subsides without intervention.

5. A quality improvement program implemented to assess the efficacy of a criteria based endoscopy discharge plan, as assessed by the nurse recovering the patient, would include predetermined discharge criteria, and documentation of the patient's achievement of each. Assessing the efficacy of discharge parameters that have been previously determined enables the nurse to determine which interventions were the most successful in achieving desired patient outcomes. Factors to be considered in an evaluation of such a program are multiple. Is the patient satisfied with the services provided? Was the quality of technical care received by the patient adequate to meet his individual needs? Was there an efficient use of personnel and resources? What are the possible risk factors that

might be generated by an entirely nurse-driven discharge program? It would involve a review of nursing care and patient outcomes performed while the patient was receiving care. It is performed through direct observation of nursing care, patient interviews, and chart reviews (the concurrent audit). It offers the advantage of immediate feedback, and thereby immediate corrective actions, as deemed necessary. It is an important tool for the evaluation of patient care, and enables the caregiver to change and improve interventions and quality of care, with the result of an immediate improvement in the quality of care and future patient interventions.

Sally's proposal will include a checklist of patient needs met, not met, and/or partially met for all of the unit's predetermined outcome criteria for discharge. From this checklist she can determine compliance with the plan of care, and where areas for improvement are required. She can then proceed further to document the patient's understanding of the discharge instructions delivered and identify any areas of learning deficits she feels could be addressed more succinctly at this juncture of care.

REVIEW TERMS

affective outcome, cognitive outcome, concurrent, audit, evaluative process, outcome criteria, psychomotor, outcome, quality of care, standards of care

REVIEW QUESTIONS

1. The reason that nursing professionals evaluate the quality of care include all of the following, except:
   (a) Nurses recognize that quality in health care is elusive and complex.
   (b) Nursing professionals aim to promote excellence in nursing care.
   (c) Nurses must be accountable to society for the quality of care they provide.
   (d) Nurses want to improve professional performance by identifying deficiencies in care provided, and therefore educational needs, and to analyze and explain the differences in patterns of practice and results of care.

2. Criteria are:
   (a) nationally recognized standards.
   (b) facts.
   (c) interventions.
   (d) measurable.

3. Examination of nursing care consists of:
   (a) examining the cost-effectiveness of nursing actions, the efficiency of admission and discharge, and the rate of patient readmission.
   (b) determining whether or not a patient has achieved outcomes or is making progress toward goals developed in the outcome identification stage of care; whether nursing interventions chosen to treat identified health problems are effective in reducing or resolving identified health problems; and whether

health care provided has been effective overall.
   (c) verifying whether policies and procedures are eliminating problems; whether the doctors are practicing according to the dictums of their specialty; and whether administrators are adequately staffing nursing units.
   (d) examining nursing values; identifying structure, process, and outcome criteria; and executing performance appraisals to correct individual resistance to quality practices.

4. Evaluative statements:
   (a) must include the patient's response to care provided.
   (b) must describe actual outcomes of care.
   (c) may decline skills developed, knowledge obtained, or changes in health status.
   (d) all of the above.

5. Changes in values, beliefs, and attitudes are difficult to evaluate because:
   (a) they are less concrete.
   (b) survey questionnaires used to evaluate them are rarely valid.
   (c) there is little value placed on casual conversation with patients.
   (d) all of the above.

6. A quality improvement review is:
   (a) an acceptable, expected level of performance established by authority, custom, or consent.
   (b) an ongoing process of review in which data collected over a period of time are used to compare actual practice against standards of practice to determine if the care actually rendered meets a level of quality deemed acceptable within a practice setting.
   (c) a review of documentation for the purpose of determining whether or not specific objectives were met during the period of time outlined.
   (d) a statement defining an actual outcome (e.g., skills developed, knowledge obtained, change in health status).

7. Which statement is least accurate concerning QI Programs?
   (a) They collect data for evaluation by evaluating past and present nursing interventions and documentation.
   (b) They conduct studies of overall effectiveness of care.
   (c) They evaluate two specific areas of practice: staff competence and risk management.
   (d) They analyze the degree to which external factors, such as different types of health services, specialized equipment or procedures, or socioeconomic factors, influence health and wellness.

8. Nurses, patients, other health care professionals, regulatory agencies, such as JCAHO and OSHA, and the community at large; all of whom are concerned with the effectiveness, efficiency, and safety of nursing care, are interested in the analysis of nursing interventions to discover:
   (a) whether nurses or other health team members are better able to provide specific kinds of care.

(b) which nursing interventions are most successful in achieving desired outcomes and what it costs to achieve them.

(c) both a and b.

(d) none of the above.

9. Cognitive outcomes:

(a) define increases in knowledge.

(b) relate to changes in the patient's values, beliefs, and attitudes

(c) address the achievement of new, learned skills.

(d) none of the above.

10. Patient teaching is the responsibility of:

(a) the doctor.

(b) the nurse who admits the patient.

(c) all health care workers.

(d) a and b only.

BIBLIOGRAPHY

Ackley, B. & Lodwig, G. (2001). *Nursing Diagnosis Handbook* (5th ed.). St. Louis, MO: Mosby.

Agency for Healthcare Research and Quality (1997). *Case Studies from the Quality Improvement Support System* (Publication No. 97-0022). Washington DC: U.S. Government Printing Office.

Alfaro, R. (1999). *Applying Nursing Process: A Step-By-Step Guide* (4th ed.). Philadelphia: J. B. Lippincott.

Alfaro-LeFevre, R. (2001). *Applying Nursing Process: Promoting Collaborative Care* (5th ed.). Philadelphia: J. B. Lippincott.

Alfaro-LeFevre, R. (1999). *Critical Thinking in Nursing: A Practical Approach* (3rd ed.). Philadelphia: W. B. Saunders Company.

Andersen, G. (1998). Assessing The Older Patient. *RN 61:3*, 47-51.

Ballard, K.A., Arborgast, D., Boeckman, J., Conlon, P., Cox, J.A., Dayhoff, N.E., Fournier, J., Hozdic, L., Murcko, A., Peters, D.A., Staudt, G.A., Stordahl, N., Waszak, L.C. (2003) ANA Standards of Clinical Nursing Practice, Draft published for Public comment. American Nurses Publishing, Washington, D.C., http://www.nursingworld.org/

Batalden, P.B. & Stoltz, P.K. (1993). A Framework for the Continual Improvement of Health Care: Building and Applying Professional and Improvement Knowledge to Test Changes in Daily Work. *Joint Commission Journal on Quality Improvement 19(10)*; 424-52.

Bender, A., Motley, R., Pierotti, R.J., Bischof, R.O. (1999). Quality and Outcomes Management in the Primary Care Practice. *Journal of Medical Practice Management 14(5)*, 236-40.

Carpenito, L. (1997). *Handbook of Nursing Diagnosis* (7th ed.). Philadelphia: J. B. Lippincott.

Carpenito, L. (1999). *Nursing Care Plans and Documentation* (3rd ed.). Philadelphia: J. B. Lippincott.

Cassidy, C. (1999). Want to Know How You're Doing? *AJN 99:9*, 51-59. American Journal of Nursing.

Christensen, R. (2000). What's Your Diagnosis? *Nursing 2000.* 32 hn 1 - 32 hn 4.

Clancy, C.M. (1998). Continuous Quality Improvement and Primary Care. *Medical Care 36(5)*, 619-20.

Doenges, M. & Moorhouse, M. (2000). *Nurses Pocket Guide, Diagnosis, Interventive, Rationale* (7th ed.). Philadelphia: F.A. Davis.

Doenges, M. & Moorhouse, M. (1997). *Nursing Care Plans: Guides for Individualizing Patient Care* (4th ed.). Philadelphia: F.A. Davis.

Gregory, K. (2000, September). Nurse the Patient. *RN 63:9*, 52-4.

Johnson, M., Bulecheck, G., McCloskey, J., Maas, M., and Morehead, S. (2001). *Nursing Diagnoses Outcomes & Interventions.* St. Louis, Missouri: Mosby.

Kozier, B., Berman, A.J., and Erb, G. (2000). *Fundamentals of Nursing* (6th ed.). Upper Saddle River, New Jersey: Prentice Hall.

Lewis, S.M., Heitkemper, M.M. and Dirksen, S.R. (2000). *Medical-Surgical Nursing* (5th ed.). St. Louis, Missouri: Mosby.

Liese, A. (2003, January). *Ways to Choose the Right Answer on the NCLEX Exam* [On-line]. Available: http://www.angelfire.com/ga/anneliese/page2.htm.

Fowler, P. (2003). *Nursing Process: Implementation and Evaluation* (Fall 2002) [On-line.]. Available: http://www.rsu.edu/faculty/PFowler/Implementation%20and%20evaluation.ppt.

Price, A. & Price, B. (2000). Problem-Based Learning in Clinical Practice Facilitating Critical Thinking. *Journal for Nursing in Staff Development 6:6*, 66-68.

Rubenfeld, M.G. & Scheffer, B.K. (1999). *Critical Thinking in Nursing: An Interactive Approach* (2nd ed.). Philadelphia: J. B. Lippincott.

Solberg, L.I., Brekke, M.L., Kottke, T.E. & Steel, R.P. (1998). Continuous Quality Improvement in Primary Care: What's Happening? *Medical Care 36(5)*: 625-35.

Tanner, C. (2000, November). Critical Thinking: Beyond Nursing Process. *Nursing Education 39:8*, 33 38.

ANATOMY, PHYSIOLOGY, AND PATHOPHYSIOLOGY

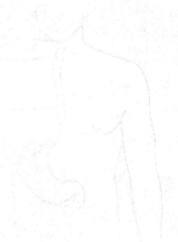

Chapter 13

ESOPHAGUS

This chapter will acquaint the gastroenterology nurse with the normal anatomy and physiology of the esophagus and the clinical features, diagnosis, and treatment of selected esophageal disorders.

Learning objectives

After reviewing the content of this chapter, the gastroenterology nurse should be able to:

1. Describe the anatomy of the esophagus, including the upper and lower esophageal sphincters and the esophageal body.
2. Explain the normal motility of the esophagus.
3. Discuss a number of pathological conditions of the esophagus and the corresponding pathophysiology, diagnosis, and treatment alternatives.

ANATOMY AND PHYSIOLOGY

The **esophagus** is a hollow, muscular tube, approximately 23 to 25 cm (10 inches) in length and 2 to 3 cm (approximately 1 inch) in diameter in adults. The esophagus serves as a channel for food going from the mouth to the stomach (Fig. 13-1).

It is considered the third organ of digestion, after the mouth and pharynx. The esophagus is located posterior to the trachea and larynx. It passes through the diaphragm and into the abdomen at an opening called the **diaphragmatic hiatus**. Almost immediately after the esophagus passes through the hiatus, it enters the stomach (Fig. 13-2).

The wall of the esophagus is made up of three layers: the mucosa, submucosa, and muscularis. Unlike most of the rest

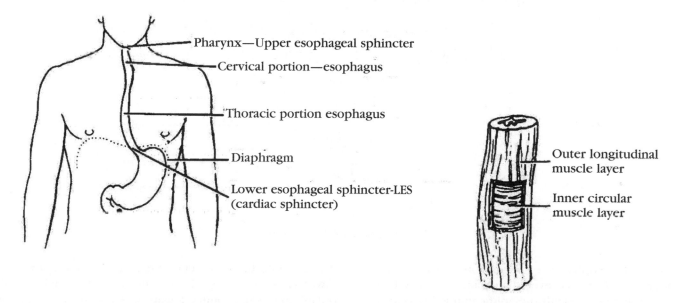

Pharynx—Upper esophageal sphincter

Cervical portion—esophagus

Thoracic portion esophagus

Diaphragm

Lower esophageal sphincter-LES (cardiac sphincter)

Outer longitudinal muscle layer

Inner circular muscle layer

Fig. 13-1. Esophageal anatomy. Insert shows muscular layers of esophagus.

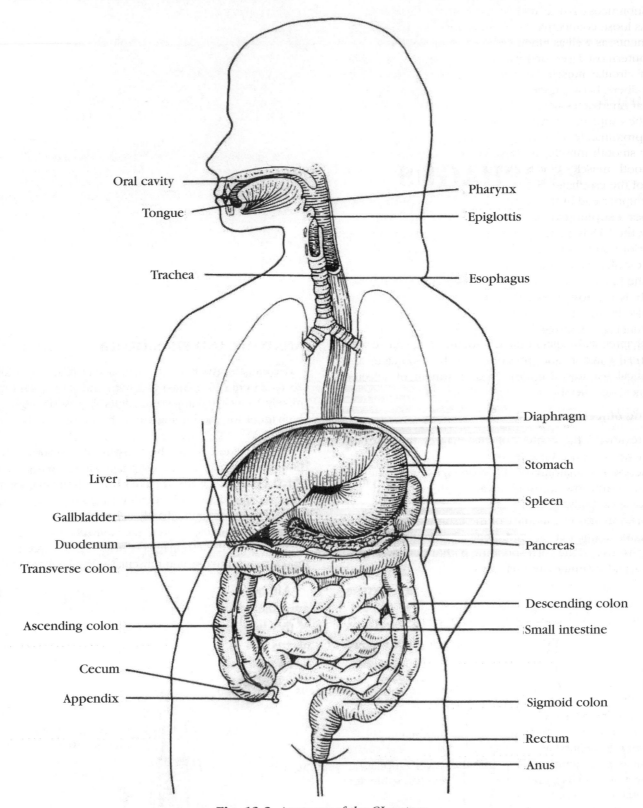

Fig. 13-2. Anatomy of the GI system.

of the GI tract, the esophagus is not surrounded by serosa.

The inner mucosal layer is covered with a layer of stratified squamous epithelium. Beneath the epithelium is the lamina propria, which consists of loose connective tissue. Extensions of the lamina propria, called the dermal pegs, protrude into the epithelium. Particularly at the upper and lower ends of the esophagus, the mucosa contains well-organized mucus-producing glands. A thin band of smooth muscle, the muscularis mucosae, separates the lamina propria from the underlying submucosa.

The submucosa is the middle layer of the esophagus. It contains loose connective tissue with both fibrous and elastic elements, as well as blood vessels and nerve fibers.

The outermost layer, or muscularis, consists of an inner layer of circular muscle and an outer layer of longitudinal muscle fibers. Between the two muscular layers is the intramuscular Auerbach's nerve plexus. Approximately the first 5% of the esophagus is made up strictly of striated muscle, and approximately 50% to 60% of the distal esophagus is entirely smooth muscle. A transition zone of both striated and smooth muscles covers as much as 35% to 40% of the length of the esophagus.

At the upper end of the esophagus is the hypopharyngeal, or **upper esophageal, sphincter (UES)**. Posteriorly and laterally, the UES is made up of the cricopharyngeal muscle; its anterior border is the cricoid cartilage. At the lower end of the esophagus, directly above the angle of His, which marks the junction between the tubular esophagus and the stomach, is the **lower esophageal sphincter (LES)**. The LES is also known as the gastroesophageal sphincter or cardiac sphincter. It controls the passage of ingested food to the stomach. The LES is a physiological rather than an anatomical sphincter, and is 2 to 4 cm in length.

The esophagus receives arterial blood via the esophageal arteries of the aorta, the inferior thyroid artery, and the left gastric artery. The gastroesophageal junction receives arterial blood from branches of the left gastric artery and the inferior phrenic arteries. Blood is returned by way of the azygos, thyroid, and left gastric veins.

The esophagus receives both sympathetic and parasympathetic innervation. The swallowing center in the medulla initiates peristaltic contractions via the vagus nerve, which innervates striated muscle in the upper esophagus. Sympathetic innervation, which controls secondary peristalsis (which arises from within the esophagus), is derived from cervical and thoracic ganglia and from preganglionic fibers of the greater and lesser splanchnic nerves. The LES is believed to receive both sympathetic and parasympathetic innervation.

Motility

At rest, both the UES and the LES are closed. When a bolus of food is pushed through the pharynx, the UES opens, allowing the bolus to pass into the esophagus. At this point, gravity and peristalsis combine to advance the bolus down through the esophagus.

Peristalsis is defined as a distally progressive band of circular muscle contraction. When it is initiated by swallowing, it is known as primary peristalsis. Secondary peristalsis originates below the hypopharynx with no antecedent swallowing movement; it is elicited by esophageal distention. In the esophagus, peristalsis begins in the pharynx and moves distally at a rate of 3 to 5 cm per second, effectively transporting material toward the stomach.

When the bolus reaches the LES, the sphincter opens to allow the bolus to enter the stomach and then closes to prevent a reflux of food and acid.

PATHOPHYSIOLOGY

Important disorders of the esophagus include gastroesophageal reflux disease (GERD), varices, tumors, diverticula, and strictures. Other noteworthy pathological conditions include esophageal rings and webs, foreign-body obstructions, infectious diseases, Mallory-Weiss tears, motility disorders, caustic injuries, Barrett's esophagus, fistulas, and congenital disorders.

Gastroesophageal reflux disease (GERD)

Gastroesophageal reflux develops when gastric or duodenal contents flow back into the esophagus. All adults and children normally have some amount of reflux, particularly after eating. Esophageal reflux is considered a pathological condition only when it causes undesirable symptoms, such as pain or respiratory distress. Patients with excessive or symptomatic esophageal reflux have an incompetent LES; that is, the LES does not have sufficient intraluminal pressure to prevent reflux. Esophageal reflux may also occur as a result of pyloric stenosis, intestinal malrotation, or a motility disorder.

The most common symptoms of esophageal reflux are **dyspepsia** (epigastric discomfort or pain), **heartburn** (pyrosis), and **regurgitation**. Other symptoms may include **dysphagia** (a sensation of difficulty in swallowing), **odynophagia** (painful swallowing), bleeding from erosions or **esophagitis**, asthma, and aspiration pneumonia.

There are three objectives in the treatment of GERD: relief of symptoms, the healing of damaged mucosa, and the prevention of complications. Diagnostic testing associated with gastroesophageal reflux includes the following:

1. **Barium swallow, or upper GI.** An upper GI series will demonstrate reflux but does not allow for evaluation of the frequency of reflux or its association with other symptoms (e.g., respiratory distress, pain). Upper GI may show inflammation associated with esophagitis but is not always a reliable test for esophagitis, especially in children. Upper GI is a valuable tool for determining if an anatomical abnormality (e.g., malrotation, stricture, obstruction) is responsible for the reflux symptoms. Upper GI also allows for evaluation of swallowing, motility, and anatomy.

2. **Esophageal manometry.** This procedure may be indicated if a motility disorder is suspected as the cause of the patient's symptoms. Manometry is sometimes a useful adjunct to evaluation for gastroesophageal reflux, but the diagnosis cannot be confirmed by manometry alone.

3. **Esophagoscopy** with biopsy. Used to determine the presence of esophagitis or Barrett's esophagus, as well as anatomical abnormalities, esophagoscopy with biopsy helps to determine the aggressiveness of medical or surgical therapy.

4. **pH study.** An extended "24-hour" esophageal pH **study** is used to determine the frequency of reflux episodes and the relationship of these episodes to symptoms as they occur (i.e., respiratory symptoms, chest

pain, bradycardia). Intraesophageal pH is recorded for 24 hours; symptoms are recorded manually on a diary or electronically, using the pH monitoring equipment. Twenty-four-hour pH monitoring is generally thought to be the most accurate test for gastroesophageal reflux.

5. A **Bernstein test.** May be ordered to differentiate between cardiac and noncardiac chest pain. A feeding tube is placed intranasally so the tip is positioned in the esophagus. Hydrochloric acid is instilled, and the resultant symptoms are compared with the patient's presenting symptoms.

6. **Nuclear scintiscan** and **gastric emptying studies.** These may be ordered to determine reflux and to observe for evidence of aspiration. With this test, a radioactive isotope is added to liquid, which is then ingested by the patient. Nuclear scanning is then carried out to detect the presence of the isotope in the esophagus (for reflux) or in the lungs (for aspiration) and to determine the length of time that passes before the liquid passes from the stomach into the intestine.

The first step in treatment of esophageal reflux is behavior modification by incorporating the following recommendations:

(a) dietary adjustment with avoidance of foods and beverages that lower LES pressure, including alcohol; tomatoes; peppermint; licorice; and caffeine-containing foods and beverages such as coffee, tea, chocolate, and colas;

(b) weight loss and avoidance of tight-fitting garments;

(c) elevation of the head of the bed on blocks; the use of pillows to elevate the patient's head causes the patient to bend at the waist, thus increasing intraabdominal pressure and thereby increasing reflux;

(d) smoking cessation; and

(e) avoidance of food or drink 2 hours before bedtime.

The next step in the treatment of esophageal reflux is drug therapy, using antacids; histamine2 (H2) blockers; sucralfate (Carafate); or one of the proton-pump inhibitors, omeprazole (Prilosec), rabeprazole (Aciphex), or lansoprazole (Prevacid). If these drugs are not helpful, the addition of a medication to increase motility and strengthen the LES, such as metoclopramide (Reglan, a dopamine antagonist), bethanechol (Urecholine, a cholinergic agent), may be useful.

In 1995 and 1996 over-the-counter histamine2-receptor antagonists were given Food and Drug Administration (FDA) clearance for use in reducing the production of gastric acid. Appropriate use of these, without a medical evaluation, offers some benefits to the patient. Inappropriate use, however, may mask a more serious disorder.

If patients are debilitated by severe esophagitis, aspiration pneumonia, or other disabling symptoms, antireflux surgery may be needed to provide an artificial closing mechanism. Surgical possibilities include invaginating the esophagus into itself (Belsey's operation) or creating a gastric wraparound with or without fixation (Hill and Nissen fundoplication procedures). Laparoscopic Nissen fundoplication is another surgical alternative for treatment of GERD. Early

studies indicate a decreased morbidity, shortened recovery period and hospital stay, minimal discomfort, and the potential for cure of GERD.

For patients with gastrostomy tubes, reflux may be decreased by elevating the head of the bed on blocks and slowing the rate of feedings.

Complications of gastroesophageal reflux may include esophageal stricture, esophageal ulcer, Barrett's esophagus, pulmonary aspiration, or upper GI bleeding.

The majority of infants manifest some symptoms of esophageal reflux up to 6 months of age. In most cases, the condition has a benign course, and symptoms improve by 18 months of age. The most common symptom in infants is recurrent vomiting or "spitting up," failure to thrive, and aspiration. Diagnosis of gastroesophageal reflux in infants is based on history; if indicated, testing is performed. Diagnostic testing for reflux in infants and children may include any of the tests performed on adults (e.g., pH monitoring, upper endoscopy, barium swallow). Infants who vomit frequently after feeding but have no respiratory symptoms and are growing well may need no testing or treatment.

If symptoms are severe, the following measures may be helpful:

(a) Limiting the volume of formula;

(b) Thickening feedings with dry rice cereal;

(c) Placing the infant in an elevated position; and

(d) Avoiding active play in the first hour after feeding.

The physician may prescribe bethanechol (Urecholine), or metoclopramide (Reglan) to improve GI motility. Histamine2 (H2) blockers are used to decrease the potential of damage from acid. Up to 15% of infants with esophageal reflux undergo surgery, most often the Nissen fundoplication, in which the fundus of the stomach is wrapped around the distal esophagus.

Gastroesophageal reflux in pregnancy is a frequent occurrence. Symptoms of heartburn begin during early pregnancy and resolve with delivery. Increased reflux symptoms coincide with intraabdominal pressure from the growing fetus and a decrease in LES pressure in early pregnancy, which both return to normal after delivery. Lifestyle modifications may be enough to manage the heartburn. Careful consideration must be given to use of systemic medications because of potential risk to the fetus.

Esophageal varices

Although varices may occur in other parts of the GI tract, they develop most commonly in the submucosal veins of the distal esophagus, the stomach, and the hemorrhoidal plexus.

Esophageal **varices** are related to portal hypertension, which is often associated with alcoholic cirrhosis, but may also be seen in patients with cirrhosis resulting from other causes, such as chronic hepatitis, portal vein thrombosis, and congenital disorders such as biliary atresia. In such cases, fibrotic liver changes and hepatic vein obstruction cause increased pressure within the portal venous system. This pressure is transmitted to preexisting collateral circulation, which results in dilatation of submucosal esophageal veins. Although varices may be asymptomatic and variceal bleeding is painless, there is a high risk of rupture of the distal esophageal veins, which causes life-threatening bleeding. In an acute episode, bright red blood gushes from the patient's mouth and the patient shows signs and symptoms of hypovolemia. An upper endoscopy is useful to diagnose esophageal varices and to evaluate the risk of bleeding. Varices can be classified on a scale of I to IV, depending on their size. Larger varices (grade III or IV) carry a higher risk of bleeding. Supportive measures are required for shock. The physician may order replacement of blood volume with packed red blood cells, albumin, and IV hydration and correction of concurrent coagulopathy with fresh frozen plasma.

Endoscopic injection of a sclerosing agent has been the historical treatment of choice for acute variceal bleeding. Potential complications of sclerotherapy include inflammation of the mediastinum secondary to extraesophageal injection or perforation; rebleeding; stricture formation; or ulceration. Following sclerotherapy, patients should be observed for any signs of complications. A newer treatment alternative for variceal bleeding is esophageal variceal ligation (EVL), which involves the endoscopic placement of rubber bands or O-rings on the target vessel(s).

Bleeding is often also controlled with a trial of IV vasopressin (Pitressin). Although vasopressin appears to stop variceal bleeding, it is also associated with serious systemic side effects, including hyponatremia, hypertension, cardiac arrhythmias, and decreased cardiac output.

A last resort may be balloon tamponade, a procedure that makes use of either a four-lumen Minnesota tube or a triple-lumen Sengstaken-Blakemore tube.

For long-term prevention of recurrent bleeding, a portal-systemic shunt may be used to divert esophageal blood from the portal circulation to the systemic circulation. Because operative morbidity and mortality are high in patients with end-stage liver disease and active variceal bleeding, this type of surgery is most useful as a long-term measure and may not be appropriate in emergency situations. The new nonsurgical procedure, transjugular intrahepatic portosystemic shunt (TIPS), is being used for control and prevention of esophageal variceal bleeding. Because this procedure stops bleeding quickly, it is becoming more common.

Overall prognosis for patients with acute variceal bleeding is poor. Approximately one third die during initial hospitalization, one third within the first 6 weeks after hemorrhage, and one third during the first year after bleeding.

Tumors

The esophagus may develop benign or cancerous tumors. The most common cancer type is squamous cell carcinoma. Adenocarcinoma occurs about 5% of the time in patients with Barrett's esophagus. Chronic irritation of the esophageal mucosa caused by caustic ingestion, chronic or persistent reflux, or excessive smoking or drinking may predispose a patient to esophageal cancer.

The most common indications of an esophageal tumor are dysphagia and odynophagia. A steady pain may be located substernally or occasionally in the back. Other symptoms may include anorexia and weight loss, anemia, hoarseness, and cough. Blood loss is usually slow and steady rather than by acute hemorrhage. The primary diagnostic method is direct-vision esophagogastroduodenoscopy (EGD) with a tissue biopsy and/or cytological examination. By the time the diagnosis is made, esophageal tumors are usually large.

The overall survival rate for patients with esophageal tumors is only 3%. Because cure is uncommon, surgery is primarily palliative and is intended to restore normal swallowing. Surgical procedures include excision and reconstruction or bypass. Endoscopic prosthetic intubation is another alternative. Radiation therapy or endoscopic laser therapy such as photodynamic therapy (PDT) may be recommended for advanced, untreatable tumors. A patient with an obstructing tumor may need dilatation or stent placement to allow limited oral nutrition and to relieve symptoms. If surgery is impossible and palliative care is unsuccessful, a gastrostomy may be initiated to bypass the esophagus and allow the patient to be fed directly into the stomach.

Psychological care is important for patients who undergo a gastrostomy or who have inoperable cancer or an esophageal obstruction. Such patients may experience feelings of grief and altered body image and should be encouraged to express them.

Diverticula

Diverticula are outpouchings of one or more layers of the esophageal wall; they probably result from esophageal motor abnormalities. Esophageal diverticula may occur immediately above the UES (Zenker's diverticulum), near the esophageal midpoint (traction diverticulum), immediately above the LES (epiphrenic diverticulum), or intramurally along the body of the esophagus (intramural diverticulosis).

Zenker's diverticulum

Zenker's diverticulum is associated with a dysfunctioning UES and is usually found in men over 50 years of age. Patients usually present with cervical dysphagia, halitosis, or aspiration pneumonia. Diagnosis is by barium swallow. Except in cases of recurrent disabling respiration pneumonia, the condition is left untreated. Patients may be encouraged to sleep with the head of the bed elevated on blocks and should not eat or drink within 3 to 4 hours of bedtime.

If surgical intervention is necessary in such cases small diverticula may be treated simply by cutting the cricopharyngeal muscle under local anesthesia (myotomy alone); by diverticulectomy; or in a two-stage operation involving both myotomy and diverticulectomy. Currently, the most common method is the one-stage diverticulectomy.

Complications of Zenker's diverticulum may include malnourishment caused by poor oral intake, aspiration pneumonia, or perforation of the diverticulum, leading to severe inflammation of the mediastinum with possibly fatal sequelae.

Traction diverticula

Traction diverticula may cause no signs or symptoms. They are commonly small and nonretentive, and they usually do not require therapy. Recent evidence suggests that they may be caused by esophageal motor dysfunction. Occasionally this underlying abnormality requires a long myotomy.

Epiphrenic diverticula

The patient with epiphrenic diverticula may regurgitate massive amounts of fluid, usually at night when lying down. Incoordination between esophageal contraction and LES relaxation may be the cause of this abnormality. If surgical intervention is indicated, epiphrenic diverticula are best treated with removal and long myotomy.

Intramural diverticulosis

Intramural diverticulosis is characterized by numerous small intramural outpouchings that probably represent dilated ducts that come from submucosal glands and are often associated with a smooth stricture in the upper esophagus. In rare cases, a Candida infection is present. Intramural diverticulosis generally responds to dilatation of the stricture.

Strictures

An esophageal **stricture** is an abnormal formation of white fibrous tissue that is usually at the lower end of the esophagus and may or may not be circumferential. Esophageal strictures are common complications of caustic injuries or may be the result of candidiasis or of prolonged and severe reflux. Progressive dysphagia is the most common clinical feature. To exclude malignancy as the cause of the stricture, endoscopic examination with multiple biopsies and a brush exfoliative cytological examination is mandatory.

In treatment of a stricture, the physician may use weighted tungsten or mercury-filled bougies, also known as Maloney or Hurst dilators; pneumatic balloon dilators; or graduated plastic Savary-Gilliard or American dilators. Many patients require follow-up with further dilatation at variable intervals, but this is easily accomplished. A long, narrow stricture is seen more often in children and may be treated surgically by colon interposition.

Perforation is the primary complication of dilatation. The most common symptom of esophageal perforation is persistent pain after dilatation; even mild pain is abnormal, although minor bleeding is common. Bacteremia, another complication, is a serious problem only in immunocompromised patients.

Rings and webs

Esophageal rings and webs are thin, circumferential, mucosal shelves within the esophagus. Webs consist of mucosa and submucosa, whereas rings, which are usually thicker than webs, consist of mucosa and muscle. Webs generally appear in the upper esophagus; rings usually arise in the lower esophagus at the gastroesophageal junction.

Esophageal webs often present as intermittent dysphagia. Although endoscopic examination can provide the diagnosis, it usually ruptures the web. If the obstruction remains after an endoscopy, bougienage with Maloney dilators may be used. In rare cases a patient may require dilatation with a pneumatic balloon. If symptoms recur, further dilatation may be necessary.

The association of a cervical esophageal web and iron deficiency anemia in middle-age women is known as Paterson-Kelly or Plummer-Vinson syndrome. In these patients the webs seem to regress spontaneously with treatment of the iron-deficiency anemia. This syndrome is also associated with an increased incidence of postcricoid carcinoma.

Lower esophageal rings, also known as **Schatzki's ring** or B-rings, are thin, concentric membranes located at the esophagogastric junction. Rings are more likely to cause symptoms than are esophageal webs. A characteristic symptom is episodic dysphagia, or food impaction, which is often related to eating rapidly. Diagnosis is by barium swallow; endoscopic investigation may also be needed to rule out the presence of a peptic stricture. To relieve symptoms, patients may need one or two esophageal bougienages with a large Maloney dilator. Occasionally, pneumatic dilatation is required.

Foreign bodies

The esophagus is the most common site of acute foreign-body obstruction. The majority of foreign-body ingestions occur in children, with coins being the most frequently ingested object. In adults, the most frequently observed foreign body is meat. Eighty to ninety percent of ingested foreign bodies pass spontaneously from the esophagus into the stomach and through the GI tract.

Patients with an acute esophageal obstruction usually experience local pain, dysphagia, or odynophagia. Plain x-ray films may be ordered to provide information on the location and size of the obstruction if the object is radiopaque. If barium x-ray films are used to visualize an obstruction, it is important to be aware of the danger that the patient may aspirate the barium.

Larger foreign bodies tend to lodge at the gastroesophageal junction. Once objects enter the stomach, most will pass uneventfully.

The treatment method used to remove the obstruction depends on the type of foreign body and the etiology of the obstruction.

1. Pharmacological agents, such as sublingual nitroglycerin or IV glucagon, may be used to relax the LES and allow passage of the item for adults.
2. Endoscopy may be used to extract the foreign body by using a snare or basket, or the object may be crushed and then pushed into the stomach. Elongated forceps are used to extract coins that have been swallowed by pediatric patients.
3. Surgery may be indicated for large or long objects that do not clear the stomach in 3 to 5 days, for sharp objects,

for bags of illegal narcotics, or when there is perforation or bleeding.

Meat boluses have been dissolved enzymatically using papain. However, the use of papain may be associated with esophageal perforation or pulmonary aspiration and is not recommended.

For pediatric patients, chronic foreign body presents itself as a recurrent cough or abdominal pain.

Potential complications of foreign-body esophageal obstructions include esophageal perforation or penetration of the aorta or its branches, followed by hemorrhage. The risk of perforation can be minimized by the use of overtubes and hoods that cover the object as it is being withdrawn.

It is not uncommon for children to ingest small alkaline batteries, such as those found in electronic equipment. Such batteries must be retrieved as soon as possible and any signs of perforation should be treated surgically, because local corrosive effects may be fatal.

If a pill is swallowed with little or no fluid intake when the patient is in a supine position or just before going to bed, it can remain in the esophagus, thus eroding the esophageal tissue and causing an ulcer. Medications known to damage the esophagus include doxycycline, tetracycline, clindamycin, potassium chloride, ferrous sulfate, quinidine, aspirin, nonsteroidal antiinflammatory drugs (NSAIDs) and Vitamin A. Treatment involves stopping medication, relieving odynophagia, providing adequate nutrition, and watching for complications. In 3 to 6 weeks, the patient's symptoms should be relieved.

Infectious diseases

Viruses, bacteria, fungi, and mycobacteria can all cause esophageal infection. The most common causes are *Candida*, herpes simplex virus, and cytomegalovirus (CMV). Infection of the esophagus is more commonly found in patients who have an underlying disease that compromises the immune system.

Esophageal candidiasis

Esophageal **candidiasis** rarely develops in patients who do not have an underlying disease, such as diabetes, immune deficiency, or malignancy. The main symptoms of esophageal candidiasis are dysphagia and odynophagia. Severe infection can destroy esophageal innervation, thus causing abnormal motility. Serious complications include hemorrhage, yeast dissemination, and, rarely, perforation. Esophagitis may be diagnosed on barium swallow, but a specific diagnosis of candidiasis is not possible using radiographic studies. An endoscopy will reveal whitish plaques with a normal mucosal pattern between the plaques. Definitive diagnosis is by demonstration of mycelial forms in tissue samples obtained from a biopsy or cytology brushings. Therapy consists of a trial of nystatin suspended in water or mixed in methyl cellulose. More severe infections may respond to ketoconazole (Nizoral) or amphotericin B (Fungi-zone).

Herpetic esophagitis

Predisposing factors to herpetic esophagitis include lymphoma, leukemia, or any immunocompromised state. Separate ulcers or shallow plaques are visible on endoscopy. Diagnosis is by virus tissue culture or by characteristic cellular changes on cytology or biopsy.

Crohn's esophagitis

Crohn's disease can produce inflammation anywhere in the GI tract. Inflammation isolated to the esophagus can occur, but is usually associated with disease elsewhere in the GI tract.

CMV esophagitis

CMV esophagitis may appear as a spectrum of lesions in the esophagus ranging from superficial mucosal inflammation to giant ulcerations. Diagnosis may be made by double contrast barium swallow, or by endoscopy. Esophageal biopsy should be performed and sent for viral culture and brushing sent for stain to detect infected cells. Symptomatic relief of CMV esophagitis can be achieved by using viscous lidocaine, histamine2 blockers, sucralfate, or antacids. Ganciclovir has been reported to be effective in the treatment of CMV esophagitis; however, there are some reports of ganciclovir-resistant strains of CMV.

Eosinophilic Esophaphagitis

Esophagitis can occur secondary to eosinophilic gastroenteritis. This is an immune-mediated reaction characterized by excessive histamine production and mast cell degradation, usually found in the upper GI tract. Patients complain of dyspepsia symptoms. Apthous ulcers in the mouth are often associated with this disease. Diagnosis is made by eosinophil counts greater than 10 per high power field on microscopic examination of biopsies. Treatment usually consists of H1 and H2 blockers (Zantac and Atarax) and may also require mast cell stabilizers such as singular or gastrochrom.

HIV esophagitis

HIV esophagitis may be present in patients who are HIV-positive with complaints of odynophagia. Endoscopy with tissue cultures can differentiate between HIV and CMV ulcers. HIV esophagitis will respond dramatically to treatment with steroids.

Mallory-Weiss tears

A **Mallory-Weiss tear** is a mucosal tear at the gastroesophageal junction. It is associated with prolonged, forceful vomiting; trauma; childbirth; or complications of EGD. Patients who have a Mallory-Weiss tear often have a history of alcohol abuse. Typically, prolonged emesis, or dry heaves, is followed by vomiting of bright red blood. The amount of blood lost is usually small and these patients are generally treated conservatively, because bleeding stops spontaneously. Profuse bleeding may be controlled endoscopically with a coagulating contact probe.

Motility disorders

Esophageal motility disorders are primary if the etiology of the abnormality is unknown but the esophagus is the site of major involvement or secondary if the esophageal abnormalities are features of a more generalized disease process. Primary esophageal motility disorders include achalasia, diffuse esophageal spasm, and nutcracker esophagus.

Achalasia

Achalasia is a combined defect of a peristalsis of the esophageal body and elevated LES pressure. Patients with achalasia present with dysphagia to solids and liquids, regurgitation, and weight loss. Diagnostic evaluation procedures may include a radiographic examination, manometric study, and EGD. On x-ray films the esophagus appears dilated, with a narrow "bird beak" at the distal end. Microscopically, a loss of nonargyrophilic ganglion cells in the myenteric plexus is evident.

Symptoms may be relieved by eating slowly, chewing well, drinking fluids with meals, and sitting up while eating. Many patients benefit from pneumatic balloon dilatation. A cardiomyotomy (Heller's operation) may be performed to reduce LES pressure in patients who experience unsuccessful treatment with pneumatic dilatation or who are poor candidates for dilatation. In patients who are not considered suitable for dilatation or surgery, long-acting nitrates such as sublingual isosorbide dinitrate (Isordil), or calcium channel blockers such as nifedipine (Adalat), may be used to reduce LES pressure. Until recently, these conventional treatments have been the only ones available to patients. The use of botulinum toxin is expected to provide a safe, alternative therapy for treatment of achalasia. Botulinum toxin is injected into the four quadrants of the LES using a sclerotherapy needle. The toxin acts as a paralytic agent, thereby reducing the LES pressure.

Complications of achalasia are related to retention and stasis in the esophagus. Esophagitis may be evident endoscopically. Aspiration of esophageal contents is a danger and may be followed by bronchopneumonia. The prevalence of esophageal carcinoma is higher than normal in achalasia patients, possibly because it may be precipitated by stasis and mucosal irritation. Regular follow-up care is recommended.

Diffuse esophageal spasm

Diffuse esophageal spasm (DES) is a motility disorder of unknown cause and pathophysiology. It is defined manometrically as repetitive or prolonged simultaneous contractions (nonperistaltic esophageal contractions that occur all at once up and down the length of the esophagus, independent of pharyngeal contractions) with intermittent normal peristalsis. One symptom may be noncardiac substernal chest pain, which may be severe and may closely mimic angina pectoris. Dysphagia may be present with both solids and liquids and is most severe when the patient ingests extremely hot or cold foods. In most cases, the distal two thirds of the esophagus show muscular thickening.

A barium swallow may show isolated, uncoordinated movements of the lower two thirds of the esophagus. The entire two thirds of the esophagus may contract as a unit, propelling barium both retrograde and into the stomach. Manometric examinations may reveal a simultaneous high-amplitude, abnormally long contraction in the lower two thirds of the esophagus.

DES may be relieved by pharmacological therapy with anticholinergics, nitrates, smooth muscle relaxants such as hydralazine, or calcium channel blockers such as nifedipine (Adalat) or verapamil. When the condition is severe and unresponsive, dilatation may be used to relieve symptoms. Some patients benefit from a long esophagomyotomy, which involves cutting the esophageal muscles to prevent peristalsis.

Nutcracker esophagus

Nutcracker esophagus, also known as symptomatic esophageal peristalsis, is the most common manometric disorder in patients presenting with noncardiac chest pain. Nutcracker esophagus is defined manometrically as peristalsis with a contractile amplitude that is two to three times the normal value. If treatment is necessary, pharmacological therapy may be tried, as described for DES.

Caustic injury

Accidental or suicidal ingestion of highly alkaline or acid compounds may result in injury to the esophagus. The most common symptom is odynophagia, but patients may also complain of dysphagia and chest pain or they may drool profusely. Prognosis depends on the depth and extent of injury. Esophageal burns may be classified as one of the following, according to Holiger's classification:

Clinical staging of esophageal burns

(a) first-degree hyperemia and edema of the mucosa; damage limited to the mucosa;

(b) second-degree exudate, erosions, shallow ulcers destructive of the mucosa and submucosa with penetration of the injury into the muscle layers;

(c) third-degree deep ulceration, circumferential necrosis, often presence of a black coagulum; and full-thickness injury with extension into the pleura and mediastinum.

Alkaline compounds, such as lye, drain cleaners, and bleaches, typically cause more damage than acidic compounds, such as toilet bowl cleaners, soldering fluxes, and battery fluids. In the case of acid ingestion, the physician may order large volumes of milk or water to dilute the acid.

Diagnostic evaluation of caustic injuries involves determining the nature of the ingested agent; radiographic examinations of the neck, chest, and abdomen to exclude perforation or pneumonia; and endoscopic examination to document the extent of injury, unless there is evidence of a perforation or extensive necrosis. Because tissue damage is usually not immediately evident, endoscopy is usually delayed for 12 to 24 hours after the ingestion. This allows the endoscopist to fully assess the extent of injury. Once an area of severe damage is visualized, the endoscopist may choose to discontinue the procedure to reduce the risk of perforation.

Treatment following caustic injury depends on the extent of the injury, but patients should always be kept NPO. Vital functions should be supported as needed, and intake and output should be carefully documented. To maintain the esophageal lumen and gastric access, a nasogastric tube should be placed. If the patient shows evidence of laryngeal involvement or respiratory difficulties, endotracheal intubation or tracheostomy may be required. The physician may also order parenteral corticosteroids and broad-spectrum antibiotics, but this type of treatment is controversial. Dilatation may be required for second-degree injury, and surgery is indicated for patients who deteriorate despite intensive medical management.

Complications of caustic ingestion may include formation of strictures or squamous cell carcinoma.

Barrett's esophagus

Barrett's esophagus is defined as epithelial metaplasia in which normal squamous epithelium is replaced by one or more of the following types of columnar epithelium: a distinctive, specialized columnar epithelium; a junctional type of epithelium; and/or a gastric fundus type of epithelium. Barrett's esophagus occurs in up to 20% of patients with chronic esophageal reflux.

Diagnosis of Barrett's esophagus is by endoscopic visualization of the mucosa, supported by examination of tissue biopsy. There is no effective medical or surgical treatment for Barrett's esophagus. Treatment is directed at the underlying reflux esophagitis and may include stricture dilatation.

The prevalence of adenocarcinoma in patients with Barrett's esophagus has been reported to be about 30 to 50 times that of the general population. Although the actual frequency with which dysplasia progresses to cancer is not known, some endoscopists continue to recommend annual screening with endoscopy and biopsy to identify early neoplastic changes.

Congenital defects

In embryonic development, the esophagus and trachea begin as one tube. If the two do not separate completely, or if they retain a communication channel, atresia and/or a fistula may develop. The most common abnormality is a tracheoesophageal **fistula**, in which the esophagus closes to form a blind sac **(atresia)** and either the upper or lower esophagus links with the trachea through a fistula (a tube-like passage between the two cavities). In another type of tracheoesophageal fistula, a normal trachea and esophagus attach to form an H-type fistula.

These anomalies become apparent shortly after birth when the infant regurgitates mucus and fluid. Atresia without tracheal involvement causes cyanotic coughing or other signs of aspiration during feeding. Fistulas may be located by cinematoradiography, which is performed during feeding.

To ensure the infant's survival, prompt surgical closure of the fistula at the communication point and anastomosis to correct atresia are required. As the child grows, stricturing of the esophageal anastomosis may occur and may result in reflux problems with respiratory involvement but can be resolved with simple dilatation.

Fistulas in adults

Bronchoesophageal or tracheoesophageal fistulas in adults are usually caused by cancer but may also be caused by a benign inflammatory process or trauma. Symptoms include chronic cough, fever, and recurrent pulmonary infections, with or without dysphagia. Diagnosis is by barium swallow. The treatment of choice for a benign fistula is surgery to remove necrotic and irreversibly damaged tissue and to close the fistula. Fistulas related to cancer cause acute episodes of coughing after eating. Surgical procedures are purely palliative in such cases.

Aortoesophageal fistulas may develop if an ingested foreign object lodges in the region above the aortic arch or if a tumor extends through the wall of the esophagus. Minor bleeding usually occurs as erosion connects the aorta and esophagus. Massive bleeding may begin at any time and almost always causes death.

CASE SITUATION

Doris Johnson is a 51-year-old woman who lives with her husband and four grown, unmarried sons on a large dairy farm in Wisconsin. For the past 4 years Mrs. Johnson has been experiencing increasing amounts of retrosternal discomfort or a burning sensation shortly after eating or on sudden bending. Recently, the discomfort, described as "heartburn," has progressed to a painful ache that radiates to her neck, shoulders, and upper arms. Because both gallbladder and coronary artery disease are in her family history, Mrs. Johnson has become concerned enough to seek medical assistance. Her physician has made a tentative diagnosis of esophageal reflux and has referred her for diagnostic workup before prescribing treatment.

Mrs. Johnson is 5'7" tall and weighs 186 pounds. Her admitting vital signs are as follows: blood pressure 170/90; pulse 90; respiration 22; temperature 99.2° F. She denies use of all habit-forming substances, including tobacco, although she admits she may have a small amount of alcohol on festive occasions. She takes no prescribed drugs regularly, but she has used an antacid to help the "burning" sensation. She is scheduled for a complete cardiac workup, barium swallow, esophageal function studies, and an EGD.

Points to think about

1. Mrs. Johnson comes to the endoscopy unit for her EGD. Besides the information on the normal assessment form, what other information would be helpful to the gastroenterology nurse?

2. What finding during EGD would help make Mrs. Johnson's diagnosis?
3. What nursing diagnosis would fit this case?
4. How might a nurse assist Mrs. Johnson in managing the stress associated with EGD?
5. What can the nurse teach Mrs. Johnson?

Suggested responses

1. Additional data about Mrs. Johnson that might be helpful would include:
   (a) whether the other studies in her recent workup were normal, including cardiac workup and upper GI studies;
   (b) whether Mrs. Johnson is currently taking any medications other than the antacid; whether she is allergic to any medications; the effectiveness of the antacid she is using, length and frequency of use, and name of drug;
   (c) the presence of symptoms specific to reflux, such as regurgitation, dysphagia, or odynophagia; duration, time, and other factors associated with discomfort/pain episodes (e.g., eating, bending over, exercise, tight clothing, pregnancy, sleeping)

2. A finding of gross esophagitis would give a definitive diagnosis of esophageal reflux; however, 40% of symptomatic patients may not have this finding with endoscopic examination.

3. An appropriate nursing diagnosis might be "altered nutrition: more than body requirements, related to caloric intake exceeding metabolic need." It is important to note that excessive weight gain can increase intraabdominal pressure and exacerbate reflux. Furthermore, eating the wrong foods can add calories, decrease LES tone, exacerbate pain, and increase gastric acid secretion rate. If a full nutritional assessment seems warranted, an appropriate referral should be provided.

4. Measures by which a nurse can help Mrs. Johnson manage stress during EGD might include:
   (a) reiteration of the procedural process, focusing on Mrs. Johnson's questions and concerns;
   (b) reexplanation of the method and type of anesthetic to be used, rationale for its use, its duration, and related postprocedural nursing precautions and measures;
   (c) periodic reassurance before and during the procedure that she will be able to breathe normally
   (d) teaching and practicing basic muscle relaxation techniques so that she can recognize tense muscles and relax them voluntarily or on request during the procedure
   (e) reassurance that salivary secretion can be managed and an explanation of how this is accomplished without swallowing or speaking; and
   (f) assignment of a nurse who can support Mrs. Johnson throughout the procedure both verbally and through touch.

5. To be sure that Mrs. Johnson has adequate knowledge about her condition and proposed treatment, the gastroenterology nurse might:

(a) use anatomical drawings to describe the physical process involved, such as LES area, hiatal hernia, location of inflammation, or strictures;
(b) explain how to use gravity to decrease reflux, by not lying down after meals and elevating the head of the bed on 6-inch blocks to decrease acid reflux at night;
(c) explain the medications the physician has prescribed for this problem, how they work, when to take them, and any side effects to watch for;
(d) review any medications Mrs. Johnson is already taking to avoid those that are potentially harmful to this condition (e.g., anticholinergics, sedatives, tranquilizers, theophylline, calcium channel blockers);
(e) explain dietary modifications that may be helpful;
(f) suggest other lifestyle modifications that may be helpful, such as cessation of smoking (cigarette smoking reduces LES tone); avoidance of clothing that is tight around the abdomen; if overweight, initiation of a supervised diet; use of proper body mechanics to avoid bending;
(g) advise Mrs. Johnson that chronic irritation of the esophagus can lead to complications, such as ulceration, stricture formation, Barrett's esophagus, and pulmonary problems; and
(h) encourage her to follow the prescribed treatment regimen carefully and to seek follow-up care

REVIEW TERMS

achalasia, atresia, Barrett's esophagus, candidiasis, diaphragmatic hiatus, diffuse esophageal spasm (DES), diverticula, dyspepsia, dysphagia, esophageal rings and webs, esophagitis, esophagus, fistula, gastroesophageal reflux, heartburn, lower esophageal sphincter (LES), Mallory-Weiss tear, nutcracker esophagus, odynophagia, peristalsis, regurgitation, Schatzki's rings, stricture, upper esophageal sphincter (UES), varices

REVIEW QUESTIONS

1. In adults, the approximate length of the esophagus is:
   (a) 15 cm.
   (b) 25 cm.
   (c) 35 cm.
   (d) 45 cm.
2. The outermost layer of the esophagus is made up of:
   (a) Mucosa.
   (b) Submucosa.
   (c) Muscularis.
   (d) Serosa.
3. The progressive circular muscle contraction initiated by esophageal distention is known as:
   (a) Achalasia.
   (b) Diffuse esophageal spasm.
   (c) Primary peristalsis.
   (d) Secondary peristalsis.

4. The first step in the treatment of esophageal reflux disease is:
   - (a) Behavior modification.
   - (b) Drug therapy.
   - (c) Dilatation.
   - (d) Antireflux surgery.

5. Life-threatening bleeding is a frequent complication of:
   - (a) Esophageal varices.
   - (b) Esophageal reflux.
   - (c) Esophageal tumors.
   - (d) Zenker's diverticulum.

6. Outpouchings of the esophageal wall located immediately above the lower esophageal sphincter are known as:
   - (a) Zenker's diverticula.
   - (b) Traction diverticula.
   - (c) Epiphrenic diverticula.
   - (d) Intramural diverticulosis.

7. The most frequently observed foreign-body obstructions in the esophagus of adults are:
   - (a) Coins.
   - (b) Pieces of bone.
   - (c) Hard candy.
   - (d) Pieces of meat.

8. The infectious disease found most often in the esophagus is:
   - (a) Cytomegalovirus.
   - (b) Herpes simplex virus.
   - (c) Candidiasis.
   - (d) Giardiasis.

9. A patient's radiographic examinations show a dilated esophageal body with a narrow "bird beak" at the end. The most likely diagnosis is:
   - (a) Achalasia.
   - (b) Diffuse esophageal spasm.
   - (c) Nutcracker esophagus.
   - (d) Caustic ingestion.

10. Esophageal fistulas in adults are most often caused by:
    - (a) Trauma.
    - (b) Foreign-body obstruction.
    - (c) Cancer.
    - (d) Congenital defects.

BIBLIOGRAPHY

Angelucci, P. (1995). TIPS for controlling bleeding. *Nursing 95 25,* 43.

Bongiovanni, G., (Ed) (1988). *Essentials of clinical gastroenterology* (2nd ed.), New York: McGraw-Hill.

Brady, P. (1994). Management of esophageal and gastric foreign bodies: Clinical Update. *ASGE 2(1),* 1-4. American Society for Gastrointestinal Endoscopy.

Casteel, D. & Richter, J. (2002). The Esophagus (2nd ed.). Philadelphia, Pennsylvania: Lippincott.

Cote, D. & Amedee, R. (1995). Zenker's diverticulum. *Otolaryngol Head Neck Surg Rep 144,.*

DeVault, K. (1996). Current management of gastroesophageal reflux disease. *Gastroenterol 4(1),* 24-32.

Dunitz, M. & Bloom, S. (Eds.) (2002). *Practical gastroenterology.* Florence, KY: Taylor & Francis.

Durkin, S. (1999). Photodynamic therapy: a cancer treatment for the 21st century. *Gastroenterology Nursing 22(3),* 115-20.

Foglia, R. (1994). Esophageal disease in the pediatric age group. *Chest Surg Clin North Am 4(4),* 785-809. Chest Surgical Clinic of North America.

Fox, D. & Bignall, S. (1996). Management of gastro-oesophageal reflux. *Paediatr Nurs 8(1),* 17-20. Paediatric Nursing.

Hyman, P. (1994). Gastroesophageal reflux: one reason why baby won't eat. *J Pediatr 125(6),* S103-S109. The Journal of Pediatrics.

Levine, M. (1995). Role of the double-contrast upper gastrointestinal series in the 1990s. *Gastroenterol Clin North Am 24(2),* 289-308. Gastroenterology Clinics of North America.

Ogilvie, J. (1995). Botulinum toxin: a new therapeutic use. *Gastroenterol Nurs 18(3),* 92-95.

Peters, J. (1996). Laparoscopic surgery for the treatment of gastroesophageal reflux disease (article 2 in the series). *Pract Gastroenterol 20(3),* 8. Practical Gastroenterology.

Robinson, M. & Garnett, W. (1996). Marketing heartburn relief: evolution in the treatment of heartburn and gastroesophageal reflux disease and its impact on patients and physicians. *Pract Gastroenterol 20(8),* 36-42.

Sleisenger, M. & Fordtran, J. (Eds.) (2002). *Gastrointestinal disease: pathophysiology, diagnosis, management* (7th ed.). Philadelphia: W.B. Saunders.

Smeltzer, S.C. & Bare, B.G. (2002). *Textbook of medical-surgical nursing* (9th ed.). Philadelphia, Pennsylvania: Lippincott.

Torbey, C. & Richter, J. (1995). Gastrointestinal motility disorders in pregnancy. *Semin Gastrointest Dis 6(4),* 203-16, Seminars in Gastrointestinal Disease.

Walker, W.A., Durie, P., Hamilton, J.R., Watkins, J.B. and Walker-Smith, J.A. (2000). *Pediatric gastrointestinal disease: pathophysiology, diagnosis, management* (3rd ed.). Ontario, Canada: Decker.

Wells, S. (1995). Gastroesophageal reflux: the use of pH monitoring. *Curr Probl Surg 30(6),* 431-558. Current Problems in Surgery.

Chapter 14

STOMACH

This chapter will acquaint the gastroenterology nurse with the normal anatomy and physiology of the stomach. The symptoms, diagnosis, and treatment options for selected gastric ailments will be reviewed.

Learning objectives

After reviewing the content of this chapter, the gastroenterology nurse should be able to:

1. Describe the anatomy of the stomach, including both macroanatomy and microanatomy.
2. Explain the normal motor and secretory functions of the stomach.
3. Discuss the pathophysiology, diagnosis, and treatment of certain pathological conditions that affect the stomach, including peptic ulcer disease, cancer, gastritis, and *Helicobacter pylori* infection.

ANATOMY AND PHYSIOLOGY

The stomach has several important physiological purposes. Through a complex combination of exocrine secretory mechanisms and smooth muscle contraction and relaxation, the stomach maintains relatively low levels of microbes in the upper digestive tract; digests food and prepares nutrients for absorption; serves as a reservoir for swallowed food, drink, and digestive secretions; mixes and delivers chyme to the small intestine for further digestion and absorption; and originates signals for hunger and satiety.

The stomach is a J-shaped, distensible organ located just below the diaphragm, between the esophagus and the duodenum (see Fig. 13-2). It is approximately 25 to 30 cm (10 to 12 inches) long and 10 to 15 cm (4 to 6 inches) wide at its widest point. The portion of the stomach that immediately adjoins the esophagus is the **cardia**. The gastric **fundus** is the dome-shaped part of the stomach that extends to the left above the cardia. Below the fundus is the gastric **body**, which extends to the incisura angularis, a notchlike indenta-

tion located on the upper lateral border of the stomach. Below the incisura angularis and extending to the narrow, tubular pylorus is the **antrum**. The upper lateral border of the stomach is called the **lesser curvature**, and the lower lateral border is called the **greater curvature** (Fig. 14-1).

The entry of food into the stomach is controlled by the lower esophageal sphincter (LES), or cardiac sphincter, which comprises a group of thickened circular muscles at the distal end of the esophagus. The LES regulates the opening and closing of the esophageal lumen. At the distal end of the stomach is the **pylorus**, which has a thick, muscular wall that forms the **pyloric sphincter**. The pyloric sphincter controls the movement of stomach contents into the duodenum.

The stomach wall consists of the following four layers: an outer serosa, a three-tiered muscular layer (muscularis propria), a submucosa, and mucosa. The outer serous layer of visceral peritoneum that covers the exterior of the stomach includes both the **greater omentum**, which hangs in a double layer from the greater curvature over the anterior side of the abdominal viscera, and the **lesser omentum**, which connects the lesser curvature to the underside of the liver.

The muscularis propria consists of an outer layer of longitudinal muscle fibers, a middle layer of circular smooth muscle fibers, and an inner layer of transverse fibers. These three muscle layers contract to produce the peristaltic motion of the stomach while it churns and compresses the food during digestion.

Below the muscular layers of the stomach lies the submucosa. The submucosa is composed mainly of areolar connective tissue. It contains the blood vessels, *lymphatics*, and nerves.

The gastric mucosa lines the interior of the stomach. When it is not filled, the stomach interior has a series of wrinkled ridges called **rugae**. The rugae allow the stomach to distend to hold a large quantity of food without any substantial

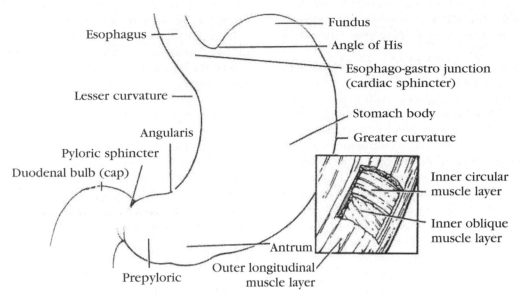

Fig. 14-1. Gastric anatomy. Insert shows muscular layers of stomach.

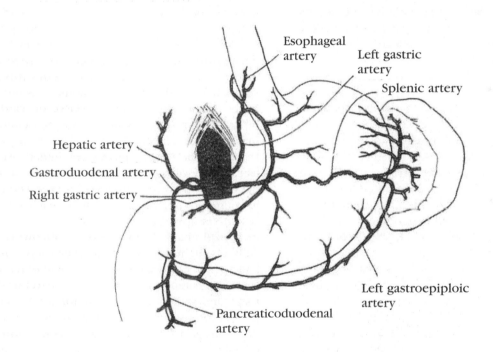

Fig. 14-2. Blood supply of the stomach and duodenum. (From Price SA, Wilson LM: *Pathophysiology: clinical concepts of disease processes*, ed 4, St. Louis, 1992, Mosby.)

increase in pressure, thus helping to control the rate at which food enters the duodenum. The gastric mucosa contains several types of epithelial cells.

The stomach receives arterial blood from the celiac axis, which sends branches to the lesser and greater curvatures. Along the lesser curvature the left gastric artery flows down from the cardia. At this point it joins with the right gastric artery, which is a branch of the hepatic artery. The greater curvature receives blood from the gastroepiploic artery, which runs from the fundus to the pylorus. In addition, short gastric arteries derived from the splenic artery supply blood to the fundus of the stomach (Fig. 14-2). Blood is drained from the stomach via the portal vein. The greater curvature is drained by the right and left gastroepiploic veins, and the lesser curvature is drained by both the right gastric vein and the coronary vein.

Parasympathetic innervation of the stomach is via the vagus nerve. Over the lower esophagus, the vagus nerves split. The anterior vagus divides into anterior gastric and hepatic branches. The posterior vagus also divides into two branches, one that supplies the posterior wall of the fundus and the body of the stomach, and another that supplies the posterior wall of the antrum. Vagal innervation to the body and fundus primarily stimulates acid secretion, whereas vagal innervation to the antrum primarily stimulates motility.

Sympathetic innervation of the stomach is derived from the greater splanchnic nerves and the celiac ganglia. The afferent fibers conduct visceral gastric pain impulses, and the efferent fibers inhibit gastric secretion and motility. Intrinsic innervation of the stomach involves Auerbach's and Meissner's plexuses. Auerbach's plexus influences gastric motility, and Meissner's plexus is believed to be involved in gastrin release.

The primary function of the stomach is to initiate digestion by using both chemical secretions and mechanical movements. Gastric secretions also promote the absorption of vitamin B_{12}. In addition, the stomach serves as a reservoir for ingested food and liquid and regulates their entry into the duodenum.

Secretion

The mucosa contains three types of glands, which differ from one region of the stomach to another. **Cardiac glands** are located just distal to the esophagogastric junction. These glands secrete mucus and pepsinogens, which are converted by hydrochloric acid to pepsin.

The proximal two thirds of the stomach is the **oxyntic gland** area. At least four types of cells have been identified in these glands: zymogen or **chief cells**, oxyntic (parietal) cells, mucous neck cells, and endocrine or endocrine-like cells. **Parietal cells** secrete hydrochloric acid and intrinsic factor, which is a glycoprotein necessary for the absorption of vitamin B_{12}. The chief cells secrete pepsinogens.

The antrum and pylorus contain the **pyloric glands**; these glands contain mucous cells, which secrete mucus and pepsinogens, and **G cells**, which secrete gastrin. The pyloric and oxyntic glands also have **enterochromaffin cells**, which secrete serotonin. In addition, the cardiac, oxyntic, and pyloric glandular mucosae contain at least nine different types of endocrine cells, which secrete hormonal products such as somatostatin and glucagon. In addition, the parietal and pyloric glands both secrete bicarbonate.

When the stomach is at rest, normal secretions occur at a rate of about 0.5 ml/min. With food in the stomach, secretions increase to about 3 ml/min. The stomach secretes approximately 1500 to 3000 ml of gastric juice daily.

Motility

The movements of the stomach serve the following two functions: mixing and grinding of food, which takes place in the distal areas; and the controlled emptying of the gastric contents into the duodenum.

The peristaltic movement of the stomach combines each bolus of food with a mixture of digestive juices to form a relatively homogeneous, semiliquid mass called **chyme**. Normally, peristalsis moves the chyme slowly toward the pylorus at a rate of about three waves per minute, as regulated by a small region in the middle of the gastric body

known as the gastric pacemaker. Before the chyme is ready to enter the duodenum, it must be of the proper consistency and acidity and the duodenum must be receptive. When these conditions are present, antral peristaltic contractions force the chyme through the pyloric sphincter and into the duodenum.

Only a portion of the chyme that is advanced toward the pylorus actually moves through the pyloric sphincter and into the duodenum. The rest is propelled backward, colliding with and further breaking down larger food particles in the antrum and body. Normally, particles passing into the duodenum have a diameter of 1 mm or less.

The gastric emptying rate is controlled by neural impulses, by the composition of the chyme, and by hormones secreted by the small intestine.

PATHOPHYSIOLOGY

Pathological conditions that are frequently seen in the stomach include ulcer disease, cancer, and gastritis. Other important gastric disorders include hiatal hernia, gastric outlet obstruction, congenital anomalies, gastric motor disorders, and bezoars.

Acid-peptic disorders

When the normal balance between factors that promote mucosal injury (e.g., gastric acid, pepsin, bile acids, ingested substances) and those that protect the mucosa (e.g., an intact epithelium, mucus, bicarbonate secretion) is upset, inflammation or **ulcers** may arise. The unique causal event may be mechanical, chemical, infectious, or ischemic in nature. In the case of **gastric ulcers**, a variety of irritants can initially disrupt the gastric mucosa. In some patients, decreased pyloric sphincter pressure may permit an increased reflux of duodenal material into the stomach, which disrupts the gastric mucosal barrier and leads to an increased back-diffusion of acid into the mucosa. Subsequent histamine release may cause mucosal damage and edema. Continued erosion may damage mucosal capillaries and submucosal blood vessels, thus leading to hemorrhage and shock. If erosion continues through the serosa, perforation and peritonitis may result.

Typical risk factors for gastric ulcer disease include the following:

(a) **Helicobacter pylori (H. pylori)** infection;
(b) chronic use of salicylates or nonsteroidal antiinflammatory drugs (NSAIDs), such as indomethacin or ibuprofen;
(c) family history of gastric ulcers; and
(d) cigarette smoking.

The roles which stress and personality type play in the development of gastric ulcers remain controversial.

Most patients with peptic ulcer disease have abdominal pain. However, the sensitivity and specificity of abdominal pain as a marker for gastric ulcer are low. In a large survey of patients in a dyspepsia clinic, abdominal pain occurred in 94% of patients with an ulcer but was also present in 82% of patients without ulcers. In general, gastric ulcer symptoms include abdominal pain that is localized to the epigastrium and does not radiate. It is most often described as having a burning quality. The most discriminating symptom, although inexact, is the presence of pain that awakens the person from sleep.

Symptoms that mimic a gastric ulcer in patients who have no objective evidence of an ulcer are called *nonulcer dyspepsia*. *Dyspepsia* is a vague term that refers to epigastric discomfort, burning or pain, nausea, belching, and bloating.

To aid in the diagnosis of peptic ulcers, the provider may order an upper GI series or an esophagogastroduodenoscopy (EGD). Gastric acid secretion tests or serum gastrin levels may be ordered to determine the cause of existing peptic ulcers, but are not helpful in the actual diagnosis of an ulcer. An EGD is the procedure of choice for a patient with active bleeding. Prepyloric ulcers are invariably benign and best diagnosed endoscopically. Gastric ulcers are potentially malignant, and therefore multiple tissue biopsies are necessary to exclude the presence of cancer. A repeat EGD must be performed in 8 weeks to document gastric ulcer healing.

Complications of a peptic ulcer include hemorrhage, perforation, penetration, and obstruction. Hemorrhage, the most common complication, occurs in approximately 15% of ulcer patients, causing hematemesis and/or melenotic stool. In some cases, life-threatening hemorrhage is the first indication of an ulcer. Perforation is less common, occurring in about 7% of peptic ulcer patients. Gastric ulcers tend to perforate along the anterior wall of the lesser curvature of the stomach. Patients who have a perforation experience upper abdominal pain, guarding, rebound tenderness, and absent bowel sounds. Surgery is often required. Penetration is pathologically similar to perforation, except that the ulcer crater extends into an adjacent organ, most commonly the left lobe of the liver. Rarely, gastric ulcers can penetrate into the colon, resulting in a gastrocolic fistula. Symptoms may include back pain, night distress, changing epigastric pain, or pain that is refractory to agents that previously provided relief. Surgical intervention is often necessary. Gastric outlet obstruction can result from impaired antral motility caused by inflammation and edema of the ulcer or from obstruction caused by scarring at the gastroduodenal junction. Symptoms of obstruction include abdominal distention, tympany, succussion splash, vomiting, and early satiety. Vague abdominal pain and early satiety may be symptoms of a partial obstruction. Diagnosis is made by EGD or an upper GI series. Obstruction must be treated by decompressing the stomach using nasogastric aspiration, restoring fluid and electrolyte balance, and administering IV histamine2 (H$_2$) blockers. Surgery may be indicated if these therapies fail.

In general, treatment for nonmalignant gastric ulcers will be pharmacological. The effectiveness of diet manipulation in ulcer healing is unknown. Foods known to increase acid secretion include milk and milk products, alcoholic and caffeinated beverages, and decaffeinated coffee. Other than encouraging patients to avoid foods that cause symptoms, dietary restrictions are not generally applied.

Drug therapy for ulcer patients without *H. pylori* centers on the following agents:

1. Proton pump inhibitors (lansoprazole and omeprazole) are effective in decreasing gastric acid by inhibiting the enzyme responsible for completing the final step of acid secretion. The name of the enzyme is hydrogen-potassium adenosinetriphosphatase.

2. H$_2$ blockers, such as cimetidine (Tagamet), famotidine (Pepcid), or ranitidine (Zantac), reduce the amount of acid produced by the stomach by binding to the histamine receptor on parietal cells and blocking histamine-stimulated acid production.

3. Sucralfate (Carafate), a complex of aluminum hydroxide and sulfated sucrose, forms a protective gel at the site of disrupted mucosa, thus providing a protective covering for the ulcer.

4. Antacids act to neutralize gastric acid, strengthen the gastric mucosal barrier, and heighten the tone of the LES. Optimally, antacids should be taken 1 and 3 hours after meals and before sleep. Most antacids contain either magnesium hydroxide (Milk of Magnesia), aluminum hydroxide (Gaviscon), or calcium carbonate (Tums). They are not recommended for maintenance treatment of gastric ulcer disease.

5. Prostaglandins (Cytotec) have antisecretory and cytoprotective effects.

6. Investigational drugs include both tricyclic compounds, which block acid production by interfering with acetylcholine-stimulated acid secretion, and colloidal bismuth compounds, which act by coating the ulcer crater.

Surgery for benign peptic ulcer disease is rare since the advent of H$_2$ blocker medications. Emergency gastric surgery is only required for uncontrolled hemorrhage from a gastric ulcer. Surgical options include vagotomy with pyloroplasty, Billroth I (gastroduodenostomy and hemigastrectomy), Billroth II (gastrojejunostomy), total gastrectomy (esophagojejunostomy), or gastric resection (antrectomy). The complications of those surgeries include dumping syndrome, hypoglycemic symptoms, nutrient deficiency states, weight loss, diarrhea, and recurrent ulceration. In addition, the risk of gastric carcinoma may be increased after certain types of surgery for peptic ulcer disease.

Helicobacter pylori

In recent years, a strong link between the bacteria *H. pylori* and peptic ulcer disease has been identified. The association was noted in 1982 when Marshall and Warren cultured a gram-negative spiral rod-shaped bacterium. The bacterium was originally thought to be *Campylobacter*-like but later was named *Helicobacter pylori*. The bacterium has many flagella on one end and therefore is highly mobile. It has adapted to and avoids the acidic nature of the stomach by burrowing beneath the mucosa of the stomach and duodenum.

The transmission of *H. pylori* is thought to be via fecal-oral or oral-oral pathways. It is found in all parts of the world but is more prevalent in third-world countries and areas with overcrowding and poor sanitation. In the U.S., incidence is directly proportional to increased age.

Consequences of *H. pylori* infection include gastritis and gastric and duodenal ulcers. It is also noted that patients with *H. pylori* have a higher rate of gastric cancer. This point is currently being investigated.

Multiple methods of diagnosis are available. Serology for antibody or antigen detection and carbon 13 or 14 urease breath testing are noninvasive methods. Invasive tests include biopsy during endoscopy for either rapid urease testing or histology. Culture has been considered the gold standard but is usually prohibited by cost and time.

Treatment for *H. pylori* continues to be debated and is ever changing. Presently, treatment may be suggested in *H. pylori*-positive patients with *nonulcer dyspepsia*. The goal of treatment is eradication of the bacteria. Eradication is associated with decrease in duodenal ulcer recurrence from 90% in untreated individuals to 5% in successfully treated patients. Therapy involves a combination of drugs ranging from dual coverage to quadruple therapy (Table 14-1). Choice of therapy depends on compliance, effectiveness, and economic considerations.

Gastric cancer

Gastric cancer tends to be hereditary and occurs more frequently in individuals with type A blood and lower socioeconomic status. Its incidence is higher in blacks than in whites, in the northern United States than the southern United States, and in men as compared to women. The incidence of gastric cancer increases with age and among those who eat foods high in starch, nitrates, pickled vegetables, and salted fish and meat. Gastric ulcers, previous gastric surgery, achlorhydria, pernicious anemia, chronic atrophic gastritis, intestinal metaplasia, and **adenomatous polyps** may also increase the risk of gastric cancer. As noted, *H. pylori* also may be linked with gastric cancer.

Ninety-seven percent of gastric cancers are adenocarcinomas; the remaining 3% are lymphomas, leiomyosarcomas, carcinoid tumors, or sarcomas.

Most gastric carcinomas develop in the antrum or along the lesser curvature, although cancer stemming from gastric atrophy tends to affect the upper portion of the stomach. Benign lesions on the greater curvature are rare; therefore, all lesions in this area should be considered malignant until proven otherwise.

Signs and symptoms of gastric cancer include epigastric discomfort, vomiting, and occult blood. Gross hematemesis is rare. Depending on the location of the lesion, patients may also present with the following symptoms:

(a) unexplained weight loss, early satiety, or anorexia;

(b) anemia;

(c) abdominal mass;

(d) gastric outlet obstruction, including nausea and vomiting;

(e) epigastric mass;

(f) ascites; and

(g) enlarged lymph nodes in the supraclavicular areas.

Gastric cancer can spread by four routes:

(a) *direct extension* to omentum, liver, pancreas, spleen, transverse colon;

(b) *lymphatics* to local perigastric nodes; regional to celiac, common hepatic, left gastric, or splenic nodes; distant to supraclavicular, left axillary, or umbilical nodes;

(c) *hematogenous* to liver, lungs, bone, or central nervous system; and

(d) *peritoneal* to pelvis (ovary or rectum) or general dissemination.

Gastric cancer may be revealed in plain stomach x-ray or chest x-ray films, double-contrast upper GI series, CT scan, or endoscopy. Patients may also have a low hematocrit, occult blood, or **hypoalbuminemia**. A double-contrast upper GI

Table 14-1. Examples of drug therapy for *H. pylori*

Regimen	Name of drugs	Dosage*	Duration
Dual therapy	Omeprazole/amoxicillin	20 mg bid/500 qid	2 weeks
	Omeprazole/clarithromycin	40 mg qd/500 tid	
Triple therapy	Bismuth subsalicylate	2 tablets qid	2 weeks
	Metronidazole	250 mg qid	
	Tetracycline or	500 mg qid	
	Amoxicillin	500 mg qid	
Quadruple therapy	Triple therapy + omeprazole	Triple therapy, 20 mg qd	
Other	Metronidazole	500 mg bid	7 days
	Omeprazole	20 mg bid	
	Clarithromycin	250-500 mg bid	
	Metronidazole	500 mg tid	12 days
	Amoxicillin	750 mg tid	
	Ranitidine	300 mg qhs	6-8 weeks

Modified from Fennerty MB, Peura DA: *Helicobacter pylori*: a primer for internal medicine physicians, *Intern Med* December:45, 1995.
*Pediatric doses are based on the child's weight.

series is about 90% sensitive, but a gastroscopy with multiple tissue biopsies and cytological examination is needed to make a definitive diagnosis. An abdominal CT scan may be ordered to determine the spread of the tumor.

The 5-year survival rate for patients with early gastric cancer that is limited to the mucosa or submucosa is 95%. This survival rate is most common in Japan, where mass screening programs make early detection more likely.

Another variation is superficial-spreading cancer, in which the cancer spreads laterally within the mucosa and submucosa without deep invasion. The 5-year survival rate for patients who have these tumors is also 95%.

Surgery is the treatment of choice for curable lesions. Patients without metastatic disease who undergo partial gastrectomy with local lymphadenectomy have a 50% or greater 5-year survival rate if lymph nodes test negative. Unfortunately, in the United States, gastric cancer is frequently diagnosed at an advanced stage and therefore prognosis is poor. Most patients survive less than 5 years.

The worst prognosis is for patients with linitis plastica, or "leather bottle stomach," which is a submucosal tumor that spreads diffusely and is associated with the formation and development of fibrous tissue. In this condition, the stomach becomes narrowed and nondistensible.

Treatment for advanced gastric cancer is largely palliative. It involves tumor resection to relieve obstruction or dysphagia or to control chronic bleeding, or gastrojejunostomy to provide temporary relief or to prevent obstruction. Following surgery, combination chemotherapy may be used alone or with local radiation therapy. Complications of metastasis, such as perforation and obstruction, should be managed as they develop. Primary nursing responsibilities include meeting patient's emotional needs, providing adequate nutrition, and assisting with pain management.

Polyps

Gastric **polyps** are defined as any circumscribed, discrete stomach tumor and are relatively uncommon. Single polyps appear more often than multiple polyps and frequently arise in the antrum and along the lesser curvature. Polyps most often develop after the age of 55; they are seldom found in young people. Types of gastric polyps include the following:

(a) hyperplastic (regenerative) polyps, which consist of normal gastric epithelium, are the most common type of gastric polyp and are always benign;

(b) adenomas;

(c) leiomyomas, or smooth muscle tumors; and

(d) adenomyomas (hamartomas), which are benign but abnormal admixtures of tissue indigenous to the organ.

Generally speaking, polyps greater than 2 cm in diameter are more likely to be malignant.

Gastric polyps are more common in patients with **achlorhydria**, atrophic gastritis, pernicious anemia, and gastric cancer or in patients who have undergone gastric resection.

Gastric polyps are usually detected by an upper GI series or endoscopy with a tissue biopsy and a cytology. Unless a polyp bleeds, it usually causes no symptoms. Endoscopic polypectomy or partial gastrectomy may be used to remove polyps.

Gastritis

Gastritis is an inflammation of the gastric mucosa. It is caused by an irritant material, such as gastric acid, bile reflux, medications, or toxins, and is often combined with an impairment of natural protective mechanisms.

Gastritis may be classified according to the inflammatory pattern as acute (erosive, hemorrhagic gastritis) or chronic (nonerosive gastritis). There are also specific forms of gastritis, including Ménétrier's disease, eosinophilic gastritis, sarcoidosis, and certain infections, but they are less common.

In acute gastritis, erosive mucosal damage occurs. Acute gastritis may be associated with serious illness, alcoholism, localized gastric trauma, and gastrectomy.

Chronic gastritis (also known as non-erosive, non-specific gastritis, or NNG) is common in adults and may be associated with normal aging, gastric ulcers, pernicious anemia, gastric cancer, or *H. pylori*. The types of NNG are superficial gastritis, atrophic gastritis, or gastric atrophy.

1. In **superficial gastritis**, pathological changes are limited to the upper one third of the mucosa.
2. **Atrophic gastritis** involves the full thickness of the mucosa, producing atrophy of gastric glands with loss of chief and parietal cells.
3. In **gastric atrophy**, there is marked or total gland loss but little inflammation and the mucosa is thinned.

Severe atrophic gastritis and gastric atrophy may be seen endoscopically as a thinned mucosa with prominent submucosal vessels.

NNG is a histological, rather than a clinical diagnosis. It has never been proven to be a cause of pain or other symptoms. It is possible that no specific treatment is necessary, except for vitamin B$_{12}$ in cases of **pernicious anemia**.

In chronic gastritis, patients may have a gradual blood loss that goes unnoticed for years. Patients may test positive for occult blood in stool, have flecks of blood in vomitus, or exhibit chronic anemia.

In patients with acute GI bleeding the most effective tool for diagnosing gastritis is an EGD. In rare instances, serum gastrin and a gastric analysis may be ordered to determine the cause of gastritis.

Treatment for gastritis without bleeding depends on the patient's signs and symptoms. Pharmacological treatment may involve the use of antacids, sucralfate (Carafate), H$_2$ blockers, or prostaglandins. Most patients who bleed from diffuse gastritis cease bleeding spontaneously. Contributing factors must be assessed, including medications, sepsis, *H. pylori*, smoking, and other illnesses.

Stress ulcers

Stress ulcers are gastric mucosal stress erosions that are associated with serious illness. They seem to arise in the following types of patients:

1. those who have sustained severe trauma, who have ongo-

ing sepsis, or who are being treated for serious illness

2. those who have significant burn injuries (**Curling's ulcer**)
3. those who sustain intracranial trauma, such as craniotomy or traumatic head injuries (**Cushing's ulcer**)
4. those who chronically ingest drugs that have adverse effects on the gastric mucosa, such as NSAIDs or alcohol

Cushing's ulcers may be located in the esophagus, stomach, or duodenum. They tend to be deep and of full-thickness and therefore are more prone to perforation than gastric mucosal ulcerations induced by trauma or sepsis.

The most common symptom of a stress ulcer is massive upper GI bleeding. Bleeding usually occurs within 3 to 7 days, but occasionally as late as 21 days, after the initial injury. Stress ulcers rarely cause classic ulcer signs and symptoms before bleeding begins. Once hemorrhage is apparent, the mortality rate is about 50%. Treatment is focused on controlling bleeding, correcting shock, and treating the underlying disorder.

Gastric varices

Portal hypertension, which is most often the result of alcoholic cirrhosis, may lead to the development of collateral circulation with formation of varices that carry blood away from the portal circulation. Esophageal varices are by far the most clinically significant type, however, two thirds of patients with esophageal varices also have gastric varices. Other less common sites of varices are the duodenum, ileum, colon, and rectum.

Upper GI bleeding from esophagogastric varices is potentially lethal. Approximately one third of deaths in cirrhotic patients are caused by variceal hemorrhage. Patients who bleed from gastric varices appear to have a higher mortality. The chances of recurrent variceal bleeding are about 9 in 10. Reducing variceal pressure by pharmacological or other means may decrease the risk of bleeding in early cirrhosis. A complete upper endoscopy is needed to diagnose variceal bleeding.

The objectives for managing esophagogastric varices are listed as follows:

(a) to hemodynamically stabilize the patient;
(b) to stop acute variceal bleeding by using octreotide or a Sengstaken-Blakemore tube; and
(c) to reduce portal pressure by surgical insertion of a shunt between the portal and systemic circulations or a transjugular intrahepatic portosystemic shunt (TIPS).

Hiatal hernia

In normal subjects, the muscle structure at the diaphragmatic hiatus anchors the stomach under the diaphragm. A **hiatal hernia** occurs when part of the stomach protrudes through the diaphragm and into the thoracic cavity. Such hernias are extremely common in older people and more common in women than in men. Most are sliding hernias, in which a portion of the stomach slides up through the opening so the gastroesophageal junction lies above the level of the diaphragm. A sliding hiatal hernia is often associated with a weakening of the LES and esophageal reflux.

In the less common rolling hiatal hernia, the gastroesophageal junction is located below the level of the diaphragm, but a part of the greater curvature of the stomach herniates through the diaphragm and into the thoracic cavity. Patients may have a feeling of fullness and discomfort after meals, but reflux is not common. Strangulation and infarction are potential complications of a rolling hiatal hernia. Ulceration may occur with either type of hiatal hernia.

Diagnostic tests for hiatal hernia include a chest x-ray examination, barium swallow, and endoscopic examination. The condition is treated in much the same way as esophageal reflux.

Complications of hiatal hernias include reflux esophagitis, heartburn, acid regurgitation, water brash, and dysphagia.

Congenital abnormalities

After inguinal hernia, the most common disorder requiring surgery in the first few months of life is **infantile hypertrophic pyloric stenosis**, which affects approximately 1 in 500 births. Boys are affected four to five times as often as girls, and the disorder seems to occur in family clusters. The first symptoms of pyloric stenosis usually occur at about 6 weeks of age. Patients have a history of progressive nonbilious vomiting, which becomes projectile. They may become dehydrated, have electrolyte disturbances, and commonly are in metabolic alkalosis with hypokalemia. An upper GI series demonstrates an unchanging elongation and narrowing of the antrum and pylorus. Pyloric stenosis may also be diagnosed by abdominal ultrasound. The treatment of choice is pyloromyotomy.

Other congenital abnormalities of the stomach include the following:

1. Gastric, antral, and pyloric atresias, in which the stomach ends blindly or is totally occluded by two apparent membranes connected by a strand each of mucosa and submucosa.
2. Pyloric or antral membranes, which may produce no obstructive symptoms until late in life.
3. Microgastria or hypoplasia, a rare condition with limited life expectancy, in which the stomach never becomes differentiated from the primitive foregut into a true fundus, body, and pylorus.
4. Gastric duplication, a rare condition in which a distinct mass lesion that contains all layers of the gastric wall develops in the stomach.
5. Neonatal perforations of the gastric wall, a rare condition associated with prematurity, peptic ulceration, and distal small intestinal obstruction.

Most gastric diverticula are also congenital and are located high on the posterior wall of the stomach, below the gastroesophageal junction. Prepyloric diverticula, which are relatively rare, are usually associated with previous peptic ulceration. Occasionally, gastric diverticula may cause *dyspepsia* or symptoms of postprandial vomiting and nausea.

Motor dysfunctions

A number of gastric motor abnormalities have been identified, ranging from conditions that are of little or no clinical importance to those that result in severe or chronic disability. Both excessively slow and excessively rapid gastric emptying can produce disabling symptoms. Symptomatic gastric motor abnormalities may be seen after vagotomy and pyloroplasty or in patients with mechanical obstructions, acute metabolic disorders and inflammatory diseases, longstanding diabetes mellitus, or as a side effect of certain medications. Serious gastric motor dysfunction may also be idiopathic, as in antral tachygastria, in which an aberrant pacemaker in the antrum cycles three to four times faster than the usual pacemaker area in the gastric body.

Management of acute gastric retention is directed at the underlying cause, if known. Gastric muscle stimulants such as metoclopramide (Reglan), cisapride (Propulsid), or bethanechol (Urecholine) may be of benefit.

Gastric surgery that includes vagotomy (e.g., gastroenterostomy, gastrojejunostomy, or Billroth II) may lead to rapid gastric emptying and a group of disabling symptoms known as **dumping syndrome**. Early symptoms appear 15 to 30 minutes after the start of a meal and include anxiety, weakness, dizziness, tachycardia with a pounding pulse, diaphoresis, flushing, abdominal cramps, and diarrhea. Approximately 90 to 120 minutes after a meal, symptoms may result from reactive **hypoglycemia**; weakness, diaphoresis, tachycardia, and sometimes a decreased level of consciousness may be experienced.

The cause of dumping syndrome is complex and may be related to rapid fluid shifts from plasma to intestinal lumen as a result of the rapid introduction of hyperosmolar solutions into the jejunum and the release of numerous hormones and vasoactive intestinal polypeptides into the bloodstream. Treatment centers on slowing the intestinal delivery of nutrients and minimizing the release of endogenous vasoactive peptides. Standard recommendations include meals high in fat and protein and low in carbohydrates, as well as minimal fluids. Fluids should be taken before or after ingestion of solid food. Use of medications to inhibit gastric emptying has had disappointing results.

Infectious diseases

The number of cases of infectious gastritis has increased in recent years. Immunocompromised patients are particularly at risk, including those with AIDS or those who have undergone transplantation or chemotherapy for cancer.

The agents implicated in infectious gastritis may be parasitic, bacterial, fungal, or viral. Bacterial inflammations besides *H. pylori* are relatively rare but may include phlegmonous and emphysematous gastritis, tuberculosis, and syphilis. Fungal infections, such as *Candida albicans* or *Torulopsis glabrata*, may be found in gastric ulcer or erosion beds in immunocompromised hosts. Gastric cytomegalovirus has been observed in transplant patients, in cytomegalovirus mononucleosis, in children, and in AIDS patients. Parasitic infestations that have been found in the stomach are infrequent but include cryptosporidiasis, anisakiasis, strongyloidiasis, and giardiasis.

Gastric outlet obstruction

Obstruction of the pyloric sphincter at the outlet of the stomach blocks the flow of gastric contents into the duodenum. Patients may vomit partially digested gastric contents and may complain of gastric pain or a feeling of fullness that is relieved only by vomiting. The pain is aggravated by eating, and as many as two thirds of patients with gastric outlet obstruction may become anorexic. Prolonged vomiting may lead to metabolic alkalosis, and the patient may complain of abdominal tenderness; a succussion splash may be noted. Abdominal x-ray films, nasogastric tube placement, an upper GI series, barium Burger test, nuclear scanning, endoscopic examination, or a saline load test may be ordered to confirm gastric retention and to rule out atony as the cause.

Treatment begins with restoration of fluid and electrolyte balance, decompression of the stomach, and correction of nutritional deficiencies. To eliminate the obstruction, the physician may use an endoscope to dilate the pylorus with a balloon. If surgery is indicated, the procedure used depends on the cause of the obstruction.

Caustic injury

The ingestion of acid or alkaline chemicals may cause tissue injury on contact with the oropharynx, esophagus, stomach, or duodenum. The severity of the tissue injury after caustic ingestion depends on the nature, concentration, and quantity of the caustic agent ingested and the duration of tissue contact. Contact with strong alkaline agents causes liquefactive necrosis, which is the complete destruction of entire cells and their membranes. In contrast, contact with strong acids promotes coagulation necrosis and the formation of a firm, protective eschar, which limits the depth, penetration, and injury produced by the acid.

The oropharynx and esophagus are most frequently injured by ingestion of alkaline agents, but 20% to 30% of patients with esophageal injury also have some extent of gastric injury. In the case of acid ingestion, the caustic agent tends to pass rapidly through the esophagus, thus producing shallow burns. In the stomach, acids usually collect in the antrum, where the most severe damage occurs. The severity of tissue injury ranges from diffuse gastritis to hemorrhagic ulceration and necrosis, thus leading to perforation of the stomach. Gastric perforation, in turn, may lead to mediastinitis, peritonitis, and shock. Patients with severe gastric injury may present with epigastric pain; retching; or emesis of tissue, blood, or material resembling coffee grounds. There is no definitive evidence of an increased risk of gastric carcinoma in patients with a history of caustic ingestion.

Stricture formation is a common late complication of caustic ingestion and is usually apparent by the eighth week following injury. Strictures in the stomach may cause gastric outlet obstruction, which leads to early satiety, postprandial vomiting, and weight loss.

Management of caustic injuries includes determining the type of agent ingested, keeping the patient NPO, performing x-ray examinations to assess signs of aspiration pneumonia or perforation, and performing cautious endoscopy to establish the extent and severity of tissue damage. Emergency surgery may be necessary in the event of perforation, peritonitis, or severe hemorrhage. If strictures develop, they may be treated by dilatation. In the case of severe gastric burns, antral and pyloric stenosis may require partial or total gastrectomy.

Bezoars

Bezoars are concretions of foreign material found in the stomach. They are usually composed of either vegetable and plant material (phytobezoars) or hair that has been chewed (trichobezoars).

Phytobezoars, which are more common, are composed of partially digested fibers, leaves, roots, and skins of almost any plant matter. Excessive ingestion of rinds from melons and oranges is a frequent cause of phytobezoars. They are most commonly seen in men over the age of 30 and may be associated with hypochlorhydria, diminished antral motility, and incomplete mastication. Recent reports describe a link between phytobezoars and partial gastrectomy, especially when accompanied by vagotomy. Diabetic persons with gastroparesis are also at risk.

Trichobezoars are composed of large quantities of hair matted together and decaying foodstuff. They are most commonly seen in females under the age of 30 and are caused by trichophagia (hair ingestion), which may represent a neuropsychiatric disturbance (trichotillomania).

Patients with bezoars may present with vague complaints of fullness in the upper quadrants, anorexia, halitosis, weight loss, epigastric pain, and periodic attacks of nausea and vomiting. A palpable mass is evident in 57% of phytobezoars and 88% of trichobezoars. Signs and symptoms depend largely on the size, location, and degree of disturbance in gastric physiology. EGD is the best technique for diagnosing and classifying bezoars, although plain films of the abdomen or an upper GI series may show evidence of an abdominal mass.

Bezoars can result in anorexia and vomiting, ulceration and bleeding, perforation, or small bowel obstruction. Phytobezoars may be disrupted endoscopically or enzymatically by using papain, acetylcysteine, or cellulase. Use of enzymatic preparations can result in gastric perforation, especially if the bezoar has caused ulceration of gastric tissue. If these methods fail, a gastrotomy may be necessary. Surgical mortality is minimal; however, the mortality of untreated bezoars may be significant. To prevent postgastrectomy phytobezoars, it may be helpful to improve dentition and counsel the patient to avoid pulpy, fibrous fruits (especially oranges) and vegetables. Trichobezoars must be treated surgically, because there is no way to dissolve the matted hair in vivo.

Lactobezoars, also known as milk curd bezoars, have been reported in infants as a result of ingesting a powdered formula diluted with an inadequate amount of water. Continuous-drip feeding of preterm infants seems to be the most important predisposing factor. Symptoms may be resolved by withholding feedings for 48 hours, implementing gastric lavage with saline solution, and using proper hydration.

CASE SITUATION

Mr. Williams, age 74, passed out during his daily walk and was brought to the emergency room (ER). Two months earlier, Mr. Williams had undergone his annual physical with flying colors. His only complaint at that time had been right arm and shoulder pain. This was attributed to the exertion of building a fence, and his physician prescribed an NSAID. Mr. Williams stopped smoking 10 years ago and drinks alcohol only at occasional social functions. He does drink two to three cups of coffee daily.

In the ER, Mr. Williams' chest x-ray films and ECG are normal. His CBC shows hemoglobin, 9 g, but he denies any abdominal pain. Mr. Williams reports having occasional black-looking bowel movements for the last 6 weeks, but he attributes them to something in his diet. A rectal examination in the ER confirms that there is blood in his stool.

Points to think about

1. Because Mr. Williams denies abdominal pain, is there any easy way to identify upper GI bleeding?
2. Mr. Williams is admitted. Before going to his room he is taken to the GI endoscopy unit for a gastroscopy. What items in this history are important?
3. Mr. Williams is found at endoscopy to have acute erosive hemorrhagic gastritis. What nursing diagnosis might apply?
4. How might the defining characteristics of the nursing diagnosis be identified?
5. What are specific expected outcomes and associated nursing interventions for this nursing diagnosis?
6. What else can the gastroenterology nurse tell Mr. Williams about treatment and follow-up care?

Suggested responses

1. In the ER, aspiration of gastric contents through a nasogastric tube reveals coffee-ground appearing material that tests positive for occult blood. Blood in the nasogastric aspirate is good evidence of an upper source of GI bleeding, but a negative test does not rule it out. Care must be taken to avoid trauma to the nares or to the esophageal or gastric mucosa, because it might cause bleeding and obscure the diagnosis.
2. Some things the gastroenterology nurse has learned about Mr. Williams that will help with the evaluation are listed as follows:
   (a) Mr. Williams was taking an NSAID, which is known to be a gastric mucosal irritant and may cause gastritis or

a gastric ulcer. Older patients are more likely to bleed from NSAID use and are more likely to suffer upper GI tract perforations.

(b) Gastritis or gastric erosions may heal very quickly when offending mucosal irritants are discontinued, often within 48 hours, so early endoscopy is important.

(c) Mr. Williams had noticed occasional black stools, which may indicate blood loss, leading to anemia, which is even more indicative of gastritis.

(d) Gastritis is an inflammation of the gastric mucosa caused by an irritant material, such as gastric acid, bile reflux, medications, or toxins, and is often combined with an impairment of natural protective mechanisms.

3. The applicable nursing diagnosis for Mr. Williams' case is: "fluid volume deficit related to blood loss."

4. The defining characteristics of this nursing diagnosis include the following:

(a) fluid volume deficit related to blood loss;
(b) decreased urine output;
(c) output greater than intake;
(d) decreased venous filling;
(e) thirst;
(f) increased pulse rate;
(g) decreased pulse amplitude;
(h) increased body temperature;
(i) dry mucous membranes;
(j) concentrated urine;
(k) hypotension;
(l) narrowed pulse pressure;
(m) decreased skin turgor;
(n) change in mental status; and
(o) weakness.

5. Some, but not necessarily all, expected outcomes and nursing interventions for this nursing diagnosis might be as follows:

Expected outcomes	Nursing interventions
There will be an adequate fluid volume	Monitor and record vital signs and central venous pressure Weigh daily Monitor intake and output Assess for signs and symptoms of hypovolemic shock Assess for signs and symptoms of dehydration Administer drugs and IV/oral fluids as ordered
Laboratory values will be within normal limits	Monitor laboratory values pertinent to fluid volume deficit

6. Because Mr. Williams' gastric mucosa is sensitive to injury, he should discontinue use of NSAIDs and aspirin-containing products. Caffeine and alcohol are also recognized as gastric irritants and should be discontinued, at least during treatment. Depending on what medication is pre-

scribed, the gastroenterology nurse should inform Mr. Williams of the following:

1. H_2 blockers inhibit the action of histamine at receptor sites in gastric parietal cells, which inhibits the production of gastric acid, thus decreasing further mucosal injury by acid contact. Tablets should be taken with meals or at bedtime if the patient is on once-daily therapy. Some H_2 blockers interact with other medications, so it is important to know all medications the patient is taking and to choose an H_2 blocker accordingly.

2. Antacids are usually taken between meals and at bedtime to neutralize gastric acid, but are rarely prescribed since the introduction of H_2 blockers. It is sometimes difficult to adhere to this regimen; if so, the patient should ask the physician for an alternative treatment. Liquid antacids should be shaken well and should be taken with a little water to ensure passage to the stomach. Some antacids can cause diarrhea or constipation and may need to be alternated. In older patients it is best to use low-sodium antacids.

3. Sucralfate (Carafate) is an oral medication that adheres to the gastric mucosa to form a protective barrier against further damage, particularly where cell protein is exposed because irritants have eroded the protective mucosa. The medication should be taken on an empty stomach for best results, 1 hour before meals and at bedtime. Since sucralfate is not readily absorbed systemically, there are few side effects. Occasionally, patients experience constipation.

4. Misoprostol (Cytotec) is a synthetic prostaglandin E, which replaces prostaglandins that are depleted by NSAIDs, and may be given concomitantly with NSAIDs to help prevent gastric mucosal damage. (This drug is strictly contraindicated in pregnant women, because it can cause spontaneous abortion.)

In addition, the gastroenterology nurse should teach Mr. Williams how to use slides to test for occult blood in his stool at home. He should be told to report any further signs of bleeding and/or epigastric pain to his physician. The nurse should provide a list of foods high in iron to help raise hemoglobin levels to normal.

REVIEW TERMS

achlorhydria, adenomatous polyps, antrum, bezoars, body, cardia, cardiac glands, chief cells, chyme, Curling's ulcer, Cushing's ulcer, dumping syndrome, enterochromaffin cells, fundus, G cells, gastric ulcers, gastritis, greater curvature, greater omentum, *Helicobacter pylori* **(H. Pylori), hiatal hernia, hypoalbuminemia, infantile hypertrophic pyloric stenosis, lesser curvature, lesser omentum, oxyntic gland, parietal cells, pernicious anemia, polyps, pyloric glands, pyloric sphincter, pylorus, rugae, stress ulcer, ulcers**

REVIEW QUESTIONS

1. Entry of food into the stomach is controlled by the:
   (a) lower esophageal sphincter.
   (b) fundus.
   (c) pyloric sphincter.
   (d) antrum.

2. The stomach wall has four layers, the mucosa, submucosa, the muscularis, and the:
   (a) rugae.
   (b) cardia.
   (c) serosa.
   (d) connective tissue.

3. The parietal cells secrete:
   (a) mucus.
   (b) hydrochloric acid and intrinsic factor.
   (c) pepsinogens.
   (d) gastrin.

4. Intrinsic factor is necessary for the:
   (a) conversion of pepsinogens to pepsin.
   (b) secretion of mucus.
   (c) absorption of vitamin B_{12}.
   (d) secretion of hormones.

5. The gastric emptying rate is controlled by neural impulses, hormones secreted by the small intestine, and:
   (a) the amount of food ingested;
   (b) the composition of the chyme;
   (c) the amount of gastric secretions;
   (d) vitamin B_{12} absorption.

6. *H. pylori* infection:
   (a) has been associated with gastric cancer.
   (b) is a virus of the stomach.
   (c) should be treated by surgical resection.
   (d) is not detectable by biopsy.

7. Most gastric cancers are of which of the following types?
   (a) adenocarcinomas.
   (b) leiomyosarcomas.
   (c) sarcomas.
   (d) lymphomas.

8. Cushing's ulcers are a form of:
   (a) specific gastritis.
   (b) nonerosive, nonspecific gastritis.
   (c) peptic ulcers.
   (d) stress ulcers.

9. Gastric surgery may lead to rapid gastric emptying and a group of disabling symptoms that can cause reactive hypoglycemia. This syndrome is called:
   (a) Curling's syndrome.
   (b) Paterson-Kelly syndrome.
   (c) Dumping syndrome.
   (d) Cushing's syndrome.

10. The best technique for diagnosing bezoars is:
   (a) plain x-rays.
   (b) palpation.
   (c) gastroscopy.
   (d) upper GI series.

BIBLIOGRAPHY

Beare, P. & Meyers, J. (1998). *Principles and practice of adult health nursing*. St. Louis, MO: Mosby.

Eisenberg, M.M., Fondacaro, P.F. & Durin, D.H. (1995). Applied anatomy and anomalies of the stomach. In Haubrich, W.S., Schaffner, F. & Berk, J.E. (Eds), *Bockus gastroenterology, Vol. 1* (5th ed.). Philadelphia: W.B. Saunders.

Fennerty, M.B. & Peura, D.A. (1995, December). Helicobacter pylori: a primer for internal medicine physicians. *Intern Med*, 32-50.

Hunt, R.H. (1996). Eradication of Helicobacter pylori infection. *Am J Med 100*, 5A42S-5A50S. American Journal of Medicine.

Isenberg, J.I. (1999). Acid peptic disorders. In Yamada, T., (Ed.), *Textbook of gastroenterology, Vol. 1* (3rd ed.). Philadelphia, Pennsylvania: Lippincott.

Martin, D. (2002). *Practical gastroenterology*. Florence, KY: Taylor and Francis.

National Institutes of Health (1994). *NIH consensus statement: Helicobacter pylori in peptic ulcer disease* 1(12), 1-22. Washington, DC: Department of Health and Human Services.

Pezzi, J.S. & Shiau, Y. (1995). Helicobacter pylori and gastrointestinal disease. *Am Fam Physician 52*, 1717-25. American Family Physician.

Price, S.A. & Wilson, L.M. (1992). *Pathophysiology: clinical concepts of disease processes* (4th ed.). St. Louis, MO: Mosby.

Sleisenger, M. & Fordtran, J. (Eds.) (2002). *Gastrointestinal disease: pathophysiology, diagnosis, management* (7th ed.). Philadelphia: W.B. Saunders.

Smeltzer, S.C. & Bare, B.G. (2000). *Textbook of Medical Surgical Nursing* (9th ed.). Philadelphia, Pennsylvania: Lippincott.

Sol, A.H. (1996). Medical treatment of peptic ulcer disease: practice guidelines. *JAMA 275*, 622-9.

Walker, W.A., Durie, P., Hamilton, J.R., Watkins, J.B. and Walker-Smith, J.A. (2000). *Pediatric gastrointestinal disease: Pathophysiology, diagnosis, management*. Ontario, Canada: Decker.

Yamada, T. Alpers, D., Laine, L., Owyang, C., Powell, D.W. (1999). *Textbook of gastroenterology, Vol. 1* (3rd ed.). Philadelphia: J.B. Lippincott.

Chapter 15

SMALL INTESTINE

This chapter will acquaint the gastroenterology nurse with the normal anatomy and physiology of the small bowel (small intestine). In addition, a number of pathological conditions of the small bowel are described in terms of their pathophysiology, diagnosis, and treatment alternatives.

Learning objectives

After reviewing the content of this chapter, the gastroenterology nurse should be able to:

1. Describe the normal anatomy of the small bowel.
2. Discuss the physiology of intestinal absorption, secretion, and motility.
3. Explain the pathophysiology, diagnosis, and treatment of a number of important disorders of the small bowel.

ANATOMY AND PHYSIOLOGY

The small intestine is a tubular structure that extends from the pyloric sphincter to the cecum (see Fig. 13-2) and has digestive, absorptive, secretory, barrier, and immunologic functions. The small intestine is approximately 275 cm in the neonate, growing to 5 to 6 m in the adult. The first 30 cm (12 inches) of the small intestine is the c-shaped, muscular **duodenum**, which begins at the pyloric sphincter and ends at the **ligament of Treitz**. The common bile duct empties into the duodenum at the **ampulla of Vater** (Figure 15-1). After the duodenum, the proximal two fifths of the small bowel is known as the **jejunum**. The distal three fifths of the small bowel, known as the **ileum**, extends from the jejunum to the **ileocecal valve**. This valve controls the flow of chyme into the large intestine and prevents reflux into the ileum.

The small intestinal wall consists of the following layers:

- An outer serous layer (serosa) composed of peritoneum and connective tissue;
- A muscular layer (muscularis) containing outer longitudinal and inner circular muscles, separated by a nerve network called the *myenteric plexus*;
- A submucous layer (submucosa) of areolar connective tissue containing blood vessels, lymphatics, and a submucosal nerve plexus; and
- An inner mucous layer (mucosa) containing simple columnar epithelium; a layer of connective tissue known as the **lamina propria**; and a thin sheet of smooth muscle, which separates the mucosa from the submucosa.

The mucosa and submucosa are arranged in circular folds called the *plicae circulares*, which provide a greater surface area for secretion and absorption during the 3 to 6 hours the chyme remains in the small intestine.

In addition, the mucosa forms an estimated 4 to 5 million small, fingerlike villi, which project into the intestinal lumen (Fig. 15-2). Each **villus** is lined with simple columnar epithelial cells. Below the epithelium, the lamina propria contains nerve fibers, smooth muscle, lymphatic vessels or lacteals, blood vessels, and connective tissue. A brush border consisting of multiple **microvilli** covers the surface of each columnar cell.

The presence of the mucosal folds, the villi, and the microvilli increases the total surface area and therefore the absorptive capacity of the small bowel by approximately 600-fold.

Between the villi are small, tubular glands known as the **crypts of Lieberkühn**. The entire intestinal epithelial surface is replaced every 32 hours. Extremely mitotic undifferentiated cells that lie deep in the crypts serve to replace the epithelium. Paneth's cells are also located at the base of the crypts. The function of **Paneth's cells** is uncertain, but it is possible that they regulate the intestinal flora.

In the proximal duodenum, the normal villous pattern is interrupted at intervals by **Brunner's glands**, which are elaborately branched acinar glands that contain both mucous cells and serous secretory cells. Brunner's glands empty into the crypts of Lieberkühn.

Lymphoid tissue makes up approximately 25% of the intes-

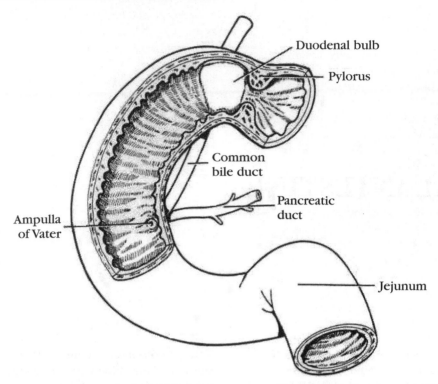

Fig. 15-1. Duodenal anatomy.

tinal mucosa. The GI-associated lymphoid tissue is made up of three distinct populations, which are listed as follows:

- **Peyer's patches** are circular, aggregated lymph nodes that lie in the mucosa and submucosa of the ileum. They participate in antibody synthesis and in the body's immune response.
- Lymphocytes and plasma cells are located in the lamina propria. Approximately 70% to 80% of these cells produce immunoglobin A (IgA), which is the major immunoglobulin in intestinal secretions. This secretory IgA plays an important role in the resistance of the mucous membranes to pathological microorganisms and dietary antigens.
- A third population of lymphocytes, known as the intraepithelial lymphocytes, lies between the intestinal epithelial cells. A large proportion of these intraepithelial lymphocytes are T cells.

The duodenum receives arterial blood from the hepatic artery, whereas the rest of the small bowel derives its blood supply from the superior mesenteric artery. Blood from the entire small bowel drains through the superior mesenteric vein.

The wall of the digestive tract is innervated by the **enteric plexus**, which is an autonomic nerve plexus made up of the submucosal plexus **(Meissner's plexus)**, myenteric plexus **(Auerbach's plexus)**, and the subserosal plexus. Parasympathetic stimulation by way of the vagus nerve increases the tone of the small bowel and the frequency, strength, and velocity of smooth muscle contractions. Vagal stimulation also enhances motor and secretory activities. Sympathetic stimulation via spinal nerves from levels T6 to

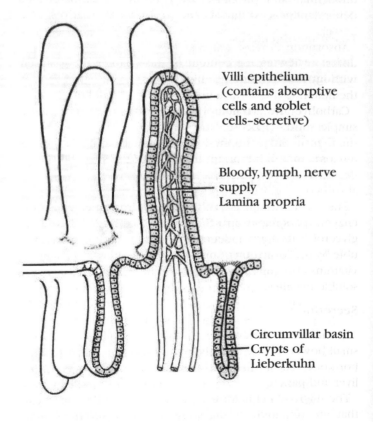

Fig. 15-2. Small bowel villi anatomy.

T12 reduces peristalsis and inhibits GI activity. The intrinsic nerve supply, which initiates motor function, passes through Auerbach's and Meissner's plexuses.

Absorption

The primary function of the small intestine is to absorb nutrients from the chyme. The small intestine receives up to 8 L of fluid per day and passes only 500 to 1000 ml to the large intestine. The rest is absorbed by the columnar cells of the villous epithelium.

Absorption of different nutrients takes place at different locations in the small intestine. The duodenum is the primary site of iron and calcium absorption, and the jejunum is the site of absorption of fats, proteins, and carbohydrates. The ileum absorbs vitamin B_{12} and bile acids.

There are five basic mechanisms for absorption in the small intestine: hydrolysis, nonionic movement, passive diffusion, facilitated diffusion, and active transport. Water, for instance, diffuses passively across the wall of the small intestine, with only a small portion left unabsorbed.

Sodium is absorbed in the jejunum through active transport. Magnesium, phosphate, and potassium are absorbed throughout the small intestine. Chloride diffuses with sodium in the jejunum; in the ileum, it is actively transported. Dietary iron is absorbed predominantly by the duodenum and proximal jejunum.

Calcium absorption occurs by each of the following mechanisms: a transcellular route that takes place largely in the duodenum and proximal jejunum, and a concentration-dependent process that occurs along the length of the small bowel.

Absorption of most water-soluble vitamins takes place by diffusion. The exception is vitamin B_{12}, which combines with intrinsic factor for active transport and is absorbed in the ileum.

Carbohydrates are hydrolyzed by intestinal enzymes into simple sugars (glucose, fructose, and galactose), which are then absorbed into the bloodstream via the intestinal mucosa, using either active transport or facilitated diffusion. Proteins are hydrolyzed into amino acids, which are absorbed by active transport.

Fats are emulsified and then broken down primarily by the enzyme pancreatic lipase into glycerides, fatty acids, and glycerol. Fatty acids and monoglycerides are made water-soluble by the formation of micelles with bile acids. Fat-soluble vitamins also combine briefly with bile salts to form water-soluble micelles.

Secretion

In addition to their absorptive function, cells located in the small bowel secrete digestive juices, mucus, and a variety of hormones. The small bowel also receives secretions from the liver and pancreas.

The microvilli contain the peptidases and disaccharidases that are required for digestion of proteins and carbohydrates.

Brunner's glands, which are located in the proximal duodenum, secrete a clear, alkaline (pH 8.2 to 9.3), viscous fluid that protects the duodenal mucosa from gastric acid secretions. **Goblet cells** located on and between the villi on the mucosa secrete a protective mucus.

The crypts of Lieberkühn secrete 2 to 3 L of succus entericus per day. This watery fluid supplies a carrier substance for absorption of nutrients when the villi come in contact with the chyme.

There are ten different types of endocrine cells located in the crypts that produce a number of peptides and hormones, including secretin, cholecystokinin, gastrin, somatostatin, enteroglucagon, motilin, neurotensin, gastrin inhibitory peptide, vasoactive intestinal peptide, and serotonin.

Motility

Within the small bowel, three types of movement contribute to the mixing of the chyme:

- Concentric, segmenting contractions, which normally take place in the jejunum, give the small intestine the look of a chain of sausage links. The concentric movement helps to mix secretions of the small intestine with the chyme particles.
- Short, propulsive contractions or peristaltic waves slowly push the chyme in the direction of the colon. Peristaltic contractions are found predominantly in the first portions of the duodenum and jejunum.
- The continuous shortening and lengthening of the villi constantly stirs the intestinal contents.

As the chyme nears the large intestine, contractions in the ileum increase. After a meal the ileocecal sphincter relaxes, allowing the chyme to move from the ileum into the cecum.

PATHOPHYSIOLOGY

Pathological conditions of the small intestine can affect absorption of nutrients in the affected area. To best understand the impact of a particular condition on nutrient absorption, consider the location of disease. Duodenal disease may lead to deficiencies in iron and calcium, whereas jejunal disease may lead to malabsorption of fats, proteins, and carbohydrates. Ileal disease may result in vitamin B_{12} deficiency and bile acid malabsorption.

Important pathological conditions of the small bowel include duodenal ulcer disease, parasitic infestations, bacterial and viral infections, Crohn's disease, Meckel's diverticulum, vitamin B_{12} deficiency, and small bowel tumors. A variety of malabsorption syndromes also affect the small bowel, such as celiac disease, Whipple's disease, short bowel syndrome, and lactose intolerance.

Common intestinal disorders affecting children include Hirschsprung's disease, appendicitis, Meckel's diverticulum, inflammatory bowel disease, intussusception, celiac disease, short bowel syndrome, acute infectious diarrhea and constipation.

Duodenal ulcers

Peptic ulcers can develop in the lower esophagus, stomach, pylorus, duodenum, or jejunum. About 80% of all peptic ulcers are duodenal ulcers. They occur when the protective mucosa of the duodenum cannot resist corrosion by above-normal hydrochloric acid levels.

Duodenal ulcers are most common in men who are between the ages of 20 and 50, and in persons with Type O blood. It is now recognized that *H. pylori*, a spiral bacteria that is most likely transmitted by the fecal-oral route, is present in almost all adults with duodenal ulcer, most with gastric ulcer, and virtually all patients with histological evidence of gastritis. *H. pylori* is associated with peptic disease much less frequently in children than adults. Children with peptic inflammation of the small bowel are also much less like to develop duodenal ulcers than adults. In peptic ulcer disease, erosion of the affected mucosa can lead to hemorrhage, perforation, and peritonitis.

Symptoms of duodenal ulcers include gnawing or burning epigastric pain occurring 1 to 3 hours after meals, heartburn, and intermittent nighttime pain or discomfort, which is localized in the epigastrium. Pain is exacerbated by fatty foods but may be relieved by other foods. Attacks usually occur about 2 hours after meals, when the stomach is empty, or after consumption of orange juice, coffee, aspirin, or alcohol. Many patients report symptoms that are unlike those expected in the classic presentation.

Diagnosis is by upper GI radiographic examination and/or upper GI endoscopy. The sensitivity of individual radiologists in detecting ulcers varies between 44% and 80%, with a double-contrast technique being somewhat more sensitive than a single-contrast technique. Endoscopy may be more sensitive than radiography, with experienced endoscopists detecting 85% to 95% of gastroduodenal lesions.

During endoscopy with biopsy, testing for the presence of *H. pylori* may be performed by placing a biopsy into a medium designed for a rapid urease test. Although several manufacturers make different types of this test, most commercially available tests show a color change in the presence of the enzyme urease, which is produced by *H. pylori*. Nonendoscopic methods of testing for this bacteria include the performance of a C-urea breath test, or measurement of *H. pylori* antibodies in the blood. Before identification of *H. pylori* as a cause of peptic ulcer disease, treatment was directed toward acid suppression. Today, treatment is directed toward eradication of the infection through the use of a combination of antibiotics, acid suppression, and bismuth.

A small percentage of patients with duodenal ulcer disease require surgical intervention because of hemorrhage, obstruction, perforation, or intractability. There are four surgical procedures in use today. The choice of procedure depends on the needs of the individual patient, the indication for the operation, and the experience of the surgeon. Surgical procedures include the following:

- Subtotal gastric resection without vagotomy, which is seldom used now because of the high incidence of side effects
- Truncal vagotomy with a drainage procedure (pyloroplasty), which is preferred in very elderly or very ill patients with hemorrhage
- Truncal vagotomy and antrectomy (Billroth I or II), which is preferred in patients with recurrent hemorrhage because of the low incidence of rebleeding; also it may

offer better long-term results in patients presenting with obstructions
- Highly selective vagotomy, which is preferred for patients with intractable ulcers because of its low mortality and morbidity and fewer postoperative side effects

Patients with perforations may undergo a simple closure or closure combined with one of the definitive operations described above.

Bacterial and viral infections

GI tract infections are a major cause of morbidity and mortality throughout the world. The small bowel may become infected by any of the following types of agents:

- Enterotoxigenic bacteria produce enterotoxins that stimulate the active secretion of electrolytes into the lumen of the proximal small bowel. The watery, voluminous diarrhea caused by these bacteria is not usually accompanied by fever, and fecal leukocytes are seldom present. Examples are toxigenic *Escherichia coli*, *Vibrio cholerae*, *Bacillus cereus*, *Clostridium perfringens*, and *Staphylococcus aureus*.
- Invasive bacteria invade and damage the intestinal mucosa of the distal small bowel and colon, often producing scant, bloody, mucoid stools; fever; and fecal polymorphonuclear leukocytes. Examples are *Salmonella* species, *Shigella* species, *E. coli*, *Vibrio parahaemolyticus*, *V. cholerae*, *Clostridium difficile*, and *S. aureus*.
- Penetrating bacteria invade the mucosa, usually in the distal small intestine, but do not produce extensive mucosal ulcerations. They often cause extraintestinal disease (e.g., sepsis), fever, and fecal leukocytes. *Yersinia enterocolitica* and *Salmonella typhi* are examples of penetrating bacteria.
- Viruses, such as coronavirus, rotavirus, Norwalk virus, and adenovirus, may also invade the small bowel mucosa, resulting in malabsorption and diarrhea.

Identification of the etiological agent in GI infections requires taking a careful history to obtain information on the symptom pattern, any recent exposure to infected individuals or contaminated food or water, or any recent history of foreign travel. Patients should be evaluated for fluid status and abdominal tenderness, and stools should be examined for the presence of fecal leukocytes.

In most cases, infectious diarrhea can be treated with rest and fluid replacement. IV fluids may be needed for patients with severe dehydration. Generally, for both adults and children with acute infectious diarrhea, consumption of an unrestricted diet should continue with additional fluids or oral rehydration solutions provided to replace increased stool water losses. Antidiarrheal medications are contraindicated as they may prolong mucosal contact with the infectious organism and exacerbate intestinal stasis, gas, and discomfort. If the etiological agent is identified, specific antibiotics may be indicated. Table 15-1 lists some of the causes of infectious diarrhea in which antibiotic treatment is indicated.

Table 15-1. Antibiotics used to treat infectious diarrhea

Infectious agent	Antibiotic(s) used
Staphylococcus aureus	Non; self-limited
Toxigenic Escherichia coli	Trimethoprimsulfamethozazole (Septra)
Vibrio cholerae	Tetracycline (Achromycin) or cloramphenicol (Chloromycetin)
Clostridium botulinum	Polyvalent antitoxin, penicillin, and colonic lavage
Clostidium perfingens	None
Vibrio Parahaemolyticus	Tetracycline
Shigella	For severe infection, ampicillin or trimethoprimsulfamethoxazole
Salmonella	For degilitated patient, ampicillin, chloramphenicol, amoxicillin, or trimethoprim-sulfamethoxazole
Clostidium difficile	Metonidazole (Flagyl) or vancomycin (Vancocin)

Parasitic diseases

There are a number of parasitic diseases that affect the small intestine, including giardiasis, coccidiosis, cryptosporidiosis, strongyloidiasis, ascariasis, and diphyllobothriasis.

Giardiasis

Giardiasis is caused by the protozoan *Giardia lamblia* and is most often associated with ingestion of contaminated food or water. Overall prevalence of giardiasis in the United States is 7% to 10%. Endemic areas include upstate New York and the Rocky Mountain region, especially Colorado.

The two forms of the parasite are cysts and trophozoites. After the cyst is ingested orally or nasally it matures, and once in the stomach, releases trophozoites. These trophozoites adhere to the wall of the proximal small intestine, causing an inflammatory response.

Most adults with giardiasis are asymptomatic, although nonbloody diarrhea and even malabsorption may occur. Clinical symptoms exhibited by children range from none at all to acute illness characterized by abdominal discomfort and distention, nonbloody diarrhea, headaches, nausea, and vomiting. Diagnosis is by examination of multiple fresh stool specimens, stool specimen for Giardia antigen, or duodenal aspiration and small intestinal biopsy examination.

If treatment is necessary, the drug of choice is metronidazole (Flagyl), which is administered in three divided doses for 1 week. Pediatric patients may be treated with metronidazole or furazolidone (Furoxone). Stools and/or duodenal aspirate may be rechecked 2 weeks after treatment in symptomatic patients. A second course of treatment is instituted if necessary. For patients who are resistant to metronidazole alone, a combined regimen of quinacrine (Atabrine) and metronidazole for 2 weeks may be effective.

Coccidiosis

Coccidiosis is caused by the intracytoplasmic protozoans *Isospora belli*, *Isospora hominis*, and *Isospora natelensis*. It is endemic throughout the world but is rarely seen in the United States. The parasite multiplies in the small bowel, causing mucosal damage. Clinical features include acute fulminant diarrhea, continuous or intermittent chronic diarrhea, and steatorrhea (fatty stools). Diagnosis is by stool examination, small intestinal biopsy examination, and blood tests for eosinophilia.

Most patients have a benign, self-limited course that lasts from a few days to 6 months. Adult patients with a mild case may be treated with fluid and electrolyte replacement only. In children, severe diarrhea with malabsorption may necessitate temporary parenteral nutrition. For severe cases, the drug of choice is furazolidone (Furoxone).

Cryptosporidiosis

Cryptosporidiosis is caused by the coccidial sporozoa *Cryptosporidium*. The colon and small bowel are the most common sites of infection, but *Cryptosporidium* has been reported in all parts of the GI and respiratory tracts. Transmission is fecal-oral; it may be transmitted between animals and humans but is rarely transmitted from human to human. Water-borne transmission has also been reported. After the oocysts are ingested they embed in the surface of the bowel, where they complete their entire life cycle. After about 12 days, oocysts are passed in the stools.

Before 1981, only eight cases had been reported in humans. However, because immunocompromised patients are particularly susceptible to *Cryptosporidium*, the beginning of the AIDS epidemic marked a noteworthy increase in its prevalence in humans. Recent evidence indicates that it may be more common than was previously supposed.

The severity of the illness ranges from self-limited diarrheal episodes lasting from 3 days to 4 weeks in immunocompetent hosts to death in immunocompromised individuals. Onset is acute, with malaise and fever, followed by abdominal pain, diarrhea, vomiting, steatorrhea, and occasionally mild rectal bleeding and nonspecific proctitis.

The diagnosis may be made by serial stool examinations or intestinal biopsy examination. The most accurate staining method for identification of the parasite is a three-step procedure that involves concentration evaluation using a sugar flotation technique, iodine staining, and a modified acid-fast stain.

Therapy focuses on correction of severe fluid and electrolyte imbalance. In complicated, life-threatening cases, conventional antiparasitics such as metronidazole (Flagyl) or thiabendazole (Mintezol) may be effective.

Strongyloidiasis

Strongyloidiasis occurs in warm, moist climates and is caused by the helminth *Strongyloides stercoralis* (S. stercoralis). Filariform larvae are the infectious form; rhabditiform larvae are noninfectious. Multiple cycles of the parasite may occur in a single host, thereby allowing some patients to harbor *S. stercoralis* for 30 to 50 years. In some patients, repeated autoinfection may produce an overwhelming fatal hyperinfective syndrome.

Early symptoms of strongyloidiasis include fever; migratory, erythematous, macular eruptions over the distal extremities; and productive or nonproductive cough. Later, GI symptoms predominate. Patients with hyperinfective syndrome may have heavy worm burdens, which are manifested by esophagitis, pneumonitis, gastritis, enterocolitis, hepatitis, myocarditis, intestinal obstruction or perforation, shock, or meningitis.

Diagnosis is by blood tests, stool examination, duodenal aspirate, chest x-ray, or upper GI series with small bowel follow-through.

For both symptomatic and asymptomatic patients, the drug of choice is thiabendazole (Mintezol). Patients with hyperinfective syndrome also require fluid and electrolyte maintenance and appropriate bacterial cultures. Stools and/or duodenal aspirate should be rechecked 1 to 2 weeks after completion of appropriate therapy, with a second course of treatment initiated if necessary.

With treatment, most patients with mild to moderate cases have an excellent prognosis. In patients with hyperinfective syndrome, however, the mortality rate approaches 50%.

Ascariasis

Ascariasis is caused by the roundworm *Ascaris lumbricoides*, which is the largest intestinal nematode. Endemic areas in the United States include the southeastern Appalachian range and the Southern states, with prevalence rates approaching 90% in some areas.

Transmission is by ingestion of eggs that are passed in the stool. The adult worms live in the small bowel for 6 months or longer and then penetrate intestinal blood vessels and lymphatics. At this point they are carried through the portal circulation and pass through the liver into the lungs.

Reactions to the larvae include high fever, frequent spasmodic coughing, and hemoptysis. Reactions to the adult worms include colicky midepigastric pain, abdominal distention, vomiting, and constipation. The most frequent complication is partial or complete intestinal obstruction.

Definitive diagnosis requires that the egg or the adult worm be identified in the stool. Uncomplicated ascariasis may be treated with mebendazole (Vermox). For patients with complete obstruction, surgical intervention may be necessary. Prognosis is usually good but is dependent on the worm burden and the presence of complications.

Diphyllobothriasis

Diphyllobothriasis is caused by the fish tapeworm *Diphyllobothrium latum*. Infection results from ingestion of infected, raw fish. Endemic areas in the United States include northern Wisconsin, Michigan, and Minnesota. The tapeworm lives with its head attached to the small intestinal mucosa and may reach 10 mm in length. Although the effects on the intestinal mucosa are minimal, profound vitamin B_{12} deficiency may develop. The majority of patients with this infection are asymptomatic. When symptoms do develop, those most often seen are abdominal pain, ataxia and paresthesia, nausea, vomiting, diarrhea, and weight loss.

Definitive diagnosis requires finding the operculated egg in the stool. Diphyllobothriasis is most often treated with niclosamide (Nicloside). With proper treatment, prognosis is excellent.

Crohn's disease

Crohn's disease, also known as **regional enteritis**, granulomatous colitis, or transmural colitis, is a transmural, predominantly submucosal inflammation that may affect any part of the GI tract but occurs most commonly in the terminal ileum. Crohn's disease and ulcerative colitis, the latter of which is discussed in Chapter 16, are both chronic intestinal disorders. The two are often grouped together under the term **inflammatory bowel disease**. The asymmetric and patchy distribution of the lesions helps to differentiate the condition from ulcerative colitis. The cause of Crohn's disease is unknown, although infectious, nutritional and immunological etiologies have been proposed as contributing factors in generally susceptible individuals.

The incidence of Crohn's disease is higher in persons of Jewish descent in Europe and North America. There is a higher incidence in caucasians than nonwhites and a higher incidence in urban than rural settings than in the general population. It most commonly afflicts people between the ages of 15 and 30. In some surveys, males and females are equally afflicted; in others, females predominate by as much as 1.6 to 1. The cause of Crohn's disease remains unknown, but possibilities include allergies and other immune disorders, abnormal response to some dietary or bacterial antigen, lymphatic obstruction, infection, and/or genetic factors.

Inflammation spreads slowly and progressively, with periods of remission often alternating with exacerbations. Segmental inflammation and rectal sparing are features that distinguish Crohn's disease from ulcerative colitis.

The disease process begins with lacteal blockage and lymphedema in the submucosa. Peyer's patches appear in the intestinal mucous membrane. Lymphatic obstruction causes edema, with inflammation; mucosal ulceration; stenosis; and development of fissures, abscesses, and possibly granulomas. Typically, deep longitudinal "rake ulcers" appear in the bowel. If deep ulcers appear between islands of edematous inflamed mucosa, the bowel wall takes on a "cobblestone" appearance. As the disease progresses, fibrosis occurs and serositis develops, causing diseased bowel loops to adhere to other normal or diseased loops. Perianal lesions may be present.

During periods of acute inflammation, patients with Crohn's disease may report lower right quadrant pain, cramping, abdominal tenderness, spasms, increased flatulence, nausea, low-grade fever, diarrhea, and **borborygmi** (abnormally loud bowel sounds). Bloody diarrhea and malabsorption may be severe, leading to malnutrition and weight loss. Growth failure or a decline in the rate of linear growth may be the presenting symptom in children and adolescents. Stress may play a role in exacerbation of symptoms but is not an identified cause of illness.

Chronic symptoms are more persistent but less severe. They include diarrhea, abdominal pain, steatorrhea, anorexia and weight loss, and nutritional deficiencies. Extraintestinal symptoms may include arthritis, spondylitis, iritis, skin involvement, renal disease, liver disease, and clubbing of the fingers.

Diagnosis of Crohn's disease is based on clinical history, physical examination and laboratory and radiologic testing. Upper GI series with small bowel x-ray are the mainstays Upper and lower GI endoscopy with biopsies is necessary to evaluate histologic evidence of the typical inflammatory process.

Dietary and drug therapy aim to reduce inflammation, maintain fluid and electrolyte balance, and relieve symptoms. Therapeutic measures may include the following:

- During exacerbation of symptoms, a diet that is high in protein, calories, vitamins, and minerals and low fiber to replace nutrient losses associated with the inflammatory process and to provide sufficient nutients to promote energy and nitrogen balance; small, frequent meals, with avoidance of lactose by patients who are lactose intolerant.
- Total parenteral nutrition for patients with severe disease or short bowel syndrome refractory to oral therapy or specialized enteral tube feeding.
- Drug therapy, including 5-aminosalicylate drugs (sulfasalazine, olsalazine, mesalamine), corticosteroids, immune modulating agents (azathioprine, mercaptopurine, cyclosporine), and/or antibiotics such as metronidazole and ciproflaxin.

Potential complications of Crohn's disease include intestinal obstruction, fistula formation between the small bowel and the bladder, perianal and perirectal abscesses and fistulas, intraabdominal abscesses, and, perforation. Malabsorption of bile acids and vitamin B_{12} is common in disease of the ileum.

More than half of all patients with Crohn's disease eventually need surgery, because the disease progression has caused permanent structural changes. Surgery may be needed to correct bowel perforation, massive hemorrhage, fistulas, or acute intestinal obstruction. The most common type of surgery performed is bowel resection with restoration of bowel continuity. Although surgery may successfully alleviate acute complications, the rate of recurrence is high.

Patients with Crohn's disease should be encouraged to rest, to reduce the tension in their lives, and to communicate their feelings about this chronic and often disabling disorder. They should be educated about the disease, its process, and its treatment and should be told how to contact community agencies and support groups that can help them adjust, such as the Crohn's and Colitis Foundation of America. Depression is a common emotion experienced by patients with Crohn's disease; therefore, the provision of emotional support is an important part of the treatment process.

Meckel's diverticulum

Meckel's diverticulum is a congenital anomaly of the GI tract, resulting from incomplete separation of the fetal gut from the yolk sac. This outpouching of the ileum is lined by typical ileal mucous membrane but may contain ectopic gastric and/or pancreatic tissue in its wall. Secretion of acid or pepsin from this ectopic tissue may cause ulceration of adjacent ileal tissue, resulting in hemorrhage. Hemorrhage usually occurs in children under 2 years of age and typically presents as painless passage of bright red blood from the rectum. Intestinal obstruction may result from Meckel's diverticulum, either from **volvulus** (twisting of the bowel) or **intussusception** (prolapse of the diverticulum into the lumen of the bowel). Symptoms of obstruction include abdominal pain, bilious or feculent vomiting, and/or passage of bright red or "currant jelly" stools. Meckel's diverticulum cannot be diagnosed by endoscopic or radiological contrast studies. A Meckel's scan allows diagnosis by administration of technetium, which is excreted by gastric mucosa, followed by a nuclear medicine scan to identify areas of excretion. Administration of cimetidine or ranitidine orally for several days before the examination or given IV before the examination increases the accuracy of this diagnostic tool. Treatment of Meckel's diverticulum requires diverticulectomy (resection of the diverticulum) or, if necessary, resection of the adjacent ileum.

Vitamin B_{12} deficiency

In the stomach, protein-bound vitamin B_{12} is freed by the action of gastric pepsin. The free B_{12} binds to two molecules of intrinsic factor, which is a glycoprotein secreted by gastric parietal cells. This complex protects vitamin B_{12} from use by bacteria and from the formation of unabsorbable aggregates while it is in the small bowel. In the ileum the complex of B_{12} and intrinsic factor binds to receptor sites on the brush border, thus facilitating B_{12} entry into the enterocytes. After passage through the enterocytes, B_{12} is transported in the blood bound to transcobalamins, which deliver the vitamin to the tissue. Intrinsic factor remains bound to the receptor site, where it may promote the uptake of more B_{12}. When the amount of ingested B_{12} is very large, absorption also occurs by diffusion, probably at all levels of the intestine.

Vitamin B_{12} deficiency may occur if any one of these steps is impaired. Disorders or conditions that may result in B_{12} deficiency include gastrectomy, pernicious anemia, pancreatic insufficiency, Zollinger-Ellison syndrome, Crohn's disease, bacterial overgrowth, ileal disease or resection, familial cobalamin malabsorption, or transcobalamin deficiency.

The source of vitamin B_{12} malabsorption may be pinpointed by using the three-part Schilling test, which traces the excretion of radiolabeled B_{12} in the urine with or without the addition of intrinsic factor or a broad-spectrum antibiotic. Treatment is directed at the underlying disease state. Parenteral vitamin B_{12} may be required in cases of severe disease or extensive ileal resection.

Malabsorption syndromes

Malabsorption syndromes include abnormalities of mucosal transport and/or intraluminal digestion of one or more dietary constituents. Because all nutrients are absorbed across the mucosa of the small bowel, disorders that affect the mucosa may affect the absorption of fat, protein, carbohydrates, vitamins, and/or minerals. The clinical significance of malabsorption depends on the site and extent of involvement. The primary feature of malabsorption syndromes is chronic diarrhea. Other symptoms may include weight loss and anorexia despite normal or high caloric intake, physical weakness, abdominal distention and cramping, and malaise.

A wide variety of disorders of the digestive organs may cause malabsorption or **maldigestion**, including pancreatic exocrine deficiency; bile acid insufficiency; lymphatic disorders; gastric hypersecretory states; postgastrectomy disorders, especially following a Billroth II operation; small bowel resection; and small bowel disease, such as celiac sprue, tropical sprue, Whipple's disease, lactase deficiency, or abetalipoproteinemia.

To pinpoint the cause of malabsorption, the physician may order laboratory blood tests and specific absorption tests. Small bowel x-ray may be used to detect mucosal disease. A small bowel biopsy may be ordered to diagnose celiac sprue, Whipple's disease, abetalipoproteinemia, or agammaglobulinemia.

Treatment of most malabsorption conditions is directed at the underlying disease.

Celiac Disease (also known as gluten sensitive enteropathy and celiac sprue)

Celiac sprue is characterized by poor food absorption and intolerance of gluten, which is a protein found in wheat, oats, rye, barley, and their products. Malabsorption in the proximal small bowel results from atrophy of the villi and a decrease in the activity and amount of enzymes in the surface epithelium.

Celiac disease most likely results from a combination of environmental factors and genetic predisposition. Risk factors for celiac sprue include female sex, family history, and northwestern European ancestry.

The typical age of onset is between 8 and 24 months, after the child has been receiving gluten in his or her diet. In some cases, clinical signs disappear during adolescence and reappear in adulthood. The second peak age of presentation is in the twenties, in adults who have been previously asymptomatic.

Symptoms of celiac disease may include the following:
- recurrent attacks of diarrhea, vomiting, steatorrhea, abdominal distention, flatulence, stomach cramps, and weakness;
- anorexia or increased appetite without weight gain;
- irritability, uncooperativeness, and/or apathy; and
- growth failure, muscle wasting, delayed development, and/or anemia.

Diagnosis is made based on clinical history, physical examination, laboratory tests and upper GI endoscopy. Elevated blood antigliaden antibodies, antireticulin antibodies, and endomycial antibodies raise suspicion for this disorder. D-xylose absorption test may be performed to determine small bowel malabsorption but is not specific to celiac disease. Definitive diagnosis requires an initial biopsy examination that shows typical characteristics of celiac disease (severe flattening or complete absence of intestinal villi and hypertrophied crypts), followed by a second biopsy examination after strict adherence to a gluten-free diet, and a third biopsy examination after gluten challenge to demonstrate a recurrence of the disease.

Treatment of celiac disease involves *lifelong* elimination of gluten from the patient's diet, which means avoidance of all wheat, barley, rye, and oats. It is important that the patient also avoid meats containing wheat fillers and certain commercially prepared foods that may use wheat as an extender, such as ice cream and candy bars. Rice, corn, soy, and the flours of these grains are acceptable. Parents and children require continuing education and support to maintain compliance with a gluten-free diet, even when overt symptoms disappear.

In addition to diet restrictions, therapy may include enteral nutrition support to correct nutritional deficiencies, including macro and micronutrients. The clinical response to treatment is often dramatic, beginning with an improved disposition and general appearance. In adults, potential complications include an increased risk of malignant small bowel lymphoma and carcinoma of the esophagus and stomach.

Tropical sprue

Tropical sprue, which is a chronic disorder acquired in endemic tropical areas, is characterized by progressively more severe alterations of the jejunum and ileum.

Histological changes associated with tropical sprue consist of lengthening of the crypt area, broadening and shortening of the villi, epithelial cell changes, and infiltration by chronic inflammatory cells. Resulting nutritional deficiencies, notably megaloblastic anemia, may be ameliorated by treatment with a 2- to 6-month course of folic acid and tetracycline (Achromycin).

Whipple's disease

Whipple's disease is a rare disorder characterized by chronic diarrhea and progressive wasting. Only about 200 cases have been reported, primarily in the United States, England, continental Europe, and South America. It is also known as intestinal lipodystrophy and lipophagia granulomatosis. The cause is unknown, but it may be caused by an infection.

Whipple's disease most often affects Caucasian men between the ages of 20 and 67. Signs and symptoms include arthralgia; vague abdominal pain; diarrhea; steatorrhea; impaired intestinal absorption; progressive weight loss; slight fever; hyperpigmentation; peripheral, mesenteric, periaortic and celiac lymphadenopathy; and occasional splenomegaly.

Diagnosis is by biopsy examination of the small intestine, which shows macrophages and large cytoplasmic granules that stain a brilliant magenta with the periodic acid-Schiff stain.

Treatment consists of hospitalization and a 14-day course of therapy with penicillin G procaine (Bicillin) and streptomycin, followed by daily administration of tetracycline (Achromycin) for 10 to 12 months. During the acute phase, corticosteroids may be administered. Patients with iron-deficiency anemia need iron supplements.

Short bowel syndrome

Short bowel syndrome (SBS) is a malabsorptive disorder that occurs as a result of decreased functional mucosal surface area, usually due to massive resection of the small bowel. The malabsorption of macro and micronutrients, fluid, and electrolytes may lead to severe undernutrition, fluid, acid/base balance and electrolyte disturbances. Malabsorption may be exacerbated by complications frequently associated with SBS, such as bacterial overgrowth and dysmotility. These problems lead to a host of symptoms including diarrhea, abdominal pain, distension and vomiting. The severity of these disturbances varies with age (if occurring in infancy or childhood), the length and location of the bowel that is removed, and the condition of the remaining bowel.

The most common causes of SBS in infants include congenital anomalies (jejunal and ileal atresia, gastroschisis); necrotizing enterocolitis; and vascular injury (volvulus). Other causes of SBS in infants and children include small bowel resection due to long-segment Hirschsprung's disease, omphalocele, Crohn's disease, and trauma. Although rare, congenital short bowel may also be a cause of SBS in a small number of infants. Radiation enteritis may lead to functional SBS if injury to small bowel mucosa is extensive. In adults, common causes of SBS include Crohn's disease, tumors and trauma.

The prognosis for children and adults has dramatically improved in the past 25 years primarily due to advances in parenteral nutrition and the understanding of the importance of enteral nutrition. The capacity for adaptation and eventual ability to absorb all nutrients necessary to sustain growth by the enteral route may not be known for weeks or months following the initial resection as attempts to feed progress.

Intestinal adaptation and long-term outcome depends, in part, on the length and location of the residual small intestine and whether or not the ileocecal valve was preserved. Before the days of adequate nutritional intervention, infants with less than 15 cm of small bowel with the ileocecal valve, or less than 40 cm of small bowel without the ileocecal valve rarely survived (Wilmore, 1972). However, more recently, the prognosis for children with even less residual small bowel without an ileocecal valve has improved. There are case reports of children with as little as 12 cm of residual small who have survived and been successfully weaned from parenteral nutrition support (Surana et. al., 1993)

Although isolated duodenal resection is uncommon, the removal or bypassing of the duodenum may result in malabsorption of micronutrients and lead to clinically significant deficiencies. Malabsorption of iron, folate and calcium may lead to anemia and osteopenia in the child who had undergone duodenal resection. Malabsorption of fat and lipid-soluble vitamins may occur in the absence of adequate digestion and absorption aided by duodenal pancreatic and biliary secretions.

Extensive jejunal resection often leads to significant carbohydrate malabsorption due to the loss of the primary intestinal site of disaccharidase activity. Undigested and malabsorbed carbohydrate contributes to osmotic diarrhea. The duodenum and jejunum are also the primary site of absorption of proteins, fats, copper and lipid-soluble vitamins. Although resection of the ileum and preservation of the jejunum may initially cause fewer complications associated with fluid and nutrient absorption, the long-term capacity for adaptation is greater in the ileum after a proximal small bowel resection than in the jejunum after a distal small bowel resection.

Extensive resection of the ileum may lead to severe, early consequences. There may be tremendous fluid and electrolyte malabsorption due to the inability of the jejunum to compensate. Bile salt malabsorption following ileal resection may also contribute to watery diarrhea and fat malabsorption. Steatorrhea, fat and lipid soluble vitamin malabsorption are the consequence.

Preservation of the ileocecal valve is a factor affecting prognosis because the ileocecal valve performs functions that ultimately influence enteral feeding tolerance. The ileocecal valve regulates the flow of fluid and nutrients from the small bowel into the colon and the rate of small bowel transit. The ileocecal valve also prevents migration of colonic bacterial flora into the small bowel. Bacterial counts in the small bowel increase dramatically increase when the ileocecal valve is resected, due to migration of colonic flora.

The combined problems of small bowel bacterial overgrowth and carbohydrate malabsorption can lead to metabolic acidosis. Acidosis occurs when bacterial fermentation of unabsorbed carbohydrates produces short chain fatty acids which are then absorbed into the circulation. Treatment should be aimed at decreasing the bacterial population in the small bowel with antibiotics, administration of low-carbohydrate formulas, and the addition of citrate or bicarbonate to the enteral or parenteral nutrition solutions.

Motility disturbances following small bowel resection occur frequently, and may compound problems associated with SBS including malabsorption and bacterial overgrowth. The condition of the remaining bowel may have a more significant impact on motility and absorption than the total length and location of bowel resected. Stasis due to fibrosis, surgical narrowing or poor perfusion can be as detrimental to enteral feeding success as is fast transit.

Gastric acid hypersecretion is a common problem associated with SBS. Treatment with H2 receptor antagonist drugs, such as ranitidine or famotidine, or more potent proton pump inhibitors, such as omeprazole may be indicated if upper gastrointestinal symptoms or biopsy proven endoscopic findings of peptic disease are present.

Following extensive small bowel resection, a marked adaptation response occurs in the residual bowel. These compensatory changes begin within days of bowel resection and last for many months. The most striking feature of adaptation is hyperplasia of the villus cells. The villus height increases with an increase in the number of epithelial cells and elongation of the crypts. The degree of hyperplasia appears to be directly proportional to the amount of small bowel resected.

Several factors appear to be trophic for small bowel adaptation, and the most important stimulus for adaptation is enteral feeding. Nutrients in the small bowel lumen stimulate mucosal adaptation through several mechanisms including: (a) direct contact and absorption of nutrients by enterocytes, (b) stimulation of pancreatic and biliary secretions, and (c) stimulation of trophic hormones and growth factors in the bowel and elsewhere.

Cholestasis is a common complication in children and adults with SBS who require long-term parenteral nutrition. Although the mechanisms contributing to this problem are not fully understood, there is evidence that both prolonged parenteral nutrition and a lack of enteral feeding play independent and significant roles.

Following the initial surgical interventions, management of nutritional therapy should become the focus of care for these children. Maintaining optimal nutritional status and growth, with a combination of parenteral and enteral nutrition support, should be a priority for all patients with SBS.

The goals of parenteral nutrition therapy include maintenance of fluid and electrolyte balance and support of rapid growth during infancy and childhood while bowel adaptation occurs. Adjustments in total caloric delivery via parenteral nutrition should be adjusted based on the child's growth or the adult's energy needs.

The first major goal for children and adults with SBS is achieved when parenteral nutrition support is no longer required, thus the goal of parenteral nutrition weaning during advancement of enteral feeding should remain a high priority.

Enteral feeding should begin as soon as possible following small bowel resection, once fluid and electrolyte balance is achieved and gastrointestinal motility has returned. During the advancement of enteral feeding, parenteral nutrition should be continued for the balance of caloric needs.

Malabsorption of protein, carbohydrate and fat all occur with SBS. Initial enteral feedings should be provided as continuous infusion via nasogastric or gastrostomy tube. A formula containing hydrolyzed protein will he optimal in most cases. Protein hydrolysates have the advantage of being more readily absorbed than whole protein.

The role of carbohydrate in dietary management of SBS requires much attention. Severe malabsorption of carbohydrate contributes to osmotic diarrhea and metabolic acidosis. In this situation, carbohydrate often needs to he restricted. Complex starches should be avoided initially because they require considerable digestion before absorption can occur.

Recently, researchers and clinicians have shown that high-fat diets resulted in improved weight gain without increased fat malabsorption or stool volume in patients with protracted diarrhea on infancy and cystic fibrosis (Jirapinyo et al., 1990; Luder et al., 1989). Even when total stool fat increases with high-fat enteral feedings, if a fraction of the increased fat is absorbed, then high-fat feedings can prove beneficial.

Medium-chain triglycerides are more readily absorbed than long-chain triglycerides in the absence of sufficient bile acids, as medium-chain triglycerides may pass directly into the portal circulation.

Advancements in enteral feeding should be made at regular intervals, as tolerated, with increased volume or concentration of formula. Once complete enteral nutrition is achieved, compression of continuous feedings can be attempted, with increased hourly infusion rates with fewer hours of feedings during the day. Oral feedings (low fructose and lactose) can be encouraged and advanced as tolerated.

Supplemental enteral mulltivitamin and mineral products should be administered. Severe deficiencies may be corrected with additional individual micronutrients administered enterally or parenterally.

Successful management of complex nutrition support has provided the opportunity for long-term survival and a desirable quality of life for many with SBS. Early and aggressive enteral feeding is the primary stimulus for intestinal adaptation, which is the key to ultimate independence from parenteral nutrition and prevention of associated complications.

Lactase deficiency

The most common disorder of carbohydrate absorption is acquired **lactase deficiency**, in which a deficiency in the brush-border enzyme lactase causes malabsorption of the disaccharide lactose. This disorder is often called lactose intolerance. Secondary lactase dcficiency can result from diseases that damage the small bowel mucosa, such as celiac disease, tropical sprue, Crohn's disease, bacterial or viral enteritis, and radiation enteritis. Congenital lactase deficiency is a rare disorder in which mucosal lactase levels are low at birth.

Patients with lactase deficiency typically experience distention, flatulence, abdominal cramps, and watery diarrhea after ingesting cow's milk or milk products. The diagnosis is suggested by relief of symptoms on a lactose-free diet and reappearance of symptoms on reintroduction of lactose. Definitive diagnosis may be made by a lactose breath hydrogen test or by biochemically assaying the lactase content of the small bowel mucosa obtained by peroral or endoscopic biopsy examination. Treatment consists of restricting milk and milk products or use of lactose enzyme (lactase) supplements.

Motility disorders: intestinal pseudoobstruction. Pseudoobstruction is a rare disorder of impaired GI motility. Symptoms, which commonly appear within the first weeks of life, include nausea, vomiting, distention, abdominal pain, and failure to thrive without evidence of anatomical obstruction. In the absence of prompt intervention, children will develop malnutrition with impaired growth and development due to enteral feeding intolerances. Diagnostic evaluation includes fluoroscopic and nuclear medicine studies, as well as antroduodenal and intestinal motility studies. Treatment is generally supportive in nature. Use of motility agents may be effective in alleviating symptoms in some patients. The mainstays of therapy include treatment for bacterial overgrowth with antibiotics and nutritional therapy. Enteral feedings may be given via nasogastric, nasojejunal, gastrostomy, or jenunostomy tube. However, many children with pseudoobstruction tolerate enteral feeding only on an intermittent basis or not at all. In these children, parenteral nutrition is required to meet nutritional needs. Gastric and/or intestinal decompression may be necessary to maintain comfort. At the present time, surgery has a limited role in the treatment of pseudoobstruction. Future progress with small bowel transplantation may provide an alternative treatment option.

Abetalipoproteinemia

Abetalipoproteinemia is another absorption defect. Lack of betalipoproteins causes accumulation of fat and consequent malabsorption, resulting in increased stool fat. A small bowel biopsy examination will show villous epithelial cells distended with fat. Fat malabsorption lessens by restricting dietary long-chain triglycerides and administering medium-chain triglycerides.

Small bowel tumors

Benign or malignant neoplasms of the small bowel make up less than 5% of GI tumors. Small bowel neoplasms may be hamartomas, lymphomas, alpha heavy chain disease, primary or secondary carcinoma, or carcinoid tumors.

- **Peutz-Jeghers syndrome** is characterized by mucocutaneous pigmentation on the face, hands and feet, and in the perianal and genital areas. GI hamartomas may appear anywhere from the cardiac sphincter to the anus but are regularly present in the small bowel.

- Lymphomas of the GI tract may be primary, with or without involvement of the adjacent mesenteric nodes, or secondary, having spread from elsewhere. In primary small bowel lymphomas, patients present with abdominal pain or obstruction. In secondary lymphomas, nonalimentary complaints usually precede involvement of the gut.

- Alpha heavy chain disease is a proliferation of lymphoid tissue that involves the IgA secretory system, thus leading to the production of incomplete immunoglobulin molecules made up of IgA heavy chains. Clinical features of alpha heavy chain disease include severe malabsorption syndrome and, frequently, finger clubbing. Histopathological features include plasma cell proliferation in the small intestinal mucosa and in the nodes, followed by the development of overt malignant lymphoma in most cases.

- Primary carcinomas of the small bowel are most likely to occur in the duodenum; virtually all are adenocarcinomas. Symptoms include pain, vomiting, anorexia, malaise, and/or nausea. Diagnosis is by barium x-ray. Small bowel carcinomas are usually flat, stenosing, ulcerative, or polypoid.

- Secondary carcinomas of the small bowel are relatively common. They most often arise from the breast or bronchus or are metastatic malignant melanomas.

- Carcinoid tumors are often found by chance during appendectomy and occur most frequently in the ileum and appendix. Carcinoid tumors that metastasize to the liver may be associated with carcinoid syndrome, which includes watery diarrhea, abdominal cramps, borborygmi, episodic flushing and lacrimation, pellagra-like skin lesions, bronchospasm, and valvular lesions of the right side of the heart.

Small bowel tumors usually only occur in patients who are over the age of 50. Presenting symptoms may include small bowel obstruction; abdominal pain and/or vomiting, GI bleeding; weight loss; distended, tympanitic abdomen; and high-pitched bowel sounds. The patient's stool may contain occult blood. The physician may order blood studies; an upright plain x-ray of the abdomen; barium contrast x rays; endoscopy and biopsy examination for lesions in the proximal duodenum; ultrasonography or CT scan; or selective arteriography of the celiac axis and superior mesenteric artery.

Most small bowel tumors are treated surgically. Even metastatic tumors may require palliative surgery to relieve obstruction or bleeding. Institutional protocols for treatment of lymphomas may include surgical resection in addition to radiotherapy and chemotherapy. Radiation and chemotherapy of other malignant small bowel tumors have been largely ineffective. In Peutz-Jeghers syndrome, multiple enterotomies are usually required over the lifetime of the patient to remove large polyps that may be responsible for severe colicky pain.

CASE SITUATION

Mrs. O'Malley, age 43, was referred to a gastroenterologist after a 2-year history of diarrhea, abdominal distention with increased flatulence, stomach cramps, and fatigue. She has experienced two to four daily stools that are usually soft and bulky and a 15-pound weight loss. She describes herself as "tense and nervous" because of family problems. Her referring physician has treated her for irritable bowel syndrome (IBS) with antispasmodics and sedatives without improvement in her symptoms. She had upper and lower GI barium studies 18 months ago, which were normal. Her blood work shows she is anemic and hypoalbuminemic, but her stool is negative for occult blood.

Points to think about

1. Given Mrs. O'Malley's symptoms, what might be possible medical diagnoses?
2. What factors point to a diagnosis of celiac disease?
3. Mrs. O'Malley had normal upper and lower GI barium studies; would further barium studies be helpful?
4. It would also be necessary to obtain stool specimens for ova and parasites to rule out infectious or parasitic causes for Mrs. O'Malley's symptoms. What should the gastroenterology nurse tell the patient about collecting stool specimens?
5. The gastroenterology nurse knows that small bowel biopsy examination of the distal duodenum/proximal jejunum is the most definitive test for celiac disease. It will show that the mucosal surface is flat with shortened villi and elongated crypts, with changes in surface epithelial cells from tall columnar to cuboidal. What can he or she tell Mrs. O'Malley to expect when she goes for her biopsy examination?
6. What is one nursing diagnosis the nurse might consider for a patient with celiac sprue?
7. What might the nurse teach Mrs. O'Malley about her follow-up care?

Suggested responses

1. Possible medical diagnoses in Mrs. O'Malley's case might include the following:
   - IBS might explain her symptoms, but weight loss, anemia, and hypoalbuminemia are not usually seen in IBS. Also, her primary physician has tried treating her for IBS without success.
   - An inflammatory bowel disease could cause these symptoms, particularly Crohn's disease.
   - Lymphoma of the small bowel can cause obstruction of lymphatic drainage necessary for fat absorption.
   - Chronic pancreatitis causing pancreatic insufficiency and inadequate amounts of lipase for fat digestion might account for steatorrhea.
   - Tropical sprue or some parasitic disorders can cause these symptoms, but Mrs. O'Malley denies any travel history.

- Celiac disease with malabsorption in the proximal small bowel and intolerance of gluten could cause these symptoms, but her age may extend beyond the typical range.
2. Factors that point to a diagnosis of celiac disease include the following:
   - female sex;
   - presentation of features of malabsorption syndrome, including anemia (iron deficiency), protein deficiency (hypoalbuminemia), and steatorrhea (excessive fat in stool); and
   - age factor: although celiac disease is often diagnosed by 2 years of age, many patients experience the onset of this disease beginning in the third or fourth decade.
3. Because celiac disease affects the small bowel, an upper GI series with small bowel follow-through should be done. This may show excessive secretions and dilatation of mucosal folds in the proximal small bowel. Regarding collection of stool specimens, Mrs. O'Malley should receive the following instructions:
   - Obtain stool specimens before barium x-ray, because barium interferes with microscopic examination.
   - Use a clean, dry container.
   - Do not use stool that has been in contact with toilet-bowl water or urine.
   - Take the specimen to the laboratory immediately to ensure accurate results.
   - It is often necessary to test several specimens; for example, the first morning stool each day for 3 days.
4. Regarding her upcoming small bowel biopsy examination, Mrs. O'Malley should be told that:
   - The physician may try to get a large enough biopsy specimen by doing a standard esophagogastroduodenoscopy (EGD). Mrs. O'Malley may have this done in the hospital endoscopy unit or in the office endoscopy setting. The gastroenterology nurse should explain this procedure to the patient, with reassurance that a gastroenterology nurse will be there to assist her through all phases of the procedure.
   - Large submucosal biopsy specimens may be obtained by suction capsules that are guided under fluoroscopic control to the proper location in the proximal jejunum. The patient is attended during the procedure by the gastroenterologist and the gastroenterology nurse. Full explanation of the procedure and complications should be provided by the physician and may be reinforced by the nurse during the procedure.
   - Normally, a submucosal biopsy examination is done as an outpatient procedure; therefore, Mrs. O'Malley will not be admitted to the hospital. The nurse should instruct her to immediately report any severe abdominal pain or distention, nausea, vomiting, or bleeding.
5. The nurse might consider the nursing diagnosis "knowledge deficit related to necessary dietary modifications for celiac disease." The nurse can begin intervention predicated on such a diagnosis in many instances; however, it is important to recognize that the act of acquiring and recall-

ing new information does not necessarily mean that the learner will change his or her behavior as a consequence.

- The "knowledge deficit" diagnosis is broad and involves three learning domains: receiving/retaining new information; responding emotionally by personalizing the information; and changing behavior by alteration in neuromuscular pathways. There may be a deficit or deficits in any one or more of these learning dimensions, although most deficits occur in the cognitive or psychomotor areas.
- Other factors that might influence the patient's response to nursing interventions based on this diagnosis include cognitive function, lack of exposure to information, visual or auditory sensory deficits, pathophysiological states or conditions, state of motivation or readiness to learn, cultural or language barriers, or coping strategies (e.g., denial, anxiety).

6. Regarding her follow-up care, the nurse should explain the following to Mrs. O'Malley:

- It will be necessary for her to make permanent, lifelong adjustments in her diet based on written gluten-free diet instructions, which the nurse will provide
- Fecal fat studies and laboratory blood studies will be required at specified intervals
- Foods containing lactose may not be tolerated well (because they may cause diarrhea and flatulence) and often must be eliminated from the diet
- Response to dietary changes can be dramatic; within a few days or weeks general appearance will improve and fatigue will lessen, stools will be more formed and less frequent, and abdominal distention will decrease
- Lost weight is usually recovered within several months
- The villous architecture in the small bowel should return to normal, and a follow-up biopsy examination might be done to confirm improvement
- There are several support groups for families with celiac disease; also, several companies produce gluten-free products

REVIEW TERMS

abetalipoproteinemia, ampulla of Vater, Auerbach's plexus, borborygmi, Brunner's glands, celiac disease, Crohn's disease, crypts of Lieberkühn, duodenum, enteric plexus, giardiasis, goblet cells, ileocecal valve, ileum, inflammatory bowel disease, intussusception, jejunum, lactase deficiency, lamina propria, ligament of Treitz, malabsorption, maldigestion, malnutrition, Meckel's diverticulum, Meissner's plexus, microvilli, Paneth's cells, peptic ulcers, Peutz-Jeghers syndrome, Peyer's patches, regional enteritis, short bowel syndrome, small bowel, steatorrhea, tropical sprue, villus, volvulus, Whipple's disease

REVIEW QUESTIONS

1. The proximal two fifths of the small bowel is known as the:
   (a) Duodenum.
   (b) Ileum.
   (c) Jejunum.
   (d) Cecum.
2. The mucous layer of the small bowel is lined with:
   (a) Squamous epithelium.
   (b) Columnar epithelium.
   (c) Connective tissue.
   (d) Peritoneum.
3. The principal function of Brunner's glands is to:
   (a) Synthesize antibodies.
   (b) Absorb nutrients.
   (c) Secrete a viscous, alkaline fluid.
   (d) Secrete hormones.
4. The primary site of absorption for vitamin B_{12} and bile acids is the:
   (a) Duodenum.
   (b) Jejunum.
   (c) Ileum.
   (d) Stomach.
5. The intestinal contents are constantly being stirred by:
   (a) Active transport.
   (b) Segmenting contractions.
   (c) Peristalsis.
   (d) Shortening and lengthening of the villi.
6. Segmental submucosal inflammation and a cobblestoned appearance of the bowel wall are associated with:
   (a) Ulcerative colitis.
   (b) Crohn's disease.
   (c) Duodenal ulcers.
   (d) Celiac sprue.
7. The most effective treatment for symptomatic Meckel's diverticulum is:
   (a) Diverticulectomy.
   (b) Antibiotic therapy.
   (c) Bowel resection.
   (d) Dietary modification.
8. About 80% of all peptic ulcers occur in the:
   (a) Stomach.
   (b) Duodenum.
   (c) Ileum.
   (d) Jejunum.
9. A malabsorption syndrome characterized by gluten intolerance is:
   (a) Cystic fibrosis.
   (b) Whipple's disease.
   (c) Tropical sprue.
   (d) Celiac sprue.
10. Primary carcinomas of the proximal small bowel are virtually all:
    (a) Lymphomas.
    (b) Melanomas.
    (c) Adenocarcinomas.
    (d) Sarcomas.

BIBLIOGRAPHY

Avunduk, C. (2002). *Manual of gastroenterology: diagnosis and therapy* (3rd ed.). Boston: Lippincott, Williams & Wilkins.

Beare, P. & Myers, J. (1994). Nursing management of adults with intestinal disorders. In Principles and practice of adult health nursing (2nd ed.). St. Louis, MO: Mosby.

Black, M. (1989). Crohn's disease: pathophysiology, diagnosis and management. *Gastroenterol Nurs 11*, 259-63.

Bongiovanni, G. (Ed.) (1988). *Essentials of clinical gastroenterology* (2nd ed.) New York: McGraw-Hill.

Coleman, D. (1987). *Anatomy and physiology of the small bowel* (2nd ed.). *SGA J 10*, 44-5. Society of Gastrointestinal Assistants.

Given, B. & Simmons, S. (1984). *Gastroenterology in clinical nursing* (4th ed.). St. Louis, MO: Mosby.

Goldberg, K. (Ed.) (1986). *Gastrointestinal problems: Nurse Review Series*. Springhouse, PA: Springhouse.

Hamilton, H. (Ed.) (1985). *Diseases, Nurse's Reference Library Series*. Springhouse, PA: Springhouse.

Hays, T.L., Saavedra, J.M., Mattis, L.E. (1995). The use of high-fat low-carbohydrate diets for advancement of enteral feedings in children with short bowel syndrome. *Top Clin Nutrition 10(4)*, 35-41.

Kirschner, B.S. (1988). Inflammatory bowel disease in children. *Pediatr Clin North America 35*, 189-208. Pediatric Clinics of North America.

MacDonald, W.C., Trier, J.S. & Everett, N.B. (1964). Cell proliferation and migration in the stomach, duodenum and rectum of man: Radioautographic studies. *Gastroenterology 46*, 405-17.

Madara, J.L. & Trier, J.S. (1994). Functional morphology of the mucosa of the small intestine. In Johnson, L.R. (Ed.), *Physiology of the gastrointestinal tract* (3rd ed.). New York: Lippincott-Raven.

Martin, D. (2002). *Practical gastroenterology*. Florence, KY: Taylor and Francis.

McFarland, G. & McFarlane, E. (1989), *Nursing diagnosis and intervention*. St. Louis, MO: Mosby.

Peck, S. & Altschuler, S. (1992). Pseudoobstruction in children. *Gastroenterol Nurs 14(4)*, 184-8.

Peterson, W.L. (1991). Helicobacter pylori and peptic ulcer disease. *N Engl J Med 324*, 1043-8, New England Journal of Medicine.

Phaosawasdi, K. LIST ALL AUTHORS (1988). Cryptosporidiosis in the immunocompetent host: a case report and an examination of an increasingly important parasite. *SGA J 11*, 80-4.

Sachar, D., Waye, J. & Lewis, B. (Eds.) (1989). *Gastroenterology for the house officer*. Baltimore, MD: Williams & Wilkins.

Sleisenger, M. & Fordtran, J. (Eds.). *Gastrointestinal disease: pathophysiology, diagnosis, management* (7th ed.). Philadelphia: W.B. Saunders.

Smeltzer, S.C. & Bare, B.G. (2002). *Textbook of medical surgical nursing* (9th ed.). Philadelphia: W.B. Saunders.

Surana, R., Quinn, F.M.J. & Puri, P. (1994). Short-gut syndrome: Intestinal adaptation in a patient with 12 cm of jejunum. *J Pediatr Gastroenterol Nutr. 19*, 246-9. Journal of Pediatric Gastroenterology and Nutrition.

Walker, W.A., Durie, P., Hamilton, J.R., Watkins, J.B. and Walker-Smith, J.A.. (2000). *Pediatric gastrointestinal disease: Pathophysiology, diagnosis, management*. Ontario, Canada: Decker.

Weaver, L.T., Austin, S. & Cole, T.J. (1991). Small intestinal length: a factor essential for gut adaptation, *GUT 32*, 1321-1523.

Wilmore, D.W. (1972). Factors correlating with a successful outcome following extensive intestinal resection in newborn infants. *J Pediatr. 80*, 88-95.

Chapter 16

LARGE INTESTINE

This chapter will acquaint the gastroenterology nurse with the normal anatomy and physiology of the large intestine. Selected diseases and disorders of the large intestine in terms of pathophysiology, diagnosis, and treatment are discussed.

Learning objectives

After reviewing the content of this chapter, the gastroenterology nurse should be able to:

1. Explain the normal macroanatomy and microanatomy of the large intestine.
2. Outline the physiology of absorption, secretion, and motility in the large intestine.
3. Discuss the pathophysiology, diagnosis, and treatment of a number of diseases and disorders of the large intestine, including intestinal polyps; anatomical, inflammatory, parasitic and diverticular diseases; cancer; and anorectal disorders.

ANATOMY AND PHYSIOLOGY

The large intestine is 90 to 150 cm (4 to 5 feet) long and approximately 4 to 6 cm (2 inches) in diameter (see Fig. 13-2). It extends from the ileocecal valve to the anus and is divided into the following five sections: the ascending, transverse, descending, and sigmoid colon, and the rectum (Fig. 16-1; see Fig. 13-2).

At the distal end of the small intestine, a flap valve known as the ileocecal valve acts as a sphincter both to control the passage of intestinal contents from the ileum to the **colon** and to prevent the reflux of bacteria from the colon back into the small bowel, thus preserving the relative sterility of the small bowel. In the adult, the resting pressure of the ileocecal valve is about 20 mm Hg above the colonic pressure, and the length of the high-pressure zone is approximately 4 cm.

The first section of the large intestine to receive material from the small bowel is the **cecum**, a short blind sac that is wider in diameter than long and to which the **vermiform appendix** is attached. The appendix itself is a thin, tubular structure that ranges from 2 to 20 cm in length, being somewhat longer in children and about 8 mm in diameter. It has no known digestive role.

Immediately above the cecum is the **ascending** (right) **colon**, which passes up the right side of the abdomen to the lower border of the liver, where it bends to the left at the right colic, or **hepatic, flexure**. The **transverse colon** is the portion of the bowel that crosses the abdomen from right to left, from the hepatic flexure to the left colic, or **splenic, flexure**. The **descending** (left) **colon** runs down the left side of the abdomen from the spleen to the iliac crest, where it makes an s-curve at midline to form the **sigmoid colon**.

The last major portion of the large intestine is the rectum, which follows the curvature of the lower sacrum and coccyx. The **rectum** length is about 9 cm in infants, increasing to 15 cm in adults. The distal portion forms the anal canal. Movement of feces through the anal canal is controlled by an inch-wide internal sphincter composed of involuntary smooth muscle, and an external sphincter made up of voluntary striated muscle. Levator ani muscles surrounding the rectum also help keep defecation under voluntary control. The actual opening is called the **anus**.

The wall of the large intestine has four layers: the serosa, the muscularis, the submucosa, and the mucosa. The outer serous layer is formed by the visceral peritoneum. The rectum does not have a serous layer.

The second layer, or muscularis, includes an inner circular layer and an outer longitudinal layer that is composed of three heavy longitudinal bands **(tenia coli)**. The tenia coli are shorter than the intestine, thus causing it to pucker and form small sacs called **haustra**. The size and shape of the haustra vary with the state of contraction of the circular and

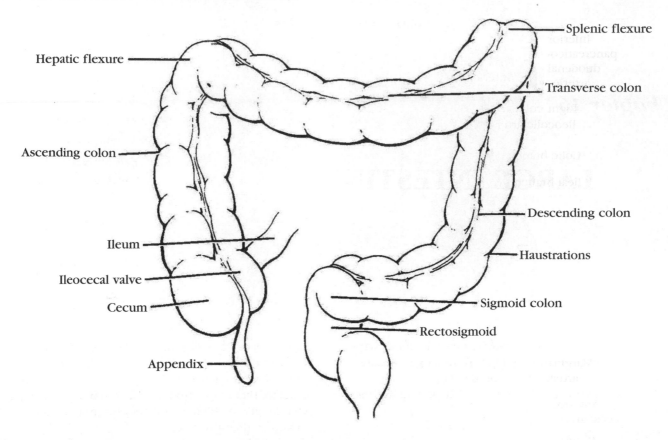

Fig. 16-1. Large bowel anatomy.

longitudinal muscle layers. Auerbach's nerve plexus is located between the circular and longitudinal muscle layers. A prominent extracellular matrix contains increased amounts of collagen and elastin than is present in the small bowel. The amount of collagen and elastin increases with advancing age.

The third layer of the large intestine is the submucosa, loose connective tissue that contains arteries, veins, and lymphatic vessels and the nerve fibers and ganglion cells that form Meissner's plexus. The submucosa is separated from the mucosa by the muscularis mucosae, a layer of smooth muscle cells.

The mucosa itself is smooth-surfaced and is arranged in folds called the *plicae semilunares*. As in the small bowel, the tubular crypts of Lieberkühn open into the lumen of the large intestine. Intestinal villi, however, are absent in the large bowel; the absorptive surface is flat and is lined by columnar epithelial cells and a number of goblet cells. There are fewer microvilli on the colonic columnar cells than in the small intestine. The epithelium in the lower half of the crypts is composed of proliferating undifferentiated columnar cells, mucus-secreting goblet cells, and a few endocrine cells.

The mucous membrane that lines the rectum is arranged in longitudinal rows called *rectal* or *anal columns*. Each rectal column contains an artery and a vein. These rectal columns end about 2 cm from the anal orifice, where they join trans-

verse tissue folds. At the anorectal line, also known as the mucocutaneous border, the colonic mucosa meets the external anal canal. The anorectal line also marks a change in nerve supply and venous drainage.

The right half of the large intestine receives arterial blood from the branches of the superior mesenteric artery, and the left or lower portion receives arterial blood from branches of the inferior mesenteric artery. Venous blood from the colon is drained mainly through the inferior and superior mesenteric veins (Fig. 16-2).

The rectum and anal canal receive arterial blood from the hemorrhoidal artery, which is a branch of the inferior mesenteric artery. The rectum is also supplied by branches of the hypogastric artery. Above the anorectal line, venous blood drains upward to the superior hemorrhoidal veins and from there to the portal veins. Below the anorectal line, venous blood drains downward to the inferior hemorrhoidal veins.

Colonic nerve supply lies close to the arterial vessels. Parasympathetic innervation of the right portion of the colon is derived from the vagus nerve. The remaining portion receives parasympathetic innervation through branches of the sacral nerves and sympathetic innervation through the spinal nerves. In general, stimulation of the parasympathetic nerves increases intestinal contraction and mucus secretion and inhibits the rectal sphincter, whereas stimulation of sympathetic fibers inhibits colonic motility and

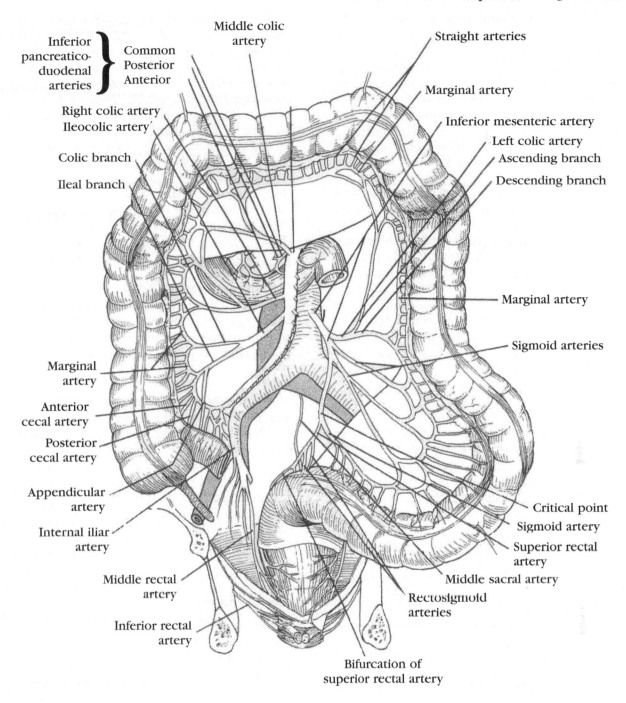

Inferior
pancreatico-
duodenal
arteries
} Common
  Posterior
  Anterior

Middle colic
artery

Straight arteries

Marginal artery

Inferior mesenteric artery

Left colic artery

Ascending branch

Descending branch

Right colic artery

Ileocolic artery

Colic branch

Ileal branch

Marginal artery

Marginal
artery

Sigmoid arteries

Anterior
cecal artery

Posterior
cecal artery

Appendicular
artery

Internal iliar
artery

Critical point

Sigmoid artery

Superior rectal
artery

Middle rectal
artery

Middle sacral artery

Rectosigmoid
arteries

Inferior rectal
artery

Bifurcation of
superior rectal artery

Fig. 16-2. Arterial and venous blood supplies to primary and accessory organs of the GI tract. (From Broadwell DC, Jackson BS: *Principles of ostomy care*, St. Louis, 1982, Mosby.)

secretions and stimulates the rectal sphincter.

The main functions of the large intestine are the storage and movement of intestinal contents; absorption of water, some electrolytes, and bile acids; and to a minor extent, the excretion of mucus, potassium, and bicarbonate.

Motility

The colon has three basic patterns of movement, which are explained as follows:

1. Periodic, uncoordinated tonic contractions or segmentations of both the longitudinal and circular muscles bunch up the folds of the mucosa, forming the haustra.

2. Phasic, random, nonpropulsive contractions last 30 seconds to 2 minutes and include peristalsis and retrograde peristalsis, which mix the stool material and help absorb its liquid contents without advancing the material toward the anus.

3. Spontaneous mass movements occur three or four times

a day when the colon becomes filled and distended. This rapid caudal movement of material is much more evident in the colon than are the phasic or mixing movements. When mass movements of the sigmoid colon move feces into the rectum, the urge to defecate is stimulated, causing peristaltic waves in the rectum and relaxation of the internal and then the external anal sphincter.

If relaxation of the internal and external sphincters is not enough to provide for defecation, a **Valsalva maneuver** assists in the process. Through the Valsalva maneuver, the involuntary movement of the bowel wall and the relaxation of the external sphincter are assisted by contraction of the diaphragm and the thoracic and abdominal muscles. This strain and downward push lasts approximately 8 seconds, thus increasing the intraabdominal pressure and frequently emptying the colon from as high as the splenic flexure.

Under normal conditions, gas moves down the colon at a rate of about 1 to 4 inches per second. Liquids are moved by gravity and peristalsis and by mass movements, but solid materials move primarily by mass movements. Overall motility of the large intestine is slow compared to the small intestine, and it can take as long as 7 days for material to clear the colon.

Secretion

Colonic secretion is scanty and consists primarily of water, mucus, potassium, and bicarbonate. The alkaline mucus secreted by goblet cells in the crypts lubricates the intestinal walls, protects the mucosa from acidic bacterial action, and helps lubricate the passage of stool.

Absorption and elimination

Of the 1000 to 2000 ml of liquid chyme that enters the colon daily, only 150 to 250 ml of fluid is evacuated in the stool. The colon is much more efficient than the small intestine in removing water, operating at 80% to 90%. The mechanisms for water and ion transport are the same as in the small intestine. The epithelial lining of the colon, however, would be considered tight relative to the small bowel, allowing less back diffusion of ions and therefore enhanced water absorption. The colon absorbs sodium, chloride, and water, with most absorption being accomplished in the ascending colon.

Normal feces contain intestinal bacteria that help break down and putrefy body wastes, trace fluids, mucus, indigestible cellulose, undigested connective tissue and toxins from meat proteins, undigested fats, and bile pigments. Feces are normally brown in color because of the metabolism of bile pigments to stercobilin. Odor is the result of indole and skatole, both of which are products of protein catabolism.

Indigenous bacteria

The colon is sterile at birth but rapidly becomes colonized by swallowed bacteria. The bacterial composition is established primarily from maternal contamination within 1 week of birth and is maintained throughout the lifetime. The normal adult colon contains approximately 10^9 to 10^{11} organisms per g of stool, which consist primarily of gram-negative anaerobic bacteria, such as *Bacteroides*, *Lactobacillus*, and *Clostridium*. The positive effects of these resident bacteria include breaking down cellulose and other waste material, deconjugating bile salts, synthesizing vitamin K, controlling the overgrowth of harmful bacteria, thickening the mucosal lining of the bowel, and destroying pancreatic enzymes that are harmful to the skin and other structures.

Indigenous bacteria also have a number of potentially harmful effects, including the manufacture of gas; production of the toxins or chemicals that produce colitis or diarrhea; invasion of the bowel wall, thereby producing infectious colitis; and the production of ammonia, which can cause hepatic encephalopathy in patients with hepatic cirrhosis.

PATHOPHYSIOLOGY

Among the diseases and disorders that affect the large intestine are intestinal polyps, angiodysplasia, colitis, irritable bowel syndrome, chronic recurrent abdominal pain syndrome, parasitic infestations, diverticular disease, tumors, obstructions, and anorectal disorders.

Polyps

Colonic **polyps** are discrete tissue masses that protrude into the lumen of the bowel. Pedunculated polyps are attached to the intestinal wall by a stem. Broad-based, sessile polyps attach directly to the intestinal wall. Diagnosis is by colonoscopy or proctosigmoidoscopy and air-contrast barium enema.

Most polyps are asymptomatic, but some patients experience bleeding. Research shows that removal of rectal polyps dramatically reduces the incidence of subsequent rectal cancer. Familial polyposis coli, Gardner's syndrome, and Peutz-Jeghers syndrome are the most common polyposis syndromes.

Juvenile polyps

Nearly all polyps found in children are benign. These are referred to as juvenile polyps, also called *retention* or *inflammatory polyps*. These types of polyps are rarely found in infants but increase in prevalence with age and reach a peak of occurrence between 5 and 6 years of age. They are uncommon after early adolescence.

Familial polyposis coli

In **familial polyposis coli**, which is inherited as an autosomal dominant trait, hundreds of adenomatous polyps develop throughout the colon. Familial polyposis is diagnosed by digital rectal examination, colonoscopy or proctosigmoidoscopy, and barium enema. Patients may also present with nonspecific symptoms, such as **hematochezia** (passage of bloody stools), **diarrhea**, abdominal pain, and intestinal obstruction. Because these polyps may become cancerous, surgery is strongly recommended; most likely total proctocolectomy with ileostomy.

Gardner's syndrome

In **Gardner's syndrome**, multiple adenomatous polyps appear along the colon or other parts of the GI tract, and osteomas appear on the mandible, skull, and long bones. Like familial polyposis coli, Gardner's syndrome is familial. Symptoms of both diseases are similar and some sources suggest that the two may be variable expressions of a single disease. Because the polyps associated with Gardner's syndrome tend to become cancerous in 10 to 15 years, surgical treatment is recommended.

Peutz-Jeghers syndrome

Peutz-Jeghers syndrome, inherited as an autosomal-dominant trait, is characterized by hamartomatous polyps and abnormal brown pigmentation of the lips, oral mucosa, and skin. Polypoid lesions have also been noted outside the GI tract, and abdominal pain caused by mechanical blockage or intussusception is the most common symptom. The freckle-like pigmentation of the lips appears in childhood and tends to fade with age. Pigmentation of the buccal mucosa is a more reliable indicator in older individuals and may appear earlier in infancy than do cutaneous lesions. Peutz-Jeghers syndrome has been associated with precocious puberty in girls, feminizing gonadal tumors in boys, hepatic cysts, and thyroid papillary adenocarcinoma. Most individuals do well over many decades, although there is a definite increased risk of developing bowel cancer.

Angiodysplasia

Angiodysplasias are vascular dilatations in the submucosa that consist of arterial, venous, and capillary elements. They are often multiple and occur most frequently in the cecum and right colon but may be found throughout the GI tract. Most are associated with normal aging, but their etiology remains uncertain. In the hereditary autosomal-dominant disorder Osler-Weber-Rendu disease, also known as hereditary hemorrhagic telangiectasia, angiodysplasias occur throughout the GI tract and on the skin, in the nail beds, and in the mucosa of the mouth and nasopharynx.

As many as 25% of individuals over the age of 60 with no history of GI bleeding may have vascular ectasias of the colon. Asymptomatic individuals require no treatment. In symptomatic individuals, the usual presentation is acute lower GI bleeding, which may be attributed to another coexisting disorder. It is not uncommon for a patient to experience several bleeding episodes before the proper diagnosis is made.

Diagnosis of angiodysplasias (arteriovenous malformations) is by colonoscopy or angiography. Treatment is by resection of the bowel segment that contains the lesion. Bleeding recurs in 15% to 37% of patients who are treated surgically. Alternative treatment methods include endoscopic treatment with a laser, heater probe, or bipolar electrocoagulation; however, these methods are attempted with caution because of poor healing and the risk of perforation.

Colitis

Colitis is broadly defined as an inflammation of the colon. Several different forms of this disorder are recognized, including ischemic colitis, necrotizing enterocolitis, ulcerative colitis, pseudomembranous colitis, Crohn's colitis, cow's milk protein-induced enterocolitis, and radiation enteritis.

Ischemic colitis

Ischemic colitis is an acute vascular insufficiency of the colon. It may occur in any portion of the small or large bowel but usually affects the descending colon (most often in the region of the splenic flexure) or the sigmoid colon, portions of the colon that are supplied by the inferior mesenteric artery.

Ischemic colitis may be either occlusive or nonocclusive. Occlusive ischemic disease represents a mechanical obstruction in the blood vessels that supply the bowel. It can often be traced to emboli from an artificial mitral valve or a fibrillating atrium or to surgical bypass, especially vascular surgery involving the distal aorta. Nonocclusive ischemia is usually related to a severe derangement in the central circulation consequent to such conditions as congestive heart failure, myocardial infarction, major hemorrhage, sepsis, or cardiac arrhythmia. Drugs causing arterial or venous thrombosis, intense arterial constriction, or hypotensive agents may also cause intestinal ischemia.

Symptoms of ischemic colitis include abrupt onset of pain at the left iliac fossa, bloody diarrhea, low-grade fever, abdominal distention, and minor abdominal tenderness. The classic radiological sign is thumbprinting in the affected area of the bowel, resulting from localized elevation of the mucosa by submucosal hemorrhage or edema. Cautious use of sigmoidoscopy may reveal nonspecific colitis, ulcerations, and/or bluish soft nodules; histology may reveal characteristic apoplosis.

Most patients recover spontaneously, although a minority develop peritoneal signs and absent bowel sounds, signifying bowel infarction and peritonitis. Such patients require surgical intervention consisting of segmental resection and either primary anastomosis or temporary colostomy. Follow-up barium enema x-rays or colonoscopy should be done 6 to 8 weeks after recovery to rule out ischemic strictures.

Necrotizing enterocolitis

Necrotizing enterocolitis (NEC) is a disease of focal or diffuse ulceration of the GI tract that usually occurs in the distal small bowel and/or colon. It occurs almost exclusively in the neonatal period, and the presentation varies from insidious to acute and fulminate. No single etiological factor has been found to be responsible for NEC. Three factors acting either individually or in concert have been associated with occurrence. These include formula feeding as opposed to breast-feeding, intestinal ischemia, and mucosal or systemic invasion of enteric bacteria. Host factors of immaturity, including an inefficient intestinal barrier, have also been implicated as a risk factor. The classic signs of NEC include abdominal distention, bilious vomiting, and bloody stools. The diagnosis of NEC is confirmed radiologically by the presence of pneumatosis intestinalis (air within the intestinal wall or air in the hepatic portal venous system). The management of a child with NEC is largely supportive. Oral feedings are withheld, a nasogastric tube placed to suction is used along with IV provision of nutrition, and broad-spectrum parenteral antibiotic therapy is utilized. Surgery involving conservative bowel resection of gangrenous bowel may be necessary in cases of perforation.

Ulcerative colitis

Ulcerative colitis (UC) is chronic, recurrent inflammation that affects the mucosa and submucosa of the large intestine. Inflammation often originates in the lower colon and then spreads proximally. The mucosa develops diffuse ulceration and hemorrhage, with congestion, edema, and exudative inflammation in the lamina propria and submucosa. Crypt abscesses form and become necrotic, leading to bloody, mucoid stools. Periods of remission often alternate with exacerbations. As crypt abscesses heal, granulation tissue forms, causing the colon to narrow, shorten, and lose its haustra. The cause of UC is unknown.

UC and Crohn's disease (see Chapter 15) are often described together as inflammatory bowel disease; signs and symptoms of the two disorders are similar. Crohn's disease, however, typically affects all layers of the bowel wall, not just the mucosa. In addition, UC is usually continuous from the rectum and is limited to the large intestine; Crohn's disease is often segmental and most often involves the small bowel, particularly the terminal ileum, but may affect any area of the GI tract.

Symptoms of UC may begin abruptly. They include the following:

(a) bloody, mucopurulent diarrhea and cramping;
(b) nausea, vomiting, and lethargy;
(c) fever, dehydration, and anemia in severe cases;
(d) decreased appetite, leading to nutritional deficiencies;
(e) lower left quadrant tenderness, guarding, and abdominal distention, although abdominal findings may be absent even in the presence of total colonic involvement; and
(f) extraintestinal symptoms involving the liver, skin, eyes, or joints.

Following a thorough history and physical examination, diagnostic sigmoidoscopy is usually performed. Findings consistent with UC include granularity and increased friability of the mucosa when wiped with a cotton swab, ulceration, and pseudopolyps. A rectosigmoid biopsy examination may provide additional histological evidence, and colonoscopy may be necessary. The physician may also order a stool analysis, stool cultures, and blood studies. A barium enema may be ordered but is contraindicated in patients with very active or fulminant colitis.

Dietary and drug therapy may be ordered to reduce inflammation, maintain fluid and electrolyte balance, and relieve symptoms. The ultimate goal is to enable the patient to return to a normal, active lifestyle. Treatment methods may include the following:

(a) In adults, avoidance of foods that appear to aggravate their symptoms;
(b) nutritional therapy in children, to correct nutritional deficiencies and provide supplemental calories, optimal healing, and growth requirements;
(c) in those with strictures, fiber restriction, and lactose avoidance in those found to be lactose intolerant;
(d) 5-aminosalicylate drugs, immunosuppressive agents, and/or antibiotics;
(e) corticosteroid therapy, administered topically (rectally), orally, or intravenously;
(f) bed rest, possibly in the hospital, for an acute exacerbation; and
(g) surgery in 20% to 25% of patients, including unresponsive patients or those with complications such as perforation and hemorrhage (if surgery is required, the physician may perform a total proctocolectomy with ileostomy.).

Arthritis is a frequent extraintestinal manifestation of UC occurring in 20% to 25% of patients and correlates with disease activity. Sacroiliitis and ankylosing spondylitis are rare and occur in patients with histocompatibility marker HLA-B27, following a course independent of intestinal disease. Minor elevations of serum transaminase or alkaline phosphatase levels are not uncommon in UC and may be secondary to hepatic steatosis. The major chronic liver disease associated with UC is sclerosing cholangitis and is generally progressive and independent of intestinal disease activity. Ophthalmological complications such as uveitis, episcleritis, and conjunctivitis may occur in children with UC. Hematological abnormalities; thromboembolic disease; dermatological manifestations such as erythema nodosum and pyoderma gangrenosum; and renal disease may also occur.

Potential minor local complications of UC include pseudopolyps, hemorrhoids, anal fissures, perianal or ischiorectal abscess, and rectal prolapse. More serious local complications may include massive colonic hemorrhage, colonic strictures, colonic perforation, and toxic megacolon. Pouchitis or inflammation of an ileal pouch after surgery for UC may occur with symptoms similar to those seen with UC. Treatment with antibiotics and antiinflammatory agents may be required.

Toxic megacolon is an acute dilatation of the diseased colon that is associated with systemic toxicity. It is the most severe, life-threatening complication of UC but may also be associated with any severe inflammatory condition of the bowel, including Crohn's disease, bacterial colitis, and amebiasis. In some patients with UC, toxic megacolon represents the first attack but is relatively rare in young patients.

Prominent symptoms of toxic megacolon are fever, abdominal pain and distention, vomiting, and fatigue. The patient may experience a progressive decrease in the frequency of stools resulting from loss of colonic propulsive activity. Leukocytosis, anemia, hypomagnesemia, and hypoalbuminemia are common laboratory findings. Clinical symptoms such as fever and abdominal tenderness may be masked by high-dose corticosteroid therapy or immunosuppressive agents. Plain films of the abdomen will reveal dilatation of the entire colon or only the transverse colon. Catastrophic complications of toxic megacolon include colonic perforation, gram-negative sepsis, and massive hemorrhage.

Treatment of toxic megacolon includes NPO status; nasogastric suction; and IV fluids, electrolytes, steroids, and broad-spectrum antibiotics. If toxic megacolon does not improve within 48 to 72 hours, total colectomy is indicated.

UC patients are also at increased risk of developing adenocarcinoma of the colon. The risk of cancer is directly related to the extent of colon involvement and duration of disease. For surveillance purposes, it is recommended that colonoscopy be performed yearly after 7 to 10 years of disease identification. However, surveillance colonoscopy is costly, entails some risk, and does not afford complete assurance that adenocarcinoma is not present.

Pseudomebranous colitis

Pseudomembranous colitis is defined as an acute inflammation of the bowel mucosa, with the formation of pseudomembranous plaques overlying an area of superficial ulceration. It is also called pseudomembranous **enterocolitis** or enteritis, antibiotic-associated colitis or diarrhea, and *clostridium difficile*-associated colitis or diarrhea. The preferred method of diagnosis of pseudomembranous colitis is endoscopy to detect typical red, edematous, fragile mucosa with yellow-white raised plaques that may extend from the rectosigmoid area to the proximal colon. Sigmoidoscopy is usually adequate, but up to one third of patients have lesions restricted to the right colon, thus necessitating colonoscopy. Biopsies identify pseudomembranes too small to visualize endoscopically.

The great majority of cases of pseudomembranous colitis involve a toxin or toxins produced by *C. difficile*, which is a spore-forming, gram-positive, anaerobic rod capable of producing many toxic factors. Pseudomembranous colitis caused by other pathogens is rare but has been attributed to organisms such as *Salmonella, Clostridium perfringens, Plesiomonas shigelloides*, and other clostridia. The most useful diagnostic test is the demonstration of this toxin in the stool, using either enzyme-linked immunosorbent assay (ELISA) or counterimmunoelectrophoresis. Pseudomembranous colitis is commonly associated with oral or IV antibiotic therapy and, less often, with chemotherapeutic agents. It should be suspected in any patient who develops diarrhea during or within 10 weeks of antibiotic therapy.

Symptoms of pseudomembranous colitis may range from mild diarrhea to fulminant colitis and include nonbloody, watery diarrhea; crampy abdominal pain; fever; and leukocytosis. Complications may include toxic megacolon, pneumoperitoneum, severe electrolyte imbalance hypoalbuminemia, and acute migratory polyarthritis.

Pseudomembranous colitis is usually self-limited, although diarrhea can last for 4 to 6 weeks. One third of patients require hospitalization. It is treated by discontinuing antibiotics and administering an agent that binds the C. difficile toxin, such as cholestyramine (Questran) or colestipol (Colestid), or one that eradicates the organism altogether, such as oral vancomycin (Vancocin), metronidazole (Flagyl), or bacitracin. Cholestyramine also binds vancomycin, so the two are not given concurrently.

Crohn's colitis

Crohn's disease may be confined to the colon (hence **Crohn's colitis**) or may be associated with small bowel disease. Clinically, Crohn's colitis may resemble UC, but the ulceration is often longitudinal and involves the full thickness of the bowel. The disease is often segmental. Stricture formation is common, and fistulas are a frequent complication, especially in the perineum. Crohn's colitis is most often diagnosed by colonoscopy. Treatment options are discussed in Chapter 15.

Radiation enteritis

When radiation injury occurs to the GI tract, it is usually a result of radiotherapy for pelvic, intraabdominal, or retroperitoneal malignancies, such as carcinoma of the cervix, prostate, bladder, testicle, or ovary. Many patients experience mild acute symptoms during treatment, but approximately 5% to 15% experience severe, chronic damage.

The acute phase of **radiation enteritis** occurs during treatment and is related to alterations in epithelial cell function. It is characterized by nausea, cramping, and altered bowel habits. If the colon is involved, there may be acute proctocolitis with diarrhea, tenesmus, and rectal bleeding. The extent of injury can be controlled by altering the size and timing of radiation dosage and by using antiemetics, bulk-forming agents, and antidiarrheal agents.

The chronic phase of radiation enteritis results from abnormalities in vascular and connective tissues. Symptoms may appear 3 months to 30 years after radiation treatment. When the colon and rectum are involved, proctocolitis, bleeding, strictures, perforation, and fistula formation may result. Chronic enteritis is often an intractable and progressive disease associated with significant morbidity and mortality. Valuable diagnostic studies include upper GI contrast study with small bowel follow-through, lactose breath hydrogen test, fecal fat collection, and small bowel biopsy. Medical management consists of administration of steroid enemas and sulfasalazine (Azulfidine) and transfusions for chronic bleeding. Strictures can be dilated manually or by using a colonoscope. Surgery may be used selectively in patients with complete obstruction, uncontrolled bleeding, perforation, or fistulas. Complications and disease progression following surgery are common. Resection is recommended for localized disease, but bypass is preferred for more extensive disease.

Cow's milk protein-induced enterocolitis

Cow's milk protein-induced enterocolitis may present soon after birth or up to 6 months of age. Classic manifestations include vomiting, diarrhea, poor weight gain, hematochezia, and irritability. The exact mechanism of the hypersensitivity reaction to cow's milk protein is not known, and there is a wide spectrum of clinical presentation. Diagnosis is made by withdrawal and challenge with the offending protein, and supportive evidence can be gained by small bowel and/or rectosigmoid biopsies revealing increased plasma cell content of the lamina propria along with eosinophilia. This syndrome has been found to occur even in breast-fed infants who are sensitized to cow's milk protein through the mother's diet. Reactivity to soy proteins may occur in as many as 50% of those with cow's milk protein-induced enterocolitis. Treatment of cow's milk protein-induced enterocolitis may involve simple measures such as switching to a hypoallergenic formula or, if severe, total parenteral nutrition with bowel rest and slow reintroduction of feedings via a nasogastric tube with a synthetic elemental formula.

Irritable bowel syndrome

Irritable bowel syndrome (IBS) is the most common GI disorder in the United States and is the most frequent reason for outpatient visits to gastroenterologists. It ranks close to the common cold as a cause of work absenteeism. Synonyms for IBS include irritable colon and spastic colon.

IBS is characterized by motility disorders of the large and small intestine, without evidence of anatomical abnormality or organic illness. Patients with IBS present with complaints of abdominal distention, pain, and constipation and/or diarrhea. Symptoms vary in pattern and intensity but usually can be traced to periods of emotional stress. Although it is associated with severe discomfort, IBS is not related to other chronic or life-threatening conditions, nor with decreased longevity.

The anatomical cause of IBS is unknown, but the most commonly accepted etiological theory is that the behavioral tendencies of these patients cause exaggerated colonic motility in response to environmental stress.

Diagnosis is by identification of the characteristic symptom complex and by careful exclusion of other, organic GI disorders.

The usual treatment for IBS involves the following regimen:
(a) sympathetic diagnosis and reassurance that organic causes have been ruled out;
(b) a high-fiber diet;
(c) anticholinergic agents to decrease abdominal pain; and
(d) psychological support aimed at decreasing stress.

IBS is more common in Jewish and white populations, but the female predominance that is found in adults does not exist in children. In 75% of children with IBS, at least one parent or sibling has a functional GI disorder.

Chronic recurrent abdominal pain syndrome

Chronic recurrent abdominal pain syndrome is a common disorder in childhood and adolescents and is thought to be a manifestation of IBS in pediatric patients. Apley first described this syndrome of intermittent abdominal pain occurring in school-age children, persisting for more than 3 months, and affecting normal activity. Children with chronic recurrent abdominal pain syndrome have the predominant symptom of abdominal pain with only occasional bloating, dyspepsia, and alteration of bowel patterns. The etiology and pathogenesis of the pain with this syndrome are unknown; however, the prevailing viewpoint revolves around a disorder of GI motility and/or visceral hypersensitivity. Associated symptoms in children with chronic recurrent abdominal pain syndrome include headache, pallor, dizziness, and nausea. In most cases, only a limited evaluation is indicated to rule out organic causes. However, treatment must follow, not precede, establishing the diagnosis. Careful counseling and explanation is often the key to success. Emphasis on acknowledging the presence and severity of the pain is important for both the parent and child. Use of a high insoluble fiber diet is somewhat controversial but has shown to be of some benefit. There are no data to support the use of drug therapy in children with chronic recurrent abdominal pain syndrome, and it may lead to hypochondriasis. Consultation with a child psychologist may be beneficial if stress or maladaptive coping mechanisms are found to exist.

Although IBS and chronic recurrent abdominal pain syndrome may be associated with severe pain and discomfort, they do not predispose to other chronic or life-threatening conditions and there is no evidence that they interfere with longevity.

Parasitic infestations

There are a number of parasitic diseases that affect the large intestine, including amebiasis, trypanosomiasis, and trichuriasis.

Amebiasis

Amebiasis is a form of colitis caused by the protozoan *Entamoeba histolytica* (E. histoytica). It is transmitted primarily by fecal contamination of food or water, but other modes of transmission include close interpersonal contact, venereal spread, and houseflies and cockroaches. Ingested cysts form trophozoites in the small bowel. The amebae penetrate host tissues, causing necrosis without inflammation. Lesions are located throughout the colon, most often in the cecum, ascending, and rectosigmoid colon areas.

Carriers of *E. histolytica* are often asymptomatic but may suffer from amebic diarrhea; amebic dysentery; amebic appendicitis; ameboma (a large, mass-like lesion in the wall of the intestine, most often in the cecum); or visceral abscess, particularly a single abscess in the right lobe of the liver. Amebic diarrhea is an afebrile illness that is usually intermittent and followed by constipation. Amebic dysentery, on the other hand, is associated with headache, nausea and vomiting, fever and chills, **tenesmus** (a felt need to urinate or defecate, combined with an ineffectual straining to do so), abdominal cramps, and stools with a large amount of blood-tinged mucus.

Diagnosis of amebiasis requires demonstration of *E. histolytica* trophozoites and cysts in the stool. Sigmoidoscopy and indirect hemagglutination titers may be useful, and a barium enema may be helpful in diagnosing amebomas. In cases of suspected liver abscess, liver-spleen scan, abdominal ultrasonography or CT scan, or percutaneous needle aspiration may be used.

Amebiasis is treated with oral antibiotics, most often diiodohydroxyquin (Yodoxin) with or without metronidazole (Flagyl). With appropriate treatment, response to therapy is often dramatic and prognosis is excellent.

Trypanosomiasis

Trypanosomiasis is a chronic illness caused by the protozoan *Trypanosoma. Trypanosoma cruzi* (T. cruzi) causes Chagas' disease, also known as South American trypanosomiasis, which is transmitted primarily by the bite of the reduviid bug but may also be transmitted by blood transfusions, damage to the placenta during delivery, or contaminated food. The parasite multiplies rapidly at the site of inoculation, producing a severe inflammatory reaction. It may be disseminated through the bloodstream to any organ, particularly the heart, esophagus, or colon. At the site of infection, the parasite causes degeneration of the intramuscular autonomic nerve plexuses, resulting in megaesophagus, **megacolon**, or dilatation of other tubular organs many years after the initial infection.

Symptomatic Chagas' disease has been confined largely to rural areas of South and Central America, but it has been found in all Western Hemisphere countries except Guyana, Surinam, and Canada. Acute Chagas' disease is most often seen in children who are under the age of 2. Symptoms include anorexia, nausea, and vomiting; generalized lymphadenopathy; diarrhea; unilateral conjunctivitis; edema of the face and eyelids; swelling of lacrimal and submaxillary glands; hepatosplenomegaly; cardiac arrhythmias; congestive heart failure; and frequently death.

Diagnosis requires identification of *T. cruzi* in blood or tissue. For active infections, prolonged oral administration of Lampit (nifurtimox) is 70% to 95% effective. Ultimately surgery may be required to correct the "mega syndromes."

Trichuriasis

Trichuriasis is caused by the nematode *Trichuris trichiura*. It is also known as whipworm because of the whiplike appearance of the parasite. Whipworm is most often found in tropical areas or in areas of poor sanitation. Transmission is fecal-oral. The ingested eggs hatch in the duodenum. When the larvae mature into adult worms, they migrate down the GI tract and accumulate in the cecum and ascending colon.

The majority of patients are asymptomatic. Heavy infestations may cause dehydration, weakness, abdominal distention and cramping, acute and chronic diarrhea, bloody mucoid stools, anemia, and occasionally rectal prolapse. In children, chronic heavy infection may be an important contributor to impairment of growth and development.

Diagnosis requires identification of the characteristic eggs in the stools or, rarely, detection of the worms by sigmoi-

doscopy or colonoscopy. After treatment with mebendazole (Vermox), prognosis is excellent.

Diverticular disease

Diverticular disease affects 30% of all adults over the age of 60. It is characterized by herniation at weak points on the intestinal mucosa and submucosa, most often in the descending and sigmoid colon. A diverticulum typically has a narrow neck that contains all four mucosal layers and a spherical sac that contains intestinal serosa and mucosa only.

Contributing factors for diverticular disease include the following:

(a) Hypertrophy of segments of the colon's circular muscle;

(b) Increased intracolonic pressure;

(c) Age-related atrophy or weakness in the bowel muscles;

(d) Chronic constipation and straining;

(e) Irregular, uncoordinated bowel contractions;

(f) Lack of dietary fiber; and

(g) Obesity.

Diverticular disease is found in approximately 10% of the population in the United States, the United Kingdom, Australia, and other developed nations. In contrast, it affects only about 1% of the population in Asian countries. In migrants from low-prevalence areas to westernized countries, diverticular disease increases within 10 years. Prevalence is strongly correlated with advancing age.

Diverticular disease may take the form of diverticulosis or diverticulitis. In children the most common diverticulum of the GI tract to become symptomatic is Meckel's diverticulum.

Diverticulosis

Diverticulosis is uncomplicated diverticular disease. Patients with diverticulosis show no signs of infection; in fact, most are asymptomatic. When symptoms are reported, they may include pain, usually in the left lower quadrant; diffuse abdominal pain that may be chronic or intermittent and is affected by eating or bowel evacuation; constipation alternating with diarrhea; and possibly lower quadrant tenderness and hypertrophic sigmoid colon. Diagnosis of diverticulosis is confirmed by barium enema or colonoscopy.

Diverticulitis

Diverticulitis is an inflammation in the wall of the diverticulum at its apex and, rarely, at its neck. It occurs most often in the sigmoid colon and adjacent structures and may last for several weeks.

The most common symptoms of diverticulitis are fever and left lower quadrant pain. Other symptoms include nausea and vomiting, constipation, left lower quadrant tenderness, and palpable sigmoid. Diagnosis is by abdominal pain, x-ray films, and proctosigmoidoscopy. Repeated attacks of diverticulitis may cause pericolic abscesses.

Possible complications of diverticular disease include rupture of an inflamed diverticulum, with localized or generalized peritonitis; abscess formation around the diverticulum; edema or spasm related to inflammation; vesicolonic fistula formation; erosion of an artery or vein; and colonic fibrosis and narrowing, possibly leading to obstruction.

Treatment of mildly symptomatic diverticular disease usually involves dietary management, most often in the form of a high-fiber diet, and use of hydrophilic colloids or bulk-forming laxatives to help maintain a regular, soft stool. Bed rest, antibiotics, and analgesics may be prescribed for acute attacks. For patients with colonic strictures or peritonitis or septicemia, surgical intervention may be necessary, in the form of a colon resection or a temporary diverting colostomy.

Colorectal cancer

Colorectal cancer is the second most common cancer type in adults, after lung cancer in men and breast cancer in women. It occurs most frequently in persons who are between the ages of 50 and 80. Approximately 95% of intestinal cancers are adenocarcinomas. Types of adenocarcinoma include mucinous or colloid varieties. In adults, mucinous tumors comprise 15% of colorectal carcinomas and as high as 40% in children. The prognosis for children with carcinoma of the colon is dismal based on delayed recognition and types of tumors found. The highest percentage of colorectal cancers in U.S. whites are currently located in the cecum and ascending colon (22% in males and 27% in females) and sigmoid colon (25% in males and 23% in females). Cancers of the colon in children tend to be more evenly distributed throughout the large intestine. Metastasis usually involves the liver.

Risk factors for colorectal cancer include the following:
(a) a diet high in fat, protein, and beef and low in fiber;
(b) increasing age;
(c) a family history of colon or rectal cancer;
(d) previous colon cancer;
(e) a personal history of adenomatous polyps;
(f) familial polyposis or Gardner's syndrome;
(g) UC for more than 7 years; and
(h) genital cancer or breast cancer (in women).

Early detection of colon cancer is of primary importance, because for patients with carcinoma limited to the bowel wall, the 5-year survival rate is 75%, compared to only 5% for patients with disseminated disease. Unfortunately, large bowel tumors often exhibit no signs or symptoms until they become rather large, thereby reducing the likelihood of early diagnosis and making surgical cure difficult.

Periodic serial stool screening for occult blood is important to detect colorectal lesions before metastasis occurs. The American Cancer Society recommends annual digital rectal examinations after age 40, annual serial stool screening for occult blood for all persons over age 50, and sigmoidoscopy every 3 to 5 years from age 50 on, after two initial negative sigmoidoscopies 1 year apart. Patients with predisposing factors for colorectal cancer should receive more frequent and lifelong surveillance, beginning at an earlier age.

The American Cancer Society guidelines on screening and surveillance for the early detection of colorectal cancer are included below for average risk women and men, 50 years of age and older, and increased or high risk women and men.

American Cancer Society Guidelines on Screening and Surveillance for the Early Detection of Colorectal Adenomas and Cancer - Average-Risk Women and Men Ages 50 and Older (Table 16.2).

The following options are acceptable choices for colorectal cancer screening in average-risk adults. Since each of the following tests has inherent characteristics related to accuracy, prevention potential, costs, and risks, individuals should have an opportunity to make an informed decision when choosing a screening test (Table 16.1).

Test	Interval (beginning at age 50)	Comment
Fecal Occult Blood Test (FOBT) & Flexible Sigmoidoscopy	FOBT annually and flexible sigmoidoscopy every 5 years	Flexible sigmoidoscopy together with FOBT is preferred compared with FOBT or flexible sigmoidoscopy alone. All positive tests should be followed up with colonoscopy.*
Flexible Sigmoidoscopy	Every 5 years	All positive tests should be followed up with colonoscopy.*
Fecal Occult Blood Test (FOBT)	Yearly	The recommended take-home multiple sample method should be used. All positive tests should be followed up with colonoscopy.*, **
Colonoscopy	Every 10 years	Colonoscopy provides an opportunity to visualize, sample and/or remove significant lesions.
Double Contrast Barium Enema (DCBE)	Every 5 years	All positive tests should be followed up with colonoscopy

*If colonoscopy is unavailable, not feasible, or not desired by the patient, double contrast barium enema (DCBE) alone, or the combination of flexible sigmoidoscopy and DCBE are acceptable alternatives. Adding flexible sigmoidoscopy to DCBE may provide a more comprehensive diagnostic evaluation than DCBE alone in finding significant lesions. A supplementary DCBE may be needed if a colonoscopic exam fails to reach the cecum, and a supplementary colonoscopy may be needed if a DCBE identifies a possible lesion, or does not adequately visualize the entire colorectum

**There is no justification for repeating FOBT in response to an initial positive finding.

Table 16-2. American Cancer Society Guidelines on Screening and Surveillance for the Early Detection of Colorectal Adenomas and Cancer — Women and Men at Increased Risk or at High Risk

Risk Category	Age to Begin	Recommendation	Comments
INCREASED RISK			
People with a single, small (< 1 cm) adenoma	3-6 years after the initial polypectomy	Colonoscopy[1]	If the exam is normal, the patient can thereafter be screened as per average risk guidelines.
People with a large (1 cm +) adenoma, multiple adenomas, or adenomas with high-grade dysplasia or villous change.	Within 3 years after the initial polypectomy	Colonoscopy[1]	If normal, repeat examination in 3 years; If normal then, the patient can thereafter be screened as per average risk guidelines.
Personal history of curative-intent resection of colorectal cancer	Within 1 year after cancer resection	Colonoscopy[1]	If normal, repeat examination in 3 years; If normal then, repeat examination every 5 years.
Either colorectal cancer or adenomatous polyps, in any first-degree relative before age 60, or in two or more first-degree relatives at any age (if not a hereditary syndrome).	Age 40, or 10 years before the youngest case in the immediate family	Colonoscopy[1]	Every 5-10 years. Colorectal cancer in relatives more distant than first-degree does not increase risk substantially above the average risk group.
HIGH RISK			
Family history of familial adenomatous polyposis (FAP)	Puberty	Early surveillance with endoscopy, and counseling to consider genetic testing	If the genetic test is positive, colectomy is indicated. These patients are best referred to a center with experience in the management of FAP.
Family history of hereditary nonpolyposis colon cancer (HNPCC)	Age 21	Colonoscopy and counseling to consider genetic testing	If the genetic test is positive or if the patient has not had genetic testing, every 1-2 years until age 40, then annually. These patients are best referred to a center with experience in the management of HNPCC.
Inflammatory bowel disease Chronic ulcerative colitis Crohn's disease	Cancer risk begins to be significant 8 years after the onset of pancolitis, or 12-15 years after the onset of left-sided colitis	Colonoscopy with biopsies for dysplasia	Every 1-2 years. These patients are best referred to a center with experience in the surveillance and management of inflammatory bowel disease.

[1]If colonoscopy is unavailable, not feasible, or not desired by the patient, double contrast barium enema (DCBE) alone, or the combination of flexible sigmoidoscopy and (DCBE) are acceptable alternatives. Adding flexible sigmoidoscopy to DCBE may provide a more comprehensive diagnostic evaluation than DCBE alone in finding significant lesions. A supplementary DCBE may be needed if a colonoscopic exam fails to reach the cecum, and a supplementary colonoscopy may be needed if a DCBE identifies a possible lesion, or does not adequately visualize the entire colorectum.

Signs and symptoms of a right-sided tumor may include melenic stools, dull abdominal pain referred to the upper abdomen and back, anorexia and weight loss, malaise, lethargy, weakness, and indigestion. Left-sided tumors frequently cause a distinct change in bowel habits, including difficulty passing stools, abdominal distention, ribbon- or pencil-shaped stools, constipation, cramping, flatulence, and a feeling of rectal pressure or incomplete stool evacuation.

To diagnose colorectal cancer, the physician may order a stool test for occult blood; sigmoidoscopy or colonoscopy with biopsy examination and brush cytology; barium enema, usually with air contrast; upper GI series if small intestine involvement is suspected; and possibly a serum carcinoembryonic antigen test, but this is less sensitive in children.

Treatment of colorectal cancer depends on the stage of the disease. Two different methods are used to stage colon cancer: Duke's classification and the tumor, nodal involvement, and metastasis (TNM) classification. Duke's classification recognizes four stages of tumor involvement.

1. Class A—limited to the mucosa and submucosa.

2. Class B—penetration of the entire bowel wall and serosa or pericolic fat.
3. Class C—Class A and B, plus invasion of the regional draining lymph node system.
4. Class D—advanced and widespread regional metastasis.

A comparison of staging of adult versus young patients with colon cancer is displayed in Table 16-3.

Table 16-3. Comparison of staging of adult versus young patients with colon cancer

Stage	Adult	Children
Limited to mucosa	60%	2.2%
Through mucosa but no nodes	60%	16.2%
Nodes involved	40%	47.6%
Distal metastasis	40%	34.0%

The TNM classification describes the anatomical extent of the primary tumor depending on its size, invasion depth, and surface spread; the extent of nodal involvement; and the presence or absence of metastasis.

Most patients with colon cancer require either curative or palliative surgery, such as bowel resection and anastomosis or stoma formation. Surgery involves resection of the tumor and associated blood vessels, lymphatic channels, and affected structures as a unit. In some cases, the physician will irrigate the peritoneum with an antineoplastic agent and will do a biopsy examination of the liver and abdominal lymph nodes.

Many patients with intestinal cancer or other intestinal disorders require formation of a permanent or temporary colostomy. Formation of a colostomy involves making an outside opening, or **stoma**, on the abdomen using a section of the colon. There are three types of stomas, which are listed as follows:

1. A **single-barrel stoma**, in which the functioning proximal end of the bowel is brought through the abdominal wall, and then folded in on itself and sutured to form a cuff.
2. A **double-barrel stoma**, in which both the active and inactive bowel ends are temporarily brought through the abdominal wall, thereby creating two stomas.
3. A **loop stoma**, which is also a temporary procedure, and is formed by bringing an intact bowel loop through the abdominal wall and making an incision in the top of the loop.

Such patients require conscientious ostomy care, with priority given to protecting the skin from corrosive enzymes and to controlling odor and fecal drainage, and emotional support and encouragement.

Additional interventions for patients with colorectal cancer may include radiation therapy, chemotherapy, and/or immunotherapy.

Intestinal obstruction

Congenital or acquired intestinal obstructions may occur in either the large or small intestine. The source of an obstruction may be mechanical, neurogenic, or vascular.

Mechanical obstruction

Mechanical obstructions that are related to congenital defects include atresia, stenosis, hernia, **malrotation**, meconium ileus, or aganglionic megacolon (Hirschsprung's disease).

Hirschsprung's disease is the congenital absence of intramural ganglia of the anorectum and variable lengths of the distal colon, resulting in failure of relaxation of the contracted segment and internal sphincter, followed by obstructive symptoms and dilatation of the more proximal normal colon. Intestinal ischemia may occur secondary to distention of the bowel wall and contribute to the development of enterocolitis, the leading cause of death in children with Hirschsprung's disease. If not diagnosed within the first 24 hours of life, other symptoms that may appear include constipation, diarrhea, vomiting, and perforation of the appendix or colon. Poor nutrient intake and growth may also be seen. It occurs in 1 of each 5000 live births, shows a male predominance of 3.8 to 1, and is familial. Approximately 2% of these patients have Down's syndrome.

Only 15% of infants are diagnosed within the first month of life. Although 80% are diagnosed by 1 year of age, as many as 8% may not be recognized until 3 to 12 years of age. Most of these children have short-segment Hirschsprung's disease. The vast majority of Hirschsprung's cases are confined to the colon. In 75% of cases the aganglionic segment is limited to the rectum and sigmoid colon. In rare cases, the aganglionic segment extends throughout the large intestine. In extremely rare cases, the aganglionic segment may extend into the small intestine, resulting in serious nutritional, medical, and surgical challenges. Hirschsprung's disease may be associated with other abnormalities involving the neurological, cardiovascular, urological, and GI systems. Most of these associated abnormalities are also associated with early errors in embryonic development.

Hirschsprung's disease becomes apparent shortly after birth when the infant passes little meconium and develops a distended colon. It is diagnosed by barium enema and anorectal manometry and confirmed by a full-thickness biopsy examination of the rectal mucosa. Surgical treatment is required, and a number of operations have been proposed to remove or to counterbalance the obstructing effect of the aganglionic segment. Obstruction in infants is relieved through creation of a stoma proximal to the aganglionic segment. In older children, however, a preliminary colostomy may not be required and a one-stage surgical procedure may be performed.

Acquired causes of mechanical intestinal obstruction include intraluminal causes such as polyps, tumors, and feces; intramural causes such as stricture or pyloric stenosis; and intrinsic causes such as postoperative adhesions or hernias.

Neurogenic obstruction (intestinal pseudoobstruction)

In neurogenic obstruction, there is no mechanical blockage; instead, this anomaly results from ineffective intestinal peristalsis. Paralysis in such patients is usually incomplete. Pain results from abdominal distention and heightens with increasing distention. Characteristic physical findings of pseudoobstruction include cachexia and variable degrees of abdominal distention. Radiographically, a paralytic ileus with dilated bowel loops and air fluid levels are intermittently present.

Chronic intestinal pseudoobstruction may be primary, associated with generalized visceral neuropathy and also known as chronic idiopathic intestinal pseudoobstruction (CIIP), or secondary, associated with identifiable smooth muscle, endocrine, neurological, or pharmacological causes. Because as many as 75% of patients have esophageal motor abnormalities, esophageal manometry shows poor peristalsis of the esophagus and incomplete relaxation of the lower esophageal sphincter.

Abdominal surgery may be a cause of neurological impairment of peristalsis (adynamic or paralytic ileus), which is a reversible, self-limited form of pseudoobstruction that usually disappears 2 to 3 days after surgery. Diagnosis is made by observation of abdominal distention, gastric aspiration, lack of flatus, and **constipation. Paralytic ileus** may be prevented by maintaining fluid and electrolyte balance and by handling the bowel gently during surgery. It is treated by nasogastric suction and IV fluid administration to correct electrolyte imbalance. In some cases, rectal tube decompression or colonoscopic decompression may be performed.

Vascular obstruction

A vascular obstruction occurs when emboli or atherosclerotic narrowing interrupts the blood supply to the bowel. This type of obstruction inhibits peristalsis and can lead to life-threatening intestinal ischemia in as little as 40 minutes.

Another source of vascular obstruction is telangiectasia, in which capillaries and venules are dilated in the mucous membranes throughout the GI system.

Symptoms of intestinal obstruction include abdominal pain, vomiting, **obstipation** (intractable constipation), failure to pass flatus, and abdominal distention. Diagnosis can be made by taking a careful history and conducting a thorough physical examination, but the physician may also order abdominal radiographic examinations; a barium enema or swallow; and blood tests to detect dehydration, tissue necrosis, and electrolyte imbalance.

Drug therapy with metoclopramide, domperidone, cisapride, and erythromycin have been tried with scattered reports of success. However, in general they have been less than successful. Dietary manipulations to lower fat, lactose, and fiber may help to prevent or control a recurrence of symptoms. Correction and prevention of specific deficiencies of vitamins and minerals is often necessary. A feeding jejunostomy, placed endoscopically, may allow for slow refeeding and tolerance of enteral nutrition without the prolonged use of parenteral nutrition that may be required in some patients, especially those with CIIP. Use of a decompressive gastrostomy or colostomy may be also beneficial during periods of exacerbation. Intervention strategies for patients with intestinal obstructions involve the following:

(a) restoring bowel patency;

(b) regulating fluids and electrolytes, often intravenously;

(c) administration of medications to control pain and nausea;

(d) administration of antibiotics to treat bacterial growth; and

(e) use of a nasogastric or intestinal tube to relieve abdominal distention

After abdominal distention and compression have been controlled, surgical intervention may be necessary. The type of surgery performed depends on the source of the obstruction but may include hernia reduction, adhesion division, intestinal bypass, lesion excision, or a diverting colostomy. After surgery the patient should be monitored for signs of recurrent obstruction or paralytic ileus. Any abdominal drain should be monitored for patency and drainage amount.

Anorectal disorders

Anorectal disorders typically cause rectal pain, rectal bleeding, and/or a change in bowel habits. The cause may be hemorrhoids, fecal impaction, encopresis, rectal cancer, trauma, anorectal abscess, fistula, or fissure and rectal prolapse.

Hemorrhoids

Hemorrhoids are vascular masses in the anal canal. Internal hemorrhoids bulge into the rectal lumen above the internal sphincter and the anorectal line. External hemorrhoids are dilatations of the inferior hemorrhoidal plexus; they lie below the anorectal line and protrude below the external sphincter. Primary internal hemorrhoids are seen in pediatric patients rarely but may be associated with portal vein obstruction. Symptoms include bright red rectal bleeding, occasionally leading to iron deficiency anemia; rectal pain, which may be severe; and in the case of external hemorrhoids, a sensation of a bulging mass on exertion. Diagnosis is by visual examination and possibly proctoscopy or anoscopy.

Medical interventions for patients with hemorrhoids may include the following:

(a) a high-fiber diet and adequate fluid intake if chronic dehydration is suspected;

(b) warm compresses, analgesic ointments, and sitz baths; and

(c) surgical intervention, such as rubber band ligation, hemorrhoidectomy, cryosurgery, or infrared photocoagulation.

Fecal impaction

Fecal impaction is the formation of a large, firm, immovable mass of stool that occurs when normal movement of the feces is impaired. This allows the bowel to absorb more water than usual, thereby hardening the fecal matter and making it difficult to pass. Fecal impaction may be caused by chronic severe dehydration, chronic constipation, inactivity, medications, anal disease that causes painful defecation, neurological problems, or barium retention after radiological studies. It is relatively common in children, resulting from voluntary withholding of stool subsequent to a painful bowel movement.

Symptoms of fecal impaction are abdominal discomfort; a sensation of rectal fullness; nausea, vomiting, and headache; passing small amounts of watery, malformed stool; or a large, firm mass in the left lower quadrant. Treatment options include breakup of low-lying impactions digitally or administration of enemas and/or fluids, or drugs to soften the stool and encourage its passage. Possible complications of an untreated impaction include intestinal or urinary tract obstruction or spontaneous perforation.

Encopresis

Encopresis is a condition of chronic constipation that results in involuntary leakage of feces, causing soiling. It is not directly related to organic illness. This problem often begins around the time of toilet training, and the ratio of boys to girls is approximately 6 to 1. Diagnosis depends on exclusion of organic causes of constipation and psychological disorders that may be associated with incontinence. Treatment involves use of non-habit-forming stool softeners and bowel habit retraining. Dietary therapy in pediatrics is rarely sufficient to overcome encopresis; however, it is used as an adjunctive therapy when stool softeners are weaned. The goal of stool softening therapy should be to promote the passage of one to two large, loose bowel movements daily. Maintenance of an empty rectal vault assists in the return of bowel tone and proper functioning. Biofeedback training in combination with stool softening may be beneficial in speeding recovery from this problem in some patients.

Anorectal abscess

Anorectal abscess occurs when infection causes localized accumulation of pus in the tissue spaces around the anorectum. In children, pruritis and perianal cellulitis and blood-streaked stools may be caused by group A beta-hemolytic streptococci. Patients with Crohn's disease are particularly susceptible to abscess formation. One symptom may be throbbing pain in the anorectum, which worsens when the patient walks or sits. Typically, the physician will drain the abscess surgically and prescribe follow-up treatment of antibiotics and analgesics, sitz baths, and stool softeners. Complications of untreated abscess may include abscess extension or anorectal fistula.

Anorectal fistula

An anorectal fistula is a hollow, fibrous tract leading from the anal canal or rectum to the perianal skin and often results from an anorectal abscess. The two main types of anorectal fistulas are an intersphincteric fistula and a transsphincteric fistula, which extends through the external sphincter muscles.

Usually, a primary drainage port drains into an anal crypt while a secondary port drains into the perianal skin or rec-

tal mucous membrane. The predominant symptom of anorectal fistula is a purulent drainage of pus, blood, mucus, or less commonly, stool. Females may complain of passage of flatus or feces through the vagina. Other symptoms may include pruritus, pain, or odor and the presence of a palpable tract on rectal examination. Anoscopy or sigmoidoscopy may locate the source of the fistula or abscess.

Anal fistulas are treated by fistulectomy to repair superficial, straight fistulas, or fistulotomy to correct deep fistulas.

Anal fissure

An anal fissure is a thin tear of the superficial anal mucosa. It occurs most commonly along the midline of the posterior anal canal. The most common cause is trauma following passage of a large, firm stool. If the fissure's edges adhere immediately after defecation, thereby preventing pus drainage, the resulting edema and fibrosis of adjacent tissue may cause the development of a sentinel pile or tag at the lower end of the fissure.

Symptoms of anal fissures include severe tearing or burning sensations after defecation, anal itching, and discharge of bright red blood. Diagnosis is by inspection, digital rectal examination, anoscopy, or sigmoidoscopy.

Most fissures can be treated with analgesic ointments, sitz baths, and bulk agents or stool softeners. Surgical excision or lateral subcutaneous sphincterotomy may be required for chronic fissures.

Rectal prolapse

Rectal prolapse occurs when rectal mucosa bulges through the anus, often as a result of increased intraabdominal pressure when straining. Prolapse may also result from relaxed anal sphincters and weak pelvic muscles. In pediatrics, both cystic fibrosis and previous imperforate anus repair have been associated with rectal prolapse. A prolapsed rectal polyp must also be distinguished from rectal prolapse in children. Symptoms are a protruding rectal mass that is apparent on defecation or other exertion, mucus discharge, rectal bleeding, and fecal incontinence.

Rectal prolapse may be prevented by avoiding constipation and prolonged straining. Primary treatment involves reduction of the prolapse. If constipation is a predisposing factor, it should be treated with non-habit-forming stool softeners titrated to a dose to maintain loose stool passage with a minimal amount of time spent sitting on the toilet. Injection treatment with a sclerosant may be used if simple measures are unsuccessful. Surgery is rarely performed.

CASE SITUATION

David Rosenstein, age 24, is a medical student who has been doing an internship rotation in pediatrics. In the last few months he has experienced fatigue and aching joints. Feeling overworked and stressed, he took a week off to go camping with his wife. During the following month he began to notice frequent episodes of bloody, mucopurulent diarrhea. He then began having abdominal cramps and more joint tenderness. He thought he must have gotten "a bug" and visited a gastroenterologist because his symptoms seemed to be getting worse. After a battery of tests and colonoscopic examination with biopsy exam, Mr. Rosenstein was diagnosed as having UC and was placed in the hospital for treatment because of his debilitated condition.

Points to think about

1. After learning of Mr. Rosenstein's diagnosis and history, what physical findings might the gastroenterology nurse expect?
2. The nurse knows that colonic biopsy can differentiate UC from Crohn's disease by showing submucosal inflammatory reactions and granuloma; what else differentiates these two types of inflammatory bowel disease?
3. Initial planning and nursing intervention for Mr. Rosenstein would, of necessity, focus on restoration of his physiological equilibrium. The nurse's data search and assessment could substantiate at least four possible nursing diagnoses in the physiological realm. What are they?
4. UC requires a great deal of reorganization of the victim's life. Establishing a trusting relationship with Mr. Rosenstein and his wife is critical if the gastroenterology nurse is to help them in these efforts. Once such a relationship is tentatively established, what is the most important psychological area to which assessment should be directed?
5. Because it is quite likely that Mr. Rosenstein is anxious, substantiation of the nursing diagnosis "anxiety," possibly related to threats to bodily health, self-concept, altered role performance, and lack of control over events, is necessary. What are the defining characteristics of this diagnosis?
6. There are three general goals for the nursing care of a patient with the nursing diagnosis "anxiety." What are they?

Suggested responses

1. Physical findings that might be expected in a patient with UC include the following:
   (a) Fever, tachycardia, signs of dehydration and hypovolemia; imminent cardiovascular collapse in severe abrupt-onset cases.
   (b) Pallor, secondary to anemia.
   (c) Tenderness on abdominal palpation and increased bowel sounds on auscultation.
   (d) Redness, swelling, and tenderness in large joints, most often unilateral.
   (e) Abdominal distention and profuse bloody mucopurulent diarrhea, vomiting, and debilitation in severe cases with toxic megacolon.
   (f) Skin manifestations on the arms and legs, such as erythema nodosum or pyoderma gangrenosum.
   (g) Ankylosing spondylitis (occurring in 6% of patients with UC), defined as an inflammation of one or more vertebrae and the sacroiliac joint.

(h) Conjunctivitis or uveitis (inflammation of the vascular middle coat of the eye) in the early course of UC.

2. Factors that differentiate UC from Crohn's disease are as follows:

Ulcerative colitis	Crohn's disease
Continuous inflammation	"Skip areas" or segmental areas of ulceration, with normal tissue between ulcerations
Mucosal ulceration only	Ulcerations typically affect all-layers of the bowel wall
Most often seen in the left colon and rectosigmoid areas, but at times may involve the entire colon	Usually seen in the right colon and involving the terminal ileum, but may involve any area of the GI tract
Characterized by exacerbations and remissions	Often slow and progressive
May cause a shortening effect on the bowel	Can narrow the lumen, with stricture formation
Cobblestoning effect less consistent	More consistent mucosal "cobblestoning" effect seen on radiographic examination
Diarrhea is bloody and mucopurulent rhea	Diarrhea is watery and sometimes associated with steator-
Pseudopolyps common	Pseudopolyps rare
Inflammatory masses rare	Inflammatory masses common

3. Possible nursing diagnoses in the physiological realm include the following:
   (a) Altered nutrition: less than body requirements.
   (b) Diarrhea related to bowel irritability.
   (c) Fluid volume deficit.
   (d) Acute pain related to bowel irritability.
   (e) Activity intolerance related to weakness, debilitated condition, and joint swelling.
4. The most important psychological priority toward which assessment should be directed is determining Mr. Rosenstein's coping mechanisms and skills. Without knowing the mechanisms by which he commonly manages problems and stresses in his daily life, a nurse cannot initiate a plan to aid him in adapting his life.
5. The defining characteristics of the nursing diagnosis "anxiety" are as follows:
   (a) reported apprehension, nervousness;
   (b) escape/avoidance behavior;
   (c) physiological arousal;
   (d) narrowed perceptual field; difficulty concentrating; self-focusing;
   (e) inappropriate behaviors, such as anger, fear, guilt, and regression;
   (f) denial;
   (g) withdrawal; and
   (h) increased wariness.
6. Three general goals for the nursing care of a patient with the nursing diagnosis "anxiety" are:
   (a) prevention of severe anxiety or panic status

(b) elimination or reduction of incapacitating anxiety status

(c) use of effective coping skills.

The nurse must realize that specific, concrete, personalized patient outcomes within these broad goals may be multiple and may be based on a variety of factors and possible patient responses.

REVIEW TERMS

amebiasis, anus, ascending colon, cecum, chronic recurrent abdominal pain syndrome, colitis, colon, constipation, cow's milk protein-induced enterocolitis, Crohn's colitis, descending colon, diarrhea, diverticulitis, diverticulosis, encopresis, enterocolitis, familial polyposis coli, Gardner's syndrome, haustra, hematochezia, hepatic flexure, Hirschsprung's disease, intestinal pseudoobstruction, irritable bowel syndrome (IBS), ischemic colitis, malrotation, megacolon, necrotizing enterocolitis (NEC), obstipation, paralytic ileus, Peutz-Jeghers syndrome, polyps, pseudomembranous colitis, radiation enteritis, rectum, sigmoid colon, splenic flexure, stoma, tenesmus, tenia coli, toxic megacolon, transverse colon, trypanosomiasis, ulcerative colitis (UC), Valsalva maneuver, vermiform appendix

REVIEW QUESTIONS

1. The first portion of the large intestine to receive material from the small bowel is the:
   (a) Ileum.
   (b) Cecum.
   (c) Appendix.
   (d) Ascending colon.
2. The small sacculations in the large intestinal wall that are formed by the tenia coli are called the:
   (a) Haustra.
   (b) Diverticula.
   (c) Crypts of Lieberkühn.
   (d) Plicae semilunares.
3. The colonic mucosa is:
   (a) Made up of thousands of finger-like projections called villi.
   (b) Covered with a layer of squamous epithelium.
   (c) Arranged in folds called the plicae circulares.
   (d) Smooth-surfaced.
4. Colonic secretion consists primarily of:
   (a) Sodium, chloride, and water.
   (b) Water, mucus, potassium, and bicarbonate.
   (c) Mucus and hormones.
   (d) Bile pigments and toxins.
5. The appearance of multiple adenomatous polyps in the GI tract and osteomas of the mandible, skull, and long bones is symptomatic of:
   (a) Osler-Weber-Rendu disease.
   (b) Colorectal cancer.
   (c) Familial polyposis.
   (d) Gardner's syndrome.
6. Toxic megacolon is a potentially serious complication of:
   (a) Ischemic colitis.
   (b) Ulcerative colitis.
   (c) Pseudomembranous colitis.
   (d) Transmural colitis.
7. The most commonly accepted cause of irritable bowel syndrome is:
   (a) An anatomical abnormality.
   (b) A high-fat, low-fiber diet.
   (c) An exaggerated motility response to environmental stress.
   (d) A parasitic infestation.
8. Mildly symptomatic diverticular disease is most often treated by:
   (a) Diverticulectomy.
   (b) Colon resection.
   (c) Dietary management and hydrophilic colloids or bulk-forming laxatives.
   (d) Colostomy.
9. Metastatic colorectal cancer most often involves the:
   (a) Small bowel.
   (b) Liver.
   (c) Pancreas.
   (d) Stomach.
10. A hollow, fibrous tract, leading from the anal canal or rectum to the perianal skin is called a(n):
    (a) Hemorrhoid.
    (b) Anorectal fissure.
    (c) Anorectal abscess.
    (d) Anorectal fistula.
11. Encopresis commonly seen in school-age children, particularly boys, is defined as:
    (a) Involuntary nocturnal passage of urine.
    (b) Involuntary leakage of stool.
    (c) Nocturnal awakening with abdominal pain.
    (d) Infectious diarrhea with fecal incontinence.

BIBLIOGRAPHY

American Cancer Society (2003). Can Colon Cancer be detected? [On-line]. Available: www.cancer.org.

Anderson, K., Keith, J. & Novak, P. (Eds.) (2001). *Mosby's Medical Nursing & Allied Health Dictionary* (6th ed.). Philadelphia: W.B. Saunders.

Avunduk, C. (2002). *Manual of gastroenterology: diagnosis and therapy* (3rd ed.). Boston: Lippincott, Williams & Wilkins.

Bahr, A. (1988). The large intestine. In Trivits, S. (Ed.), *SGA Journal Reprints*. Rochester, NY: Society of Gastrointestinal Assistants.

Bongiovanni, G. (Ed.) (1988). *Essentials of clinical gastroenterology* (2nd ed.). New York: McGraw-Hill.

Broadwell, D.C. & Jackson, B.S. (1982). *Principles of ostomy care.* St. Louis, MO: Mosby.

Chobanian, S. & Van Ness, M. (Eds) (1988). *Manual of clinical problems in gastroenterology.* Boston: Little, Brown.

Chopra, S. & May, R. (Eds.) (1989). *Pathophysiology of gastrointestinal diseases.* Boston: Little, Brown.

Gardner, S. (1988). Colorectal cancer. In Trivits, S. (Ed.), *SGA Journal Reprints.* Rochester, NY: Society of Gastrointestinal Assistants.

Given, B. & Simmons, S. (1984). *Gastroenterology in clinical nursing* (4th ed.). St. Louis, MO: Mosby.

Goldberg, K., (Ed.) (1986). *Gastrointestinal problems: Nurse Review Series.* Springhouse, PA: Springhouse.

Kraft, S. (1988). Ulcerative colitis. In Trivits, S. (Ed.), *SGA Journal Reprints.* Rochester, NY: Society of Gastrointestinal Assistants.

Larson, D. (1987). Advanced anatomy and physiology of the colon. *SGA J 10,* 92-97.

Martin, D. (2002). *Practical Gastroenterology.* Florence, KY: Taylor and Francis.

Rayhorn, N. (1992). Colonoscopy and the pediatric patient. *Gastroenterol Nurs 15(1),* 18-22.

Roy, C.C., Silverman, A. & Alagille, D. (Eds.) (1995). *Pediatric clinical gastroenterology* (4th ed.). St. Louis, MO: Mosby.

Ryan, E.T. (1992). Hirschsprung's disease: associated abnormalities and demography. *J Pediatr Surg 27(1),* 76-81. Journal of Pediatric Surgery.

Sleisenger, M. & Fordtran, J., (Eds.) (2002). *Gastrointestinal diseases: pathophysiology, diagnosis, management* (7th ed.). Philadelphia: W.B. Saunders.

Smeltzer, S.C. & Bare, B.G. (2000). *Textbook of medical surgical nursing* (9th ed.). Philadelphia, Pennsylvannia: Lippincott.

Suchy, F.J. (Ed.) (2001). *Liver disease in children* (2nd ed.). St. Louis, MO: Lippincott, Williams & Wilkins.

Swartz, M. (1989). Beyond the scope: a nursing view of the extraintestinal manifestations of inflammatory bowel disease. *Gastroenterol Nurs 12,* 172-8.

Walker, W.A. & Watkins, J.B. (Eds.) (1996). *Nutrition in pediatrics* (2nd ed.). Hamilton, British Columbia: Decker.

Walker, W.A., Durie, P., Hamilton, J.R., Watkins, J.B. and Walker-Smith, J.A.. (2000). *Pediatric gastrointestinal disease: Pathophysiology, diagnosis, management.* Ontario, Canada: Decker.

Young, R.J. (1996). Pediatric constipation: an overview of gastroenterology nursing. *Gastroenterol Nurs 19,* 88-95.

Chapter 17

BILIARY SYSTEM

This chapter will acquaint the gastroenterology nurse with the normal anatomy and physiology of the biliary system. In addition, selected pathological conditions of the gallbladder and its associated duct system are described with respect to pathophysiology, diagnosis, and treatment.

Learning objectives

After reviewing the content of this chapter, the gastroenterology nurse should be able to:

1. Describe the normal gross structure and histology of the biliary system, including the gallbladder and its associated duct system.
2. Explain the motility and secretory functions of the gallbladder.
3. Discuss a number of pathological conditions that affect the biliary system in terms of pathophysiology, diagnosis, and treatment.

ANATOMY

The biliary system consists of the gallbladder and its associated duct system; that is, the hepatic, cystic, and common bile ducts (Fig. 17-1). The **gallbladder** itself is a pear-shaped, saclike bile storage structure. It is attached to the undersurface of the liver by connective tissue, peritoneum, and blood vessels (see Fig. 13-2). The gallbladder is approximately 7 to 10 cm (3 inches) long and 2.5 to 3.5 cm (about 1 inch) wide and is capable of holding up to 50 ml of bile.

The four anatomical divisions of the gallbladder are as follows:

1. The distal blind sac, or fundus;
2. The funnel-shaped body, which connects the fundus and the infundibulum;
3. The infundibulum, which connects the body to the neck; and
4. The neck, which narrows into the cystic duct.

As it emerges from the gallbladder, the **cystic duct** combines with the **hepatic duct** to form the **common bile duct,** which joins with the main pancreatic duct to form the ampulla of Vater. The ampulla empties into the duodenum at an orifice called the papilla of Vater, or major papilla. During their passage through the duodenal wall, the common bile duct, the pancreatic duct, and the ampulla of Vater are surrounded by a complex arrangement of smooth muscles called the **sphincter of Oddi.**

The functions of the sphincter of Oddi are to (a) regulate the flow of bile and pancreatic juices into the intestine; (b) inhibit entry of bile into the pancreatic duct; and (c) prevent reflux of intestinal contents into the ducts. The gallbladder is not an essential organ; if it is removed, bile flow continues to be regulated by the sphincter of Oddi.

The walls of the gallbladder have three layers, which are listed as follows:

(a) An outer serosa that is derived from the peritoneum;
(b) A fibromuscular layer that contains longitudinal and spiral smooth muscle and fibrous tissue; and
(c) An inner mucosa that is made up of simple columnar epithelium and is arranged in folds or rugae similar to those of the stomach.

Blood supply to the biliary system is delivered by the hepatic artery and is drained through the cystic vein. Sympathetic innervation is derived from the splanchnic nerve and the seventh through tenth thoracic segments. Sympathetic stimulation inhibits smooth muscle gallbladder contraction. Parasympathetic innervation is derived from the right branch of the vagus nerve. Mild parasympathetic stimulation causes the gallbladder to contract and relaxes the sphincter of Oddi at the duodenal junction.

PHYSIOLOGY

The functions of the biliary system are to collect, concentrate, and store bile and to release it into the duodenum when it is needed for digestion.

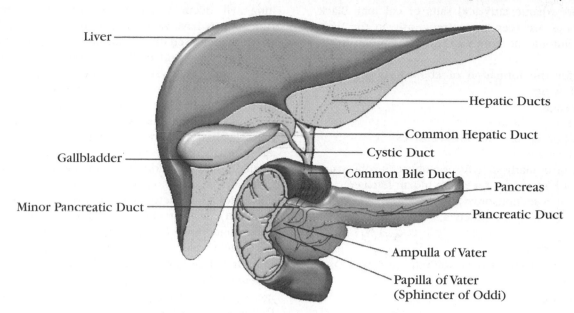

Fig. 17-1. Anatomy of liver, biliary, and pancreatic ductal systems.

Motility

Under normal conditions the sphincter of Oddi remains slightly opened, thereby allowing for a constant but miniscule amount of bile to enter the duodenum. During normal digestion as food enters the duodenum, the hormone cholecystokinin-pancreozymin is released, thus causing the gallbladder to contract, which in turn pushes increased amounts of bile into the duodenum. Other factors, such as certain drugs, sensory input, disease, and emotional states, may also affect the filling and contracting of the gallbladder.

Secretion

Bile is an alkaline, greenish-yellow fluid that is secreted continuously by the liver. Its major components are water, which makes up 97% of hepatic bile; bile salts; fatty acids; lipids, mainly cholesterol and lecithin; inorganic electrolytes; conjugated bilirubin; and other organic substances. When bile flows from the liver through the cystic duct and into the gallbladder for storage, up to 90% of the water is removed.

Bile has a variety of functions, which include: the emulsification of undigested fats; the facilitation of the absorption of fat-soluble vitamins; the activation of intestinal and pancreatic enzymes; and the provision of a route for the excretion of bilirubin, cholesterol, and certain sex, thyroid, and adrenal hormones. Bile also affects the absorption of certain minerals and helps to neutralize gastric acid in the duodenum.

If the flow of bile through the common bile duct or hepatic ducts is obstructed by gallstones or other abnormalities, bile builds up in the blood, resulting in hyperbilirubinemia. Bile pigments, mainly bilirubin, are deposited in the skin, mucous membranes, and sclera, causing a yellow discoloration of these areas that is commonly known as **jaundice.** Jaundice may also result from destruction of red blood cells or from liver cell dysfunction.

PATHOPHYSIOLOGY

Gallbladder and duct diseases may be short-term and easily correctable or may be long-term and debilitating. Generally, they present during middle age and incidence increases with age. In persons who are between the ages of 20 and 50, gallbladder and duct diseases are six times more common in women than in men, but after age 50 the incidence in men and women becomes equal.

Biliary tract disorders include cholelithiasis, choledocholithiasis, cholecystitis, cholangitis, carcinoma, various congenital anomalies, and sphincter of Oddi disease.

Cholelithiasis

Cholelithiasis is the presence of stones or calculi in the gallbladder. As many as 1 million new cases of cholelithiasis are diagnosed each year, and approximately half of those patients undergo biliary surgery. Cholelithiasis is the fifth leading cause of hospitalization among adults and accounts for 90% of all diseases of the biliary system.

There are two types of gallstones: cholesterol stones and pigment stones. Cholesterol stones, including both pure cholesterol stones and mixed stones, make up three fourths of all gallstones. They contain cholesterol, calcium salts, bile acids, fatty acids, protein, and phospholipids. Cholesterol stones are associated with either the hepatic production of bile that is supersaturated with cholesterol or with reduced bile-salt secretion. When cholesterol is no longer soluble in this supersaturated system, it forms crystal nucleates, which grow and cluster with each other and with other bile constituents to form recognizable stones in the gallbladder.

Pigment stones are less common than cholesterol stones. They include black pigment stones, which are made up of bilirubin polymers and inorganic calcium salts, and brown pigment stones, which are composed principally of calcium bilirubinate and organic fatty-acid salts of calcium. Black, radiopaque stones are seen more frequently in the West, while brown, radiolucent stones are more common in the Orient.

Risk factors for the formation of cholesterol gallstones include the following:

(a) increasing age;
(b) female sex;
(c) pregnancy or use of oral contraceptives;
(d) estrogen therapy;
(e) ethnicity, particularly specific non-obese European and Chilean patients; obese American-Indian females;
(f) ileal disease, resection, or bypass;
(g) certain forms of hyperlipidemia;
(h) obesity;
(i) weight-reduction diets;
(j) use of certain drugs, such as clofibrate (Atromid-S);
(k) gallbladder stasis; and
(l) spinal cord injury.

The prevalence of pigment stones is not influenced by gender. Risk factors for the formation of pigment stones include the following:

(a) increasing age;
(b) chronic hemolysis, such as sickle cell disease or thalassemia;
(c) alcoholism or alcoholic cirrhosis;
(d) biliary infection, usually *Escherichia coli (E. coli),* or parasitic infestation, such as *Clonorchis sinensis* or *Ascaris lumbricoides;*
(e) total parenteral nutrition;
(f) vagotomy;
(g) periampullary diverticula; and
(h) gallbladder stasis.

Gallstones may move around in the gallbladder as it empties and refills. If they remain in one place they may be asymptomatic. However, stones that move to the neck, cystic duct, or common duct may obstruct those passages, thus resulting in mucosal irritation and subsequent bacterial invasion. Stones may also pass through the biliary ducts, causing pain, or they may obstruct the flow of bile if they become lodged there. It is possible for small stones to be located in any part of the biliary system without causing distress or even to pass into the duodenum and be discharged in the stool.

Gallstones are asymptomatic in at least 50% of patients. Even in symptomatic patients, the severity, extent, and nature of the symptoms vary considerably depending on the movement of the stones, the degree of obstruction, if any, and the presence or absence of inflammation.

Symptomatic patients usually complain of a steady pain, which often stems from gallbladder distention or spasm of the sphincter of Oddi or ductal muscles. This pain is referred to as **biliary colic.** Pain most often occurs 3 to 6 hours after the heaviest meal of the day, frequently during the early hours of the night. Pain often radiates to other parts of the abdomen or back and sometimes to the scapula, the middle of the back, or the tip of the right shoulder. Nausea and vomiting may occur, and pain may be relieved by vomiting. Patients may have vague symptoms of upper abdominal discomfort, increased eructation, and dyspepsia. Some patients also have fever and chills resulting from a common duct stone, acute cholecystitis, or associated pancreatitis.

In children, mild to moderate jaundice is a common symptom, but gallbladder enlargement is infrequent. Because the diagnosis of cholelithiasis is seldom considered in children, the delay between onset of symptoms and diagnosis in this age-group may be from 1 to 5 years. Stones are generally found in the gallbladder, and they seldom occlude either the cystic or the common bile duct. Most children have a specific etiological factor, such as prolonged total parenteral nutrition, congenital hemolytic disease, or ileal disease.

Ultrasonography is the most effective diagnostic technique for cholelithiasis; it can identify stones that are as small as 2 mm. Oral cholecystography or cholangiography may also be ordered. If both oral cholecystography and ultrasonography are negative and symptoms are suggestive of cholelithiasis, the next test should be endoscopic retrograde cholangiopancreatography (ERCP) and/or examination of duodenal bile for cholesterol crystals or bilirubinate granules.

Noninterventional "expectant" management is preferred for asymptomatic patients, because neither medical dissolution therapy nor elective cholecystectomy is warranted in such cases. Management of patients with minor symptoms may include pain relief and dietary control to reduce fat intake. Small, frequent meals can sometimes help to prevent future attacks. In children, cholecystectomy is probably indicated, regardless of the severity of symptoms.

Surgery is the treatment of choice for most symptomatic patients. Typically, a cholecystectomy is used to excise the gallbladder and ligate the cystic duct. Prognosis is generally good but may vary depending on the patient's age; sex; and the presence of complicating conditions such as cholecystitis, cholangitis, or pancreatitis.

In addition to cholecystectomy, a variety of newer techniques exist for the dissolution or removal of cholesterol stones, including the following:

1. Dissolution of gallstones using ursodeoxycholic acid (UDCA, Actigall), which is a naturally occurring bile salt. This alternative is successful in 50% of patients. Patients who are considered for medical dissolution therapy must have patent cystic ducts and radiolucent small stones. Use of this agent is not recommended for women taking oral contraceptives.
2. Continuous infusion of methyl tert-butyl ether into the gallbladder to dissolve stones.
3. Infusion of substances such as cholate sodium and heparin through a T-tube to dissolve stones.
4. Biliary lithotripsy, which involves fragmentation of gallstones by use of extracorporeal acoustic shock waves and is often combined with dissolution therapy. This experimental treatment method can be used on an outpatient basis. Patients have less pain, a shorter recovery period, and less chance of infection than those who have cholecystectomies.

The disadvantages of all of these medical therapies are the probability of recurrence of cholelithiasis after cessation of the therapeutic modality and concerns regarding the effects of long-term use.

No medical intervention options exist for pigment stones. Surgery is the only alternative for symptomatic patients with stones of this type.

Approximately 5% to 8% of cholecystectomy patients later exhibit postcholecystectomy syndrome, defined as abdominal pain or dyspepsia in patients who have had a cholecystectomy. Postcholecystectomy syndrome is most often seen in women who are between the ages of 40 and 49. Their distress cannot be attributed to the surgical procedure itself. Potential causes include residual biliary tract disease, nonbiliary digestive disease, nonspecific digestion dysfunction, and psychiatric disorders. Treatment is determined by the specific diagnosis. Retained common bile duct stones, for example, are not uncommon following cholecystectomy. These stones may be removed by endoscopic introduction of a basket or balloon into the common bile duct, by a second surgical procedure, or through nonoperative manipulation of a basket inserted through a T-tube.

Potential complications of cholelithiasis include cholecystitis, cholangitis, abscess or fistula formation, perforation of the gallbladder, gangrene, and hepatic damage. Cholelithiasis has also been linked to gallbladder cancer.

Choledocholithiasis

The presence of gallstones in the common bile duct or the hepatic duct is called **choledocholithiasis.** This problem occurs when stones passed out of the gallbladder lodge in the hepatic duct or the common bile duct and obstruct the flow of bile into the duodenum. In about 5% of cases, common duct stones are primary stones that form in the common bile duct. Such stones are always pigment stones; in fact, about 40% of common bile duct stones are pigment stones. The available evidence suggests that cholesterol stones in the duct are always secondary stones that were formed in the gallbladder, whereas pigment stones can be either primary or secondary.

Patients with choledocholithiasis may have no symptoms or may present with any combination of the following:

(a) Biliary colic, with constant epigastric or right upper quadrant pain or tenderness;

(b) Obstructive jaundice and pruritus;

(c) Cholangitis, with fever, right upper quadrant pain, jaundice (known as Charcot triad), and often, rigor; and

(d) Acute gallstone pancreatitis, manifested by severe abdominal pain that radiates into the back.

Differential diagnosis may require laboratory blood and liver function tests, ultrasonography, radioisotope imaging, oral cholecystography, ERCP, or percutaneous transhepatic cholangiography (PTC).

Patients with choledocholithiasis should be kept NPO. They should be stabilized by IV maintenance of fluid and electrolyte balance. Analgesia should be provided, nasogastric suction may be used, and antibiotics may be prescribed if there is evidence of sepsis or cholangitis. Therapeutic ERCP is the preferred method of treatment. During ERCP, endoscopic sphincterotomy and stone removal can be done. This involves cutting the muscle fiber of the sphincter of Oddi and using a balloon catheter or basket to extract the stones. Large stones may be broken up using mechanical or laser lithotripsy before removal. Alternatively, the common bile duct may be explored surgically, through a choledochotomy.

Acalculous cholecystitis

Acute cholecystitis in the absence of stones is relatively rare and usually occurs in otherwise severely ill hospitalized patients. Intercurrent illnesses include bacterial enteric infections, such as typhoid fever, shigellosis, or E. coli; viral gastroenteritis; scarlet fever; respiratory infections; or pneumonia. Parasitic infestations with Giardia or Ascaris have also been found in the gallbladders of some patients. Acalculous cholecystitis also occurs in patients who have been hospitalized for burns, trauma, or major surgery. Most of these patients have been receiving total parenteral nutrition. Absence of oral intake associated with gallbladder stasis, sludge formation, and increased biliary pressure caused by narcotic drugs that increase the tone at the sphincter of Oddi may contribute to its pathogenesis.

Symptoms of acute acalculous cholecystitis include an acute onset of abdominal pain on the right side, abdominal tenderness and guarding, vomiting, and nausea. Usually, the diagnosis is made by abdominal ultrasonography. The incidence of gangrene, necrosis, and perforation is high in this group of patients, and mortality may be as high as 50%. Because of the high incidence of complications, the treatment of choice for acalculous cholecystitis is urgent cholecystectomy or cholecystostomy. Patients should also be treated with antibiotics to cover enteric organisms and enterococcus, and other supportive measures should be taken as needed.

Emphysematous cholecystitis

In emphysematous cholecystitis, the gallbladder walls and bile ducts contain gas that has been produced by infective organisms such as *E. coli, Clostridium*, and other anaerobes. Acute cholecystectomy is performed in these cases.

Cholangitis

Cholangitis is a rare bacterial infection of the bile duct that is often associated with choledocholithiasis or with obstruction of the bile duct by strictures, cysts, fistulas, neoplasms, or parasites. Widespread inflammation may cause fibrosis and stenosis of the common bile duct. Most patients experience a transient, self-limited illness that is characterized by a fever spike, chills, dark urine, and abdominal pain. In other patients, however, the illness is devastating, consistent with profound toxic sepsis with shock and impaired mental function. Prognosis for these patients is poor.

Bacteremia is present in 40% of these patients. The organisms responsible are most often E. coli and Klebsiella. When bacterial infection is severe, invasion of the liver parenchyma may occur, resulting in abscess formation.

Cholangitis is a medical and surgical emergency. The patient should be stabilized with IV hydration and antibiotics, which should be followed by prompt surgical or endoscopic decompression of the common bile duct. Drainage of the biliary tree should produce immediately beneficial results.

If the common bile duct is explored surgically to remove retained stones, a T—tube is inserted to provide a means of decompressing the biliary ducts. The tube can be removed in the clinician's office 3 weeks after surgery. Before postoperative extraction of the T-tube, a cholangiogram should be performed to detect residual stones. About 2% of patients undergoing choledochotomy have residual stones.

Retained common bile duct stones can be removed by inserting a basket through the T-tube or by endoscopically introducing a basket or balloon for extraction. Large stones that are difficult to remove may be fragmented by a mechanical lithotripter basket and the fragments pulled out by a balloon. Another alternative is to place a nasobiliary catheter into the duct and infuse a cholesterol solvent to dissolve the stone or shrink its size for easier mechanical removal. Attempted dissolution of retained common duct stones with T-tube infusion of other cholesterol solvents is not recommended.

Complications of choledocholithiasis may include cholangitis, cirrhosis with hepatic failure, portal hypertension, hepatic abscess formation, or gallstone pancreatitis.

Cholecystitis

Cholecystitis is an acute or chronic inflammation that causes painful distention of the gallbladder. Ten to twenty-five percent of patients who require surgery for gallbladder disease have cholecystitis. Most cholecystitits in the pediatric population is chronic and associated with gallstones and the presenting symptom is right upper quadrant abdominal pain, sometimes radiating to the back with complaints of vomiting. In 25-30% of children, jaundice and fever are seen and are more common in young infants.

Cholecystitis can also occur without evidence or presence of gallstones; this is rare in adults but occurs with surprising frequency in children. The cause is not known but has been associated with immediate postoperative states, traumas or burns. This condition usually presents with fever, abdominal pain and jaundice.

Acute calculous cholecystitis

More than 90% of the time, cholecystitis is associated with a gallstone that is impacted in the cystic duct, a condition known as acute calculous cholecystitis. The obstructed gallbladder becomes distended, and the walls become edematous, ischemic, and inflamed. Secondary infections with enteric organisms may compound the inflammation, leading to cholangitis and sepsis.

Predisposing factors to acute cholecystitis include older age, ethnicity (especially persons of Italian, Jewish, or Chinese descent), obesity, a sedentary lifestyle, pregnancy, hemolytic anemias, and insulin-dependent diabetes mellitus.

Acute cholecystitis produces the following symptoms, which are similar to those of cholelithiasis:

(a) acute abdominal pain, usually midepigastric or localized to the right upper quadrant, with radiation to the shoulders and back;

(b) nausea, vomiting, and anorexia;

(c) fever, headache, leukocytosis;

(d) tachycardia and tachypnea;

(e) tenderness, guarding, and rebound tenderness in the right upper quadrant; and

(f) intolerance of fatty foods and heavy meals.

To confirm the diagnosis, the physician may order blood tests, ultrasonography, and radioisotope imaging.

Patients with acute cholecystitis should be stabilized with nasogastric suctioning, IV fluid and electrolyte replacement, and analgesia. Antibiotics should be given in cases of severe illness, sepsis, or complications. Early cholecystectomy is the preferred treatment approach.

If cholecystectomy is contraindicated by the patient's condition, an operative or percutaneous cholecystostomy may be performed. In this procedure the gallbladder is evacuated of stones and infected bile, and a Foley catheter drains to the outside. Temporary or short-term biliary decompression can also be accomplished by using ERCP to place a nasobiliary catheter (NBC) or internal stent above the impacted stone. An NBC catheter consists of a long polyethylene tube, one end of which is placed inside the biliary tree with the other end exiting through the nostril and connecting to a bile drainage bag, thereby allowing the NBC to function as a T-tube. An internal stent consists of a plastic tube being placed into the biliary tree, which allows bile to flow into the duodenum without the patient having a tube in the nose.

Potential complications of acute cholecystitis include perforation with subsequent peritonitis or cholecystenteric fistula, or gallstone ileus, which is a form of intermittent or permanent intestinal obstruction that is caused by the impaction of a large gallstone that has entered the intestine through a cholecystenteric fistula. Such obstructions are most often found in the ileum because of its relatively small diameter compared to the rest of the intestine. Gallstone ileus requires an emergency laparotomy.

Primary sclerosing cholangitis

Primary sclerosing cholangitis (PSC) is a rare inflammatory process that results in multiple strictures of the bile ducts, thus causing chronic cholestatic liver disease. Its etiology is unknown. Fifty to seventy-five percent of patients with PSC have ulcerative colitis (UC) or have had it in the past. Primary sclerosing cholangitis has also been associated with Crohn's disease. Men are affected twice as often as women, and two thirds of the patients are younger than 45 years old.

Clinical manifestations of PSC are progressive fatigue, jaundice, pruritis, abdominal pain, and elevated serum alkaline phosphatase. Diagnosis is by ultrasonography, ERCP or PTC, and liver biopsy examination. ERCP might show strictured areas in the intrahepatic and extrahepatic ducts with areas of dilatation between the strictures, thus producing a beaded appearance to the ducts.

Subclinical PSC requires no treatment. If pruritis occurs, it can be treated with bile-salt binding agents such as cholestyramine (Questran). To bypass tight strictures, surgery or endoscopic balloon dilatation and/or placement of biliary stents may be required. Liver transplant may be the only viable treatment in the advanced stages of the disease and is the third most common reason for transplant in the United States. Progression to cirrhosis and portal hypertension is expected, and death occurs from liver failure. Cholangiocarcinoma may develop in 7% to 15% of these patients. Median survival after the onset of symptoms is 12 years.

Carcinoma

Cancer of the biliary system may involve the gallbladder or, less often, the bile ducts.

Gallbladder cancer

Carcinoma of the gallbladder accounts for approximately 3% of all cancers. It occurs more frequently in women than in men, and incidence peaks at age 70. Approximately 80% of patients with gallbladder carcinoma also have gallstones.

Patients with gallbladder cancer usually present with vague abdominal symptoms, including nausea, vomiting, substantial weight loss, anorexia, fat intolerance, and right upper quadrant pain. If a palpable right upper quadrant mass can be felt, the lesion is almost always incurable.

Diagnostic tests that are used include cholecystograms, cholangiograms, PTC, and ERCP. Scanning and ultrasonography may also be done. In practice, cancer of the gallbladder is rarely diagnosed preoperatively because signs and symptoms are similar to those for cancer of the liver or pancreas or for obstructive cholelithiasis.

Approximately 80% of gallbladder cancers are adenocarcinomas. The remainder is squamous cell carcinomas, adenocanthomas, and others. Benign tumors are rare. Most patients have evidence of local or metastatic spread, often through the lymph nodes, at the time of diagnosis. The majority survive less than 1 year following diagnosis; the 5-year survival rate is approximately 5%, and in most of these patients the tumor was discovered incidentally.

Medical treatment should be supportive and symptomatic, with the goals of comfort and short-term rehabilitation. For most patients, neither resection, radiotherapy, nor chemotherapy seems to prolong survival. If surgery is performed, the average postoperative survival time is only 8 months. Cholecystectomy is indicated only for patients with small, localized tumors. If the lesion is inoperable, an internal bile drainage system may be inserted to permit the flow of bile directly from the liver into the intestine. The objectives of this procedure are to relieve symptoms and to prolong the quality and length of life.

To minimize malnutrition and dehydration problems, the patient may be given antiemetics or small sips of carbonated beverages to control nausea; vitamin and mineral replacements; frequent small meals; small amounts of pain medication before meals; and, if necessary, tube feeding. In the terminal stages of the disease, skin care, pain relief, and emotional support are of vital importance.

Bile duct cancers

Cancer of the extrahepatic biliary tree is associated with gallstones in only 30% of patients. It may also be associated with long-standing UC, Crohn's, PSC, and/or congenital dilatations of the bile ducts (e.g., choledochal cysts). Often, the patient presents with painless obstructive jaundice. Later, pruritus, nausea, vomiting, weight loss, and intermittent or steady right upper quadrant pain may develop. Serum alkaline phosphatase is always elevated.

Adenocarcinoma is the most common form of cancer in the biliary tree. Benign neoplasms are relatively rare. This type of cancer is most often diagnosed at the time of laparotomy for other biliary tract disease. Most patients have localized extension or metastatic disease at the time of diagnosis.

Ultrasonography or CT scan may be used to visualize dilated intrahepatic bile ducts, and PTC or ERCP should be used preoperatively to define the level and cause of the obstruction.

The treatment of choice for patients with localized carcinoma of the proximal biliary tree is surgery, consisting of pancreaticoduodenectomy. Five-year survival rates are less than 20%. For distal common duct or hepatic duct carcinomas, treatment is basically palliative. These patients often survive less than 1 year.

The most common pediatric neoplasm of the biliary tract is botryoid embryonal rhabdomyosarcoma. Symptoms include pruritus, jaundice, right upper quadrant and epigastric abdominal pain, and sometimes a palpable mass. The tumor is usually locally invasive. Even with a large surgical resection and radiation and drug therapy, prognosis is extremely poor.

Congenital abnormalities

Congenital anomalies may occur in either the gallbladder or the bile ducts.

Gallbladder anomalies

Congenital anomalies of the gallbladder include the following:

1. Agenesis, or congenital absence of the gallbladder, which most likely occurs as a result of embryonic maldevelopment.
2. Anomalies of location (ectopic gallbladder), which may occur anywhere in the abdomen, and often, require cholecystectomy.
3. Anomalies of form, in which more than one cystic structure is found in the gallbladder fossa, suggesting either double gallbladder, bilobed gallbladder, folded fundus, or Ladd's bands across a normal gallbladder. If one of the

two organs is found to be diseased at the time of surgery, both should be removed.

4. Anomalies of fixation, which occur when the mesenteric supporting structures of the gallbladder are elongated, thus leaving a normally functioning gallbladder to "float" below the inferior surface of the liver and occasionally into the pelvis. If this floating gallbladder twists, vascular occlusion, ischemic necrosis, or perforation may occur, requiring cholecystectomy.

Bile duct anomalies

Congenital anomalies of the bile ducts include the following:

1. Anomalies of extrahepatic duct configuration, such as atresia, accessory ducts, abnormal lengths of ducts, and variations in the junction of the cystic and hepatic ducts. Liver transplantation has greatly improved the survival rate of children with biliary atresia.

2. Cystic anomalies of the common bile duct, including cystic dilatation of the common bile duct (choledochal cyst), which makes up 85% of these anomalies; congenital choledochocele; and congenital diverticulum of the common bile duct. In patients with choledochal cyst, symptoms generally appear after age 17. Diagnosis is by ultrasonography, and the recommended treatment is Roux-en-Y choledochocystojejnostomy with cholecystotomy. Complete excision of the cyst is recommended.

3. Cystic dilatation of the intrahepatic ducts, or Caroli's disease, which is a rare disorder that most often occurs in young adults. Symptoms include bile stasis, cholangitis, and intrahepatic stone or abscess formation.

Anomalies of either the gallbladder or the bile ducts may impair the normal flow of bile, resulting in **cholestasis,** which leads to sludging—(the formation in the gallbladder of an amorphous material consisting of cholesterol monohydrate crystals and bilirubin granules embedded in a matrix of mucous gel).

Congenital anomalies of the bile ducts often present in infancy, whereas congenital gallbladder anomalies are rarely of clinical significance until adulthood. Biliary anomalies do not follow recognizable patterns of genetic inheritance, nor are they associated with other developmental abnormalities, which suggest that they may be caused by pathogenic factors, such as viruses, drugs, or toxins transmitted by the mother.

CASE SITUATION

Dr. David Rosenstein, a pediatrician, was diagnosed with UC at age 24. In the following 5 years, he had two exacerbations of the disease that required medication, but they were not as serious as his first attack. For the last 13 years, the disease has been in remission and Dr. Rosenstein has required no medication.

Now, at age 42, Dr. Rosenstein has experienced fatigue and pruritus for several months. Last week, he began to notice yellowing of his skin and eyes and sought out the gastroenterologist again. He says he has been feeling fine for the last 13 years, except for the recent fatigue and itching. He denies any pain, gallbladder disease, hepatitis, IV drug use, or alcohol abuse. He has had no blood transfusions. His blood work shows elevated total bilirubin and alkaline phosphatase, with normal serum transaminases. His hepatitis panel is all negative. Ultrasonography shows that the biliary system and pancreas are normal.

Points to think about

1. Because of the negative hepatitis panel and normal ultrasonography, and given the past history of UC, what might be the diagnosis for Dr. Rosenstein?

2. Dr. Rosenstein will undergo an ERCP to visualize the biliary tree. The ERCP should show strictured areas in the intrahepatic and extrahepatic ducts, with areas of dilatation between the strictures, which can produce a beaded appearance to the ducts. How can the gastroenterology nurse help Dr. Rosenstein through this procedure?

3. What data are available in relation to the nursing diagnosis "alteration in comfort?"

4. What outcome criteria and associated nursing interventions may be devised for this diagnosis?

Suggested responses

1. Based on Dr. Rosenstein's negative hepatitis panel, normal ultrasound examination, and past history of UC, PSC might be the diagnosis. Up to 5% of patients with UC develop PSC, but PSC has no correlation with UC exacerbations or remissions. Males who are under the age of 45 account for 60% to 70% of patients with PSC. It can be diagnosed before or after a diagnosis of UC and can occur even after a total colectomy.

2. Educational endeavors by nurses must take into account an individual patient's current level of understanding and his or her readiness to learn. In this example, there are two possible inferences about Dr. Rosenstein's level of understanding:

   (a) Dr. Rosenstein has the usual medical school foundation in reference to UC and its accompanying problems and diagnostic procedures; or

   (b) because he has lived with the diagnosis of UC for many years, Dr. Rosenstein has a near-exhaustive knowledge of UC and its accompanying problems and diagnostic tests (He had probably already made a tentative diagnosis of PSC before he consulted the gastroenterologist.)

Although the second inference would seem the most likely, it should not be assumed without testing its truth. In regard to the ERCP procedure, testing can be conducted through the use of straightforward or open-ended questions, such as those that follow:

   (a) "Do you have any questions about the ERCP procedure?"

(b) "Are you aware of what happens during the ERCP procedure?"

If responses do not elicit sufficient details, leading statements and other open-ended questions can focus on specific aspects of the procedure. The nurse must be aware that Dr. Rosenstein may choose not to respond.

For a patient who does not have a medical background, the nurse might consider the following preprocedural activities:

(a) Assess the patient's knowledge and offer any necessary explanations of what will happen during the procedure.

(b) Encourage questions.

(c) Explain the duration of the procedure.

(d) Explain about the x-ray room and that radiographic examinations will be taken during the procedure.

(e) Explain the medications given and their expected effects.

(f) Reinforce awareness that he or she will be with the patient during the entire procedure and will be monitoring his or her response to sedative drugs and to the procedure itself and will be taking vital signs regularly.

(g) Review the record before the procedure to refresh recall of laboratory data so he or she will be aware of incipient problems during the procedure.

(h) Review probable postprocedural events with the patient.

3. Data are available to indicate that Dr. Rosenstein is still experiencing pruritus. The gastroenterology nurse does not know whether it is severe nor whether it is confined to limited skin areas or more widespread. Furthermore, Dr. Rosenstein may have open lesions that are associated with severe scratching on areas of his skin. The nursing diagnosis "alteration in comfort related to pruritus caused by PSC" seems applicable.

4. Outcome criteria and associated nursing interventions for the diagnosis "alteration in comfort related to pruritus caused by PSC" are as follows:

Outcome criteria	Nursing interventions
Patient will experience some relief from pruritus	Cool skin with wet compresses or baths
	Pat skin dry after bathing
	Apply prescribed antipruritic drugs
	Apply pressure to itchy areas instead of scratching
Patient will sleep for at least 2- to 3-hour intervals during night	Encourage therapeutic bath before retiring
	Have patient keep a log of sleeping/waking periods
	Place a clock and writing material at bedside

REVIEW TERMS

bile, biliary colic, cholangitis, cholecystitis, choledocholithiasis, cholelithiasis, cholestasis, common bile duct, cystic duct, gallbladder, hepatic duct, jaundice, primary sclerosing cholangitis (PSC), sphincter of Oddi

REVIEW QUESTIONS

1. The gallbladder wall is made up of:
   (a) Serosa, muscularis, submucosa, and mucosa.
   (b) Serosa, a fibromuscular layer, and mucosa.
   (c) Muscularis, submucosa, and mucosa.
   (d) Serosa, a fibromuscular layer, submucosa, and mucosa.

2. Blood is supplied to the gallbladder by the:
   (a) Superior mesenteric artery.
   (b) Hepatic artery.
   (c) Celiac artery.
   (d) Inferior phrenic artery.

3. What is the maximum amount of bile that can be stored in the gallbladder?
   (a) 5 ml.
   (b) 10 ml.
   (c) 50 ml.
   (d) 500 ml.

4. What is the major component of the bile that is produced by the liver?
   (a) Cholesterol.
   (b) Bilirubin.
   (c) Bile salts.
   (d) Water.

5. By far the most common disease affecting the biliary system is:
   (a) Choledocholithiasis.
   (b) Cholecystitis.
   (c) Cholelithiasis.
   (d) Cholangitis.

6. Chronic hemolytic disease, total parenteral nutrition, and alcoholism are among the risk factors for the formation of:
   (a) Cholesterol gallstones.
   (b) Pigment gallstones.
   (c) Cholangitis.
   (d) Gallbladder cancer.

7. The primary disadvantage of most nonsurgical treatment alternatives to cholecystectomy is:
   (a) Potential recurrence of cholelithiasis after cessation of treatment.
   (b) Unpleasant side effects.
   (c) The need for specialized equipment.
   (d) The need for specially trained personnel.

8. For most patients, the treatment of choice for choledocholithiasis is:
   (a) Sphincteroplasty.

(b) Cholecystectomy.

(c) Endoscopic papillotomy.

(d) Endoscopic retrograde cholangiopancreatography.

9. The most common cause of cholecystitis is:

(a) Cholecystenteric fistula.

(b) Bacterial infection.

(c) A gallstone impacted in the cystic duct.

(d) Gallstone ileus.

10. Treatment for cancer of the gallbladder most often involves:

(a) Supportive and symptomatic measures only.

(b) Cholecystectomy.

(c) Pancreaticoduodenectomy.

(d) Insertion of an internal drainage system.

11. The sphincter of Oddi functions to:

(a) Regulate bile flow.

(b) Regulate pancreatic juice flow.

(c) Inhibit entry of bile into the pancreatic duct.

(d) Prevent reflux of intestinal content into biliary duct.

(e) All of the above.

BIBLIOGRAPHY

Chobanian, S. & Van Ness, M. (Eds.) (1994). *Manual of clinical problems in gastroenterology.* Boston: Little, Brown.

Chopra, S. & May, R. (Eds.) (1988). *Pathophysiology of gastrointestinal diseases.* Boston: Little, Brown.

Eastwood, G. & Avunduk, C. (1988). *Manual of gastroenterology: diagnosis and therapy.* Boston: Little, Brown.

Given, B., Simmons, S. (1984). *Gastroenterology in clinical nursing* (4th ed.). St. Louis, MO: Mosby.

Meenan, J., Rauws, E. & Huibretse, K. (1996). Benign biliary strictures and sclerosing cholangitis. *Gastrointest Endosc Clin North Am 6(1),* 127-38.

Silverman, A. & Roy, C. (1983). *Pediatric clinical gastroenterology* (3rd ed.). St. Louis, MO: Mosby.

Sleisenger, M. & Fordtran, J. (Eds.) (2002). *Gastrointestinal disease: pathophysiology, diagnosis, management* (7th ed.). Philadelphia: W.B. Saunders.

Waye, J. Geenen, J.E., and Fleischer, D. (1987). *Techniques in therapeutic endoscopy.* Philadelphia: W.B. Saunders.

Weinstock, D., Andrews, M. & Cray, J. (Eds.) (1998). *Nurse's Reference Library Series: Diseases* (6th ed.). Springhouse, PA: Springhouse.

Wyllie, R. & Hyams, J.S. (1999). Diseases of the gallbladder. In *Pediatric Gastrointestinal Disease; Pathophysiology, Diagnosis, Management* (2nd ed.). Philadelphia: W. B. Saunders.

Yamada, T. Alpers, D., Laine, L., Owyang, C., Powell, D.W. (1999). *Textbook of gastroenterology, Vol. 1* (3rd ed.). Philadelphia: J.B. Lippincott.

Chapter 18

PANCREAS

This chapter will acquaint the gastroenterology nurse with the normal anatomy and physiology of the pancreas and will discuss selected pancreatic disorders in terms of pathophysiology, diagnosis, and treatment.

Learning objectives

After reviewing the content of this chapter, the gastroenterology nurse should be able to:

1. Describe the normal gross structure and histology of the pancreas.
2. Explain the normal physiological functions of the pancreas, including both endocrine and exocrine secretions.
3. Discuss pathological conditions of the pancreas, including selected diseases, disorders, and congenital anomalies.

ANATOMY

The **pancreas** is a fish-shaped, lobulated gland that lies behind the stomach (see Fig. 13-2). It is approximately 15 to 20 cm (6 to 8 inches) long and 5 cm (2 inches) wide, and it has an average weight of less than 110 g (about 4 ounces). The pancreas has three segments: the head, which lies over the vena cava in the c-shaped curve of the duodenum; the body, which lies behind the duodenum, extends across the abdomen behind the stomach and across the spine; and the thin, narrow tail, which is situated under the spleen.

The pancreas contains two basic cell types, exocrine cells and endocrine cells. The pyramidal acinar cells are exocrine cells that make up the majority of the pancreatic tissue. Groups of acinar cells form an **acinus,** and groups of acini form grape-like lobules. The lobules, in turn, are joined together by connective tissue into lobes, which unite to form the entire gland.

The acini are arranged around a small, central lumen into which they drain their enzymes. The central lumina are drained by means of ductules, the most proximal portion of

which is lined by clear, cuboidal cells called *centroacinar cells.* The ductules drain into multiple intralobular ducts; these join the interlobular ducts, which in turn drain into the **duct of Wirsung,** the main pancreatic duct. The duct of Wirsung runs the whole length of the pancreas from left to right and joins the common bile duct, emptying into the duodenum at the **papilla of Vater.** Most individuals have an accessory duct called the **duct of Santorini,** which leads from the head of the pancreas and drains into the duodenum at an accessory or minor papilla that lies just proximal and anterior to the papilla of Vater.

Endocrine cells make up the remaining 1% of the pancreatic cells. They are located in the **islets of Langerhans,** which are embedded in the loose connective tissue between the lobules, mainly in the tail.

Branches of the splenic, superior mesenteric, and celiac arteries supply blood to the pancreas. Blood is drained away from the pancreas into the portal or splenic circulation by the superior mesenteric and splenic veins.

Sympathetic nerve fibers control pain sensation, blood flow, and enzyme secretion in the pancreas. Parasympathetic fibers control exocrine and endocrine function.

PHYSIOLOGY

The pancreas is both an exocrine and an endocrine organ. The three types of endocrine cells in the pancreas are **alpha cells,** which produce glucagon; **beta cells,** which produce insulin; and **delta cells,** which produce somatostatin. These endocrine products are released directly into the circulation. When the blood sugar level falls below normal, the alpha cells are stimulated to secrete glucagon, which accelerates the conversion of glycogen to glucose in the liver. When the blood sugar level is above normal, the beta cells secrete insulin, which promotes both the metabolism of glucose by the tissue cells and the conversion of glucose to glycogen, which is then stored in the liver and muscles.

The exocrine acinar cells secrete 500 to 1000 ml of pancreatic juice daily. This colorless fluid has a pH of 8.3 and consists of water, bicarbonate, enzymes, potassium, sodium, chloride, and calcium. The three major types of enzymes secreted by the pancreas include the following:

(a) amylases (predominantly α-amylase), which hydrolyze carbohydrates into glucose and maltose;

(b) lipases (including pancreatic lipase and phospholipase A), which are important in early stages of fat digestion; and

(c) proteases (including trypsinogen, the precursor of trypsin), which break amino acid bonds of protein chains and also convert other proenzymes to their active forms.

Pancreatic secretions are controlled by the hormones **secretin** and **cholecystokinin-pancreozymin (CCK-PZ).** When the chyme is made up predominantly of undigested proteins and fats, the duodenum releases CCK-PZ, which stimulates the release of enzyme-rich pancreatic juice. When the chyme is mainly acidic, secretin stimulates the release of pancreatic juice that is rich in bicarbonate and water. Pancreatic juice enters the duodenum with the biliary secretions at the papilla of Vater.

Pancreatic secretion occurs in the following four phases:

1. At rest, the pancreas secretes bicarbonate at about 2% of the maximal rate and enzymes at about 15% of the maximal rate.

2. The cephalic phase of pancreatic secretion occurs when the sight and smell of food stimulates a modest output of enzyme-rich pancreatic juice.

3. In the gastric phase, distention of the stomach stimulates secretion of a moderate amount of pancreatic juice that is rich in enzymes but low in bicarbonate.

4. In the intestinal phase, the delivery of food into the proximal intestine evokes secretion of pancreatic enzymes at about 70% of the maximal rate. The volume of pancreatic juice and bicarbonate output increases as the pH of the meal decreases and the acid load increases.

In the absence of pancreatic enzymes, up to 40% of dietary fat and protein may be assimilated using other, less efficient pathways of digestion, such as salivary amylase, pharyngeal lipase, and peptidases from the brush borders of the gut mucosa. It has been estimated that pancreatic enzyme secretion must fall below 10% of normal before maldigestion or malabsorption occurs.

PATHOPHYSIOLOGY

Noteworthy pathological conditions that affect the pancreas (not in order of frequency) include acute and chronic pancreatitis, Zollinger-Ellison syndrome, malignant and benign tumors, congenital defects, and cystic fibrosis.

Pancreatitis

Pancreatitis is an inflammatory condition of the pancreas that can result from obstruction of the pancreatic duct and other mechanisms such as trauma, toxicity from alcohol, infections and drugs. It may be acute or chronic and represents a wide spectrum of severity and clinical presentations. Many aspects of the pathogenesis of acute and chronic pancreatitis are poorly understood. Therapy is often supportive, may be directed at a specific etiology or at morphological changes in the pancreatic duct (stricture, obstruction, disruption, stones, dilatation).

Acute pancreatitis

Acute pancreatitis is caused by alcohol use, gallstones, abdominal trauma, hyperparathyroidism, hyperlipidemia, infections and drugs (Lankisch 1998; Bank 1999). It also occurs after endoscopic retrograde cholangiopancreatography (ERCP) in about 7% of all cases but higher rates occur in certain high risk groups such as sphincter of Oddi dysnfunction. A less common association of acute pancreatitis is pancreas divisum (Carr-Locke, 1991).

The characteristic anatomical changes associated with acute pancreatitis are the results of enzymatic digestion of the pancreatic parenchyma and peripancreatic tissues by enzymes that are normally present in the pancreas in their inactive proenzyme form. This produces varying degrees of edema, necrosis, hemorrhage and the release of harmful substances (cytokines) which can injure distant organs and lead to severe complications including death.

The most severe form of acute pancreatitis is **necrotizing pancreatitis** (Baron, 1999). The morphological findings include destruction (necrosis) of pancreatic tissue, blood vessels and fat with extensive fluid accumulation in the retroperitoneum. If this collection of tissues becomes infected during the course of the disease, it is termed **infected** necrosis. The mass of inflamed pancreas was formerly called a '**phlegmon**' but this term is less used today as it does not carry any prognostic significance. It has been replaced by 'inflammatory mass' where this is appropriate. Massive necrosis frequently leads to the formation of large pancreatic and peripancreatic collections of fluid, blood, and necrotic debris which are initially diffuse. If the fluid collection persists beyond four weeks after the attack and becomes walled off by adjacent anatomical structures, it is called a pseudocyst and if this contained significant debris, it is termed organized necrosis. Overall mortality in patients with necrotizing pancreatitis is at least 30% irrespective of etiology with infected necrosis carrying the highest mortality.

Interstitial pancreatitis is a milder form of acute pancreatitis that is characterized by pancreatic interstitial edema with intact pancreatic acini and ducts without necrosis. Mortality from this form is less than that of necrotizing pancreatitis but requires the same degree of intensive care when severe. Pseudocyst formation can also occur after interstitial pancreatitis.

Symptoms and signs of acute pancreatitis include:

(a) pain in the midepigastrium, left chest, shoulder, and back;

(b) nausea and vomiting;

(c) low-grade fever;

(d) abdominal swelling and tenderness;

(e)   shock, hypovolemia, and hypotension;

(f)   anorexia and weight loss;

(g)   hypocalcemia;

(h)   hypoxia; and

Grey Turner's sign, a bluish flank discoloration, or Cullen's sign, a bluish periumbilical discoloration caused by blood tracking from the retroperitoneum to these sites (very rare).

Diagnosis of acute pancreatitis is made by detecting an elevation of serum amylase and lipase more than three times the upper normal limits. An etiology may be identified by a combination of laboratory tests, radiological evaluations (CT, MRI, MRCP), abdominal and/or endoscopic ultrasonography, and ERCP.

Treatment of acute pancreatitis (Toouli, 2002) is aimed at hemodynamic stabilization, correction of metabolic abnormalities, and reducing the risk of organ failure. Medical treatment includes:

(a)   adequate pain relief

(b)   withholding of foods and fluids by mouth

(c)   nasogastric suctioning if there is significant vomiting

(d)   bed rest

(e)   electrolyte/fluid replacement, which may be massive

(f)   blood transfusions as required

(g)   insulin to control hyperglycemia or florid diabetes

(h)   antibiotics as determined by clinical trials

(i)   full intensive care support as appropriate, endotracheal intubation and ventilation, renal dialysis, coagulation support, sedation, CT-guided fine needle aspiration of the pancreas if infected necrosis is suspected, emergency ERCP for severe gallstone pancreatitis, pressor support, etc.

The majority of patients have interstitial pancreatitis and improve with supportive care alone within several days.

When the cause is gallstones, surgery is recommended (laparoscopic cholecystectomy) during the same admission but if there is evidence of biliary tract obstruction from stones, or the attack is severe, urgent ERCP is indicated with endoscopic sphincterotomy where necessary (Sharma, 1999). ERCP by an experienced endoscopist is no longer contraindicated in acute pancreatitis if there is a chance of reducing the risk of complications and saving life.

Complications of pancreatitis within the first 30 days include secondary infection of pancreatic necrosis, pulmonary infections, pleural effusion, adult respiratory distress syndrome, multiple organ dysfunction syndrome (MODS), renal failure, cardiac dysfunction, 'third spacing', coagulopathy, persistent hypotension, encephalopathy, liver failure, immunocompromise with opportunistic infections, ischemia of limbs and internal organs and malnutrition. New complications occurring later than 30 days are mostly in or around the pancreas and include pseudocyst, organized necrosis, abscess, pancreatic fistula, and duodenal and bile duct stricture.

Chronic pancreatitis

In the Western world, 75% of chronic pancreatitis is associated with long-term, heavy alcohol use (Lankisch, 1998, Lankisch, 2001). Worldwide it may also be the result of protein calorie malnutrition, cystic fibrosis, obstruction of the pancreatic duct by tumor, tropical pancreatitis and familial pancreatitis. It is generally found in male patients who are between the ages of 40 and 60. Typically, persistent inflammation produces irreversible morphological changes by fibrosis and atrophy in the pancreas resulting in exocrine and endocrine functional loss. At least 90% of the exocrine function must be lost before significant malabsorption is noticed and diabetes develops late in the disease.

Hereditary pancreatitis, although rare, may be symptomatic by the age of 10 to 12 (Whitcomb, 2000). Chronic obstructive pancreatitis can be caused by tumor, post-traumatic stricture, pancreatic calculi, especially in tropical pancreatitis, and, possibly pancreas divisum.

Symptoms and signs of chronic pancreatitis may include:

(a)   epigastric, subcostal, or umbilical pain radiating to the back;

(b)   weight loss and debilitation;

(c)   steatorrhea;

(d)   diabetes mellitus;

(e)   obstructive jaundice from bile duct stricture; and

(f)   epigastric mass.

Diagnosis is usually made by having a high index of suspicion, the appropriate imaging examinations (CT, MRI, MRCP, ERCP, US and EUS), laboratory tests during acute exacerbations, malabsorption tests, and tests of pancreatic function. The main value of ERCP is the identification of the extent of the disease, anatomy, and the presence of potentially correctable lesions. EUS may be the most sensitive test for detecting early changes of chronic pancreatitis.

Treatment for chronic pancreatitis is initially non-surgical and includes abstention from alcohol, acute and chronic pain relief, nutritional support, and oral replacement of pancreatic enzymes when steatorrhea is detected. Use of pancreatic enzymes for pain relief has been disappointing. Endoscopic intervention has gained in popularity although scientific evidence for long-term benefit is only now emerging (ASGE, 2000; Rosch, 2002). Such endoscopic procedures as pancreatic sphincterotomy, stent placement and stone extraction should be confined to expert centers studying this form of therapy. Surgical intervention may be necessary in situations where symptoms, such as pain and/or recurrent attacks of pancreatitis, are uncontrolled. Many operations have been designed to solve different problems, but there are basically two types of surgery either involving resection (Whipple, pylorus-preserving pancreaticoduodenectomy, duodenum-preserving head resection (Beger operation), total or subtotal pancreatectomy) or drainage (lateral pancreaticojejunostomy (Puestow operation), extended pancreaticojejunostomy (Frey operation). Celiac plexus block to relieve chronic pain can be achieved percutaneously or by endoscopic ultrasound. Many patients with chronic pancreatitis in permanent pain become addicted to narcotics and require the support of pain services and psychiatry.

Pseudocyst

A pseudocyst is an encapsulated sac that is lined by granulation tissue but no epithelium (thus making it a 'pseudocyst' rather than a true cyst) and is filled with pancreatic fluid and sometimes blood. A pseudocyst is diagnosed four or more weeks after an attack of pancreatitis, since before this time it is termed an acute pancreatic fluid collection. Pseudocysts may be single or multiple and are associated with all forms of acute and chronic pancreatitis. Symptoms include epigastric pain, persistent nausea and vomiting, an inability to eat, weight loss, occasionally jaundice, and low-grade fever. In 30 to 40% of patients, the cyst may be palpated. Abdominal ultrasonography, endoscopic ultrasonography (EUS), MRI and CT scan are the methods for identifying a pseudocyst that is greater than 1 cm in diameter.

At least 60% of all pseudocysts resolve spontaneously after diagnosis. If conservative treatment for pancreatitis does not resolve the cyst or associated symptoms, a drainage procedure may be required. Pseudocysts may be drained surgically, percutaneously, or endoscopically. The choice between techniques depends on local expertise, anatomical factors, making one approach more feasible than another, and the presence of significant debris within the cyst fluid (organized necrosis, see above). Pseudocyst drainage by the three alternatives is equally effective in the short term but recurrence is higher with percutaneous drainage and there is always the risk of creating an external fistula. Urgent intervention is required if there is infection of a pseudocyst, free pseudocyst rupture into the peritoneal cavity or chest, or massive pseudocyst hemorrhage from a pseudoaneurysm within the cystic cavity.

Pancreatic fistulas

The majority of clinically significant **pancreatic fistulas** are external but internal fistulas can cause massive ascites (pancreaticoperitoneal fistula), pleural effusion (pancreaticopleural fistula) or pseudocysts. Causes of pancreatic fistulas include:

(a) trauma with pancreatic duct injury;
(b) external drainage of a pseudocyst;
(c) pancreatic surgery involving a ductal anastomsosis; and
(d) spontaneous pancreatic duct disruption complicating pancreatitis.

About 75% of pancreatic fistulas will close spontaneously within a few months, but persistence is unpleasant, and high output (greater than 200 ml per day) fistulas should always be treated. When gut rest and octreotide (octapeptide of somatostatin) suppression of pancreatic secretion fail, endoscopic therapy can be very effective (Telford, 2002). Surgery should be reserved for complex fistulas, those with additional indications for surgery or those not responding to less invasive treatment.

Carcinoma

Ninety per cent of pancreatic tumors are solid malignant adenocarcinomas and arise from the ductal epithelium. Benign and malignant cystic tumors and endocrine tumors that involve the islet cells are discussed later.

Pancreatic cancer often presents with pain that is experienced as back or spinal pain, anorexia, weight loss, an abdominal mass, and commonly jaundice when the tumor arises in the head of the gland. Dark urine and light-colored stools appear in about 75% of patients with pancreatic carcinoma, and mental depression is found in 50% to 75% of these patients. Vomiting and weakness occur in one third of patients.

Diagnosis is made by US, CT, or MRI scanning with tissue confirmation by percutaneous CT-guided biopsy, ERCP, or EUS. Staging is usually accomplished by the same tests, and laparotomy for diagnosis and staging is now rarely needed. Laparoscopy prior to a planned resection may reveal additional metastatic spread not identified by other imaging. Diagnostic ERCP is becoming rare with improvements in CT and MRI.

Therapy for pancreatic cancer is intended to be curative in a very small proportion of patients with small tumors at presentation, but more than 85% of patients will require palliation and supportive care. In operable cases, a form of pancreaticoduodenectomy (Whipple operation and variants) is usually performed. For relief of biliary obstruction and its consequences, endoscopic stent placement is the most effective approach and, if patients survive longer than three months, self-expanding metal stents are superior to plastic (Wong, 1998). Planned palliative surgery is now rarely performed as even the problem of duodenal obstruction can now be palliated by endoscopic enteral stent insertion (Yim, 2001). The rare patient with pancreatic pain or pancreatitis from malignant duct obstruction may benefit from pancreatic stent drainage (Tham, 2000).

Pancreatic cystic tumors

A different spectrum of tumors, called cystic neoplasms, involve any part of the pancreas, but most commonly the head, and contain fluid (Brugge, 2002). They range from benign to malignant and from very small to massive. They may be indistinguishable from pseudocysts on CT scan, and an absence of a history of pancreatitis should therefore raise suspicion. Terminology is complex but serous cystadenoma/cystadenocarcinoma and mucinous cystadenoma/cystadenocarcinoma are the dominant types. A variant involving the ducts and causing them to dilate and fill with mucus is now called intraductal papillary mucinous tumor (IPMT) and carries a better prognosis than the more common ductal adenocarcinoma described above.

Endocrine tumors

Islet cell tumors are classified on the basis of the predominant hormone they secrete, although most secrete more than one hormone. Types of islet cell tumors include gastrinomas, insulinomas, glucagonomas, somatostatinomas, and VIPomas. They may be benign or malignant.

In the rare **Zollinger-Ellison syndrome (ZES),** a gastrinoma, or non-beta islet cell tumor of the pancreas, releases the hormone gastrin into the circulation, which stimulates gastric acid hypersecretion and, in turn, leads to severe ulcers in the upper GI tract, predominantly in the distal duodenum or jejunum, and often severe diarrhea. The disease has two common variants, a sporadic type, which is usually malignant and is seen later in life, and a genetic type, which is associated with multiple endocrine neoplasia type 1 (MEN1) and causes tumors or hyperplasia of the parathyroid, pancreatic islet, and pituitary glands. ZES occurs most frequently between the ages of 35 and 65 and is more common in men than in women (Jensen, 1996).

Patients with ZES have pain as the predominant symptom from peptic ulcer disease and sometimes diarrhea and steatorrhea.

The hypergastrinemia of atrophic gastritis and pernicious anemia is due to loss of feedback inhibition of gastrin secretion which therefore rises unchecked. Fasting serum gastrin level is elevated in 99% to 100% of patients with ZES (Jensen, 1996). If elevated, the next step is to check the fasting gastric pH to exclude achlorhydria.

Confirmatory diagnostic tests may include secretin and/or calcium infusion to stimulate gastrin levels further when the fasting level is equivocal. The best methods for tumor localization are CT scanning, endoscopic ultrasonography, and octreotide nuclear scanning. Tumors are usually located in the pancreas and duodenum. One third of ZES patients have metastatic liver disease on presentation with metastasis to regional lymph nodes, later to the liver, and very late to the bone. It is a slowly progressive disease (Jensen, 1996).

Medical treatment of ZES is now highly effective and involves long-term administration of proton-pump inhibitors often at doses much larger than normally prescribed. Total gastrectomy to control acid secretion is now very rarely needed.

For metastatic disease, chemotherapy is promising. When medical treatment fails, surgery may be recommended to remove the primary tumor if it can be located. In patients who do not have MEN1, approximately 25% of gastrinomas can be completely resected with resultant cure; if resection is possible, this is the optimal treatment.

The extent of morbidity and mortality in patients with ZES is related principally to ulcer complications, fistulas, hemorrhage, or perforation. Complications of ulcer disease, such as bleeding or perforation, occur in 40% to 50% of patients at sometime during the course of their disease (Jensen, 1996).

The most common type of islet cell tumor is an **insulinoma,** which arises from the beta cells. The tumor is typically round, firm, and encapsulated and is most frequently located in the body or tail of the pancreas. Seventy to eighty percent are solitary benign tumors. Patients with insulinomas present with symptoms of hypoglycemia on fasting or after exercise. These patients may also exhibit neuropsychiatric manifestations, ranging from subtle personality changes to confusion, coma, or seizure disorders. Insulin-to-glucose ratio is also elevated in these patients.

Glucagon-secreting tumors of the alpha islet cells are called **glucagonomas.** They are far less common than insulinomas or gastrinomas. The most distinctive feature is a skin disorder, necrolytic migratory erythema, which appears as an erythematous area that develops a central blister and is followed by crusting, healing, and sometimes bronze hyperpigmentation. Most patients also have diabetes mellitus. Because of the catabolic activity of glucagon, patients with glucagonomas often exhibit profound weight loss and anemia. More than 50% of patients have metastases at the time of diagnosis.

Patients who have **somatostatinomas** may present with steatorrhea, mild diabetes mellitus, and/or cholelithiasis. These symptoms are consistent with somatostatin's inhibitory effect on the secretion of gastrin, secretin, insulin, glucagon, and cholecystokinin.

Patients with tumors that produce vasoactive intestinal peptide (**VIPomas**) generally experience profuse watery diarrhea, hypokalemia, and hypochlorhydria or achlorhydria, also known as the pancreatic cholera or Verner Morrison syndrome.

The treatment of choice for most islet cell tumors is surgical excision. Patients with metastatic disease may improve after surgical reduction of the tumor mass. Streptozocin has been shown to decrease tumor size and prolong survival. A long-acting analog of somatostatin effectively controls symptoms in patients with several types of islet cell tumors.

Pancreatic enzyme insufficiency

Pancreatic exocrine insufficiency generally results from chronic pancreatitis leading to acinar loss. Pancreatic duct obstruction should be excluded since this may be a correctable cause. Because pancreatic enzymes are necessary for the digestion of fat, protein, and carbohydrates, pancreatic insufficiency leads to pan-malabsorption and steatorrhea. Weight loss is a common symptom. Plain x-ray films may show calcification of the pancreas but CT is more sensitive. Fat malabsorption also may be quantified by using a 72-hour fecal fat analysis when the stool fat output will be greater than 7% of intake.

Exocrine insufficiency is treated with adequate amounts of oral enzyme preparations and concomitant acid suppresion to improve delivery of sufficient enzyme into the small bowel. In some patients, supplemental calcium, vitamin D, and other fat-soluble vitamins may be needed.

Cystic fibrosis

Cystic fibrosis is the most common lethal genetic defect in Caucasian populations, occurring in 1 out of every 2000 live births. It is an autosomal-recessive disease of the exocrine glands that affects not only the pancreas but also the respiratory system, the sweat glands, and the reproductive system. The genetic mutations for this disease have been identified and can be measured. The dysfunction of pancreatic exocrine function forces the patient to rely on oral pancreatic enzymes. The disease also affects the mucus-producing organs, making their secretions excessively viscous. Mucus may block the bronchi, small intestine, bile ducts, and pancreas.

Conflicting pathogenetic mechanisms for cystic fibrosis have been suggested, but none of these theories satisfactorily reconcile the unique sweat gland defect with the abnormal characteristics of mucus secretion. The most promising avenue of research centers on electrolyte secretion and chloride channel regulation. Elevation of sodium and chloride concentrations in the sweat is the most characteristic finding in cystic fibrosis. Obtaining sputum cultures has also become an integral part of evaluating patients with cystic fibrosis, because *Staphylcoccus aureus, Pseudomonas aeruginosa,* and *Pseudomonas cepacia* are consistently associated with morbidity and mortality in the disease (Bone, 1996). It is possible that in affected tissues of cystic fibrosis patients, alteration in a common intracellular mediator or inhibitor protein distal to the site of generation of cyclic adenosine monophosphate is likely to be the underlying abnormality.

Cystic fibrosis is frequently diagnosed in the first year of life; about 90% of affected children have obvious clinical signs and symptoms resulting from both pulmonary and pancreatic involvement. Approximately 10% to 15% of patients with cystic fibrosis present at birth or shortly thereafter with symptoms of small bowel obstruction. The cause is a plug of meconium in the terminal ileum, which is acquired in utero and is perhaps the first overt manifestation of diminished pancreatic function. Symptoms of cystic fibrosis include poor fat and protein digestion, leading to oily and foul-smelling stools; weight loss despite an increased appetite; repeated episodes of pneumonia and bronchitis; diminished or absent pancreatic enzymes; and pulmonary changes. The infant's production of thick, sticky, dry mucus leads to noisy respirations; intermittent wheezing; and coughing, particularly when lying down.

GI complications include intestinal obstruction (meconium ileus equivalent), intussusception, constipation, and rectal prolapse. Biliary cirrhosis occurs in 2% to 5% of patients. Liver disease, esophageal varices, hyperglycemia, and diabetes mellitus may also be encountered (Bone, 1996).

Approximately 80% of patients with cystic fibrosis have pancreatic insufficiency at birth, although the extent of pancreatic involvement is highly variable. The definitive diagnostic test for cystic fibrosis is the sweat electrolyte test where quantitative pilocarpine iontophoresis shows elevated sodium and chloride levels in affected patients. Sweat electrolyte testing may not be reliable in neonates and in individuals with edema. DNA testing can now be performed to identify victims and carriers of the cystic fibrosis gene.

Cystic fibrosis is managed by controlling respiratory complications and by aiding digestion through dietary regulation and pancreatic enzyme replacement, as well as supplements of vitamins A, D, E, and K. Gene therapy is promising.

Much of the morbidity and virtually all of the mortality beyond the neonatal period in cystic fibrosis patients is attributable to chronic obstructive pulmonary disease. In 1960, the mean survival age after diagnosis was less than 5 years. Since then it has increased to over 20 years. This prolongation of life can be attributed largely to the development of pancreatic replacement therapy, use of antibiotics, and vigorous pulmonary hygiene.

Congenital anomalies

Congenital anomalies of the pancreas may include pancreatic rest, pancreas divisum, and annular pancreas.

Pancreatic rest

A **pancreatic rest** is an uncommon condition that is defined as the presence of ectopic pancreatic tissue usually in the gastric antrum. It is usually an incidental finding during an upper GI endoscopy. When symptomatic, it may produce ulceration, bleeding or clinical pancreatitis. Symptomatic lesions are treated with simple excision which can be accomplished by endoscopic mucosectomy.

Pancreas divisum

Pancreas divisum is a congenital anomaly that occurs when the two embryonic precursors of the pancreas, ventral and dorsal buds, fail to fuse, thereby resulting in separate dorsal and ventral pancreatic ducts. The dorsal gland is drained by the duct of Santorini through the minor or accessory papilla into the duodenum, whereas the ventral gland is drained by an abnormally short duct of Wirsung and enters the duodenum through the major papilla together with the bile duct. Pancreas divisum is present in about 5% of the population and up to 15% in patients with unexplained pancreatitis.

Clinical pancreatic disease is an uncommon sequela of this anomaly, although the risk of developing acute pancreatitis is increased (Carr-Locke, 1991). It may be that both pancreas divisum and a stenotic accessory papilla must be present for clinically evident pancreatitis to occur. Recurrent acute pancreatitis may be attributable to divisum and the pancreatic ducts appear normal but chronic pancreatitis may occur coincidentally and often affects both ducts.

For patients with frequent episodes of recurrent acute pancreatitis, intervention may be considered. Alternatives include surgical sphincterotomy or sphincteroplasty of the accessory papilla and endoscopic sphincterotomy of the minor papilla with a temporary protective stent, both of which give similar results.

Annular pancreas

Annular pancreas occurs when the embryonic dorsal and ventral glands fail to fuse and part of the ventral pancreas encircles the duodenum, often resulting in duodenal obstruction. Annular pancreas is the most common anomaly obstructing the duodenum in infancy and may also be associated with other congenital anomalies, such as atresia of the duodenum and Down's syndrome. Annular pancreas may not cause any symptoms until adulthood. At that time, presenting complaints include intermittent epigastric discomfort, which is relieved by vomiting. Upper GI x-ray films show a narrowing of the second portion of the duodenum. Symptomatic cases are best treated by surgical bypass using a duodenojejunostomy.

Pancreatic insufficiency in children

Pancreatic diseases in children are rare and may prove to be a diagnostic challenge. These disorders occur with less frequency in the pediatric age group compared to the adult population. A well-documented symptomatology is needed to reveal the occurrence of pancreatic diseases. Pancreatic insufficiency should be considered in children with weight loss, failure to thrive, malabsorption, or steatorrhea. The most common causes of pancreatic insufficiency in children are cystic fibrosis and Schwachman-Diamond syndrome (Lerner, 1996).

Schwachman-Diamond syndrome

The **Schwachman-Diamond syndrome,** first described in 1964, represents the second most common cause of pancreatic insufficiency. The main features presented are pancreatic insufficiency, cyclic neutropenia, metaphyseal dysostosis, and growth retardation. Associated manifestations include dental abnormalities, renal dysfunction, hepatomegaly, abnormal lung function, delayed puberty, and ichthyosis. The estimated incidence is 1 in 10,000 to 20,000 live births, with no sex predominance; the suggested mode of inheritance is autosomal recessive (Gaskin, 1996; Lerner, 1996).

Stunted growth was seen as the most prevalent clinical feature in Schwachman-Diamond syndrome. This is related to metaphyseal dysphasia of the long bone. There is a noted delay in the growth spurt of preadolescence, which resolves during puberty. These patients are usually below the 3rd percentile for height, but linear growth is maintained. As adults, rarely do they reach above the 25th percentile for height (Gaskin, 1996). Another clinical feature is malabsorption, which is manifested during infancy with steatorrhea. Stools are greasy, pale, and foul smelling. A negative sweat test excludes cystic fibrosis. The diagnosis is confirmed by performing a pancreozymin/secretin stimulation test, which results in a very low or absent pancreatic zymogen enzyme or an elevation in stool fat content. An increased stool fat excretion or pancreozymin/secretin stimulation test that reveals very low or nonexistent pancreatic zymogen enzymes confirms the diagnosis (Gaskin, 1996; Lerner, 1996). Patients with steatorrhea have less than 1% of normal colipase and less than 2% of normal lipase secretion. Patients without steatorrhea have diminished lipase activity that is more than 10% of normal. In contrast to cystic fibrosis, the volume and bicarbonate content of the stimulated pancreatic fluid are usually normal, as is its viscosity. In some patients, spontaneous improvement occurs with disappearance of steatorrhea, whereas in others, steatorrhea persists into adulthood (Gaskin, 1996; Lerner, 1996).

There are clearly significant hematological changes noted in patients with Schwachman-Diamond syndrome. Neutro-

penia, thrombocytopenia, and anemia are present in 95%, 70%, and 50% of patients, respectively. These hematological changes make the patient susceptible to infection and bleeding tendencies. Blood counts are performed twice weekly for 3 weeks as a confirmation of diagnosis.

Malnutrition and growth failure are the result of pancreatic insufficiency. The patients are susceptible to bacterial infections and predisposed to orthopedic complications. They are at risk for aplastic anemia and leukemia, which contribute further to their morbidity and mortality. There is a prevalent association of pancreatic insufficiency with hematopoietic manifestations and leukemia.

The treatment of Schwachman-Diamond syndrome at this time is primarily symptomatic and supportive. Pancreatic enzyme replacement is often the treatment of choice for patients with pancreatic insufficiency. Fat-soluble vitamins may be needed as a replacement because of severe malabsorption. Because the increased susceptibility to infections is an obvious concern, antibiotic therapy must be considered. The patient's orthopedic and hematological needs are monitored and treated as necessary.

Acute pancreatitis in children

Acute pancreatitis is the same acute inflammatory process of the pancreas as in adults with the same risks for complications. The difference, however, is the incidence of different etiologies. Acute pancreatitis is not a common cause of abdominal pain in the pediatric population and presents a challenge in this age group (Lerner, 1996). Biliary tract disease and alcohol abuse account for 60% to 80% of acute pancreatitis in the adult population but alcohol is rarely heard or seen as a cause in the pediatric age group (Robertson, 1996). The three leading causes of acute pancreatitis in children are trauma (accidental and non-accidental), drugs, and viral infections with a long list of rarer causes (Lerner, 1996):

Often the symptoms of acute pancreatitis will mimic other emergency situations. A mild disease might be confused with gastritis, whereas severe disease may be presented as small bowel obstruction or perforation. The patient may have midepigastric tenderness and/or pain with a sudden onset, increasing gradually and changing in severity. This adds to the challenges in diagnosis. A careful history of possible trauma, exposure to viral infection, or drug ingestion must be obtained. Any family history of metabolic or other conditions associated with pancreatitis should be investigated.

The most frequently used diagnostic tools are serum and urinary amylase and abdominal ultrasonography (Robertson, 1996). CT scan of the abdomen is more sensitive for diagnosis of acute pancreatitis compared to abdominal ultrasound. However, children with recurring episodes of pancreatitis should undergo ERCP to assess for congenital anomalies such as pancreas divisum, sphincter of Oddi dysfunction, and microlithiasis as in the adult population. It is important to note that although serum amylase is the most frequently used diagnostic tool, normal serum amylase can be seen in patients with severe pancreatitis.

CASE HISTORY

A 55-year-old female went to her doctor because of severe epigastric pain. For three days she had endured the pain, along with nausea and vomiting, thinking she had "stomach flu." Her doctor noted that she was dehydrated and put her in the hospital for a further workup. He suspects she has acute pancreatitis.

Points to think about

1. In making a nursing assessment, what questions might the gastroenterology nurse ask the patient about her pain to support the physician's tentative diagnosis of acute pancreatitis?
2. Mrs. Jones is scheduled for an ultrasonogram and a CT scan. What might be found on these tests?
3. Under what circumstances might the nurse expect to do an ERCP on this patient?
4. What nursing interventions would be appropriate for the desired outcome "this patient will have no increase in pain or fever after the ERCP"?
5. What can the nurse teach this patient to help her avoid future attacks of acute pancreatitis?

Suggested responses

1. In performing a nursing assessment, the gastroenterology nurse might ask this patient the following questions about her epigastric pain:
   (a) "How long have you had the pain? Can you describe it?" Onset, duration, and character of pain is always an important factor. The pain of pancreatitis can be gradual or sudden and usually becomes severe, constant, and boring.
   (b) "Can you point to where the pain is?" Pancreatic pain usually localizes in the left epigastric area and often radiates to the back and left shoulder. The pancreas is located in the left epigastric area and lies posterior to the stomach, which accounts for radiation of pain to the back and left shoulder.
   (c) "Does it hurt to touch there?" The inflamed pancreas is often tender to palpation.
   (d) "Does the pain come and go or is it there all the time; do you notice that it is worse at certain times?" Pain is usually constant and is worse several hours after eating a large meal or ingesting alcohol.
   (e) "Is the pain better after you vomit?" Vomiting does not relieve the pain of pancreatitis as it might for patients with intestinal obstruction.
   (f) "Is there anything you do that helps relieve the pain?" Patients with pancreatitis often assume a characteristic position of bending over at the torso with hands over the left epigastric area.
2. Most of the time, pancreatitis in women of this age-group is a result of gallstones. The second leading cause of pancreatitis is alcohol abuse. You might expect the following findings when Mrs. Jones undergoes ultrasonography

and CT scan:
   (a) Ultrasonography would be a first-line test for cholelithiasis. It may also identify pseudocysts, abscesses, common duct dilatation, and calcifications.
   (b) CT scan may further define and evaluate the above findings and may also evaluate the architecture of the liver, biliary tree, and pancreas.
3. At present the only indication for ERCP in acute pancreatitis is relief of gallstone-related pancreatitis in selected patients with severe indicators or evidence of concomitant biliary obstruction. In such cases, a sphincterotomy may be done to drain the common bile duct and remove any stones that may be causing an obstruction. This allows drainage of the pancreatic duct to resume, and pancreatitis will usually subside uneventfully.

   In patients who have had two or more attacks of acute pancreatitis, ERCP should be considered when looking for potentially correctable lesions, such as stones (biliary and pancreatic), strictures, obstructions of the main duct (benign and malignant) or pseudocysts.
4. To ensure that this patient will have no increase in pain or fever after ERCP, appropriate nursing interventions might include:
   (a) Be aware of the increased risk of causing pancreatitis after ERCP;
   (b) Watch the x-ray monitor while injecting contrast to confirm cannulation of the pancreatic duct;
   (c) Slowly and carefully inject the minimal amount of dye, taking care not to produce acinar filling of the pancreas;
   (d) Use sterile accessory equipment; and
   (e) Instruct the patient to report any chills, fever, or increase in pain.
5. To avoid future attacks of pancreatitis, this patient should be instructed to adhere to the following instructions:
   (a) Avoid alcohol completely until an etiology is established;
   (b) Follow a diet that is low in fat and avoid large meals;
   (c) Avoid drugs that are known to cause pancreatitis, including estrogens, birth control pills, tetracycline, furosemide, thiazide diuretics, azathioprine, and sulfonamides; and
   (d) Be reassured that if a cause can be found, future attacks may be eliminated by its treatment.

REVIEW TERMS

acinus, alpha cells, annular pancreas, beta cells, cholecystokinin-pancreozymin (CCK-PZ), cystic fibrosis, delta cells, duct of Santorini, duct of Wirsung, ERCP, endoscopic sphincterotomy, endoscopic stents, infected necrosis, interstitial pancreatitis, islets of Langerhans, multiple organ dysfunction syndrome, necrotizing pancreatitis, organized necrosis, pancreas, pancreas divisum, pancreatic exocrine insufficiency, pancreatic fistulas, pancreatic rest, pancreatitis, pseudocyst, Schwachman-Diamond syndrome, secretin, Zollinger-Ellison syndrome (ZES).

REVIEW QUESTIONS

1. The majority of the pancreatic tissue is made up of:
   (a) Acinar cells.
   (b) Alpha cells.
   (c) Beta cells.
   (d) Delta cells.
2. The endocrine cells of the pancreas are located in the:
   (a) Crypts of Lieberkühn.
   (b) Islets of Langerhans.
   (c) Duct of Wirsung.
   (d) Pancreatic lobules.
3. The beta cells secrete:
   (a) Somatostatin.
   (b) Glucagon.
   (c) Vasoactive intestinal peptide.
   (d) Insulin.
4. The cephalic phase of pancreatic secretion is stimulated by:
   (a) Gastric distention.
   (b) The sight and smell of food.
   (c) The presence of acidic chyme in the small intestine.
   (d) The presence of alkaline chyme in the small intestine.
5. The most severe form of pancreatitis is:
   (a) Chronic pancreatitis.
   (b) Necrotizing pancreatitis.
   (c) Interstitial pancreatitis.
   (d) Alcoholic pancreatitis.
6. A sac-like structure that is filled with pancreatic fluid six weeks after an attack of pancreatitis is called a:
   (a) Pancreatic rest.
   (b) Pancreas divisum.
   (c) Annular pancreas.
   (d) Pseudocyst.
7. The most specific test for pancreatic cancer is:
   (a) ERCP.
   (b) PTC.
   (c) Ultrasound.
   (d) Plain x-rays.
8. Zollinger-Ellison syndrome often results in what clinical manifestation?
   (a) Peptic ulcer disease.
   (b) Steatorrhea.
   (c) Necrolytic migratory erythema.
   (d) Pancreatic cholera syndrome.
9. The preferred treatment for most islet cell tumors is:
   (a) Supportive and palliative measures only.
   (b) Radiotherapy.
   (c) Chemotherapy.
   (d) Surgical excision.
10. The definitive diagnostic test for cystic fibrosis is the:
   (a) Sweat electrolyte test.
   (b) Schilling test.
   (c) Bernstein test.
   (d) Serum amylase and lipase level.

11. The most common cause of pancreatic insufficiency in children is:
   (a) Malabsorption.
   (b) Steatorrhea.
   (c) Maldigestion.
   (d) Cystic fibrosis.
12. The most prevalent clinical feature of Schwachman-Diamond syndrome is:
   (a) Stunted growth.
   (b) Jaundice.
   (c) Pigmented retinopathy.
   (d) Edematous extremities.
13. The three leading causes of acute pancreatitis in children are:
   (a) Malabsorption, steatorrhea, and maldigestion.
   (b) High-fat diet, high potassium level, and high sugar consumption.
   (c) Trauma, drugs, and viral infections.
   (d) Parasitic diseases, immunocompromised state, and congenital defects.
14. Emergency ERCP is indicated in acute gallstone pancreatitis in:
   (a) All patients.
   (b) Patients with stones in the gallbladder on ultrasound.
   (c) Patients classified as mild who have recovered.
   (d) Patients with severe pancreatitis within 72 hours of onset of the attack.
15. A 3 cm diameter cystic lesion in the pancreas found incidentally on CT scan is most likely to be a:
   (a) Pseudocyst.
   (b) Cystic neoplasm.
   (c) Insulinoma.
   (d) Endometrioma.
16. Palliation of biliary obstruction caused by advanced pancreatic cancer is best achieved by:
   (a) Cholecystectomy.
   (b) Whipple operation.
   (c) Enteral Wallstent.
   (d) Biliary stent.
17. Which of the following statements is true about post-ERCP pancreatitis?
   (a) All cases are mild and do not require specific treatment.
   (b) It is worse after therapeutic ERCP compared with diagnostic ERCP.
   (c) Steroids are protective if given the day before.
   (d) The risk is higher in young women with suspected sphincter of Oddi dysfunction.

BIBLIOGRAPHY

American Society of Gastroenterological Endocopists (2000). Endoscopic therapy of chronic pancreatitis. *Gastrointestinal Endoscopy 52,* 843-8.
Bank, S. & Indaram, A. (1999). Causes of acute and recurrent pancreatitis: clinical considerations and clues to diagnosis. *Gastroenterology Clinics of North America 28,* 571-89.
Baron, T.H. & Morgan, D.E. (1999). Acute necrotizing pancreatitis. *New England Journal of Medicine 340,* 1412-1417.

Bone, R. (1996). Cystic fibrosis. In Bennet, J.C., Plum, F. (Eds). *Cecil textbook of medicine* (20th ed.). Philadelphia: W.B. Saunders.

Bongiovanni, G. (Ed.) (1988). *Essentials of clinical gastroenterology* (2nd ed.). New York: McGraw-Hill.

Brewer, J. (1988). The anatomy and physiology of the pancreas. In Trivits, S. (Ed). *SGA Journal Reprints.* Rochester, NY: Society of Gastrointestinal Assistants.

Brugge, W.R., (Ed.) (2002). Cystic Diseases of the Pancreas. *Gastrointestinal Endoscopy Clinics of North America 12,* 1-828.

Carr-Locke, D.L. (1991). Pancreas divisum: the controversy goes on. *Endoscopy 23,* 105-10.

Chobanian, S. & Van Ness, M. (Eds.) (1988). *Manual of clinical problems in gastroenterology.* Boston: Little, Brown.

Chopra, S. & May, R., (Eds.) (1989). *Pathophysiology of gastrointestinal diseases.* Boston: Little, Brown.

Damsgard, C. (1988). Pancreatic disorders: an overview. *SGA J 11,* 117-19.

Davis, P., Drumm, M. & Konstan, M. (1996). Cystic fibrosis. *Am J Resp Crit Care Med 154(5),* 1229-56. American Journal of Respiratory Critical Care Medicine.

DiMagno, E. (1996). Carcinoma of the pancreas. In Bennet, J.C., Plum, F., (Eds.), *Cecil textbook of medicine* (20th ed.). Philadelphia: W.B. Saunders.

Eastwood, G. & Avunduk, C. (1988). *Manual of gastroenterology: diagnosis and therapy.* Boston: Little, Brown.

Gaskin, K.J. (1996). Hereditary disorders of the pancreas. *In Pediatric Gastrointestinal Disease* (2nd ed.). St Louis: Mosby.

Goldberg, K. (Ed.) (1986). *Gastrointestinal problems: Nurse Review Series.* Springhouse, PA: Springhouse.

Haught, J. (1988). Zollinger-Ellison syndrome: an overview. In Trivits, S. (Ed.), *SGA Journal Reprints.* Rochester, NY: Society of Gastrointestinal Assistants.

Jensen, R. (1996). Zollinger-Ellison syndrome. In Bennet, J.C. & Plum, F. (Eds.), *Cecil textbook of medicine* (20th ed.) Philadelphia: W.B. Saunders.

Lankisch, P. (2001). Natural course of chronic pancreatitis. Pancreatology 1, 3-14.

Lankisch, P.G., Banks, P.A. (1998). *Pancreatitis.* New York: Springer-Verlag.

Lerner, A., Branski, D. & Lebenthal, E. (1996). Pancreatic diseases in children. *Pediatr Gastroenterol 3(1),* 125-37. Pediatric Gastroenterology.

Matthews, J., Maher, K., & Cattau, E. Jr. (1990). The role of endoscopic retrograde cholangiopancreatography injection training sessions for the gastroenterology nurse and associate. In Trivits, S. (Ed.) *SGA Journal Reprints II,* Rochester, NY: Society of Gastroenterology Nurses and Associates.

Mills, A. (1989). Pancreatitis: disruption in structure and function. *Gastroenterol Nurs 12,* 63-5.

Palmieri, M. (1988). Pathophysiology of the pancreas. In Trivits, S. (Ed.) *SGA Journal Reprints,* Rochester, NY, Society of Gastrointestinal Assistants.

Robertson, M.A. & Durie, P.R. (1996). Pancreatitis. *Pediatric gastrointestinal disease* (2nd ed.). St. Louis, MO: Mosby.

Rosch Endoscopy paper on 1001 cases of CP

Sharma, V.K. & Howden, C.W. (1999). Meta-analysis of randomized controlled trials of ERCP and endoscopic sphincterotomy for the treatment of acute biliary pancreatitis. *American Journal of Gastroenterology 94,* 3211-4.

Silverman, A. & Roy, C. (1983). *Pediatric clinical gastroenterology* (3rd ed.). St. Louis, MO: Mosby.

Sleisenger, M., Fordtran, J., (Eds.) (2002). *Gastrointestinal disease: pathophysiology, diagnosis, management* (7th ed.). Philadelphia: W.B. Saunders.

Soergel, K. (1996). Pancreatitis. In Bennet, J.C. & Plum, F. (Eds.). *Cecil textbook of medicine* (20th ed.). Philadelphia: W.B. Saunders.

Telford, J., Farrell, J., Saltzman, J., Shields, S., Banks, P., Lichtenstein, D., Johannes, R., Kelsey, P. & Carr-Locke, D.L., (2002). Pancreatic stent placement for duct disruption. *Gastrointestinal Endoscopy 56,* 18-24.

Tham, T.C.K., Lichtenstein, D.R., Vandervoort, J., Wong, R.C.K., Slivka, A., Banks, P.A., Yim, H.B. & Carr-Locke, D.L. (2000, April). Pancreatic Duct Stents for "Obstructive Type" Pain in Pancreatic Malignancy. *The American Journal of Gastroenterology 95,* 956-60.

Toouli, J., Brooke-Smith, M., Bassi, C., Carr-Locke, D.L., Telford, INITIAL, Freeny, P., Imrie, C. & Tandon, R. (2002). Working Party Report from the 2002 World Congresses of Gastroenterology: Guidelines for the Management of Acute Pancreatitis. *Journal of Gastroenterology and Hepatology 17 (Suppl.),* 15-39.

Walker, W. Durie, P.R., Hamilton, J.R., Watkins, J.B., and Walker-Smith. (Eds.) (1996). *Pediatric gastrointestinal disease* (2nd ed.). St. Louis, MO: Mosby.

Waye, J.D., Geenen, J.E., Fleischer, D. (1987). *Techniques in therapeutic endoscopy.* Philadelphia: W.B. Saunders.

Whitcomb, D.C. (2000). Genetic predispositions to acute and chronic pancreatitis. *Medical Clinics of North America 84,* 531-47.

Wong, R.C.K., Carr-Locke, D.L. (1998). Endoscopic stents for palliation in patients with pancreatic cancer. In Reber, E.H. (Ed.), *Pancreatic Cancer.* Totowa, NJ: Humana Press.

Yim, H.B., Jacobson, B.C., Saltzman, J.R., Johannes, R.S., Bounds, B.C., Lee, J.H., Shields, S.J., Ruymann, F.W., Van Dam, J. & Carr-Locke, D.L. (2001). Clinical outcome of the use of enteral stents for palliation of patients with malignant upper GI obstruction. *Gastrointestinal Endoscopy 53,* 329-32.

Young, H.S. (1994). Diseases of the pancreas. *Scientific American 4,* 1-15.

Chapter 19

LIVER

This chapter will acquaint the gastroenterology nurse with the normal anatomy and physiology of the liver and with certain pathological conditions that affect this organ.

Learning objectives

After reviewing the content of this chapter, the gastroenterology nurse should be able to:

1. Describe the normal anatomy of the liver.
2. Explain the normal physiological functions of the liver, including its role in bile formation and secretion, metabolism, vitamin storage, coagulation, and detoxification.
3. Discuss the pathophysiology, diagnosis, and treatment of a number of pathological conditions that affect the liver, including cirrhosis, hepatitis, carcinoma, Wilson's disease, porphyria, and intrahepatic biliary dysplasia.

ANATOMY

The liver is the single largest organ in the body, weighing from 1200 to 1600 g (3 to 4 pounds). It is located in the right upper quadrant of the abdomen, immediately below the diaphragm (see Fig. 13-2). The normal liver extends from the right fifth intercostal space in the midclavicular line down to the right costal margin.

A thick capsule of connective tissue called Glisson's capsule, which contains blood vessels and lymphatics, covers the entire surface of the liver. A layer of serosa covers the capsule.

The liver is divided into a right and a left lobe by the falciform ligament. This ligament also attaches the liver to the abdominal wall and to the diaphragm. The right lobe is six times larger than the left and may be further divided into the right lobe proper, the caudate lobe, and the quadrate lobe. Each lobe is further divided into lobules that are approximately 2 mm high and 1 mm in circumference.

The hepatic lobule is the functioning unit of the liver. Approximately 1 million lobules form the principal mass of the liver parenchyma. Each lobule consists of a hexagonal row of hepatic cells called **hepatocytes.** The hepatocytes secrete bile into the bile canaliculi and also perform a number of metabolic functions. In the surrounding connective tissue, each lobule has a hepatic artery, a portal vein, and a bile duct, which are known collectively as the **portal triad.**

Between each row of cells are intralobular cavities called **sinusoids.** Each sinusoid is lined with **Kupffer cells,** which are phagocytic cells that belong to the reticuloendothelial system. The Kupffer cells remove amino acids, nutrients, sugars, old erythrocytes, bacteria, and debris from the blood that is flowing through the sinusoids. The main functions of the sinusoids are to destroy old or defective red blood cells, to remove bacteria and foreign particles from the blood, and to detoxify harmful substances.

As much as 1500 ml of blood enters the liver each minute, making the liver one of the most vascular organs in the body (Fig. 19-1). The portal vein supplies about 75% of this blood, bringing in about 50% of the oxygen supply to the liver and bringing in nutrients that are absorbed from the GI system. The hepatic artery supplies the other 25% of the blood flow and supplies the other 50% of the oxygen to the liver.

Liver cells have the ability to regenerate themselves within 3 weeks. Normal liver function can be restored within 4 months in conditions that do not lead to progressive damage to the liver. It is possible for the liver to function even with damage to 90% of its mass, but liver removal or total destruction leads to death within about 10 hours.

Blood leaves the sinusoids by entering the central lobule vein. It then enters the hepatic veins and follows the normal venous circuit into the inferior vena cava.

Nerve fibers to the liver come from the vagus nerve and the thoracolumbar system. Sympathetic nervous stimulation may cause hepatic artery and portal vein vasoconstriction and a dull pain over the area of the liver. Bile ducts receive sensory nerves, as well as sympathetic and parasympathetic innervation.

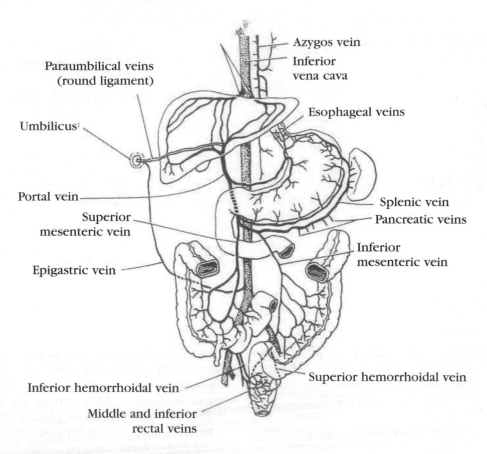

Fig. 19-1. Hepatic portal system. Blood is carried from the stomach, intestines, spleen, and pancreas into the liver sinusoids. Hepatic veins convey it to the inferior vena cava. Clinically significant sites of anastomosis between the hepatic and systemic circulations are (1) the esophageal veins (portal tributary), which anastomose with the azygos veins; (2) the paraumbilical veins in the round ligament originate in the left branch of the portal vein and connect with the superficial veins of the anterior abdominal wall (systemic tributaries) in the area of the umbilicus; (3) the superior rectal or hemmorrhoidal veins (portal tributaries), which anastomose with the middle and inferior rectal veins; (4) the portal tributaries to the intestines, pancreas, and liver, which anastomose with the phrenic, renal, and lumbar veins (systemic tributaries not shown). In portal hypertension and chronic liver disease, blood may be backed up in these veins and shunted around the liver through the points of anastomosis. (From Price SA, Wilson, LM: *Pathophysiology: clinical concepts of disease processes*, ed 4, St. Louis, 1992, Mosby.)

PHYSIOLOGY

Following are the major physiological functions of the liver:
  (a) bile formation and secretion;
  (b) metabolism of carbohydrates, proteins, fats, and steroids;
  (c) vitamin storage;
  (d) manufacture of substances necessary for coagulation and anticoagulation; and
  (e) detoxification of foreign and toxic substances.

Bile formation and secretion

The liver synthesizes and transports the bile pigments and bile salts that are necessary for fat digestion. Bile is a combination of water, bile acids, bile pigments, cholesterol, bilirubin, phospholipids, potassium, sodium, and chloride. Primary bile acids are produced from cholesterol. When bile acids are conjugated in the liver, they become bile salts. Bile pigments are formed from the breakdown of erythrocytes by the cells of the reticuloendothelial system. In this process, heme is converted to biliverdin and then to bilirubin, the main bile pigment. The water-insoluble, indirect (unconjugated) bilirubin formed in this manner is released into the blood, where it is bound to albumin. In the hepatocytes, indirect bilirubin is conjugated with glucuronic acid to form water-soluble, direct (conjugated) bilirubin, which is secreted into the bile canaliculi and excreted in bile.

The bile canaliculi branch and combine and eventually form the right and left hepatic ducts, which merge to form the common hepatic duct. As described in Chapter 17, the cystic duct of the gallbladder joins the common hepatic duct to form the common bile duct. The common bile duct then joins the duct of Wirsung at the ampulla of Vater just before entering the duodenum.

Metabolism

Carbohydrate and protein metabolism are important functions of the liver. Specific functions of the liver in carbohydrate metabolism include the following:

(a) converting glucose, fructose, and galactose to glycogen (glycogenesis) for storage in the liver;

(b) breaking down glycogen to glucose (glycogenolysis) to maintain blood glucose levels when there is a decrease in carbohydrate intake; and

(c) synthesizing glucose from noncarbohydrate nutrients (gluconeogenesis) to maintain blood glucose levels (e.g., proteins or fats).

Liver cells also deaminate amino acids to produce ketoacids and ammonia, from which urea is formed and excreted in the urine. In addition, the liver synthesizes about 50 g of new protein daily, including most of the plasma proteins, such as albumin, fibrinogen, transferrin, ceruloplasmin, haptoglobin, and the lipoproteins.

Digested fat is converted in the intestine to triglycerides, cholesterol, phospholipids, and lipoproteins. These substances are then taken up by the liver and hydrolyzed to glycerol and fatty acids, through a process known as ketogenesis.

The liver also metabolizes adrenocortical steroids, glucocorticoids, estrogens, testosterone, progesterones, and aldosterone.

Coagulation

Most of the clotting factors used in the body are produced in the liver, including prothrombin and fibrinogen. The liver also produces the anticoagulant heparin and releases vasopressor substances after hemorrhage.

Detoxification

Detoxification is another unique function of the liver. The hepatocytes attempt to make medications, foreign and toxic substances, and certain endogenous substances more water-soluble so they can be eliminated in the urine or in bile. Mechanisms of detoxification include: reduction; hydrolysis; conjugation; oxidation; excretion in bile; degradation; and storage of certain substances, such as morphine, curare, and strychnine, to be released at a later time into the circulation. In this way, the hepatocytes protect the body from drug-related hepatic injury. The reticuloendothelial system also protects the body by phagocytosis of viruses, bacteria, dyes, and foreign proteins.

Vitamin storage

High concentrations of riboflavin (vitamin B_2) are found in the liver, as are nicotinic acid and pyridoxine. Also found in the liver are small amounts of vitamin C, most of the body's vitamin D stores, vitamin E, and vitamin K. Vitamin E is excreted in bile, which is required for vitamin K absorption. Ninety-five percent of vitamin A stores are also concentrated in the liver.

PATHOPHYSIOLOGY

Some of the pathological conditions that affect the liver are cirrhosis, hepatitis, tumors, Wilson's disease, porphyria, and intrahepatic biliary dysplasia.

GLYCOGEN STORAGE DISEASES

Cirrhosis

Cirrhosis of the liver is associated with the death of liver cells and concomitant fibrosis and regeneration. The process of regeneration alters the normal vasculature, leading to impaired blood flow and ultimately to hepatic insufficiency. One of the key changes is the diversion of blood flow from the hepatic parenchyma. The anatomical hallmarks of this disorder are hepatic parenchymal inflammation and necrosis, nodular regeneration, loss of the centrilobular vein, and formation of new connective tissue (fibrosis).

There are three major etiological types of cirrhosis:

1. Alcoholic cirrhosis, also known as micronodular, portal, or Laennec's cirrhosis, accounts for up to 50% of adult patients with cirrhosis. In these patients the liver becomes enlarged and altered lipid metabolism leads to fatty infiltrates. Prognosis depends largely on the patient's ability to abstain from alcohol and the extent of damage to the liver at the time of diagnosis.

2. Immune-related bile duct injuries, including primary biliary cirrhosis and sclerosing cholangitis, are diseases of uncertain etiology that primarily affect middle-age women. Liver disease in this case is primarily cholestatic, which leads to jaundice, pruritus, steatorrhea, and death from hepatic failure. Fibrosis, ductal cell destruction, and inflammation make the liver enlarged, firm, and green. The disease usually follows a slow, steady downhill course. Primary sclerosing cholangitis is an immune-related disease, commonly associated with inflammatory bowel disease, that injures the large bile ducts and results in cirrhosis and recurrent infection.

3. Postnecrotic cirrhosis is caused by hepatic necrosis and may be related to hepatitis, infection, metabolic liver disease, or exposure to hepatotoxins or industrial chemicals. In patients with this type of cirrhosis, the liver becomes small and distorted.

Cirrhosis may also be classified on the basis of morphology into the following three categories: micronodular cirrhosis, in which regenerative nodules are uniform in size and less than 3 mm in diameter; macronodular cirrhosis, in which the regenerative nodules are variable in size but greater than 3 mm in diameter; or mixed cirrhosis, in which both types of nodules are present in approximately equal proportions.

Signs and symptoms of cirrhosis include weight loss, anorexia, abdominal pain, jaundice, and bruising. Definitive diagnosis requires histological confirmation of altered hepatic architecture, which is obtained at biopsy examination of the liver.

Most well-established cases of cirrhosis are irreversible, but the progress of the disease may be halted by managing its cause and any complications. Prognosis is grave for cirrhotic patients with persistent jaundice, intractable ascites, coagulopathy, bleeding esophageal varices, or hypoalbuminemia. Liver transplantation may be offered to patients with irreversible liver damage.

Child devised a system that is useful when assessing the severity and prognosis of patients with cirrhosis or other forms of chronic liver disease. This system of classification is detailed in Table 19-1.

Table 19.1. Childe's classification of liver failure

Group designation	A	B	C
Serum bilirubin (mg/100/ml)	Below 2.	2.0-3.0	Over 3.0
Serum albumin (g/100 ml)	Over 3.5	3.0-3.5	Under 3.0
Ascites	None	Easily controlled	Poorly controlled
Neurological disorder	None	Minimal	Advanced
Nutrition	Excelent	Good	Poor

Complications of cirrhosis

Complications of cirrhosis may include portal hypertension, varices with GI bleeding, ascites, hepatorenal syndrome, or hepatic encephalopathy. Many of these complications can also be seen with other forms of severe hepatic injury.

In addition, cirrhosis, regardless of cause, is associated with an increased risk of primary hepatocellular carcinoma (PHCC). The mechanism of development of PHCC in patients with cirrhotic livers is unknown, but geographical factors may be important. In South Africa, PHCC is found in more than 30% of cirrhotic livers, whereas in southern California it is found in only 10%.

Portal hypertension

When liver blockage leads to increased portal vein resistance and backflow, portal vein pressure increases. To redirect blood flow and relieve hypertension, collateral circulation channels may develop (Fig. 19-2). Symptoms of **portal hypertension** include splenomegaly, varices, hemorrhoids, and caput medusae (dilated cutaneous veins in the umbilical area). Physical findings may include jaundice; bleeding tendencies; peripheral edema; palmar erythema; fetor hepaticus (a sweet, fetid breath odor); and symptoms of increased estrogen levels, such as spider nevi, altered hair distribution, gynecomastia in men, testicular atrophy, or menstrual disorders.

The best way of assessing portal hypertension in cirrhosis of the liver is to measure the portal vein pressure gradient (PVPG). To measure PVPG it is necessary to do simultaneous invasive procedures that measure both the portal pressure and the pressure in the inferior vena cava.

Portal hypertension may be treated by radiological proce-

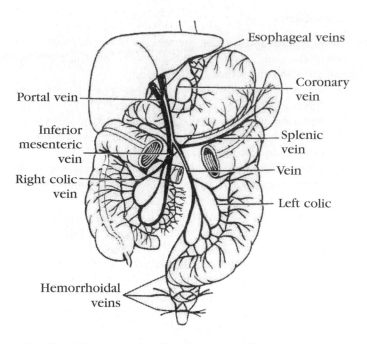

Fig. 19-2. Portal circulation showing collateral circulation.

dures or surgery that diverts blood flow around the liver and away from collateral vessels but allows some blood into the liver. Several types of shunt procedures are available, including the following:

(a) portacaval shunt, the most common shunt procedure, which joins the portal vein and inferior vena cava by using either an end-to-side or side-to-side technique;

(b) splenorenal shunt, which joins the splenic vein and left renal vein by using either an end-to-side or side-to-side technique;

(c) mesocaval shunt, which joins the superior mesenteric vein to the inferior vena cava; and

(d) transjugular intrahepatic portosystemic shunt (TIPS), a vascular radiological procedure that places an expandable wire tube in a created tract between the hepatic veins and the portal veins.

Varices

As blood enters the liver through the portal vein, the connective tissue and liver nodules compressing the blood vessels cause resistance, thereby forcing the blood back into collateral vessels that may be formed in the esophagus, umbilical area, duodenum, abdomen, or rectum, thus producing varices (Fig. 19-3). The diagnosis and treatment of esophageal varices are discussed in Chapter 13.

Ascites

When fibrotic tissue prohibits blood from leaving the liver via the vena cava, the liver begins to expand beyond its normal capacity. When this happens, fluid (mostly plasma) leaks through the surface of the liver into the peritoneal cavity, thus causing an accumulation of serous fluid that is known as **ascites.**

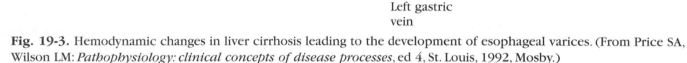

Fig. 19-3. Hemodynamic changes in liver cirrhosis leading to the development of esophageal varices. (From Price SA, Wilson LM: *Pathophysiology: clinical concepts of disease processes*, ed 4, St. Louis, 1992, Mosby.)

In some cases, ascites may be controlled by salt restriction, administration of diuretics, and bed rest. Occasionally, a peritoneojugular venous (LeVeen) shunt is inserted to divert ascitic fluid from the abdominal cavity into the superior vena cava. However, successful use of this procedure requires the patient's cooperation, and complications are not uncommon. Paracentesis is done only to relieve acute respiratory or abdominal distress or for diagnostic purposes.

Hepatorenal syndrome

Hepatorenal syndrome is a progressive, functional form of renal failure that occurs in patients with severe liver disease, in the absence of clinical or anatomical evidence of other causes to explain the degree or persistence of renal failure. Most of these patients have cirrhosis, tense ascites, and encephalopathy. It seems most likely that hepatorenal syndrome starts with subclinical renal dysfunction caused by decreased or unstable perfusion of the kidneys in patients with severe liver disease. There is no evidence of renal parenchymal damage.

Hepatorenal syndrome is characterized by progressive azotemia, urine volume less than normal in ml/kg/day in pediatric patients (or less than 500 ml/day in adult patients), concentrated urine, and urinary sodium concentration less than 10 mEq/L. Urinalysis may show a few hyaline or granular casts, minimal proteinuria, and microscopical hematuria. Hyponatremia, hyperkalemia, hepatic encephalopathy, and coma frequently precede or accompany the renal functional deterioration. Prognosis is very poor, with an associated mortality greater than 90%. Most patients die of hemorrhage, infection, hypotension, or hepatic failure.

Management should include the identification, removal, and treatment of any factors known to precipitate renal fail-

ure. A high-calorie, low-protein, low-sodium diet is advisable. All patients should undergo a trial of fluid challenge using saline with salt-poor albumin or plasma to increase the effective plasma volume. Dialysis may be helpful in patients with reversible forms of liver disease. Liver transplantation will cure hepatorenal syndrome in appropriate candidates.

Hepatic encephalopathy

Hepatic encephalopathy, or the more severe form, hepatic coma, is a major neuropsychiatric complication of chronic liver disease. It is conceivably related to the accumulation of large amounts of ammonia within the brain tissue. Ammonia is normally produced by the breakdown of protein in the bowel, and in healthy individuals it is metabolized by the liver to form urea. In patients with portal hypertension, the blood cannot pass into the liver and the ammonia enters the systemic circulation and flows to the brain.

Symptoms of hepatic encephalopathy usually progress in four stages.

Stage 1. Mild confusion, mood changes, inability to concentrate, sleep disturbances, and mild asterixis (rapid wrist flapping or liver flap).

Stage 2. Confusion, apathy, aberrant behavior, asterixis, and apraxia (loss of ability to carry out familiar, purposeful movements).

Stage 3. Severe confusion, incoherence, diminished responsiveness to verbal stimuli, hyperactive deep-tendon reflexes.

Stage 4. No reaction to stimuli, no corneal reflex, dilated pupils, flexion or extension posture.

Hepatic encephalopathy is treated by correcting pH and electrolyte disturbances, restricting dietary protein, preventing constipation, and taking measures to prevent GI bleeding, because intestinal blood breakdown also results in ammonia production. Administration of neomycin sulfate (Mycifradin) may decrease the number of bacteria that break down amino acids. Lactulose (Cephulac) may be given to promote ammonia retention and excretion through the intestinal tract.

Hepatitis

Hepatitis is defined as an inflammation of the liver that may be accompanied by parenchymal liver damage. It may be acute or chronic. Signs and symptoms vary depending on etiology. The most prevalent type of hepatitis is viral hepatitis, which may be caused by many different viruses, including Epstein-Barr virus (EBV), cytomegalovirus (CMV), rubella, herpes simplex, varicella, and others. Viral forms of hepatitis include hepatitis A (infectious hepatitis), hepatitis B (serum hepatitis), hepatitis C (parenterally transmitted non-A, non-B hepatitis), hepatitis D (delta hepatitis), and hepatitis E (epidemic or enterically transmitted, non-A, non-B hepatitis); the letter F has not been assigned to a hepatotropic virus at this time; and hepatitis G, a virus that is occasionally associated with elevated liver enzymes, has not been proven to lead to cirrhosis or acute liver failure. In addition to these viral forms, other types of hepatitis include alcoholic hepatitis, drug-induced hepatitis, and autoimmune hepatitis.

Hepatitis A

Hepatitis A virus (HAV) is the most common type of hepatitis. The virus involved is an RNA virus of the enterovirus family. HAV is usually a mild disease and is spread by the fecal-oral route, either through oral-anal sexual practices or by contaminated food, water, or shellfish. Exposed household or sexual contacts should receive prophylactic doses of immune globulin (formerly called ISG or gammaglobulin), which provide passive immunity for 2 to 3 months. Hepatitis A vaccine is now available. This vaccine is indicated for individuals at increased risk for acquiring hepatitis A, including those traveling to foreign countries, day care workers, individuals exposed to hepatitis A, military personnel, persons who live in endemic areas, IV drug users, and persons with high-risk sexual practices.

Most HAV infections, especially those acquired during childhood, are subclinical. Symptomatic patients experience early low-grade fever, fatigue, nausea, anorexia, myalgia, and malaise, followed by dark urine, light stools, and right upper quadrant discomfort. Physical findings include jaundice, tender hepatomegaly and, rarely, splenomegaly.

Most patients with HAV recover uneventfully after a period of rest from strenuous activity. HAV does not progress to chronic hepatitis, although 3% to 5% of patients with HAV infections develop a protracted cholestatic hepatitis characterized by elevated alkaline phosphatase and jaundice. In certain high-risk patients, particularly those over 60 years of age, fulminant hepatic failure is possible, but rare.

Hepatitis B

The hepatitis B virus (HBV) is a DNA virus that consists of an inner core and a surrounding envelope. It is transmitted via blood but can also be transmitted by semen or saliva. A major route of transmission is through perinatal infection ("horizontal transmission") of infants born to women who are carriers of the virus ("vertical transmission").

The serological tests that are currently used to diagnose, evaluate, and treat patients with HBV infection include hepatitis B surface antigen (HBsAg), hepatitis B surface antibody (anti-HBs), hepatitis B core antibody (anti-HBc), hepatitis B e antigen (HBeAg), hepatitis B e antibody (anti-HBe), and hepatitis B DNA. A decrease in serum levels of HBV DNA and the conversion from HBeAg to anti-HBe are the initial events in the process of natural or therapeutic viral clearance. These changes signal the decline in HBV replication and precede viral clearance. HBV is a DNA virus that utilizes a polymerase enzyme (reverse transcriptase) to undergo viral replication. HBV DNA polymerase (HBV DNAp), which can also be measured in blood, is able to use both RNA and DNA as a template for DNA synthesis. A test for DNAp was originally used as a marker of HBV replication but has been replaced by the direct measurement of HBV DNA.

Fortunately, protection against hepatitis B is available in the form of immunization. The American Academy of Pediatrics now recommends that *all* infants receive immunization for hepatitis B shortly after birth. The immunization is then repeated at 1 and 6 months of age. Infants born to mothers who test positive for HBsAg should also receive hepatitis B immune globulin (HBIG) within 12 hours of birth. Children and adolescents who have not been vaccinated against hepatitis B in infancy should begin the series at any time during childhood. Adults who are at risk for hepatitis B should receive the vaccine. At-risk populations include healthcare workers, hemodialysis patients, homosexual men, those who use illicit IV drugs, household or sexual contacts of HBV carriers, refugees from endemic areas, and prison inmates. The duration of active immunity from the vaccine is unknown but is thought to be at least 15 years.

In uncomplicated cases, hepatitis B begins with a prodrome; followed by a period of jaundice, which may last from 1 week to 1 month; and then a period of recovery. Common symptoms include dark urine, pale stools, malaise, nausea, fever, headache, anorexia, vomiting, and abdominal pain. Physical signs include jaundice and hepatomegaly with some tenderness. Some patients exhibit splenomegaly, diffuse adenopathy, and/or a maculopapular rash. Diagnosis is usually by finding HBsAg in serum.

Ninety-five percent of adults who acquire HBV recover uneventfully. Treatment entails 1 to 2 weeks of rest from strenuous physical activity. In-hospital management may be required for elderly patients and for patients who develop ascites or encephalopathy. In-hospital treatment should include a nutritionally balanced diet, IV hydration and electrolyte management if necessary, and in some cases, subcutaneous vitamin K and fresh frozen plasma. Medications should be used sparingly, and alcohol should be avoided. Liver transplantation may be an option, although the risk of damage to the transplanted organ (from the hepatitis B virus) is high.

Complications of HBV may include chronic hepatitis, which develops in about 10% of HBV patients, and fulminant hepatic failure, which occurs in only 0.1% of these patients and usually leads to death. By definition, chronic hepatitis is an inflammatory reaction of the liver that lasts for more than 6 months. Chronic hepatitis may manifest itself in several different ways.

1. Mild hepatitis has a protracted course. Cirrhosis is rare in patients with mild hepatitis, but the incidence of hepatocellular carcinoma is increased after the age of 50 years. Symptoms are usually mild, if any. No therapy is needed, and prognosis is generally good.

2. Up to 3% of patients with HBV progress to moderate to severe hepatitis. Compared to mild hepatitis, moderate to severe hepatitis is associated with higher levels of serum transaminases, along with mild hyperbilirubinemia and more severe portal and periportal inflammation with erosion of the limiting plate of peripheral hepatocytes (piecemeal necrosis). In more severe cases, necrosis may span the lobules (bridging necrosis) or multilobular collapse may be seen, thus starting a progressive process that leads to fibrosis, scar formation, and cirrhosis.

The goals of treatment of HBV infection include decreasing serum HBV DNA levels in the blood; lessening infectivity; decreasing the level of hepatic inflammation; and preventing or slowing the development of cirrhosis, liver failure, and liver cancer. The ultimate goal in the treatment of HBV infection is the clearance of HBV from the liver and from sites of extrahepatic infection. This treatment process is completed when the patient clears HBsAg and develops detectable anti-HBs. Only a few medical therapies have been found that are effective in decreasing the level of HBV replication or that result in the clearance of HBV from the blood or liver. There is no documentation that any antiviral therapy against HBV leads to the prevention of cirrhosis, liver failure, or liver cancer. Compounding problems in the development of effective therapy of HBV infection include the presence of mutant forms of HBV, an altered immune system in immunosuppressed patients, consumption of alcohol, and coinfection with other viruses.

Interferon is used for patients with HBV infection and is usually administered to patients with measurable HBV DNA levels and ongoing inflammation. About 30% to 40% of patients clear HBV DNA and HBsAg and are cured of the HBV infection.

Fulminant hepatic failure is defined as massive liver cell death within 2 months of the development of hepatitis. Other causes include poisoning or metabolic diseases. Patients with fulminant hepatic failure are confused, somnolent, or comatose and usually have ascites, edema, coagulopathy, and a shrinking liver. Death occurs in 80% of these patients as a result of GI bleeding, sepsis, brainstem compression from cerebral edema, or multisystem failure. There is only one therapy for fulminant hepatic failure: liver transplantation. The high mortality rate can be decreased with continuous supportive therapy administered in an intensive care unit without transplantation.

Hepatitis C

With the development of tests for the diagnosis of hepatitis A and B, and subsequently hepatitis C virus (HCV), the incidence and natural history of HCV (formerly called non-A, non-B hepatitis) has been defined. The discovery of HCV took place utilizing advanced molecular biological techniques such as the polymerase chain reaction (PCR). The subsequent development of antibody tests and the sequencing of HCV RNA allowed the detailed descriptions of the epidemiology, transmission, and treatment of HCV to be published. The presence of antibody to HCV, implicating HCV infection, was found in over 90% of patients with non-A, non-B hepatitis. The leading causes of transmission include IV drug use, blood transfusions, and other blood and blood-product exposure. Sexual, family, and mother-to-infant transmission is rare. Once infection with HCV occurs, the rate of chronicity exceeds 90%. More than 150,000 people are infected with HCV each year in the United States, and approximately 20% of these patients are at risk of developing cirrhosis. The current estimated prevalence of HCV is 2% of the U.S. population, with a larger variation in prevalence worldwide.

Hepatitis C is also associated with extrahepatic disease. The most important of these is cryoglobulinemia. This immune-related disease can cause kidney failure and a rash on the lower legs. Alcohol increases the risk of developing cirrhosis and accelerates the time to cirrhosis. Patients who have HCV infection and cirrhosis are at a markedly increased risk of developing liver cancer.

The only current Food and Drug Administration (FDA)-approved interferons for chronic HCV infection are interferon alfa-2b (Schering, Kenilworth, NJ) and alfa-2a (Roferon; Roche, Nutley, NJ). These recombinant interferons are produced in *Escherichia coli* and have the same sequence as naturally occurring human interferon alpha. Ribavirin, an agent that does not inhibit HCV replication alone, appears to enhance interferon effects and may be approved for combined treatment for chronic HCV infection. The evaluation and treatment of patients acutely infected with HCV is still controversial, although most hepatologists would probably do advanced testing for HCV infection early in the course of disease and offer treatment with interferon if infection is discovered. The risk of HCV after a needlestick injury is only about 3%. Healthcare workers do not appear to be at increased risk of HCV infection compared to the "normal population."

Interferon directly inhibits viral replication, decreases fibrosis, lowers inflammatory activity, and activates the immune system to aid in clearance of HCV from infected hepatocytes. Twelve to twenty percent of patients clear HCV RNA from blood and liver tissue long-term after completing 6 months of therapy at 3 million units three times a week with subcutaneous injection. Longer treatment intervals may allow a higher initial rate of viral clearance and a longer period of sustained remission and are now the standard of care. The exact group of patients who would benefit the most from interferon therapy remains controversial, although the recent National Institutes of Health consensus conference clearly identified that patients with evidence of progressive liver disease by liver biopsy should be offered treatment.

Hepatitis D

The delta agent, hepatitis D virus (HDV), is a simple parasite, a single stranded RNA virus without enzymes or protein coat, that preys on the hepatitis B virus. HDV is endemic in Italy and other Mediterranean countries and several regions of South America. In nonendemic areas, such as North America and northern Europe, HDV is transmitted primarily by serum and is found primarily in polytransfused children, homosexual men, and IV drug users.

Delta infections can occur only in patients with HBV infection, as either a coinfection or a superinfection. As a coinfection, the HBV is usually eliminated and chronic hepatitis does not ensue. Superinfection with HDV, however, often leads to rapidly progressive liver damage and a more serious prognosis. In general, HDV tends to increase the virulence and severity of HBV infection. The only promising therapeutic approach in chronic hepatitis D has been the use of α-interferon, which has been beneficial in approximately 50% of treated patients.

Hepatitis E

Hepatitis E is an epidemic or enterically transmitted form of viral hepatitis that was first identified in early 1988. It is transmitted by fecal-oral contact or contaminated food and water and is most prevalent in regions with poor sanitation systems. In India, hepatitis E is the leading cause of acute viral hepatitis in young and middle-age adults. The incubation period is 6 to 8 weeks.

Alcoholic hepatitis

Biopsy of the liver in patients with a history of alcoholism may show scattered fatty deposition, hepatocyte degeneration and necrosis, pericellular fibrosis and inflammation, cholestasis, and cirrhosis. Hepatitis is considered a precirrhotic lesion.

Symptoms of alcoholic hepatitis include right upper quadrant abdominal pain, fever, vomiting, anorexia, and dark urine. Unlike other forms of hepatitis, patients do not present with jaundice. Physical signs include an enlarged and tender liver, splenomegaly, signs of chronic alcohol abuse and cirrhosis, and mental status abnormalities.

Treatment is based on supportive care, identification and correction of metabolic abnormalities, and avoidance of factors that are known to worsen hepatic function. It is reversible with abstinence from alcohol.

Drug-induced hepatitis

Drugs can cause a wide range of hepatic injuries, including the following:
(a) A predictable dose-related hepatotoxic reaction, such as that produced by acetaminophen (Tylenol), carbon tetrachloride, and methotrexate;
(b) An unpredictable, non-dose-related viral-like hepatitis, with or without cholestasis, which is produced by such drugs as isoniazid, flurazepam, methyldopa, and IV tetracycline (Achromycin); and
(c) Cholestasis, related to the use of anabolic steroids, birth control pills, and haloperidol (Haldol).

The clinical presentation ranges from asymptomatic persons with transaminase elevations to patients who develop fulminant hepatic failure. Most patients recover within 1 to 2 weeks of discontinuing the offending agent.

Patients who ingest massive doses of acetaminophen (Tylenol) are at risk for fulminant hepatic failure. Appropriate therapy must be instituted within 24 hours of ingestion, including ipecac-induced emesis and administration of *N*-acetylcysteine in a loading dose, followed by maintenance doses until plasma acetaminophen falls below hepatotoxic levels.

Autoimmune hepatitis

Patients with autoimmune chronic active hepatitis (CAH) demonstrate a significant T-cell reactivity to autologous liver antigens. Before the advent of corticosteroid therapy, 80% of patients with autoimmune CAH died of rapidly progressive liver disease within 3 years of diagnosis. Now, patients with autoimmune CAH are treated with daily doses of prednisone or prednisolone (Hydeltrasol), which are gradually reduced and finally withdrawn altogether, and azathioprine (Imuran), which is commonly reduced to low levels. Eighty percent of patients with autoimmune CAH will need these medications for periods of up to 1 to 2 decades. Prognosis is generally favorable with treatment, and patients may pursue a nearly normal lifestyle, although frequent relapses are possible.

Non-alcoholic steatohepatitis

Non-alcoholic steatohepatitis (NASH) is not caused by alcohol consumption but does carry a worse prognosis than steatosis. NASH can progress to cirrhosis and is only diagnosed by liver biopsy. Common causes of NASH are obesity and diabetes mellitus, but NASH can occur in patients without these conditions. Treatment is to remove the cause of the fatty infiltration of the liver and remove exposure to factors that may worsen the condition. These include weight loss (even if slightly overweight), control of blood sugar level, low fat diet, aerobic exercise and strict limit or avoidance of alcohol. NASH can develop into cirrhosis without reducing the cause.

Tumors

Most benign liver tumors are hemangiomas that consist of blood vessels. Diagnosis is by ultrasonography, CT scan, or arteriography. Treatment for very large tumors involves tumor excision to reduce the risk of tumor rupture and hemorrhage. Most patients with hemangiomas are asymptomatic and rarely require any form of therapy.

Primary cancerous liver tumors originate in either the hepatocytes or bile duct cells. Predisposing factors include a history of cirrhosis, hepatitis B, hepatitis C, alcohol, androgen therapy, and exposure to hepatotoxic chemicals. Metastasis is generally to the regional lymph nodes, lungs, and peritoneum. Metastatic or secondary liver tumors are far more common than primary liver tumors, often spreading from the lungs, breasts, GI tract, thyroid, prostate, or skin.

Most patients with liver cancer are asymptomatic until the disease is well advanced. Presenting complaints include right upper quadrant pain, weight loss, and weakness. Physical signs include an enlarged and tender liver and a bruit, or friction rub over the liver. Screening of individuals in high-risk groups for liver cancer using ultrasound and serum levels of α-fetoprotein (AFP) is essential to find small tumors and apply curative procedures such as liver transplantation.

Diagnosis is by scans, angiography, and needle biopsy examination. Large elevations in serum AFP are virtually diagnostic for primary hepatocellular carcinoma. Prognosis is grim if the patient has a large tumor or has evidence of metastatic disease. For patients with a localized mass without lymph node, bile duct, or blood vessel involvement or distal metastases, up to 80% of the liver may be resected. Pain may be relieved with chemotherapeutic liver perfusion via the hepatic artery. Ligation or occlusion of the hepatic artery may temporarily slow cell growth and activity.

If the tumor obstructs the bile duct, endoscopic or transhepatic insertion of a biliary decompression catheter or stent may provide some relief.

Wilson's disease

Wilson's disease is a rare autosomal-recessive disorder that is characterized by defective excretion of copper into bile, thus leading to excessive amounts of copper accumulating in the brain, liver, kidneys, and cornea. This accumulation of copper causes tissue necrosis, hepatic disease, and potential hepatic failure. Fifty percent of all patients have symptoms before the age of 15.

Patients with Wilson's disease have a characteristic rusty brown ring of pigment, called a Kayser-Fleischer ring, around the periphery of the cornea. Kayser-Fleischer rings may be accompanied by neurological signs, such as prominent dysarthria, dystonia, and ataxia; emotional change; tremors; and/or seizures. Hepatic involvement may be minor or may be manifested by acute or chronic hepatitis, sometimes progressing to cirrhosis.

Once the diagnosis is confirmed, all family members should be screened for the disease. Treatment of Wilson's disease involves lifelong therapy with D-penicillamine (Cuprimine). Therapy has been most successful in precirrhotic asymptomatic siblings. Without treatment, patients invariably succumb to liver disease or neurological complications.

Porphyria

Porphyria is defined as a hereditary or acquired enzyme defect in which the biosynthesis of heme, in either the bone marrow or liver, leads to an overproduction of porphyrins or their precursors. Porphyrias are classified as either erythropoietic, hepatic, or erythrohepatic. The four hepatic porphyrias are listed as follows:

(a) acute intermittent porphyria;
(b) hereditary coproporphyria, which is characterized by large amounts of coproporphyrin III in the feces and lesser amounts in the urine;
(c) variegate porphyria, which is characterized by large amounts of protoporphyrin in the feces, with smaller amounts of coproporphyrin in the feces and urine; and
(d) porphyria cutanea tarda (PCT), which is the most common form of hepatic porphyria and is characterized by chronic skin lesions with fragility, blistering, poor healing, and scar formation, especially on light-exposed skin; increased hair growth, especially on the face; and mild liver disease with fatty infiltration, focal necrosis, or hepatic siderosis.

The first three hepatic porphyrias are similar clinically, with acute attacks of abdominal pain, peripheral neuropathy, and psychiatric symptoms. Attacks may be precipitated by drugs, alcohol, fasting, or infection. Inheritance is autosomal dominant. Urinary porphobilinogen and δ-aminolevulinic acid are elevated in acute attacks and can be measured using the Watson-Schwartz test. Treatment consists of IV glucose and/or hematin and supportive care with avoidance of precipitating factors.

PCT may be hereditary or acquired. Acquired PCT may be associated with alcohol abuse, estrogen, or polychlorinated hydrocarbons. Urinary uroporphyrin and urinary coproporphyrin are elevated. No acute abdominal or neuropsychiatric attacks are apparent.

Protoporphyria is an autosomal-dominant erythrohepatic porphyria that is characterized by solar urticaria, which is burning and tingling on exposure to light, and solar eczema, which is cutaneous thickening on repeated exposure. Liver involvement may progress to fibrosis or cirrhosis. Free erythrocyte protoporphyrin is elevated. Birefringent protoporphyrin pigment deposits are present in hepatocytes, Kupffer cells, and bile canaliculi.

Cholestyramine (Questran) has been used to reduce the protoporphyrin pool and thereby halt the progression of liver disease or even reverse the process. Patients are also treated with β-carotene.

Patients with PCT or protoporphyria should avoid porphyrin-stimulating agents, such as estrogen-containing oral contraceptives, chloroquine (Aralen, an antimalarial amebicidal agent), griseofulvin (Fulvicin, a fungicide), iron compounds, and alcohol.

Hemochromatosis

Hemochromatosis is a recessively inherited disorder of iron metabolism and is characterized by excessive tissue iron deposition. It is the third most common inherited disorder of metabolism in whites, after cystic fibrosis and α1-antitrypsin deficiency.

Hemochromatosis usually occurs in patients who are in middle age. Complaints of weakness, malaise, loss of libido, weight loss, change in skin color, abdominal pain, joint pain, or symptoms related to diabetes mellitus are presenting symptoms. Males are 10 times more likely to be diagnosed with hemochromatosis than females are. Hepatomegaly is found in 95% of symptomatic patients. Skin pigmentation, testicular atrophy, loss of body hair, arthropathy, and congestive heart failure are other prominent physical signs. Hepatocellular carcinoma develops in approximately 30% of symptomatic patients. Although generally not common in infants, if so presented hemochromatosis can lead to the need for a transplant.

In diagnosing hemochromatosis, a high index of suspicion is required. Serum ferritin is usually grossly elevated, and serum iron concentration is usually elevated. Plain x-ray films of the hands may show chondrocalcinosis, sclerosis of subchondral bone, loss of articular cartilage, and subchondral cyst formation. CT scans of the liver show marked increases in density, but needle biopsy examination of the liver is needed to confirm the diagnosis. Biopsy of the liver permits estimation of tissue irons by histochemical staining, chemical analysis of hepatic iron concentration, and histological assessment of liver damage.

All first-generation relatives should be screened for iron overload. The mainstay of therapy is removal of iron from the body by phlebotomy. Phlebotomy should be performed weekly or biweekly for approximately 2 years until hemoglobin, ferritin, and iron levels become normal, at which time the frequency of phlebotomy can be reduced to every 1 to 3 months.

α_1 -Antitrypsin deficiency

With an incidence of approximately 1:2000 live births in the United States, α_1 -antitrypsin (AAT) deficiency is the most common cause of liver disease in children. Fortunately, only 10% to 20% of the babies born with the deficiency will have liver disease. Adults are also affected and may have lung involvement with emphysema, as well as liver disease. The protein AAT is a substance made in the liver and plays an important role in preventing the breakdown of enzymes in various organs of the body. Deficiency of AAT can lead to liver damage with cirrhosis and abnormal liver function. An autosomal-recessive trait, AAT deficiency is inherited from both parents. The most common phenotype is PiMM, which is associated with normal circulating levels of AAT. The homozygous PiZZ phenotype and most likely the heterozygous PiMZ play an important role in the development of this disease. Currently there is no cure for this disease. Treatment is aimed at maintenance of nutrition and early identification of complications. Long-term outcomes vary. Approximately 25% of affected patients will develop cirrhosis and its complications. Liver transplantation may be performed if liver failure develops.

Intrahepatic biliary dysplasia

Intrahepatic biliary dysplasia (IHBD), also known as Alagille syndrome, is a unique, autosomal-dominant liver disease that appears in approximately 1 in 100,000 live births.

It incorporates a combination of anomalies that occur in conjunction with chronic cholestasis. Patients with IHBD display characteristic facial features; vertebral malformations; retarded physical, mental, and sexual development; and various cardiac anomalies, most often peripheral pulmonic stenosis. Liver changes progress from a decrease in the number of portal zones to bile plugging small interlobular bile ducts, hepatocytes, and small canaliculi; absence or decrease in portal bile ducts; and collapsed portal bile ducts.

Children with IHBD frequently have cholestatic jaundice in the neonatal period, often accompanied by failure to thrive, prematurity, or small size for gestational age. The liver is enlarged and firm or hard on palpation. Most infants and children with IHBD are more affected by their cardiac abnormalities than by their liver disease.

Treatment of IHBD involves symptomatic and supportive care, including good nutrition and fat-soluble vitamin supplementation. Cholestyramine (Questran) and phenobarbital may be given to relieve pruritus.

Liver transplantation is considered when cirrhosis and liver failure develop. The overall life expectancy for children with Alagille syndrome is unknown but depends on several factors, including the severity of scarring in the liver, whether heart or lung problems develop, and nutritional status. Many adults with Alagille syndrome lead normal lives.

Biliary atresia

One in 8000 to 1 in 15,000 infants born in the United States are diagnosed with biliary atresia. Biliary atresia is a bile duct disorder that results in rapid and progressive scarring, leading to obstruction of the flow of bile through the extrahepatic bile duct system. On diagnosis of biliary atresia, the Kasai surgical procedure is performed. In approximately 50% of cases the Kasai procedure allows excretion of bile from the liver into the intestine via a duct created from a length of the infant's small intestine. In the remaining 50% of cases, poor response to the procedure often occurs because obstructed bile ducts are both intrahepatic and extrahepatic. No procedure has yet been developed to correct this problem, except for transplantation. The Kasai procedure is often not effective in restoring bile flow for infants over 2 months of age, so early diagnosis of biliary atresia is critical. Unfortunately, despite bile flow, the Kasai procedure is not a cure for biliary atresia. Liver damage often continues, leading to cirrhosis and the need for transplantation. Biliary atresia is the most common indication for liver transplantation in young children.

Neonatal hepatitis

Neonatal hepatitis is inflammation of the liver that occurs only in early infancy, usually between 1 and 2 months of age. About 20% of infants with neonatal hepatitis were infected by a virus that caused the inflammation before or shortly after birth. These viruses include CMV; rubella; and hepatitis A, B, or C and result in the possibility of transmission of the infection to others who come in close contact with the infant. The remaining 80% of cases of neonatal hepatitis have no identifiable virus. Neonatal hepatitis caused by rubella or CMV may lead to mental retardation and cirrhosis. Neonatal hepatitis caused by hepatitis A usually resolves within 6 months, but cases that are the result of the hepatitis B or C viruses will most likely result in chronic liver disease. There is no specific treatment for neonatal hepatitis. Attention to normal nutrition and growth and development is essential to the long-term prognosis. Infants who develop cirrhosis may require liver transplantation.

Gilbert syndrome

Gilbert syndrome is a relatively common and benign congenital (probably hereditary) disorder found more frequently in males. The disorder is characterized by a mild, fluctuating increase in serum bilirubin. It is estimated that from 3% to 7% of the adult population has Gilbert syndrome. There are rarely significant symptoms, but occasionally, jaundice may occur. Except for elevated serum bilirubin, liver tests are normal, as is cholangiography. The diagnosis of Gilbert syndrome is established primarily by documenting the persistence of an increased serum bilirubin when other liver function tests are repeatedly normal. A liver biopsy may occasionally be necessary to rule out other liver diseases. There is no treatment necessary for Gilbert syndrome, and it will not interfere with a normal lifestyle.

Orthotopic liver transplantation

As indicated in the discussion of the various pathological conditions affecting the liver, transplantation may be an option in the treatment of fulminant liver failure and chronic liver disease. Since the enactment by Congress of the National Organ Transplant Act (NOTA) in 1984, the Organ Procurement and Transplantation Network (OPTN) manages and directs the allocation and distribution of lifesaving organs within the United States. The United Network for Organ Sharing (UNOS) is the nonprofit policy-making organization that administers the OPTN. Membership includes transplant centers, organ procurement organizations, transplant recipients, and patients awaiting transplants. After evaluation by the transplant physician, a patient is added to the national UNOS waiting list by the transplant center. Lists are specific to both geographical area and organ type. Each time a donor organ becomes available, a list of potential recipients is generated, based on factors that include genetic similarity, organ size, and medical urgency. Although most liver transplants are performed using organs from cadaver donors, "living related donor" programs have been created at some centers, utilizing a portion of the liver from a living donor for transplant in small children and having nonrelated adult-to-adult transplants

Following transplantation, the organ recipient will require medications that suppress the immune system (e.g., cyclosporin, tacrolimus) for his or her lifetime to prevent rejection of the transplanted organ. The posttransplant patient is monitored closely for organ rejection. Other potential complications include infection, hemorrhage, liver function problems, vascular graft obstruction, graft-versus-host disease, and complications from medications.

CASE SITUATION

Mr. Rudy Stern, age 34, was admitted to the emergency room for GI bleeding. His routine blood work showed a prolonged prothrombin time and elevated transaminase values. A hepatitis screen and an emergency gastroscopy are ordered to determine the cause of his GI bleeding. He has a large-bore nasogastric tube in place, which is draining copious amounts of dark red blood. In the endoscopy room, the gastroenterology nurse sets up equipment for gastric lavage and proceeds to lavage Mr. Stern's stomach until the return is clear enough to begin the endoscopy.

Mr. Stern is found to have a large gastric ulcer with an oozing visible vessel, which the physician cauterizes with a bipolar probe. The bleeding stops and Mr. Stern is moved to the intensive care unit. The next, day, however, he shows signs of rebleeding. He is taken to surgery and a partial gastrectomy is performed.

When Mr. Stern's hepatitis screen comes back, it is positive for HBsAg, anti-HBc, and hepatitis A IgG antibody (IgG-anti-HAV).

Points to think about

1. Before the nurse was able to put on gloves, she had significant contact with Mr. Stern's blood when he vomited before the lavage. Because the nurse had severe dermatitis on her hands, would she have been exposed to HAV or HBV?
2. Healthcare personnel in high-risk areas for HBV (i.e., those personnel who are in frequent contact with blood and body fluids) should be vaccinated against HBV. However, if a nurse has put off this important vaccination, what prophylaxis is available?
3. It is possible the nurse may never have been informed of Mr. Stern's hepatitis and subsequent possible exposure. What symptoms would alert the nurse to HBV infection?
4. The law requires that certain communicable diseases be reported. The nurse should determine who in the institution is responsible for reporting a communicable disease, to whom it should be reported, and what information is required in the report.
5. Although precise data are not available, the prolonged prothrombin time, Mr. Stern's tendency to bleed, and his diagnosis of viral hepatitis would lead the nurse to tentatively consider what nursing diagnosis?
6. What is an appropriate outcome criterion for this diagnosis? What nursing interventions will lead to this outcome?
7. What special infection-control precautions should the nurse take in the endoscopy setting?

Suggested responses

1. The nurse has been exposed to HBV, which is a major nosocomial problem that can have serious sequelae. Finding HBsAg in the blood is diagnostic of HBV infection. HBsAg is first detectable in serum 30 to 60 days after

exposure, during the incubation period. This marker will usually be present in the blood until the end of the acute phase of the illness, or longer. Patients are considered infectious as long as HBsAg is detectable in serum. HBV is transmitted via serum, semen, and saliva. Anti-HBc appears in the blood about the same time as serum transaminase levels rise.

The presence of IgG-anti-HAV is indicative of prior infection with HAV and a naturally acquired immunity. Mr. Stern had HAV in the past and is now immune, so this is not a contagious disease. HAV is transmitted by the fecal-oral route and not in the blood, although dirty needles can serve as a means of transmission.

2. If the nurse has not been vaccinated against HBV, the treatment of choice is HBIG, given within 1 week of exposure for passive immunity. It is recommended that HBV vaccine (Heptavax-B or Recombivax HB) be given in conjunction with the HBIG. The injections are given at different sites. Either HBV vaccine is safe in healthy adults and is given in three serial intramuscular doses of 1.0 ml within 1 week of exposure, 1 month later, and 6 months later.

3. If the nurse has been infected with HBV, the incubation period is 6 weeks to 6 months, with an average of 12 weeks. Symptoms may be relatively mild or quite severe. If symptoms are mild they can mimic a flu-like syndrome. Symptoms may include fatigue, malaise, joint or muscle pain, anorexia, nausea, vomiting, fever and chills, jaundice, clay-colored stools, dark urine, and pruritus. There may be abdominal pain and tenderness in the right upper quadrant. Even though signs and symptoms may be absent during the incubation period, the person with hepatitis is contagious.

4. Ordinarily, the patient's physician is responsible for reporting both HAV and HBV infections to the state health department. The Centers for Disease Control and Prevention (CDC) will include the case in its national statistics.

The gastroenterology nurse should know what diseases are required by law to be reported. Such cases should be reported to the infection-control nurse in the hospital (or a counterpart), and that person can make certain the state health department has been informed. The health department may refer the case to its nursing division for postdischarge follow-up, or the gastroenterology nurse may refer the patient to the visiting nurse service of a local health department, if available. The information to be reported may vary from state to state. Usually a health department will want, at a minimum, the patient's name, age, address, any possible contacts, the diagnosis, and the physician treating the patient.

5. These data would permit the nurse to consider the nursing diagnosis "potential for injury: bleeding, related to altered clotting mechanisms."

6. An appropriate outcome in relation to this nursing diagnosis would be "Mr. Stern will experience a resolution of bleeding episodes." Related nursing interventions would include the following:

(a) administer prescribed drugs;

(b) observe incision and nasogastric drainage every 2 hrs;

(c) take vital signs every hour;

(d) check the IV site for bleeding, proper cannulation, and flow every 2 hours; and

(e) monitor neurological vital signs every 4 hours;

7. Special infection-control practices that should be used by gastroenterology nurses in the endoscopy setting include the following:

(a) Following standard precautions with *all* patients. When there is a potential for coming in contact with the blood or body fluids of any patient, the nurse should wear gloves, protective gowns, masks, and eyewear.

(b) Cleaning and disinfecting equipment following accepted hospital policy (SGNA, 2002).

(c) Using information obtained in the nursing assessment to help identify patients at risk for hepatitis. High-risk patients include those who have recently had procedures using piercing instruments, such as ear piercing, tattooing, acupuncture, dental work, or blood transfusions. HBV is also common among dialysis patients; drug abusers; male homosexuals; AIDS patients; retarded people; and those with Hodgkin's disease, leukemia, or hemophilia.

REVIEW TERMS

α_1-antitrypsin (AAT) deficiency, ascites, cirrhosis, fulminant hepatic failure, hemochromatosis, hepatic encephalopathy, hepatitis, hepatocytes, hepatorenal syndrome, intrahepatic biliary dysplasia (IHBD), Kupffer cells, porphyria, portal hypertension, portal triad, sinusoids, Wilson's disease

REVIEW QUESTIONS

1. In the liver, bile is produced and secreted by:
   (a) Sinusoids.
   (b) Hepatocytes.
   (c) Glisson's capsule.
   (d) Kupffer cells.

2. Seventy-five percent of the blood that flows into the liver is delivered via the:
   (a) Inferior vena cava.
   (b) Hepatic artery.
   (c) Portal vein.
   (d) Splenic artery.

3. In the liver, carbohydrates are metabolized to:
   (a) Glycogen.
   (b) Amino acids.
   (c) Ammonia.
   (d) Glycerol.

4. The primary physiological function of the Kupffer cells is:
   (a) Metabolism.
   (b) Production of prothrombin and fibrinogen.
   (c) Vitamin storage.
   (d) Phagocytosis of harmful substances.

5. A definitive diagnosis of cirrhosis is obtained through:
   (a) Observation of a Kayser-Fleischer ring on the cornea.
   (b) Ultrasonography or CT scan.
   (c) Palpation of the liver.
   (d) Biopsy of the liver.

6. The first line of treatment for ascites is:
   (a) Dietary restrictions, diuretics, and bed rest.
   (b) Shunt placement.
   (c) Paracentesis.
   (d) Liver transplantation.

7. The most common form of chronic hepatitis liver disease is:
   (a) Hepatitis A virus.
   (b) Hepatitis B virus.
   (c) Hepatitis C virus.
   (d) Alcoholic hepatitis.

8. Most patients with HBV are treated with:
   (a) α-Interferon.
   (b) Rest from strenuous physical activity.
   (c) The hepatitis B vaccine.
   (d) IV hydration and electrolyte management.

9. Accumulation of excessive amounts of copper in certain body tissues is characteristic of:
   (a) Alagille syndrome.
   (b) Primary liver cancer.
   (c) Wilson's disease.
   (d) Porphyria.

10. Chronic skin lesions, increased hair growth, mild liver disease, and a lack of neuropsychiatric manifestations are characteristic of:
    (a) Acute intermittent porphyria.
    (b) Hereditary coproporphyria.
    (c) Variegate porphyria.
    (d) Porphyria cutanea tarda.

BIBLIOGRAPHY

Alter, M.J. (1995). Epidemiology of hepatitis C in the West. *Semin Liver Dis 15*, 5-14.

Alter, M.J. (1993). Community acquired viral hepatitis B and C in the United States. *Gut 34 (Suppl. 1)*, S17-S19.

Alter, M.J. (1991). Hepatitis C: a sleeping giant? *Am J Med 91*, 112S-115S.

Alter, M.J. (1990). The hepatitis C virus and its relationship to the clinical spectrum of NANB hepatitis, *J Gastroenterol Hepatol 5(Suppl 1)*, 78-94.

Alter, M.J. (1992). The natural history of community-acquired hepatitis C in the United States: The sentinel counties chronic non-A, non-B hepatitis study team, *N Engl J Med 327*, 1899-1905.

Alter, M.J. (1990). Risk factors for acute non-A, non-B hepatitis in the United States and association with hepatitis C virus infection. *JAMA 264*, 2231-5.

American Academy of Pediatrics. (1997). *Recommended childhood immunization schedule: United States*. (Position Statement 99(1) pp.136-137). Elk Grove Village, Illinois.

Castilla, A. (1993). Lymphoblastoid alpha-interferon for chronic hepatitis C: a randomized controlled study. *Am J Gastroenterol 88*, 233-9.

Choo, Q.L. (1989). Isolation of a cDNA clone derived from a blood-borne non-A, non-B viral hepatitis genome. *Science 244*, 359-62.

Craxi, A. (1994). Third-generation hepatitis C virus tests in asymptomatic anti-HCV-positive blood donors. *J Hepatol 21*, 730-4.

Davis, G.L. (1994). Interferon treatment of chronic hepatitis C. *Am J Med 96*, 41S-46S.

De Medina, M. & Schiff, E.R. (1995). Hepatitis C: diagnostic assays. *Semin Liver Dis 15*, 33-40.

Di Bisceglie, A.M. (1991). Long-term clinical and histopathological follow-up of chronic posttransfusion hepatitis. *Hepatology 14*, 969-74.

Esteban, J.I., Genesca, J. & Alter, H.J. (1992). Hepatitis C: molecular biology, pathogenesis, epidemiology, clinical features, and prevention. *Prog Liver Dis 10*, 253-82.

Fried, M.W. & Hoofnagle, J.H. (1995). Therapy of hepatitis C. *Semin Liver Dis 15*, 82-91.

Garcia-Samaniego, J. (1994). Hepatitis B and C virus infections among African immigrants in Spain. *Am J Gastroenterol 89*, 1918-9.

Han, J.H. (1991). Characterization of the terminal regions of hepatitis C viral RNA: identification of conserved sequences in the 5` untranslated region and poly(A) tails at the 3` end. *Proc Natl Acad Sci USA 88*, 1711-5.

Hino, K. (1994). Genotypes and titers of hepatitis C virus for predicting response to interferon-alfa. *J Med Virol 42*, 299-305.

Kato, N. (1990). Molecular cloning of the human hepatitis C virus genome from Japanese patients with non-A, non-B hepatitis. *Proc Natl Acad Sci USA 87*, 9524-8.

Kobayashi, Y. (1993). Quantitation and typing of serum hepatitis C virus RNA in patients with chronic hepatitis C treated with interferon-beta. *Hepatology 18*, 1319-25.

Konishi, M. (1994). Titration and genotyping of hepatitis C virus RNA in chronic hepatitis C patients treated with interferon. *Nippon Shokakibyo Gakkai Zasshi 91*, 147-53.

Kuo, G. (1989). An assay for circulating antibodies to a major etiologic virus of human non-A, non-B hepatitis. *Science 244*, 362-4.

Mansell, C.J. & Locarnini, S.A. (1995). Epidemiology of hepatitis C in the East. *Semin Liver Dis 15*, 15-32.

Marcellin, P. (1991). Second generation (RIBA) test in diagnosis of chronic hepatitis C. *Lancet 337*, 551-2.

Matsumoto, A. (1994). Viral and host factors that contribute to efficacy of interferon-alpha 2a therapy in patients with chronic hepatitis C. *Dig Dis Sci 39*, 1273-80.

Mattsson, L., Weiland, O. & Glaumann, H. (1988). Long-term follow-up of chronic post-transfusion non-A, non-B hepatitis: clinical and histological outcome. *Liver 8*, 184-8.

Mattsson, L. (1991). Antibodies to recombinant and synthetic peptides derived from the hepatitis C virus genome in long-term-studied patients with posttransfusion hepatitis C. *Scandanavian Journal of Gastroenterol 26*, 1257-62.

Mita, E. (1994). Predicting interferon therapy efficacy from hepatitis C virus genotype and RNA titer. *Dig Dis Sci 39*, 977-82.

Osmond, D.H. (1993). Risk factors for hepatitis C virus seropositivity in heterosexual couples, *JAMA 269*, 361-5.

Price, S.A. & Wilson, L.M. (1992). *Pathophysiology: clinical concepts of disease processes* (4th ed.). St. Louis, MO: Mosby.

Schiff, E.R., Sorrett, M.R. & Maddrey, W.S. (Eds.) (1999). *Schiff's Diseases of the Liver* (8th ed.). Philadelphia: Lippincott-Raven.

Seeff, L.B. (1992). Long-term mortality after transfusion-associated non-A, non-B hepatitis: The National Heart, Lung, and Blood Institute Study Group. *N Engl J Med 327*, 1906-11.

Takahashi, M. (1993). Natural course of chronic hepatitis C. *Am J Gastroenterol 88*, 240-3.

Tremolada, F. (1992). Long-term follow-up of non-A, non-B (type C) post-transfusion hepatitis. *J Hepatol 16*, 273-81.

Tsubota, A. (1994). Factors predictive of response to interferon-alpha therapy in hepatitis C virus infection. *Hepatology 19*, 1088-94.

Tsubota, A. (1993). Factors useful in predicting the response to interferon therapy in chronic hepatitis C. *J Gastroenterol Hepatol 8*, 535-9.

Walker, W. Durie, P.R., Hamilton, J.R., Watkins, J.B., and Walker-Smith. (1996). *Pediatric gastrointestinal disease*. St. Louis, MO: Mosby.

Weiner, A.J. (1991). Variable and hypervariable domains are found in the regions of HCV corresponding to the flavivirus envelope and NS1 proteins and the pestivirus envelope glycoproteins. *Virology 180*, 842-8.

Widell, A. (1991). Hepatitis C virus RNA in blood donor sera detected by the polymerase chain reaction: comparison with supplementary hepatitis C antibody assays. *J Med Virol 35*, 253-8.

Worman, H.J. (1999). *The Liver Disorders Sourcebook*. Chicago: Lowell House 1999.

PHARMACOLOGY, INTRAVENOUS THERAPY, AND NUTRITION

Chapter 20

PHARMACOLOGY

The primary goal of this chapter is to provide the gastroenterology nurse with the critical thinking necessary to effectively use pharmacotherapeutics in the delivery of medications that are commonly used to diagnose and treat GI disorders. It is important that nurses know not only the names, actions and uses of drugs, but that they also can employ effective clinical decision-making when monitoring drug therapy. General information is provided on techniques and routes of drug administration, dosage calculations, patient education, and documentation. The classes of drugs used most often in gastroenterology practice are described in general terms, including indications, contraindications, and possible side effects. An extended table is provided with the generic and trade names of representative medications, including primary use, usual adult and pediatric doses, and common adverse effects.

Learning objectives

After reviewing the content of this chapter, the gastroenterology nurse should be able to:

1. Discuss general aspects of drug therapy that are relevant to nursing practice, including techniques and routes of administration, dosage calculations and conversions, patient education, and documentation.
2. Describe the general classes of medications that are important in gastroenterology, including general indications, contraindications, and potential adverse effects.
3. Identify representative drugs used in gastroenterology practice, their respective generic and trade names, indications, usual adult dosages, and possible side effects.

BASIC PRINCIPLES

Gastroenterology nurses should be able to recognize expected actions of drugs prescribed, be confident that ordered dosages are within the safe range for a particular patient, and have knowledge of possible adverse effects or undesirable drug interactions. If, based on knowledge and experience, nurses have any questions about medication or dosage ordered, or if serious adverse effects are noted, the physician should be consulted immediately. The gastroenterology nurse should be cognizant of the differences in medication administration; dosing; and effects specific to differences in the pediatric, adult, and geriatric patients. The pediatric patient requires frequent review of medication treatment and therapies because of the rapid changes throughout childhood. A child who is ill can experience growth spurts with rapid weight gain or acute weight loss. Geriatric patients present special concerns because they are prone to drug-drug interactions caused by poly- medication regimens for multiple system problems (e.g., heart disease, arthritis). The geriatric patient may have a gradual decline in vision, hearing, and memory loss, making medication compliance difficult. The reduction of renal function is of particular concern for all patients but more so with the aging population and must be considered with all medication interventions and gastroenterology procedures. In addition over-the-counter medications, herbs, and vitamins may affect drug therapy in all age groups.

Patient education

Patient education is another important aspect of drug therapy. The patient and/or the responsible party should understand the purpose of any medication that is ordered. If there is a change in medication or dosage, the patient should be informed. He or she should be instructed, as appropriate, about possible side effects and should be encouraged to report any symptoms that may indicate adverse effects.

Patient education should also encompass drug-diet and drug-drug interaction. Unless gastric irritation is a problem, it is usually best for the patient to take medications on an empty stomach because food can interfere with drug absorption. In addition, most drugs are more efficiently absorbed if taken with 100 to 250 ml of fluid. Smaller amounts of fluid are used for children and should be based on the size of the child. Antacids, on the other hand, should not be taken with water. It is important that the patient be aware of these considerations to maximize the effectiveness of drug therapy.

The issue of drug-drug interactions is another significant and increasingly complex area of concern. Generally speaking, drugs that increase GI motility, such as stimulant cathartics, decrease the rate and extent of absorption of time-released drugs and drugs that require prolonged intestinal contact. Drugs that decrease motility, such as anticholinergics, may alter the absorption of certain drugs. Medications that alter gastric pH, such as antacids, decrease the absorption of some weakly acidic drugs, such as phenobarbital and aspirin. Patients must be cautioned to report all of the prescription and over-the-counter medications they are taking to their physician, and they should be informed of any potentially problematic interactions. They should also be encouraged to report any known drug allergies.

Techniques and routes of administration

Medications may be administered orally, parenterally, or topically. The route of administration is determined by the required speed of onset of the drug's effect, patient comfort and safety considerations, and the organ or system targeted by the drug. Intravenous injections, for example, take effect quickly because they are immediately accessible in the bloodstream, whereas drugs administered by topical routes must be absorbed before they can be effective. However, injections are more uncomfortable for the patient than oral or topical drugs and carry a greater risk of side effects. When the GI system is the target of drug therapy, oral administration may be the most effective.

The **oral** route is the most common route of drug administration. Oral medications may take the form of tablets, capsules, syrups, elixirs, oils, liquids, suspensions, powders, or granules. Most oral medications are swallowed by mouth, but they may also be given through a nasogastric or gastrostomy tube or may be dissolved between the cheek and gum or under the tongue. Nausea, vomiting, inability to swallow, or unconsciousness may contraindicate oral administration of medications.

Parenteral medications are administered by injection, using a subcutaneous (SC), intramuscular (IM), or intravenous (IV) route. SC injections are administered into the adipose tissue (the fatty layer) beneath the skin. The SC route is faster than oral administration but allows slower, more sustained drug action than an IM injection. SC injections also cause minimal tissue trauma and carry little risk of striking large blood vessels and nerves. The most common SC injection sites are the outer aspect of the upper arm, anterior thigh, buttocks, upper back, and loose tissue of the lower abdomen.

IM injections deposit medication deep into muscle tissue, where it can be readily absorbed. Muscles used for IM injections include the deltoids, dorsogluteal and ventrogluteal

areas, and vastus lateralis (lateral muscle of the quadriceps group). The addition of drugs to IV solutions and IV push administration are discussed in Chapter 21.

If the volume of medication to be injected is not excessive, the combination of two drugs in one syringe avoids the discomfort of two injections. Drugs can be combined from two multidose vials, from one multidose vial and one ampule, or from two ampules. Drugs may be combined only if their compatibility has been documented. Rarely are more than two drugs combined in one syringe. One exception is the administration of sedative medications in younger pediatric patients. To avoid giving two injections, meperidine (Demerol), promethazine (Phenergan), and chlorpromazine (Thorazine) are routinely combined in one syringe.

Depending on their purpose, **topical** drugs may be administered to gastroenterology patients in the form of ointments or sprays (e.g., antiseptics, anesthetics), transdermal patches, rectal suppositories , or rectally administered foams or enemas. Medicated shampoos, eye medications, ear drops, nasal sprays and drops, vaginal medications, and inhaled products are also considered topical medications. The site of topical drug application should be inspected frequently for side effects, such as skin irritation or an allergic reaction.

Before administering any medication, it is important that the nurse compare the physician's order with the patient's medication record. There should be a written order for every medication given. If the medication order is verbal, institutional policies and state laws will determine the time frame in which verbal orders must be signed by the physician. Verification of the patient's identity, the drug to be administered, the dose, the route, and the time of administration is essential. It is also important to check that the label on the medication matches the medication order and that the expiration date has not passed. Privacy should be provided as needed for injections and for application of topical drugs. The procedure should be explained to the patient. Regardless of the route of administration, prior hand washing is essential.

Calculations and conversions

To administer the correct dose of a medication, it may be necessary for the nurse to convert the physician's order to a different unit of measure or to dilute available doses. Usually, physicians order medications in grains, grams, milligrams, or other units of *weight*. Before the medication can be administered to the patient, the order may need to be converted to the corresponding number of tablets, capsules, minims, drams, ounces, milliliters, or other units of *volume*. Abbreviations for these units and for other terms used in drug administration are given in Table 20-1.

Doses may be specified in any one of three different systems of measurement:

(a) metric units (e.g., milliliters, grams);

(b) apothecary units (e.g., ounces, drams, minims); and

(c) household units (e.g., teaspoons, drops, cups).

Some of the more common equivalents are contained in

Table 20-1. Abbreviations used in drug administration

Abbreviation	Definition
ac	Before meals
ad lib	As desired
bid	Twice a day
caps	Capsules
fld or fl	Fluid
g, gm	Gram
gr	Grain
gtt	Drop
h or hr	Hour
hs	At bedtime
IM	Intramuscular
IV	Intravenous
kg	Kilogram
μg, ug, mcg	Microgram
mEq	Milliequivalent
mg	Milligram
m	Minim
pc	After meals
per os, po	By month
pr	By rectum
prn	When required
qd	Every day
qh	Every hour
q2h	Every 2 hours
qid	Four times/day
SC	Subcutaneous
SL	Sublingual
tab	Pill
tid	Three times/day
u	units

Table 20-2. It is important that nurses memorize the equivalents necessary to convert between these three systems of measurement. By applying these conversion factors to simple arithmetic calculations involving ratios and proportions, any dosage problem can be easily solved.

In addition to the metric, apothecary, or household systems of measurement, some drugs are measured in milliequivalents (mEq) or units (U). A milliequivalent refers to the number of ionic charges of an element or a compound. It is a measure of the chemical combining power of a substance. Units mean something different for every drug. One *United States Pharmacopeia* (USP) unit of insulin, for example, is

defined as the quantity that promotes the metabolism of about 1.5 g of dextrose. Labels on drugs that are measured in this way indicate the number of milliequivalents or units in a particular volume measure (e.g., 400,000 U/ml or 20 mEq/15 ml).

When administering medications in tablet or capsule form, it is important to remember that only scored or marked tablets can be divided accurately; capsules cannot be divided. It is best to look for tablets or capsules of the desired dose.

Most volume doses of oral medications can be measured out in medicine cups, which are frequently marked in drams, ounces, milliliters (or cubic centimeters), teaspoons, and tablespoons. Smaller volume amounts, such as minims and drops, must be measured by using droppers, calibrated pipettes, or syringes. Drops are an approximate household unit of measure that can be safely measured by using a medicine dropper. A minim is a more accurate apothecary unit of measure and must be measured by using a minim pipette or syringe.

Solutions for parenteral administration may be ordered in units of volume but are more frequently ordered in units of weight, such as grams or milligrams. The nurse must then convert the weight ordered to a unit of volume, such as drams, ounces, or milliliters. In many cases, labels on drugs in solution indicate a certain weight measure in a particular volume (e.g., 500 mg/5 ml). Labels may also state a percentage or ratio strength of the solution (e.g., a 5% or 1:20 solution).

Occasionally it may be necessary to prepare oral or topical solutions from crystals, powder, or stock solutions or to prepare children's doses from adult dose tablets. Preparation of solutions is a simple problem in proportions. For pediatric doses, tablets that are soluble in water can be dissolved in a specified amount of water and the ordered dose measured by using a syringe. Although such preparations are acceptable, commercially prepared liquid medications are more accurately measured and should be used whenever possible.

Most drug references include pediatric dose ranges for drugs that are approved for use in children. Doses are given in milligrams per kilogram of body weight. Pediatric dosages may be calculated based on the child's weight in kilograms. Consideration of body surface area can also be used. Use of surface area requires consultation of one of the various charts or nomograms used to determine body surface area

Table 20-2. Approximate equivalents

Weight units			Fluid units		
Metric	**Apothecary**	**Household**	**Metric**	**Apothecary**	**Household**
1 gram	15-16 grains		1 ml or 1 cc	15-16 minims	15-16 drops
30-32 grams	1 ounce	2 tablespoons	30-32 ml	1 fluid ounce	2 tablespoons
	8 drams	8 teaspoons	30 ml	8 fluid drams	8 teaspoons
1 kilogram	2.2 pounds (avoirdupois)		240 ml	8 ounces	1 cup
			1000 ml		4 cups or 1 quar
			4000 ml		1 gallon

from height and weight. If surface area can be determined, the following formulas are used to calculate the pediatric dosage from the usual adult dosage:

(a) (Surface area in m^2 × Adult dose)/1.7 = Child's dose
(b) Surface area in m^2 × 60 = Percentage of adult dose

If surface area is not known, the most commonly used procedures for determining approximate pediatric dosages include the following:

(a) **Young's rule (children from 1 or 2 to 12 years)**
(Age in years/age + 12) × Adult dose = Child's dose
(b) **Fried's rule (infants and children up to 1 or 2 years)**
(Age in months/150) × Adult dose = Child's dose
(c) **Clark's rule (infants or children)**
(Weight in pounds/150) × Adult dose = Child's dose

Again, if there is any question about the appropriateness of the ordered dosage for any patient, the physician or pharmacist should be consulted.

Documentation

Documentation describes the care of service provided for a patient. In addition, documentation facilitates communication and is a valuable source of data for making decisions about funding and resource management as well as facilitating nursing research, which has the potential to improve the quality of nursing practice and client care. Medical records must reflect care and services provided. Requirements for documentation of medication administration are drawn from federal and state legislation, case law, professional standards of practice, regulating agencies, and facility policies and procedures. The key principles of documentation remain the same whether nurses use the traditional (e.g., paper) or electronically generated (e.g., computer) documentation methods. Nurses are accountable for safeguarding the confidentiality of client information regardless of which method is used.

Documentation must includes name of the drug administered, person administering the drug, dose and route of administration, date and time, and the patient's response or adverse reaction. Parenteral medications requires documentation of injection site. If the patient refuses a drug, the refusal should be documented, and the charge nurse and the patient's doctor should be notified. If a drug is omitted or withheld for other reasons, such as radiology or laboratory tests, that omission and the reason should be documented according to institutional policy.

If the patient's intake and output are being monitored, the fluid volume of any medications administered orally, intravenously, or through a nasogastric or enteral tube should be noted on the intake and output sheet. In the case of topical administration, the nurse should note the condition of the skin at the time of application.

DRUGS COMMONLY USED FOR PATIENTS

With Gastrointestinal Disorders

It is important that the gastroenterology nurse has a work-ing knowledge of the various classes of drugs used in the practice of gastroenterology endoscopy. Some of the medications prescribed for gastroenterology patients are intended to alter GI secretions and/or motility, including anticholinergics and cholinergics, some laxatives, and certain antiulcer agents. Others are prescribed for their antacid, antiinflammatory, antiemetic, or antidiarrheal effects. Still other medications are used in diagnostic testing or to facilitate endoscopic or invasive procedures, which often require the use of topical anesthetics, sedatives, and/or narcotics. In addition, prophylactic antibiotics and therapeutic antiparasitic agents may be prescribed.

The following pages outline the general characteristics of various drug classifications that should be familiar to gastroenterology nurses. Table 20-3 lists specific medications from these categories, with their respective trade names, indications, adult dosages, pediatric dosages, and adverse effects.

Antacids

Antacids still have a place in the treatment of acid-peptic disease even with the widespread availability of proton pump inhibitors, H2-receptor antagonists, and sucralfate. Antacids usually contain combinations of aluminum hydroxide, aluminum phosphate, calcium carbonate, and magnesium salts. Unlike other antiulcer agents, they have no direct effect on gastric acid secretion and they do not coat or protect the mucous lining. Instead, antacids neutralize gastric acid there by reducing the total acid load in the GI tract. This leads to transient raising of gastric pH, reducing peptic activity and strengthening the gastric mucosal barrier.

Antacids are indicated in the treatment of common heartburn (pyrosis), peptic ulcer disease, esophagitis (gastroesophageal reflux), gastritis, symptomatic hiatal hernia, dyspepsia, and acid indigestion. Research studies demonstrate that antacids are clearly superior to placebos in healing duodenal ulcers. Studies of efficacy in healing gastric ulcers are equivocal. Antacids may also be used to reduce gastric acidity in patients with upper GI bleeding that stems from peptic ulcer.

Because antacids leave the stomach rapidly, they are best used for intermittent symptoms. Taken on an empty stomach, the effects of antacids last less than 1 hour; after meals, the buffering effect may last as long as 3 hours. For optimal effect, antacids should be given about 1 hour after meals or feedings and during periods of acid rebound. Their effect can be enhanced if the patient remains recumbent after eating.

Antacid suspensions have a longer action than tablets or solutions. Tablets should be chewed and followed with a glass of water to help them dissolve.

Prolonged use of magnesium- or calcium-containing antacids may cause systemic absorption of toxic quantities of these ions. Magnesium-containing antacids can precipitate hypermagnesemia in patients with chronic renal failure and should be avoided in these patients, since central nervous depression, skin irritation, and rarely, but reported mus-

Table 20-3. Representative pharmacological agents used in gastroenterology

Agent	Trade name	Indications	Adult dosage	Pediatric dosage	Adverse effects
Antacids					
Aluminum hydroxide	Gaviscon	Heartburn, sour stomach, acid indigestion	2-4 tablets 4x/day		Not to be taken with tetracycline or by patients on a sodium-restricted diet.
Aluminum OH+ Magnesium OH+ Simethicone	Mylanta; Maalox	Temporary gastric hyperacidity and gas	2-4 tsp or 2-4 tablets between meals and hs		CNS depression and other symptoms of hypermagnesemiam in patients with renal insufficiency.
Calcium carbonate	Tums	Hyperacidity and acid indigestion	1 g po, 46 x/day		Constipation; hypercalcemia; hypophosphatemia.
Magnesium hydroxide	Phillip's Milk of Magnesia (suspension)	Acid indigestion: sour stomach; heartburn; constipation	Antacid dose: 1-3 tsp up to 4x/day laxative dose: 2-4 tsp	Peptic ulcer disease: 5-15 ml/dose q3-6h; laxative dose: 0.5 ml/kg/dose	Contraindicated for patients with kidney disease.
Magaldrate	Ricpan (suspension)	Hyperacidity; heartburn; sour stomach; acid indigestion	1-2 tsp between meals and hs		Not to be taken with tetracycline or by patients with kidney disease.
Antibiotics					
Ampicillin	Ampicillin	Antibiotic prophylaxis; *Salmonella* infections; shigellosis	Prophylaxis: 250-400 mg 4x/day; *Salmonella*: 6-8 g/day IV; shigel-losis: 1 g po q6h for 5 days	100-200 mg/kg/day IV, up to 10 gm/24 hr	Most frequent are nausea, vomiting, and diarrhea. Laryngeal edema and anaphylaxis may occur in sensitive patients.
Gentamicin	Garamycin	Antibiotic prophylaxis	3 mg/kg 3x/day	1.5-2.5 mg/kg/dose IV, q8h	Most frequent are ototoxicity and nephrotoxicity.
Tetracycline	Tetracycline, Achromycin	Shigellosis; cholera	Shigellosis: 2.5 g/day po or 500 mg po q6h for 5 mdays; cholera: 500 mg q6h for 3 days	>8 yrs old po 25-50/kg/day; do not exceed 3 g/day	Dental staining in children under age 10.
Tobramycin	Nebcin	Antibiotic prophylaxis for serious infections caused by susceptible aerobic gram-negative bacilli	Normal renal function: 3-5 mg/kg IV, IM in 3 equal doses q8h. Impaired renal function: modify, individualize dose; duration: no more than 10 days	2.5 mg/kg/dose IV, q8h	Irreversible ototoxicity, both cochlear and vestibular. Nephrotoxicity usually mild and reversible. Classified FDA Pregnancy Category D.
Vancomycin	Vancocin	Antibiotic prophylaxis in patients allergic to penicillin; pseudomembranous colitis	Colitis: 125 mg po q6h for 1-2 weeks for 1 g IV q12h slow infusion ≤ 10 mg/min	40 mg/kg/24 hr IV	Bad taste, toxicity in patients with renal failure, flushing of upper body.

Continued

Table 20-3. Representative pharmacological agents used in gastroenterology—cont'd

Agent	Trade name	Indications	Adult dosage	Pediatric dosage	Adverse effects
Antibiotics – cont'd					
Metronidazole	Flagyl	Antibiotic prophylaxis; Crohn's disease; pseudomembranous colitis	250 mg po qid	5 mg/kg/dose qid	Metallic taste; peripheral paresthesia; bad taste.
Anticholinergics					
Atropine sulfate	Atropine	Premedication for endoscopic procedures; to avert vasovagal reactions, arrhythmia, and bradycardia and to reduce bowel motility and secretion	0.4 mg IM/IV	0.01-0.02 mg/kg/dose iV, up to 0.4 mg/dose	Tachycardia; use caution with patients with bladder outlet obstruction; increases intraocular pressure in patients with narrowangle glaucoma.
Dicyclomine HCl	Bentyl	Antispasmodic for treatment of IBS	80-160 mg/day in 4 equally divided doses	10 mg/dose 3-4 x/day	Dry mouth; dizziness; blurred vision; nausea; lightheadedness.
Glycopyrrolate	Robinul	Adjunctive therapy of peptic ulcer disease; premedication for endoscopic procedures	2-8 mg/day in 2 or 3 equally divided doses	Premedication: 4.4 µg/kg 30-60 min before procedur	Headache; dizziness; palpitations; constipation; urine retention.
Hyoscyamine	Levsin	Treatment of GI spasms and hypermotility; conjunct therapy for peptic ulcer disease	IV/IM/SC: 0.25 mg q6h; PO/SL: 0.125-0.25 mg tid or qid prn		
Methantheline Br	Banthine	Adjunctive therapy for peptic ulcer disease; pylorospasm; spastic colon; pancreatitis; gastritis	50-100 mg po q6h	12.5-50 mg 4 x/day	Palpitations; blurred vision; dry mouth; paralytic ileus; urinary hesitancy or retention.
Propantheline Br	Pro-Banthine	Adjunctive therapy for peptic ulcer disease; IBS; reduction of GI motility for diagnostic testing	15 mg 30 min before each meal and 30 mg hs	1-2 mg/kg/day in 3 or 4 divided doses	Dry mouth; decreased sweating; blurred vision; tachycardia.
Cholinergics					
Bethanechol Cl	Urecholine	Cholinergic drug that relieves urinary retention, stimulates gastric motility, restores impaired peristalsis	10-50 mg po, 3-4 x/day or 5 mg SC, 3-4 x/day	0.6 mg/kg/day divided 3-4 x/day	Dizziness; lightheadedness; abdominal discomfort; urinary urgency.
Edrophonium	Tensilon	Cholinergic used in provocative tests of esophageal motility disorders that present as chest pain	provoca- 0.08 mg/kg IV	Diagnosis: initial 0.04 mg/kg followed by 0.16 mg/kg if no response, to a maximum of 5-10 mg	Lacrimation; dizziness; GI discomfort; rarely, bradycardia; papillary constriction; laryngospasm.

Antidiarrheals

Generic	Brand	Indication	Adult Dose	Pediatric Dose	Side Effects/Comments
Bismuth subsalicylate	Pepto-Bismol	Diarrhea; heartburn; indigestion; upset stomach; nausea	Two 262-mg tablets or 2 Tbs (262 mg each) every 30-60 min, up to 8 doses/24 hr	Age 9-12: 1 Tbs; age 6-9: ⅔ tsp; 3-6: 1 tsp	Contraindicated for patients who are allergic to aspirin or salicylates.
Difenoxin HCl† with atropine sulfate	Motofen	Acute, nonspecific diarrhea and acute exacerbations of chronic diarrhea	2 mg, then 1 mg after each loose stool or 1 mg q3-4h as needed, up to 8 mg/24 hr	0.3-0.4 mg/kg/day	Nausea; vomiting; dry mouth; dizziness and lightheadedness; drowsiness.
Diphenoxylate HCl† with atropine sulfate	Lomotil	Diarrhea	Up to 5 mg 4 x/day	0.3-0.4 mg/kg/day	Sedation; dizziness; dry mouth; paralytic ileus.
Kaolin + pectin	Kaopectate	Mild, nonspecific diarrhea	60-120 ml po after each bowel movement	Age 6-12: 1 Tbs; age 3-6: ½ Tbs	Absorbs nutrients, drugs, and enzymes; constipation.
Loperamide HCl	Imodium	Acute, nonspecific diarrhea and chronic diarrhea associated with IBS	4 mg after the first loose bowel movement, plus 2 mg after each subsequent loose movement, up to 16 mg/24 hr	0.4-0.8 mg/kg/day divided q6-12h; maximum 2mg/dose, 2 days maximum	Hypersensitivity reactions; abdominal pain; distention or discomfort, nausea and vomiting; constipation.

Antiemetics

Generic	Brand	Indication	Adult Dose	Pediatric Dose	Side Effects/Comments
Chlorpromazine	Thorazine	Control of nausea and vomiting	10-25 mg po prn; 25-50 mg IM q3-4h prn; one 100-mg suppository q6-8h prn	IV or po 0.5-1 mg/kg/dose q4-6h as needed	Tardive dyskinesia.
Dimenhydrinate	Dramamine	Prevention and treatment of motion sickness	1-2 50 mg tablets q4-6h, up to 8 tablets/24 hr; 4-8 tsp q4-6h, up to 32 tsp/24 hr	IM or po 5 mg/kg/day in 4 divided doses, not to exceed 75 mg/day for 2-6 yrs old, max 150 mg for 6-12 yrs old	Drowsiness, especially with alcohol, sedatives, or tranquilizers.
Metoclopramide HDl	Reglan	Short-term therapy for esophageal reflux; enhances gastric emptying; facilitates small bowel intubation	10-15 mg qid	0.1 mg/kg/dose po 3-4 x/day; maximum dose: 5 mg/kg/day	Restlessness; drowsiness; fatigue; and lassitude.
Prochlorperazine	Compazine	Control of severe nausea and vomiting	Not to exceed 40 mg/day	IM 0.1-0.15 mg/kg/dose up to 10 mg; po or pr: 0.4 mg/kg/24 hr in 3-4 divided doses; maximum 10 mg dose	Dizziness; extrapyramidal symptoms; blurred vision; skin reactions; and hypotension.
Trimethobenzamide HCl	Tigan	Control of nausea and vomiting	One 250 mg capsule, 200 mg suppository, or 200 mg (2 ml) IM injection tid or qid	pr <14 kg 100 mg/dose; po or pr 14-40 kg 100-200 mg/dose 3-4 x/day	Hypersensitivity reactions; Parkinson-like symptoms; drowsiness; Reye's syndrome.
Ondansetron hydrochloride	Zofran	Prevention of nausea and vomiting; postprocedure nausea	IV: 0.4 mg slow IV push tid prn; po 8 mg 1 hr before procedure	Not established in children under 4; age 4-18 yrs IV: up to 4 mg slow IV push tid prn; age 4-18 yrs po: 4-8 mg tid	Dizziness; diarrhea; constipation; dry mouth.

Continued

Table 20-3. Representative pharmacological agents used in gastroenterology—cont'd

Agent	Trade name	Indications	Adult dosage	Pediatric dosage	Adverse effect
Antiflatulants					
Simethicone	Mylicon	Relief of painful symptoms of excess gas in the digestive tract	1 40 mg tablet po after meals and hs or as needed, up to 12 tablets daily	40 mg 4 x/day	
Antiparasitic agentsx					
Metronidazole	Flagyl	Giardiasis	250 mg po 3 x/day for 1 week	15-30 mg/kd/day q8h	Convulsive seizures; peripheral neuropathy.
Antiulcer agents					
Cimetidine	Tagamet	Short-term treatment of duodenal ulcers	300 mg po qid with meals and hs 300 mg IV/IM q6h continuous IV 37.5 mg/hr; total 900 mg/day	20-30 mg/kg/day q6h	Headache, malaise, myalgia, diarrhea, skin rash, pruritis, gynecomastia.
Cisapride	Propulsid	Adjunctive therapy for symptom relief of reflux esophagitis and nocturnal heartburn by lowering esophageal sphincter pressure, increasing the movement of the esophagus, and increasing contractions in the stomach accelerating gastric emptying time	10 mg po qid 15 min ac and hs	0.2 mg-0.3 mg/kg tid to qid	Diarrhea; abdominal pain; nausea; vomiting; epigastric pain. Rare: palpitations; elevated liver enzymes.
Famotidine	Pepcid	Duodenal ulcer; pathopological hypersecretory conditions	Acute therapy: 40 mg po once daily hs; maintenance: 20 mg po once daily hs	0.5 mg/kg q8-12h	Headache; diarrhea; constipation.
Misoprostol	Cytotec	Prevention of NSAID-induced ulcers	200 μg po qid with food	Safety has not been established	Diarrhea; abdominal pain; contraindicated in pregnancy.
Nizatidine	Axid	Duodenal ulcers	Acute therapy: 300 mg po hs or 150 mg bid; maintenance therapy; 150 mg po hs	Not recommended	Headache.
Omeprazole	Prilosec	Gastroesophageal reflux disease; erosive esophagitis; duodenal ulcers; long-term treatment erosive esophagitis; hypersecretory conditions	Esophageal reflux: 20 mg po/day Hypersecretory states: 60 mg po daily	Safety has not been established	Headache; diarrhea; abdominal pain; nausea; dizziness; vomiting; rash; constipation.

	Trade name	Indication	Adult dosage	Pediatric dosage	Side effects
Ranitidine HCl	Zantac	Duodenal and gastric ulcers; hypersecretory conditions; esophageal reflux	150 mg po bid or 300 po mg once daily hs; 150 mg po once daily for maintenance therapy 50 mg IM q6h; 50 mg continuous IV at 6.25 mg/hr	IM/IV 0.75-1.5 mg/kg/dose q6-8h; po 1.5-2 mg/kg/dose q12h maximum daily dose 400 mg	Headache.
Sucralfate	Carafate	Short-term treatment of duodenal ulcer	1 g po qid 1 hr ac or 2 hrs pc	<6 yrs old 0.5 g/dose qid >6 yrs old 1 g/dose qid	Constipation; dizziness; sleepiness. Must separate concurrent drugs by at least 2 hrs.
Corticosteroids					
Hydrocortisone	Hydrocortone	Ulcerative colitis; Crohn's disease	Approximately 120-240 mg po/day, depending on the severity of the disease and the patient's response	Antiinflammatory 1-5 mg/kg/day	Acne; Cushingoid changes; fluid and electrolyte disturbances; osteoporosis; pancreatitis; gastric ulcer.
Methylprednisolone	Medrol	Ulcerative colitis; Crohn's disease	4-8 mg po.day, depending on the severity of the disease and the patient's response	Antiinflammatory 0.16-0.8 mg/kg/day, divided doses q6-12h	Acne; Cushingoid changes; fluid and electrolyte disturbances; osteoporosis; gastric ulcer.
Prednisolone sodium phosphate	Hydeltrasol injection	Ulcerative colitis; Crohn's disease	4-60 mg/day, depending on the severity of the disease and the patient's response		Fluid and electrolyte disturbances; peptic ulcer; menstrual irregularities; Cushingoid changes; osteoporosis.
Triamcinolone acetonide	Kenalog	Relief of dysphagia in patients with benign esophageal strictures.	5 mg injections in each quadrant of the narrowest region of the stricture; adult dosage: 2.5-15 mg		Myopathy; anorexia with weight loss; sedation, and depression.
Agents used in diagnostic tests					
Bentiromide	Chymex	Screening for pancreatic exocrine insufficiency	500 mg po, followed by 250 ml water	Ages 6-12 14 mg po/kg, maximum 500 mg	Diarrhea; headache; flatulence; nausea.
Glucagon	Glucagon	Inhibition of GI motility; especially in conjunction with ERCP	Increments of 0.2-0.4 mg IV	0.03-0.1 mg/kg IV/dose, maximum 1 mg	Nausea, vomiting.
Pentagastrin	Peptavlon	Stimulates gastric acid secretion	6 µg/kg SC	Safety has not been established	Abdominal discomfort; nausea; flushing; light-headedness.
Secretin	Secretin	Stimulates pancreatic exocrine secretion; diagnosis of gastrinoma	2 units/kg IV over a 1 min period	Not recommended for pediatric use	Clinically significant side effects are unusual.

Continued

Table 20-3. Representative pharmacological agents used in gastroenterology

Agent	Trade name	Indications	Adult dosage	Pediatric dosage	Adverse effects
Gallbladder therapeutic agents					
Chenodiol (chenodeoxycholic acid)	Chenix	Dissolution of radiolucent cholesterol stones	250 mg po bid for the first 2 weeks, followed by weekly increases of 250 mg/day, up to 13-16 mg/kg/day for up to 24 months	Not recommended for pediatric use	Diarrhea; cramps; heartburn; reversible elevated hepatic enzymes.
Monooctanoin	Moctanin	Dissolution of cholesterol stones retained in the biliary tract after cholecystectomy	Continuous infusion (3-5 ml/hr) directly into the common bile duct for 7-21 day	Not recommended for pediatric use	GI pain and discomfort; nausea; vomiting.
Ursodiol (ursodeoxycholic acid)	Actigall	Dissolution of radiolucent cholesterol stones less than 20 mm in diameter	8-10 mg/kg po daily in 2 or 3 divided doeses for up to 12 months	Chronic cholestasis: 10-20 mg/kg/day; biliary artresia: 15 mg/kg/day	Rarely, diarrhea; pruritus; cough; headache; nausea.
Laxatives, cathartics, and bulk agents					
Bisacodyl	Dulcolax; Correctol Stimulant	Acute or chronic constipation; preoperative preparation or postoperative care	2-3 5 mg po or 1 10 mg suppository	pr >2 yrs old 10 mg; po >2 yrs old 5-10 mg as a single dose	Abdominal cramping.
Docusate sodium	Modane Soft; Ex-Lax; Correctol	Constipation, especially to lessen the strain of defecation	1-3 100 mg capsules daily	<3 yrs old: 10-40 mg/24 hr; age 3-6: 20-60 mg/24 hr; age 6-12: 40-150 mg/24 hr	Diarrhea; nausea; cramping pains; and rash (all uncommon).
Lactulose	Chronulac; Cephulac; Duphalac	Constipation (Duphalac, Chronulac); portal-systemic encephalopathy (Cephulac)	Constipation: 15-30 ml po daily; portal-systemic encephalopathy; 20-30 g po (30-45 ml) tid or qid, or as a retention enema to reverse hepatic coma	pO 40-90 ml/day	Abdominal cramps; belching; diarrhea; hypernatremia.
Magnesium citrate	Citrate of Magnesia	Bowel evacuation before GI examination; after treatment with a vermifuge used to evacuate parasites and toxic materials from the colon	240 ml once	<6 yrs old 2-4 ml/kg; age 6-12: 50-100 ml	Abdominal cramps; nausea; fluid and electrolyte imbalance.
Methylcellulose	Citrucel	Chronic constipation	5-20 ml liquid pot id with a glass of water or 15 ml syrup po morning and evening	Age 6-11 ½1 tsp 1-3 x/day	Nausea; abdominal cramps.
Evacuation polyethylene glycol	Colyte; GoLYTELY	Bowel evacuation before GI examination	240 ml po q 10 min until 4 L is consumed	25-40 ml/kg/hr until rectal effluent is clear	Nausea; bloating; cramps; vomiting.
Psyllium	Metamucil	Constipation; bowel management	1-2 rounded tsp po in full glass of liquid daily, bid or tid, followed by a second glass of liquid	Age 6-11 ½1 tsp 1-3 x/day	Nausea; vomiting; diarrhea with excessive use; contraindicated in intestinal obstruction or fecal impaction.

Narcotics and antagonists

Generic name	Brand name	Indication	Dosage (adult)	Dosage (pediatric)	Side effects
Fentanyl citrate	Sublimaze	Premedication and conscious sedation for endoscopic procedures; postprocedural analgesia	2 µg/kg	IM/IV 1-2 µg/kg/dose	Respiratory depression; apnea; rigidity; and bradycardia.
Meperidine HCl	Demerol	Relief of moderate to severe pain; preoperative medication	For pain relief 50-150 mg IM SC, or po q3-4h; for preoperative medication: 50-100 mg IM or SC	Pain relief: 1-1.5 mg/kg/dose q 3-4 h; preoperative: 1-2 mg/kg maximum 100mg	Respiratory depression and, to a lesser extent, circulatory depression; nausea and vomiting.
Morphine sulfate	Roxanol	Relief of severe, acute or chronic pain	10-30 mg q4h	IM/IV 0.1-0.2 mg/kg/dose q2-4h; maximum 15 mg/dose	Respiratory depression and, to a lesser extent, circulatory depression; nausea and vomiting.
Naloxone HCl	Narcan	Reversal of narcotic depression	0.2-0.4 mg IV every 2-3 min; may also given IM or SC	0.01 mg/kg; may repeat q2-3 min based on response	Nausea; vomiting; sweating; tachycardia; hypertension; tremulousness; seizures and cardiac arrest.

Sclerosing agents

Generic name	Brand name	Indication	Dosage (adult)	Dosage (pediatric)	Side effects
Ethanol 100%		Variceal bleeding	0.1 ml/injection	Safety and efficacy have not been established	
Ethanolamine oleate	Ethamolin	Esophageal varices that have recently bled, to prevent rebleeding	1.5-5 ml varix; maximum total dose per treatment session not to exceed 20 ml	2-3 ml of 5% solution; maximum 10 ml	Pleural effusion and /or infiltration; esophageal ulcer; pyrexia; retrosternal pain; esophageal stricture; pneumonia.
Morrhuate sodium (5% or 1%)	Scleromate	Obliteration of esophageal varices; varicose veins	1-2 ml per varix	5% solution 2-4 ml	Esophageal ulceration; allergic reactions; stricture; chest pain.
Sodium tetradecyl sulfate (1% or 3%)	Sotradecol	Obliteration of esophageal varices; varicose veins	1-2 ml per varix; not to exceed 15 ml per session	Safety and efficacy have not been established	Esophageal ulceration; allergic reactions; stricture; chest pain.

Sedatives and antagonists

Generic name	Brand name	Indication	Dosage (adult)	Dosage (pediatric)	Side effects
Diazepam	Valium	Relief of preprocedural anxiety and tension and reduction of recall of the procedure	5-15 mg IV immediately before the procedure and prn during the procedure; titrate individually	po 0.12-0.8 mg/kg/day; IM/IV 0.04-0.3 mg/kg/dose	Respiratory depression and arrest, especially when used for conscious sedation.
Flumazenil	Mazicon	Reversal of sedation from use of benzodiazepines (Valium, Versed)	0.2-1.0 mg given at 0.2 mg/min IV; no more than 1 mg should be given at once; no more than 3.0 mg/hr	5-10 µg/kg	Dizziness; injection site pain; blurred vision; headache; flushing; sweating; nausea and vomiting; agitation; dry mouth; tachycardia.

Continued

Table 20-3. Representative pharmacological agents used in gastroenterology—cont'd

Agent	Trade name	Indications	Adult dosage	Pediatric dosage	Adverse effects
Sedatives and antagonists –cont'd					
Midazolam HCl	Versed	Premedication for anxiety relief and reduced recall; conscious sedation	Conscious sedation: titrate individually, beginning with 0.5 mg (usual dose does not exceed 5 mg)	Preoperative sedation: IM 0.07-0.08 mg/kg; IV 0.035 mg/kg/dose, repeat until desired sedation effect is achieved, up to 0.1-0.2 mg/kg Conscious sedation for procedures: IV 0.05 mg/kg 3 min before procedure loading dose; follow with infusion of 1-2 μg/kg/min and titrate	Respiratory depression and arrest, especially when used for conscious sedation.
Smooth muscle relaxants					
Isosorbide dinitrate	Isordil	Achalasia	5-10 mg before meals, sublingually	Safety and efficacy have not been established	Headache.
Nifedipine	Procardia, Adalat	Achalasia	10-20 mg, capsule broken in patient's mouth	0.25-0.5 mg/kg/dose	Light-headedness; flushing; headache.
Topical anesthetics					
Benzocaine	Hurricaine; Cetacaine	Suppresses gag reflex and controls pain	2 oz aerosol spray, 1 oz liquid, or 1 oz gel; liquid may be used as a gargle, gel as a lubricant	Administered as spray	No significant adverse effects.
Dyclonine HCl	Dyclone	Topical anesthetic for mucous membranes; blocks gag reflex	Lowest dose needed to provide effective anesthesia, up to 30 ml of 1% solution	2 ml of the 1% solution until reflex has been abolished	Excitatory and/or depressant CNS effects; drowsiness; cardiovascular depression; allergic reactions.
Lidocaine HCl	Xylocaine	Topical anesthesia in spray or gel form for use in the oral cavity	10% oral spray: up to 2 metered doses per quadrant; 2% viscous solution: 4.5 mg/kg	Topical: apply as needed, maximum 3 mg/kg/dose	Excitatory and/or depressant CNS effects; drowsiness; cardiovascular depression; allergic reactions.
Other agents					
Mesalamine (5-ASA)	Rowasa	Suspension retention enema for distal ulcerative colitis, proctosigmoiditis, or proctitis	1 enema daily hs, retained for approximately 8 hr; course of therapy, 3-6 wks.	Safety has not been established	Cramping; acute abdominal pain; bloody diarrhea; sometimes fever, headache, and rash.

Mesalamine	Asacol	Treatment of ulcerative colitis; delayed release tablet that reaches the terminal ileum and beyond	800 mg tid for 6 wks	Abdominal pain; cramps; nausea; diarrhea; headache; malaise.
Cholestyramine	Questran powder	Relief of pruritus in patients with partial biliary obstruction	9 g powder (4 g cholestyramine) mixed with 2-6 oz fluid po 1-6 times daily	Constipation; nausea.
Interferon alfa	Intron-a	Hepatitis C	3 million units SC, 3x/week for at least 6 months; Hepatitis B 5 million units/square meter/day	Mild to moderate flulike symptoms; reactions at the injection site.
Olsalazine sodium	Dipentum	Remission maintenance in sulfasalazine-intolerant patients with ulcerative colitis	1.0 g/day in 2 divided doses, preferably with food	Transient diarrhea; abdominal pain; rash and/or itching.
Pancreatin	Donnazyme	Steatorrhea; pyrosis; flatulence; belching	2 tablets with each meal and 1 or 2 tablets with each snack; swallowed whole	Safety has not been established
Pancrelipase	Cotazym	Pancreatic enzyme replacement for treatment of exocrine insufficiency	1-3 capsules or tablets po before or with meals and 1 capsule or tablet with snacks	As above
Neomycin sulfate	Mycifradin Sulfate	Hepatic encephalopathy	Age 1-6 yrs 4000-8000 units of lipase with meals; 4000 units with snacks Age 7-12 yrs 4000-12000 units of lipase with meals and snacks	Skin rash; laxative effect at excessively high doses
Penicillamine	Cuprimine	Wilson's disease	50-100 mg/kg/day divided doses q6-8h	Nausea; diarrhea with high doses.
Sulfasalazine	Azulfidine	Ulcerative colitis; Crohn's disease	1-2 g/day po, in divided doses, on an empty stomach	Diarrhea; malabsorption; ototoxicity; nephrotoxicity
Vasopressin	Pitressin	Variceal bleeding	250 mg/dose 2-3 x/day	Fever; rash; leukopenia; thrombocytopenia.
			40-75 mg/kg/day in 3-6 divided doses, not to exceed 6 g/day; maintenance 20-40 mg/kg/day in 4 divided doses	Hypersensitivity; abdominal discomfort; nausea; vomiting; headache.
			0.01 unit/kg/min IV	Bradycardia; coronary vasoconstriction; bowel ischemia; water retention.

cle paralysis with respiratory failure can occur. In chronic renal failure patients, administration of aluminum-containing antacids is best at mealtime. Excessive use of aluminum-containing antacids may lead to hypophosphatemia. Antacids containing sodium can precipitate edema in patients with cirrhosis, hypertension, or renal or congestive heart failure. Aluminum and calcium preparations tend to be constipating, whereas magnesium preparations tend to produce a laxative effect.

The use of antacids with tetracycline, iron, or H_2-receptor antagonists is contraindicated. Calcium binds and prevents the absorption of tetracycline whereas antacids decrease the absorption of iron and H_2-blockers.

ANTIBIOTICS

Antibiotics, commonly called antimicrobial agents, may be prescribed for gastroenterology patients in ambulatory and hospital care of children and adults. The gastroenterology nurse must have basic knowledge of mechanism of action, antimicrobial spectrum, typical uses, and toxicities of commonly used antibiotics. Cost and dosing schedules must be considered in the decision-making process when prescribing to enhance patient compliance. Knowledge of drug allergies, recommended dosages, and bacterial taxonomy is of clinical importance for gastroenterology nurses in order to provide safe medical care and promote patient and family education.

Antibiotics may be prescribed for gastrointestinal disorders such as infectious diarrhea, treatment of strictures in Crohn's disease, diverticulitis, cholangitis, viral, bacterial and parasitic infections, viral hepatitis and *Helicobacter Pylori*. Example of antibiotics that may be prescribed include ampicillin, tetracycline (Achromycin), Ciprofloxacin, Norfloxacin, tremethoprim/sulfamethoxazole (Bactrim DS), Doxycline, Erythromycin, Vancomycin (Vancocin) and Paromomycin. The specific antibiotic drug selection depends on the pathogen, drug adverse-effect profile, patient drug allergies, age of patient and co-morbid illness involved.

Prophylactic antibiotics may be prescribed for at-risk patients undergoing endoscopic procedures that may produce bacteremia as well as for some subgroups of patients, notably those with mitral valve prolapse. Guidelines for antibiotic prophylaxis during endoscopic procedures have been published by American Society of Gastrointestinal Endoscopy (ASGE) and the American Heart Association (AHA). In most individuals, bacteremia is transient and resolves without complications. Bacterial endocarditis is a concern in patients with valvular heart disease, internal prosthetic devices, or a previous episode of endocarditis. Antibiotics ordered for prophylaxis against endocarditis include amoxicillin, ampicillin, gentamicin (Garamycin), vancomycin (Vancocin), tobramycin (Nebcin) and ciprofloxacin. It is important to recognize that the criteria for the use of prophylactic antibiotics continue to be controversial.

Anticholinergics and cholinergics

Anticholinergic medications, such as atropine and dicyclomine hydrochloride (Bentyl) inhibit gastric acid secretion at its source by blocking the acetylcholine receptor on gastric parietal cells. These medications decrease the output of pepsin and block vagal stimulation of smooth muscle, thus decreasing gastrointestinal tone and motility. They also decrease gastric emptying time, presumably through their inhibition of vagal and cholinergic-mediated motility.

Anticholinergics may be used in the treatment of diffuse esophageal spasm, peptic ulcer disease, ileitis, irritable bowel syndrome (IBS), pancreatitis, gastritis, and ulcerative colitis. They can help to relieve the gastric distress caused by gastric spasms, hyperperistalsis, and rapid emptying of the stomach. Anticholinergic medications are contraindicated in patients who experience bleeding or who have tachycardia, glaucoma, achalasia, obstruction, or suspected toxic megacolon.

Anticholinergics are best given about 1 hour after meals, when food-stimulated acid is at its peak. Their effects persist for 4 to 5 hours.

Adverse effects of anticholinergics include: dryness of the lips, nose, and throat; hoarseness; tachycardia; blurred vision; urinary hesitancy or retention; headache and dizziness; flushing of the skin; and constipation. Because of their side effects, they are used primarily as an adjunctive therapy for peptic ulcer disease, in combination with antacids or histamine$_2$ (H_2) blockers.

In contrast to anticholinergics, **cholinergic** agents increase GI tone and motility. They produce the same effects as stimulation of the parasympathetic nervous system, thereby stimulating GI secretion and motility, diaphoresis, and bladder contractions. Bethanechol (Urecholine) may be used to increase lower esophageal sphincter (LES) pressure in patients suffering from gastroesophageal reflux. It is also used in children with gastroesophageal reflux who are unresponsive to metoclopramide (Reglan). Cholinergics are contraindicated in the presence of peptic ulcer or possible GI obstruction. Side effects, such as abdominal cramping, blurred vision, and other cholinergic symptoms, have limited the use of this agent as well. Domperidone is a peripheral dopamine antagonist that has a safety profile similar to metoclopramide used to enhance gastric emptying. There have been only a few large studies performed to determine its efficacy but has shown promise. The drug is not FDA approved in the United States. Cisapride (Propulsid) was introduced into the American drug market in 1993 to relieve symptoms of reflux esophagitis by increasing contractions in the stomach for improved stomach emptying. The drug was removed in late 2000 with much controversy for post-market reports of cardiac dysrhythmias and fatalities associated with the combination of cisapride and several agents that are metabolized by the cytochrome P-450 system (particularly antifungal agents and some antimicrobials). The drug is available under a strict controlled access plan for extreme medical necessity.

Antidiarrheals

Antidiarrheal agents are used for symptomatic relief of diarrhea. They include drugs that decrease intestinal motility (opium alkaloids and synthetic opium alkaloids) and drugs that decrease the fluid content of the stool or inhibit intestinal secretions. Antidiarrheal agents may also be used judiciously to decrease the frequency of bowel movements in patients with ulcerative colitis or Crohn's disease.

(a) Opium alkaloids, such as morphine, methylmorphine, and camphorated tincture of opium, and synthetic opium alkaloids, such as loperamide (Imodium) and diphenoxylate hydrochloride (Lomotil), may be used as antidiarrheal agents. These agents act primarily by inhibiting intestinal motility. Because these drugs may be habit-forming, patients must be cautioned not to exceed the recommended dosage. Opium alkaloids are contraindicated in patients with toxic causes of diarrhea and should be used cautiously by patients with asthma, liver disease, prostatic hypertrophy, and narcotic dependence.

(b) Some antidiarrheal preparations are inert powders that act by decreasing the fluid content of the stool. They are most effective for acute short-term treatment of diarrhea. Kaolin and pectin (Kaopectate) fall in this category.

(c) Bismuth subsalicylate (Pepto-Bismol) is useful for mild diarrhea and upset stomach. It acts by inhibiting intestinal secretions. In addition, it may absorb toxins and provide a protective coating for the mucosa. Bismuth may also be used in combination with antibiotics for the treatment of *H. pylori* infection.

In general, antidiarrheal agents delay the intestinal clearance of pathogens. They are not recommended for patients with fever or bloody diarrhea or in patients younger than 2 years old. Agents that inhibit intestinal motility may develop toxic megacolon in patients suffering from pseudomembranous enterocolitis, acute dysentery, and acute ulcerative colitis. They should be used in acute exacerbation of inflammatory bowel disease *only* after an infectious cause of the symptoms has been ruled out.

Even in suitable patients, continued use of antidiarrheal agents over an extended period is not recommended. If it is not possible to control diarrhea promptly, diagnostic tests should be ordered. In seriously ill patients the etiological agent should be isolated, and specific antimicrobial therapy should be started.

Antiemetics

Antiemetics produce symptomatic relief of nausea and vomiting. They include both phenothiazines and antihistamines, as well as trimethobenzamide hydrochloride (Tigan). Phenothiazines are the most common type of antiemetic drugs. They appear to exert their effects on the cells of the chemoreceptor trigger zone (CTZ), located in the medulla of the brain stem, which prevents the vomiting center from being activated. Phenothiazines such as prochlorperazine (Compazine) and chlorpromazine (Thorazine) are effective in relieving vomiting associated with gastroenteritis, radiation sickness, and drug therapy, but they do not relieve motion sickness. Adverse effects of phenothiazines include sedation, hypotension, restlessness, dry mouth, blurred vision, constipation, and muscle twitching. They should be used only when nondrug antiemetic measures or other drugs fail.

Certain antihistamines, such as dimenhydrinate (Dramamine), act on the CTZ to suppress centrally mediated nausea and vomiting associated with motion sickness or drug or radiation therapy, or following surgery. The primary side effect of antihistamines is drowsiness.

The mechanism of action of trimethobenzamide hydrochloride is unknown, but it may act on the CTZ.

Metoclopramide (Reglan) may also be considered an antiemetic drug, although its principal function is to increase LES pressure and the rate of gastric emptying. Metoclopramide appears to produce its antiemetic effects as a result of its antagonism of central and peripheral dopamine receptors.

Antiflatulents

Antiflatulent agents, such as simethicone (Mylicon), are used to relieve painful symptoms of excess gas in the GI tract that may be caused by air swallowing, postoperative gaseous distention, peptic ulcers, spastic or irritable colon, diverticulosis, or infantile colic. The agents act by dispersing and preventing the formation of mucus-surrounded air or gas pockets in the GI tract. Simethicone is also added to some antacid preparations.

Antiparasitic/antifungal agents

There are a number of agents available to combat the effects of intestinal parasites and fungi. One important agent is metronidazole (Flagyl), which demonstrates antimicrobial activity with antibacterial, antiprotozoal, and anti-inflammatory effects against a wide variety of bacterial and protozoal infections including *B. fragilis* infections, *C. difficile* – associated colitis, and as surgical prophylaxis. Indications for use of metronidazole in Crohn's disease include perineal disease, Crohn's colitis, and sulfasalazine intolerance or allergy. Metronidazole has shown no benefit in therapy of ulcerative colitis. A common organism of the gastrointestinal tract that can invade tissues when the host defenses are altered is *Candida albicans*. Disease and drugs have potential to predispose oral pharynx, esophageal or vaginal infections. Antifungal treatments can be topical, oral systemic or intravenous. Examples of commonly prescribed antifungals are Nystatin, Clotrimazole, Ketoconazole, Diflucan, Nizoral, Sporonax and Amphotericin – B. Neurological side effects are the most serious and warrant discontinuation of drug.

Antiulcer agents

The various drugs prescribed for peptic ulcer disease promote healing by reducing gastric acid secretion, buffering secreted gastric acid, and/or enhancing intrinsic mucosal defenses. The classes of drugs used for these purposes include antacids, anticholinergic agents, H_2 blockers, sucralfate (Carafate), prostaglandins and proton-pump inhibitors. Antacids and anticholinergics have been discussed previously.

Histamine$_2$ (H$_2$) blockers include cimetidine (Tagamet), famotidine (Pepcid), nizatidine (Axid), and ranitidine (Zantac). They reduce the secretion of gastric acid by blocking histamine's action on the H_2 receptors in the parietal cells. H_2 blockers may also be used to reduce gastric acidity in patients with upper GI bleeding that stems from a peptic ulcer.

The most common side effects of H_2 blockers are diarrhea, headaches, dizziness, fatigue, muscle pain, rash, impotence and mild gynecomastia, leukopenia, and thrombocytopenia.

Sucralfate (Carafate) is a basic aluminum salt of sucrose octasulfate which forms a viscous adhesive gel that adheres to the ulcer crater, thereby preventing further digestive action by both acid and pepsin. It has been approved for the treatment of duodenal ulcers but not for gastric ulcers. The main side effect of sucralfate is constipation, which occurs in approximately 10% of patients who take this drug. Other rarely occurring side effects include dizziness, vertigo, sleepiness, dry mouth, skin rashes, pruritus, back pain, diarrhea, nausea, gastric discomfort, and indigestion.

Synthetic **prostaglandins,** such as misoprostol (Cytotec), have both antisecretory and cytoprotective effects. They may be used to prevent the gastric ulcers and mucosal injury that have been associated with the use of nonsteroidal anti-inflammatory drugs (NSAIDs). The most common side effect is diarrhea, followed by abdominal pain. Because of its abortifacient properties, misoprostol is contraindicated in pregnant women and generally is not recommended for women of child-bearing age.

Proton pump inhibitors (PPIs) provide more complete control of acid than H_2 blockers and are the most effective agents in the therapy of GERD. The agents available in the United States are omeprazole, lansoprazole, pantoprazole, rabeprazole, and esomeprazole. PPIs are pro-drugs and need to be administered thirty (30) minutes prior to eating in order to maximally activate proton pump blockade. Use of these agents is indicated for the treatment of patients with erosive esophagitis or active duodenal ulcers. Long-term treatment may be indicated in some hypersecretory conditions such as Zollinger-Ellison syndrome, systemic mastocytosis, and chronic erosive esophagitis. Omeprazole and lansoprazole may be used in combination therapy with clarithromycin (Biaxin) in patients with positive *H. pylori*. Patients taking anticoagulants, anticonvulsants, or diazepam will require special monitoring because of drug-drug interactions. Adverse reactions may include abdominal pain, asthenia, constipation, diarrhea, nausea, vomiting, and headaches.

Corticosteroids

Corticosteroids are used in gastroenterology practice primarily for their anti-inflammatory properties in the treatment of inflammatory bowel disease, autoimmune hepatitis,

collagenous sprue, severe cases of celiac disease, collagenous colitis, and radiation injury. They include hydrocortisone (Hydrocortone); prednisone; and synthetic analogs, such as prednisolone (Hydeltrasol) and methylprednisolone (Medrol). In addition, injection of the synthetic corticosteroid triamcinolone acetonide (Kenalog) and triamcinolone hexacetionide (Aristospan) may relieve dysphagia in patients with benign esophageal strictures of various causes following intralesional injection therapy.

In patients with Crohn's disease, proctitis, or distal colitis, corticosteroids may be administered topically (by rectal suppository, foam, or retention enema). Oral administration is effective for patients with more extensive disease and more prominent symptoms. For patients with severe and fulminant forms of the disease, IV hydrocortisone, methylprednisolone, or prednisolone may alter the course of the disease and avert colectomy.

Patients on prolonged corticosteroid therapy should be monitored for signs of Cushing's syndrome, which is characterized by rapidly developing adipose deposition of the face, neck, and trunk; kyphosis; hypertension; diabetes mellitus; amenorrhea; hypertrichosis; impotence; osteoporosis; and muscular wasting and weakness.

Because of the immunosuppressive nature of corticosteroids, the patient must be monitored for infection and cautioned to avoid exposure to infectious disease. The physician should be notified of such exposures (such as chicken pox). The physician should be consulted before the patient considers receiving immunizations prepared with live virus (e.g., measles, oral polio vaccine).

Immune modulating agents

Immune modulating agents are used in inflammatory bowel disease when the patient is unable to wean or discontinue corticosteroids without exacerbation of symptoms. These agents have a "steroid-sparing" effect, allowing the patient to eventually discontinue the corticosteroid. Commonly used immune modulating agents include mercaptopurine (6-MP), azathioprine (Imuran), cyclosporine, and methotrexate. Because of the tendency for these medications to suppress bone marrow activity, it is vital that patients be instructed to keep all follow-up appointments with their physician and to have laboratory studies drawn when requested. Patients should avoid exposure to communicable illness and should see a physician promptly when ill. Annual flu shots are a must for people who take these medications. Other immunizations should be discussed with the patient's physician because immunizations prepared with live virus should be avoided. Parents who are taking immune modulating agents should check with their child's pediatrician before their child receives oral polio vaccine because the virus is shed in stool and urine for a period of time following immunization. Some immune modulating agents have a teratogenic effect; women of child-bearing age should consult their physician before considering pregnancy while taking these drugs.

Agents used in diagnostic tests

A number of different pharmacological agents may be used in the diagnosis of GI disorders, including pentagastrin (Peptavlon), which stimulates gastric acid secretion, and bentiromide (Chymex) and secretin, which are used in tests of pancreatic exocrine secretion. The cholinergic agent edrophonium chloride (Tensilon) is used for provocative testing in patients with noncardiac chest pain. Glucagon is also used in diagnostic and therapeutic procedures, primarily to reduce GI motility. Exogenous administration of the GI hormone cholecystokinin (Kinevac) may be used in diagnostic procedures in which gallbladder contraction is desired.

Gallstone therapeutic agents

A number of chemical agents are available that may be used to dissolve gallstones, including monooctanoin (Moctanin) and the bile salts chenodeoxycholic acid (CDCA, Chenix) and ursodeoxycholic acid (UDCA, Actigall).

Both CDCA and UDCA are used to dissolve cholesterol gallstones. They decrease the rate of secretion of cholesterol into bile, thus causing the bile to become desaturated with cholesterol. This unsaturated bile dissolves cholesterol molecules from gallstones and holds them in micellar or vesicular solution until gallbladder contraction discharges them into the duodenum. Therapy must be continued until the stones dissolve completely, typically 6 to 24 months.

Medical dissolution therapy dissolves gallstones completely in up to 50% of selected patients with cholesterol stones. Urosodeoxycholic acid studies have shown clinical significance in treatment of microlithiasis post-cholestectomy. Microlithiasis is referred to as sludge, biliary sand, biliary sediment, and reversible cholelithiasis. Clinical conditions associated with the formation of microlithiasis are prolonged fasting, total parenteral nutrition, rapid weight loss, pregnancy and chronic illness. It is contraindicated for patients without patent cystic ducts, patients with radiopaque (pigment) stones, women who are or may be pregnant, and patients with stones that are larger than 15 mm in diameter. Contraindications to CDCA, but not UDCA, include severe obesity, liver disease, and inflammatory bowel disease. Potential adverse effects of CDCA include hepatic toxicity, diarrhea, and increases in serum LDL cholesterol. These adverse effects are not associated with UDCA.

Monooctanoin is used to dissolve cholesterol stones that are retained in the biliary tract after cholecystectomy. It is administered as a continuous infusion through a catheter inserted directly into the common bile duct via a T-tube or through a nasobiliary catheter. Administration of monooctanoin is contraindicated in patients with clinical jaundice, significant biliary tract infection, or a history of recent duodenal ulcer or jejunitis. Adverse reactions, including GI pain and discomfort, nausea, and vomiting, may be relieved by slowing the infusion rate or discontinuing infusion between meals.

Laxatives, cathartics, and bulk agents

Laxatives and **cathartics** are used to induce defecation. They are most commonly classified by their mechanisms of action.

1. Hyperosmotic colonic lavage solutions act by increasing intraluminal pressure, which stimulates peristalsis. These solutions are used primarily to cleanse the bowel in preparation for GI examination. Polyethylene glycol (Colyte, Golytely, Nulytely) is an example of a colon electrolyte lavage preparation. It can be administered orally or by nasogastric tube infusion. Polyethylene glycol (PEG-3350) without added electrolytes, in the form of a virtually tasteless powder (Miralax) mixed with water or juice is available for daily dose treatment of slow transit constipation in adults and encopresis in children

2. Stimulant cathartics act by producing local irritation or by stimulating Auerbach's plexus, resulting in increased intestinal motility. They are contraindicated in the presence of obstruction or peritonitis or immediately after bowel surgery. Bisacodyl (Dulcolax) is an example of a stimulant cathartic.

3. Bulk-forming cathartics are composed of natural or synthetic polysaccharides or cellulose derivatives that expand in the intestine without being absorbed and thus facilitate normal elimination. They are used to relieve chronic constipation and to ease passage of stool in patients with anorectal disorders. Psyllium (Metamucil) is an example of a bulk-forming laxative. The addition of fruits and natural fiber to the diet has the same effect.

4. Lubricant cathartics soften the stool by acting as wetting agents. The most common drug in this category is mineral oil.

5. Emollient laxatives act as surfactants that soften the fecal mass by facilitating the mixture of aqueous and fatty substances. They increase the secretion of water in both the small bowel and the colon. Docusate sodium (Modane) is an emollient laxative.

Laxatives may be used to cleanse the bowel before radiographic examination, colonoscopy, flexible or rigid sigmoidoscopy, or surgery; to eliminate a substance or organism from the GI tract; or to prevent hardened stools in patients with a colostomy or hemorrhoids. They may also be used to prevent straining, to obtain a stool specimen, or simply to treat constipation.

Narcotics and antagonists

Narcotic analgesics, particularly meperidine (Demerol) and sublimaze (Fentanyl) may be used for premedication of patients undergoing endoscopic procedures. They may also be used for postoperative pain relief.

Narcotics should be used sparingly, because they tend to mask symptoms and complications and may cause physical and psychological dependence. Abrupt discontinuance of the drug may precipitate withdrawal symptoms, including convulsions and a decrease in bowel motility.

Morphine should not be given to patients with biliary or

pancreatic problems, either preoperatively or postoperatively, because it may increase smooth muscle spasm. Meperidine is usually the drug of choice for these patients. Morphine must also be restricted in patients with severe liver disease.

Fentanyl citrate (Sublimaze) appears to have less emetic activity than either morphine or meperidine. In addition, clinically significant histamine release rarely occurs with fentanyl.

The most dangerous side effect of narcotic medications is respiratory depression. Respiratory depression and sedation and hypotension can be reversed by administration of naloxone (Narcan), which is thought to antagonize the opioid effects by competing for the same receptor sites.

Sclerosing agents

Sclerotherapy is used to stop bleeding from esophageal varies or to obliterate varices that previously bled. Sclerosing agents, such as morrhuate sodium (Scleromate), sodium tetradecyl sulfate (Sotradecol), ethanolamine oleate (Ethamolin), and 100% ethanol are injected intravariceally or paravariceally to promote intima inflammation and thrombus formation in patients with esophageal varices. The subsequent formation of fibrous tissue results in partial or complete vein obliteration. Potential complications post-procedure for scleortherpy may be various degrees of bleeding, esophageal ulcers, esophageal perforation, esophagopleural fistula, sepsis and precipitate or increase in hepatic encephalopathy.

Sedatives and antagonists

Sedatives and antianxiety agents, such as diazepam (Valium) and midazolam (Versed) are used in the practice of gastroenterology primarily to medicate patients before and during endoscopic or invasive procedures. They may be used to relieve preprocedural anxiety and tension and to decrease recall of the procedure. Sedatives are most commonly used to achieve conscious sedation for the patient during an endoscopic examination. The use of sedatives to achieve conscious sedation requires specialized training and competency of the gastroenterology nurse. Patients will require uninterrupted monitoring throughout the procedure as conscious sedation is initiated, achieved, and resolved. Resuscitative equipment must be readily available.

The most serious side effect of conscious sedation with diazepam or midazolam is a centrally mediated respiratory depression, which seems to occur in at least 1% of patients. Apnea is associated with rapid IV injection of either drug. The extent of respiratory depression is dependent on dosage, rate of administration, and individual susceptibility. Sedative effects are accentuated by the concomitant administration of other central nervous system depressants, such as opiates, barbiturates, or alcohol. Compared with diazepam, midazolam is more potent and faster acting and has a greater amnesic effect. Diazepam is associated with more injection site complications, such as thrombophlebitis.

Reversal agents

Sedative effects of benzodiazepines (i.e., diazepam, midazolam) may be reversed with flumazenil (Romazicon). Respiratory depression from benzodiazepines will not be reversed with this agent. Flumazenil is given intravenously in individualized doses (0.2 mg/min), not to exceed 1 mg at a time and not more than 3 mg/hr. The drug acts in minutes, but its duration is considerably shorter than that of the benzodiazepines. Careful monitoring for "resedation" must be carried out.

Naloxone (Narcan) reverses both sedation and respiratory depression associated with administration of opioids. As with flumazenil, multiple doses may be necessary, because the drug's duration is shorter than that of the opioid. Careful monitoring for "resedation" must be carried out.

When given a reversal agent, outpatients in the endoscopy unit should not be discharged home until the nurse is reasonably certain that the effect of the reversal agent has worn off (usually a minimum of 1 hour).

Smooth muscle relaxants

Agents that have a direct relaxant effect on the smooth muscle fibers of the LES can alleviate esophageal symptoms of achalasia and diffuse esophageal spasm in some patients. Sublingual isosorbide dinitrate (Isordil) can improve symptoms and radionuclide transit time. Calcium channel blockers, such as nifedipine (Procardia), also have recognized relaxant effects on LES muscle.

Topical anesthetics

Topical **anesthetics,** such as benzocaine (Cetacaine), lidocaine (Xylocaine), and dyclonine (Dyclone), are used in gastroenterology to suppress the gag reflex and to control pain for upper GI endoscopic procedures.

Other agents

Other drugs used in the treatment of GI disorders include 5-aminosalicylic acid (Rowasa), sulfasalazine (Azulfidine), pancrelipase (Cotazym), cholestyramine (Questran), penicillamine (Cuprimine), vasopressin (Pitressin), neomycin (Mycifradin), lactulose (Cephulac), and interferon alfa (Intron-a).

Mesalamine, or 5-aminosalicylic acid (5-ASA), may be administered in the form of a suspension retention enema for patients with distal ulcerative colitis; proctosigmoiditis or proctitis; and radiation enteritis and colitis. The suspension enema also contains potassium metabisulfite, which may cause life-threatening allergic reactions in patients with sulfite sensitivity. Epinephrine is the preferred treatment for serious allergic or emergency situations.

Sulfasalazine, which is a complex of sulfapyridine and 5-ASA, has been proven effective in the maintenance of clinical remission and in the treatment of mildly to moderately severe attacks of ulcerative colitis. It is also effective in active Crohn's colitis and ileocolitis, although it does not appear to be as effective in ileitis alone. Side effects are common and include nausea, vomiting, headache, rash, and skin sensitivity to sun exposure.

5-ASA may also be administered orally as olsalazine sodium (Dipentum) and oral mesalamine (Asacol, Pentasa). These drugs have proven as effective as sulfasalazine in preventing relapse of ulcerative colitis, but without the side effects associated with the sulfapyridine moiety. Research has demonstrated that some forms (Asacol, Pentasa) are effective when disease is proximal to the colon.

Pancrelipase is a combination of digestive enzymes, including lipase, protease, and amylase. It is used to decrease the number of bowel movements and improve stool consistency in patients with pancreatic exocrine insufficiency, cystic fibrosis, steatorrhea, and other disorders of fat metabolism. Pancreatin (Donnazyme) is also prescribed to relieve steatorrhea, pyrosis, flatulence, and belching associated with incomplete digestion of food caused by a deficiency of digestive enzymes.

Cholestyramine is an anion exchange resin that is used to lower plasma cholesterol levels. It adsorbs and combines with bile acids in the intestine to form an insoluble complex that is excreted in the feces. This increased fecal loss of bile acids leads to an increased oxidation of cholesterol to bile acids, a decrease in plasma LDLs, and a decrease in serum cholesterol. In patients with partial biliary obstruction, the reduction of serum bile acid levels reduces excess bile acids deposited in the skin, resulting in a decrease in pruritus. Cholestyramine is contraindicated in patients with complete biliary obstruction. The most common adverse reactions are constipation, abdominal discomfort, and nausea.

Penicillamine is the drug of choice for patients with Wilson's disease, which is a hereditary disorder of copper metabolism. Patients with Wilson's disease must be committed to lifelong administration of a daily dose of penicillamine, which chelates to copper and then is excreted in the urine. Complete reversal or improvement of hepatic, neurological, and psychiatric abnormalities can be expected in most patients, although a small proportion develop serious toxic reactions and may require administration of an alternative chelating agent.

IV vasopressin is used to stop variceal bleeding. Studies have shown that approximately 52% of patients stop bleeding when treated with vasopressin. The preferred method of administration is by constant IV infusion. Side effects include an increase in peripheral vascular resistance, bradycardia, coronary vasoconstriction (which may precipitate myocardial infarction in patients with coronary artery disease), and bowel ischemia. Vasopressin should be used only in intensive care settings with close cardiac monitoring.

Neomycin and lactulose are both used in the treatment of hepatic encephalopathy. Neomycin acts by reducing the production of the nitrogenous breakdown products that cause encephalopathy. Bacterial breakdown of lactulose acidifies the colonic contents, resulting in the retention of ammonia in the colon and a concomitant reduction in blood ammonia levels.

Recent research has shown that hepatitis C (non-A, non-B hepatitis) is the most common infectious cause of chronic liver disease. Several kinds of interferon products have been developed to fight Hepatitis C virus (HCV). The most commonly used ones are shown on Table 20–3. Interferon works against the hepatitis C virus by: (1) preventing the virus from entering into cells; (2) interfering with the virus's ability to make the proteins it needs to live; (3) stimulating the production of other immune system defenders; and (4) increasing the immune system's ability to recognize viral cells so that it can be destroy them. Ribavirin is an oral antiviral agent that is used in combination with interferon. Ribavirin is a nucleoside analogue that does not work when used alone against HCV. The length of treatment course depends on viral genotype. Both interferon and ribavirin can cause side effects, some of the more common are listed on Table 20–3.

CASE SITUATION

Davy Simms is admitted to the endoscopy unit with a persistent reflux problem manifested by vomiting or "spitting up." Regurgitation occurs within $1^1/_2$ to 2 hours following ingestion of food or fluids. Davy is 6 months old and was diagnosed as having a patent ductus arteriosus at the age of 4 weeks. He is a poor feeder, is highly irritable and fussy, and is on the low borderline developmental scale for his age. He weighs $13^1/_2$ pounds (6.1 kg), is $24^1/_2$ inches in length, and has a body surface area of 0.33 meters (based on a precalculated approximation). Because he lives in a high streptococcus incident area of the country and has two siblings, ages 5 and 7, he is on a daily dose of prophylactic ampicillin (20 mg). He is to have general anesthesia for the endoscopic procedure. His pediatrician orders 65 mg of ampicillin and 12 mg of gentamicin to be given by IV drip over a 1-hour period. Sedation will be by diazepam (Valium), given orally 1 hour before the procedure.

Points to think about

1. What might be the rationale for not using the drug Versed (midazolam) to sedate this patient?
2. What are the benefits of using diazepam as an adjunct to an anesthetic agent?
3. Why would diazepam be given orally in this patient rather than intravenously or intramuscularly?

Suggested responses

1. Conscious sedation in a 6 month old is risky because of the inherent danger associated with esophagoscopy in an infant who cannot be sedated enough or cannot understand the need to remain still during the procedure. Although general anesthesia has its own associated difficulties, it precludes movement during the procedure.
2. The benefits of diazepam as a premedication include the following:
   (a) reduction of fear and anxiety resulting from the

unknown and, in this case, parental separation;

(b) sedation and amnesia;

(c) probable better acceptance of face mask;

(d) few nightmares; and

(e) not likely to cause hypotension, tachycardia, dizziness, excitement, and/or postoperative nausea and vomiting.

3. Diazepam probably would be given orally to this patient for the following reasons:

(a) It absorbs rapidly from the GI tract.

(b) The rate of absorption from the IM route is erratic and absorption depends on the muscle into which the drug is injected (deltoid and upper thigh preferred rather than buttock). These muscles are relatively small in an infant.

(c) The drug cannot be mixed with other drugs for IV use.

(d) The drug may cause persistent pain at the injection site if given intramuscularly and may cause superficial, painless venous thrombosis when given intravenously in small veins.

CASE SITUATION

Susan Jones is a 35-year-old, 165-pound (77 kg) female who underwent an upper endoscopy. She received 7.5 mg of midazolam (Versed) during the procedure in titrated doses for conscious sedation. Ms. Jones was highly agitated throughout the endoscopic procedure. Her first postoperative vital signs were blood pressure 120/82, pulse 80, respirations 14, oxygen level 98%.

Points to think about

1. What should the postprocedure nurse anticipate in the course of recovery for Ms. Jones?

2. Why was a reversal agent not used immediately postprocedure?

3. What are the responsibilities of the gastroenterology nurse when conscious sedation is used on an adult patient?

Suggested responses

1. The usual dose of midazolam (Versed) for conscious sedation does not normally exceed 5 mg titrated throughout the procedure. Ms. Jones was highly agitated throughout the procedure, requiring continuous titration of midazolam for a total of 7.5 mg. The postoperative nurse should expect Ms. Jones to be highly sedated once the stimulus of the endoscopy is concluded.

2. A reversal agent for midazolam (Versed) is not necessarily warranted in a patient who is hemodynamically stable but sedated. Some physicians will order the reversal agent flumazenil (Romazicon) immediately postprocedure to block any further uptake of the benzodiazepine Versed, which will generally reverse the effects of the midazolam in 1 to 3 minutes and cause the patient to awaken from

sedation. Most physicians will not use a reversal agent if vital signs are stable with oxygen saturations above 90% to 92% and allow the patient to awaken slowly.

3. The responsibilities of the registered nurse in the gastroenterology laboratory when conscious sedation is used for an adult are as follows.

Preoperative phase:

(a) Perform a nursing assessment.

(b) Verify presence of signed, informed consent.

(c) Establish venous access.

(d) Explain procedure; medications; what patient can expect before, during, and after procedure; and review postendoscopy instructions.

Intraoperative phase:

(a) Monitor the patient's physical parameters.

(b) Document all events occurring during the procedure and patient's status on completion.

(c) Reassure patient verbally and by touch.

Postoperative phase:

(a) Monitor patient's condition and level of consciousness.

(b) Document all findings and events.

(c) Provide verbal and written instructions regarding diet, medications, activities, and signs and symptoms of complications with action to take if complications develop.

(d) Ensure that the patient meets institutional discharge criteria.

REVIEW TERMS

anesthetics, antacids, antibiotics, anticholinergic, antidiarrheal, antiemetics, antiflatulent, cathartics, cholinergic, corticosteroids, histamine₂ (H₂) blockers, laxatives, narcotics, oral, parenteral, prostaglandins, sedatives, topical

REVIEW QUESTIONS

1. When used in a medication order, the abbreviation "ac" indicates that the drug is to be administered:

(a) At mealtime.

(b) At bedtime.

(c) Before meals.

(d) As needed.

2. One kilogram is equivalent to approximately:

(a) 2.2 pounds.

(b) 22 ounces.

(c) 20 pounds.

(d) 1000 ounces.

3. Pediatric dosages are usually calculated based on the child's:

(a) Weight in kilograms.

(b) Height and weight.

(c) Age.

(d) Surface area.

4. For optimal effect, antacids should be given:

(a) Before meals.

(b) Immediately after meals.

(c) 1 hour after meals.

(d) At bedtime.

5. Antacids work by:

(a) Decreasing acid secretion.

(b) Coating or protecting mucous lining.

(c) Reducing total acid load.

(d) Decreasing gastric pH.

6. Anticholinergics are primarily used as adjunct therapy for peptic ulcer disease in combination with:

(a) Cholinergics.

(b) Sedatives.

(c) Antacids or H_2 blockers.

(d) Antiflatulents or antiemetics.

7. Corticosteroids are used most often in gastroenterology in patients who have:

(a) Inflammatory bowel disease.

(b) Peptic ulcers.

(c) Pancreatic exocrine insufficiency.

(d) Cholelithiasis.

8. The purpose of glucagon in GI diagnostic testing is to:

(a) Reduce GI motility.

(b) Stimulate gastric acid secretion.

(c) Stimulate production of bile.

(d) Increase GI motility.

9. The use of sedatives for endoscopic procedures to achieve conscious sedation requires:

(a) Ability to continuously monitor the patient.

(b) Sedation competency by the practitioners.

(c) Resuscitative equipment readily available.

(d) All of the above.

10. Omeprazole (Prilosec) is a proton pump inhibitor that:

(a) Inhibits production of stomach acid.

(b) Can cause bleeding.

(c) Increases the production of stomach acid.

(d) Is used to treat ulcerative colitis.

BIBLIOGRAPHY

Albanese, J. (1982). *Nurses' drug reference* (2nd ed.). New York: McGraw Hill.

Arky, R. (1996). *Physician's desk reference*. Montvale, NJ: Medical Economics.

Aronson, B. (1998). Update on peptic ulcer drugs, *American Journal of Nursing 98*(1), 41-7.

ASHP Therapeutic Guidelines for nonsurgical antimicrobial prophylaxis. (1999). *Ameri JourHealth Syst Pharma 56*, 1201-50.

Barnhart, F. (Ed.) (1997). *Physicians' desk reference* (51st ed.) Oradell, NJ: Medical Economics.

Benitz, W.E. & Tatro, D.S. (1995). *The pediatric drug handbook* (3rd edition). St. Louis MO: Mosby.

Bharucha, A.E. (2001, March). Slow transit constipation. *Gastroenterol Clin North Am 30*(1), 77-95.

Blume, D. (1980). *Dosages and solution* (3rd ed.). Philadelphia: F.A. Davis.

Bongiovanni, G. (Ed.) (1988). *Essentials of clinical gastroenterology* (2nd ed.). New York: McGraw-Hill.

Cappell, M.S. & Abdullah, M. (2000). High risk, underappreciated, obscure, or preventable causes of gastrointestinal bleeding. *Gastroentero Clinics 29*(1), 125-67.

Chopra, S. & May, R. (Eds.) (1989). *Pathophysiology of gastrointestinal diseases*. Boston: Little, Brown.

Clark, C.H. (1999). Hepatitis C: Role of the advanced practice nurse. *AACN Clinical Issues 10*, 455-63.

Claussen, D.S. (1995). The newest proton pump inhibitor. *Gastroenterol Nurs 18*(6), 235-6.

Claussen, D.S. (1994). Versed administration for IV conscious sedation. *Gastroenterol Nurs 17*(2), 80-4.

Damsgard, C. (1985). *Gastrointestinal Assistant certification review manual*. Rochester, NY: Society of Gastrointestinal Assistants.

Davis, G. (1989). Treatment of chronic hepatitis C with recombinant Interferon alfa: a multicenter randomized controlled trial. *New Engl J Med 321*, 1501-6.

De Vault, K.R. (1999, December). Overview of medical therapy for gastroesophageal reflux disease. *Gastroenterol Clinics 28*, 831-48.

Dewalt, S. (2002, April). *Interferons: what are the differences? Hepatitis*, 26-9.

Franciscus, A. (2003). *How does interferon work?* [On-line.] Available: http://www.hcvadvocate.org/Oldsite/200205/interferon.htm.

Given, B. & Simmons, S. (1984). *Gastroenterology in clinical nursing* (4th ed.). St. Louis, MO: Mosby.

Gruber, M. & Camara, D. (1988). Injection sclerotherapy: seven years' experience. In Trivits, S. (Ed.), *SGA Journal Reprints*, Rochester, NY: Society of Gastrointestinal Assistants.

Hamilton. H. (Ed.) (1983). *Procedures, Nurse's Reference Library*. Springhouse, PA: Intermed Communications.

Joint Commission on Accreditation of Healthcare Organizations (2002, August). *The 2003 National Patient Safety Goals*. [On-line.] Available: www.JCAHO.org.

Kirby, D. (1989). Management of esophageal varices: a review of treatment options and the role of the gastroenterology nurse and associate. *Gastroenterol Nurs 12*, 10-4.

Kirsch, M. (1991). Intralesional steroid injections for peptic esophageal strictures. *Gastrointest Endosc 37*, 180-2.

Kochhar, R. (1999, April). Intralesional steroids augment the effects of endoscopic dilation in corrosive esophageal strictures. *Gastrointest Endosc 49*,.

Levy, M. (2002, February). The hunt for microlithiasis in idiopathic pancreatitis: Shold we abandon the search or intensify our efforts? *Gastrointest Endosc 49*,.

Masci, E., Testoni, P.A., Passaretti, S. (1985). Compararison of ranitidine, domperidone maceate and ranitidine and domperidone maleate in the short term treatment of reflux esophagitis. *Drugs EXP Clin Res 11*, 687-92.

National Digestive Diseases Information Clearinghouse (2002, May 11). *Chronic hepatitis C: current disease management*. [On-line.] Available: http://www.niddk.gov/health.digest/pubs/chrnhepc/chrnhepc.htm.

Springhouse. (1990). *Nursing90 Books: Nursing90 drug handbook*, Springhouse, PA: Springhouse.

Pashankar, D.S. & Bishop, W.P. (2001, September). Efficacy and optimal dose of daily polyethylene glycol 3350 for treatment of constipation and encopresis in children. *JPediatrc 139*(3), 428-32.

Physicians' Desk Reference (55th ed.) (2001). Montvale, NJ: Medical Economics.

Remington's pharmaceutical sciences (1995). Easton, PA: Mark Publishing.

Rybacki, J.J. & Long, J.W. (1997). *The essential guide to prescription drugs*. New York: Harper Perennial-Harper Collins Publishers.

Schroeder, S., Krupp, M. & Tierney, L. Jr. (Eds.) (1988). *Current medical diagnosis and treatment*. Norwalk, CN: Appleton and Lange.

Shannon, J.T., Wilson, B.A. & Stang, C.L. (1995). *Gouani and Hayes drugs and nursing implications* (8th ed.). Stamford, CN: Appleton and Lange.

Sievert, W. (2002). Management issues in chronic viral hepatitis: hepatitis C. *J Gastrenterol Hepatol 17*, 415-22.

Swartz, M. (1990). Cytotec (misoprostol). *Gastroenterol Nurs 13*, 37-9.

Swartz, M. (1990). Losec (omeprazole/MSD). *Gastroenterol Nurs 12*, 274-6.

Taketomo, C., Hodding, J. & Kraus, D. (1996). *Pediatric dosage handbook*. Washington, DC: American Association for Clinical Chemistry.

Van Ness, M. & Gurney, M. (Eds.) (1989). *Handbook of gastrointestinal drug therapy*. Boston: Little, Brown.

U.S. Veterans Affairs (2002, November 17). *Treatment Recommendations for Patients with Chronic Hepatitis C 2002* (version 1.0). [On-line.]

Available: http://www.va.gov/hepatitisc.

Wallace, M.R. & Oldfield, E.C (2001, September). The role of antibiotics in the treatment of infectious diarrhea. *Gastoenterol Clin North Am 30*(3), 817-36.

Williams, S. & DiPalma, J. (1990). Constipation in the long-term care facility. *Gastroenterol Nurs 12,* 179-82.

Chapter 21

INTRAVENOUS THERAPY

This chapter will acquaint the gastroenterology nurse with the principles of intravenous (IV) therapy. In addition to parenteral hyperalimentation, which is discussed in Chapter 22, IV lines are used in gastroenterology practice to administer **crystalloids** for the maintenance of fluid and electrolyte balance; to administer certain drugs; and to transfuse **colloids,** such as whole blood, packed red blood cells, fresh frozen plasma, platelets, and albumin. Current issues on minimizing the risks and complications to the patient such as medication errors, infection, speedshock and infiltration will be discussed. Gastroenterology nurses must have a working knowledge of standards of practice, principles and application in IV therapy to ensure a safe working environment for themselves, colleagues and patients.

The complexity of IV therapy practice demands a higher level of expertise and training than ever before. To maximize continuity and quality of care, many institutions have designated trained IV teams, including registered nurses and pharmacists, who manage specific aspects of IV therapy. However, gastroenterology clinicians are often responsible for patient observation and for routine IV care, such as tubing changes, site care, and dressing changes. Most importantly, the aim of nurses administering any form of IV care, medications, or infusion must be to ensure safety for patient and themselves.

Learning objectives

After reviewing the content of this chapter, the gastroenterology nurse should be able to:

1. Discuss the nurse's role in IV therapy care.
2. Discuss the basic principles of fluid and electrolytes balance, early detection and reporting of imbalances, and correct method of administration of IV solutions.
3. Describe IV administration risks both to nurse and patient.
4. Explain IV equipment and administration of IV drug therapy in gastroenterology patients.
5. Describe techniques for transfusing blood and blood products in gastroenterology patients, along with signs, symptoms, and treatment of adverse reactions.

GASTROENTEROLOGY NURSE'S ROLE IN IV THERAPY

The overall role for gastroenterology nurses during IV therapy is to enhance the patient's experience and provide holistic care by using the nursing process (chapters 8, 11, 12, 13). The first step is patient assessment that includes patient's knowledge and experiences of intravenous therapy, diagnosis, activity level and mental state, as well as duration and type of therapy. Planning requires identification of the appropriate person to place the vascular access device (VAD), type of VAD and dressing. Implementation includes preparing the patient, environment and the equipment. Gastroenterology nurse's responsibilities for IV therapy is to have: (a) knowledge of the VAD used, (b) skills in performing the procedure competently and safely, (c) inspecting the insertion site, (d) problem solve as necessary, (e) monitor the patient's condition and report changes and (f) maintain recording keeping.

FLUIDS AND ELECTROLYTES

One important nursing goal for gastroenterology nurses is to maintain the patient's fluid and electrolyte balance.

Basic principles

A solution is a liquid that contains dissolved substances. The liquid portion of a solution is the *solvent;* the substance that is dissolved in the solvent is called the *solute.* **Osmosis** is the passage of a solvent, usually water, through a selectively permeable membrane that separates solutions of different concentrations. The solvent passes through the membrane from the region of lower concentration of solute to that of higher concentration of solute, thus tending to equalize the concentration of the two solutions.

Electrolytes are salts that dissociate in solution into electrically charged particles (ions), including: anions (negative ions) such as chloride, sulfate, bicarbonate, phosphate, organic acids, and proteins; and cations (positive ions) such as sodium, potassium, calcium, and magnesium. Electrolytes help to maintain osmotic pressure within cells. The concentration of particles is expressed as milliequivalents per milliliter (mEq/ml). One milliequivalent of any cation is able to react with one milliequivalent of any anion. Ordinarily, electrolyte solutes are balanced so there is an equal distribution of cations and anions.

Nonelectrolytes, such as glucose, urea, bile salts, creatinine, and cholesterol, do not dissociate in water into anions and cations, but they do affect the acid-base balance and osmotic pressure gradients.

The osmolality of a solution is determined by the concentration of solute in that solution. Osmotic pressure develops because of the differing concentrations of solute on either side of a membrane, expressed in units called osmols (Osm). One osmol is the number of particles in 1 g molecular weight of undissociated solute. One thousandth of an osmol is a milliosmol (mOsm).

Body fluid makes up about 60% of the average adult's body weight. It consists largely of water (45% to 70%) and dissolved minerals, proteins, and other nutrients and gases that are necessary for normal cell function. Body fluid exists in two main compartments: the intracellular compartment (within the cells) and the extracellular compartment (outside the cells). The extracellular compartment includes the plasma, the interstitial fluid (the fluid around the cells), and the fluid and electrolytes from certain secreting and excreting organs and tissues. Usually, two thirds of body fluid is in the intracellular compartment, and one third is in the extracellular compartment.

Water moves freely between the intracellular and extracellular compartments, maintaining an osmotic equilibrium. Thus, if the extracellular electrolyte concentration increases, water diffuses from the intracellular compartment to the extracellular compartment, thereby increasing cellular tonicity and diluting the extracellular compartment and vice versa.

Fluid and electrolyte imbalances

The body receives water through the oral intake of fluids and solid foods. Water is also produced by the chemical oxidation of nutrients. In addition, approximately 8 L of water is secreted daily via saliva, gastric juice, bile, pancreatic secretions, and enteric fluids by the GI organs.

Under normal conditions, the body loses water daily in the urine and feces, by perspiration, and via insensible (immeasurable) losses through the skin and the lungs. Patients may also lose fluids and electrolytes during surgery or through vomiting, diarrhea, suction, draining wounds, intestinal obstructions, draining fistulas, hemorrhage, infections, or prolonged use of enemas and laxatives. Infants are especially vulnerable to fluid loss because of their high proportion of body fluid, immature kidneys, increased heat production, and rapid growth.

Excessive loss of body water can result in dehydration. The goal of nursing in dehydrated patients is to restore the circulating volume of fluid without causing an overload. Careful observation, recording, and reporting of the patient's signs and symptoms and fluid intake and output are essential in such patients.

In addition to fluid imbalances, patients should be monitored for possible electrolyte disturbances. The most common imbalances of electrolytes in the GI tract are excesses or deficits of chloride, magnesium, sodium, potassium, bicarbonate, calcium, or hydrogen ions.

Systematic observations to detect fluid and electrolyte imbalances include changes in temperature, pulse rate, respirations, and blood pressure. Fatigue and changes in skin and in mucous membranes and/or in speech, behavior, facial appearance, skeletal muscle, sensations, and body weight are also significant. Desire for food and water, anorexia, and thirst are important signs in detecting imbalances. Observations of importance relative to urine output include the specific gravity, pH, volume, and character. Significant observations should be relayed to the physician to facilitate early diagnosis and treatment before serious imbalances occur.

Administration of fluids and electrolytes

One way of correcting fluid and electrolyte disturbances is by IV administration of solutions containing the necessary electrolytes and nutrients. All IV solutions are considered medications, and their infusion requires a physician's order. The order should include the name of the solution/medication, volume/dose, rate, frequency, and route of administration. Consent of the patient or a legally authorized representative and the patient's identity must be confirmed before initiation of IV therapy.

IV therapy Administration Risks

Primary risks to the gastroenterology nurse are injury and disease transmission due to needlestick injury. Spills and splashes also pose a threat. Because universal precautions require the use of gloves when dealing with blood and body fluids, development of latex allergies pose concern for healthcare workers and patients. IV therapy administration complications risk for patients include, but not limited to: infiltration/extravasation, hematoma, vascular irritation, pyrogenic infections, air embolism, catheter embolism, pulmonary edema, and speedshock/overloading of vascular system (Table 21.1). Other potential risks for patients are drug incompatibilities and medication errors.

The United States (US) introduced groundbreaking legislation in November 2000 which resulted in the Needlestick Safety and Prevention Act (HR5178), which became part of US law in April 2001, requiring healthcare facilities to select and implement safer medical devices, such as sharps with engineered sharps injury protections and needleless systems to protect healthcare workers from needlestick injuries. Diseases most often transmitted to the nurse through exposure to the blood of an infected patient include viral hepatitis (B and C), as well as HIV. The risk of all infections increases if the needlestick injury involves deep penetration with a blood-filled hollow bore needle, such as those used to establish venous access. The risk of acquiring infection for a single needlestick is 30% for Hepatitis B, 3% for Hepatitis C and 0.3% for HIV. There are a number of sharps used in IV practice, such as needles, suture needles, cannulae and introducers, scalpels, glass tubes and glass medication vials/ampoules or bottles. As a result, a variety of needleless systems have been developed to limit needle exposure in the workplace.

Latex allergies have become a serious health issue among healthcare workers at all levels. Nurses must also be aware that patients have the potential of being allergic to or developing latex allergy. A large number of products contain latex, each of which presents a potential hazard for people with latex allergies. Patients must be screened for previous sensitivity. Several studies suggest that the most important factor in latex sensitization is the degree of exposure.

Healthcare professionals who use gloves frequently or for long periods face a high risk to develop allergy from latex products. Symptoms of latex sensitivity can range from mild local reaction to systemic anaphylaxis. Most common objective symptoms are; (a) erythema, itching, hives after donning gloves, (b) chest tightness, wheezing, cough, shortness of breath, (c) nasal rhinorrhea, sneezing, lacrimation, ocular itching with potential progression to systemic anaphylaxis. Latex reactions can occur within minutes of an exposure and up to 36-48 hours afterwards followed by recovery 4 to 12 hours after leaving the work environment. The risk from gloves increases as a result of modified starch powder used in some gloves.

The Medical Devices Agency (MDA) has issued guidelines outlining the risk of powered gloves to the wearer and to others in the surrounding area. All healthcare facilities must have polices and procedures in place to protect staff and patients from latex exposure and outline a treatment plan for latex exposure. Many manufactures have eliminated latex entirely from their products.

Equipment

The equipment needed for IV therapy generally includes needles and/or catheters, containers, tubing, filters, tourniquets, tape, antimicrobial agents, stands, clamps, and sometimes, electronic pumps and controllers. The method of IV administration and choice of equipment depends on patient's condition and desired effects of therapy. The three main methods for delivering fluids and/or drugs in the gastroenterology setting are: continuous infusion, intermittent infusion, and intermittent injection.

1. **Needles should be used only when absolutely necessary.** While it is not possible to eliminate needles completely, it is possible to minimize the use of needles to prevent needlestick injuries. When **needles** must be used the favorable choice is stainless steel coated with silicone. Because **needles** tend to dislodge and infil-

trate more frequently than catheters, the use of stainless-steel needles should be limited to single-dose or short-term therapy. Winged infusion sets (Butterfly needles) are used for short-term therapy in cooperative adult patients and for therapy in infants and children or in elderly patients with veins that are fragile or sclerotic (hardened and thickened).

2. **Catheters** are made of plastic, such as polyvinyl chloride, Teflon, or Silastic. They are generally considered better than needles alone for long-term therapy. Over-the-needle catheters that are radiopaque (appear light or white on x-ray films) should be used for routine IV therapy. Over-the-needle catheters are routinely used for IV infusion or IV medication administration and are commonly called *angiocatheters.* They are composed of a metal stylet that is used to pierce the skin and a plastic catheter that is threaded into the vein and remains for the instillation of fluid or medications. The flexible catheters are associated with lower infection rates, are the most reliable stable venous access, and should be used for IV therapy.

3. A **20- to 22-gauge flexible catheter** is used in most situations for adults, whereas a 22- to 24-gauge catheter can be used for small or fragile veins such as those seen in pediatric and geriatric patients. An 18- to 19-gauge catheter is recommended when large volumes of IV fluids, blood, or blood products are to be administered.

4. **Vascular access devices (VADs)** are catheters, cannulas, or infusion ports designed for long-term or repeated access to the venous or arterial systems. The most common use of a VAD is to deliver IV fluids and medications. There are two categories of VADs designated for IV access: central venous catheters and implanted infusion ports. Central venous catheters are inserted into large veins (cephalic, internal/external jugular, or subclavian) and threaded into the right atrium or to the tip of the right atrium. If the antecubital fossa is accessed with the catheter threaded into the tip of the right atrium, it is called a *peripherally inserted central catheter (PICC) line.* The second category of centrally placed IV access lines is called *infusion ports.* An infusion port is a surgically placed IV access line. Infusion ports consist of a self-sealing injection port housed in a plastic or metal case connected to a silicone venous catheter. The infusion port is usually implanted in the subcutaneous pocket in the infraclavicular fossa, and the catheter is inserted into a large vein and threaded into the right atrium.

5. The word **cannula** may be used to refer either to a stainless-steel needle or to a catheter. The cannula selected for peripheral insertion should be of the smallest diameter and shortest length that will accommodate the prescribed therapy.

6. Before use, IV fluid containers should be checked for cracks or tears, foreign matter, cloudiness, precipitation (settling out of solid particles), any other signs of contamination, and the expiration date.

7. IV tubing may be a regular (macrodrip) solution administration set that delivers 10 to 20 drops per ml or a microdrip set that delivers 60 drops per ml. Tubing with a secondary injection port permits separate or simultaneous infusion of two solutions; tubing with a piggyback port and a back-check valve permits intermittent infusion of a secondary solution. Vented tubing is used for solutions contained in a nonvented bottle, and nonvented tubing is used for solutions in vented bottles or containers.

8. A reduced-volume chamber (e.g., Buretrol) and/or infusion pump may be used in pediatric patients to prevent accidental fluid overload and to provide greater accuracy in rate of delivery of fluids.

9. Intermittent infusion sets (saline locks) consist of a flexible catheter with tubing ending in a resealable rubber injection port. The device is flushed with saline to prevent blood clot formation. Saline locks are used both to provide immediate access in case IV therapy is needed during a procedure and to maintain venous access in patients who are receiving IV medication regularly or intermittently but do not require continuous infusion of fluids.

10. Several different types of filters are utilized in IV therapy, including 0.2-μm bacteria-retentive, air-eliminating filters, which are recommended for routine use to decrease the complications of infection and air embolism; particulate-matter filters of 1 or 5 μm, which are used to remove particulate matter in situations where bacteria-retentive filters are contraindicated; and blood filters, which range from microaggregate filters that are 20 to 40 μm in size to standard 170-μm filters.

11. Tourniquets are applied above the intended insertion site to distend a vein with a larger-than-average amount of blood. Vein distention may also be enhanced by application of warm, moist heat; light tapping or massage of the skin over the veins; or having the patient open and close a fist several times. The tourniquet should impede venous, but not arterial, flow. This can be assessed by palpating for a radial pulse after applying the tourniquet. Tourniquets should be routinely discarded or disinfected after every procedure. To avoid circulatory impairment, they should be applied only for the short time needed to perform the venipuncture.

12. Half-inch tape or a transparent semipermeable membrane dressing may be used to anchor the needle or catheter on the skin. One-inch tape is used to secure the armboard or handboard, to secure a loop of tubing, and to secure the site dressing. When tape is used, it must not be applied directly to the skin-cannula junction site. Instead, an adhesive bandage with a gauze pad may be used. Hypoallergenic tape is available for patients who have tape allergies.

13. An antimicrobial agent, such as povidone-iodine (Betadine), is used to cleanse the IV site before venipuncture.

14. IV stands may be portable or may be attached to the bed or wall. To achieve the maximum flow rate, the infusion tubing drip chamber should be suspended approximately 3 feet above the injection site.

15. Mechanical flow-control clamps, including roller, screw, and slide clamps, are suitable for the regulation of most infusions, but electronic infusion pumps or controllers should be used when warranted by the patient's age and condition, the setting in which the therapy is delivered, and the prescribed therapy. Controllers regulate gravity flow either by counting drops or by measuring volume. Infusion pumps generate flow under positive pressure; they operate independently of gravity flow.

16. Patient-controlled analgesia (PCA) devices may be used to deliver IV analgesic agents. When these devices are used, patients must be educated as to the purpose of the PCA therapy, operating instructions, expected outcomes, precautions, and potential side effects. Medications administered through PCA devices are controlled substances, therefore, must be obtained, delivered, administered, documented, and discarded in accordance with state and federal regulations.

Intravenous solutions

The **tonicity** of body fluids refers to the effective osmotic pressure equivalent. IV fluids may be categorized as **isotonic** (having the same tonicity as the extracellular fluid), **hypotonic** (having a tonicity lower than the extracellular fluid), or **hypertonic** (having a tonicity greater than the extracellular fluid).

1. The **tonicity** of plasma is approximately 290 mOsm; this is considered isotonic. Isotonic solutions are considered to be compatible with body fluids when introduced into the vascular system.

2. Solutions less than 240 mOsm are considered hypotonic. Hypotonic solutions, (e.g., NaCl in water 0.45%), unless they are balanced with sufficient numbers of electrolytes, can flood the red blood cells, causing them to burst, a condition known as **hemolysis.**

3. Solutions with a tonicity greater than 340 mOsm are considered hypertonic. Improperly balanced hypertonic solutions (e.g., 10% dextrose in water) can cause red blood cells to shrink, a condition known as **crenation.**

IV fluids may be administered for maintenance or replacement purposes. Maintenance therapy meets the patient's ordinary needs by providing approximately 3000 ml of fluid per 24 hours, along with added electrolytes, nutrients, and vitamins. Replacement therapy restores lost fluids on a volume-to-volume basis, often in excess of 3000 ml/24 hr. The electrolyte concentration of replacement therapy is generally equal to the concentration of electrolytes in the extracellular fluid.

For maintenance therapy, a balanced hypotonic electrolyte solution with the addition of 5% dextrose for calories is ideal. This balanced electrolyte solution typically contains sodium, potassium, magnesium, chloride, and acetate. These solutions are available in concentrations appropriate for pediatric and adult patients.

Ideally, replacement therapy solutions should contain ions in the same composition as that of the plasma and interstitial fluid. Five-percent dextrose may or may not be included, depending on the caloric and fluid needs of the patient. A balanced isotonic multiple-electrolyte solution would include sodium, potassium, magnesium, chloride, acetate, and gluconate, with an average pH of 6.2. Most IV solutions have an acid pH, thus making them more stable and better able to withstand the effects of bacterial overgrowth.

The IV fluids administered most often are 5% dextrose in water (**D5W**), **normal saline** solution, and lactated **Ringer's solution.** Other IV solutions include carbohydrate in water, carbohydrate in sodium chloride, isotonic sodium chloride, potassium, vitamins, protein hydrolysates, and alcohol solutions. Fructose may be added instead of dextrose, because fructose is more rapidly metabolized and converted to glycogen.

Insertion sites

Selection of an insertion site for IV therapy depends on the type of solution; the type, frequency, and duration of therapy; the patient's age, size, diagnosis, and condition; and the patency, size, and location of available veins. The vessel chosen must accommodate the size of the catheter. When a heparin or saline lock is used to administer conscious sedation during endoscopic procedures, it is usually placed in a large vessel in the right arm. A large vessel is more appropriate, because the medications used to produce sedation can irritate the vessel wall.

When choosing an insertion site it is important to distinguish between veins and arteries. If a vessel pulsates, it is an artery. Puncture and the inadvertent injection of certain medications into arteries can lead to complications such as inflammation, necrosis, sloughing, and even gangrene and loss of function of the affected part.

Peripheral IV infusions are typically inserted in a superficial vein on the nondominant arm, including but not limited to the metacarpal, cephalic, basilic, and median veins. Jointed areas, thrombosed veins, varicosed veins, shunted areas, veins over joints, and traumatized or heavily scarred areas should be avoided. It is best to begin with distal veins and then proceed to more central venous access sites as warranted. If an infiltration occurs, cannulation must always be performed proximal to the previously cannulated site.

Generally, cannulation of the lower extremities should be avoided in adults because it increases the risk of thrombophlebitis and embolism. If an IV cannula must be placed in a lower extremity, it should be changed as soon as an alternative site can be established.

In infants and children, lower extremities may be used safely and effectively. These sites generally allow for access to the IV site even when the child has been "bundled" to provide restraint. Scalp veins are acceptable IV sites for infants.

Insertion technique

Before insertion the selected site should be cleansed with soap and water, if necessary. Then the site should be swabbed with an antimicrobial agent, most often povidone-iodine (Betadine), and permitted to air dry. A tourniquet should be applied above the intended insertion site. The use of intradermal lidocaine to numb the insertion site is controversial, and it need not be used routinely for cannula insertion.

For peripheral insertion, the skin is held taut and the vein is anchored with the thumb below the injection site. The needle is inserted slowly into the vein until blood return is noted, the needle or catheter is advanced, and the tourniquet is released. Primed tubing is connected and fluid is run at a fast rate to flush blood from the tubing. Once blood is cleared, the IV drip is regulated at the prescribed rate.

The cannula should be stabilized so it does not interfere with assessment and monitoring of the IV site or impede delivery of the prescribed therapy. An antimicrobial ointment is applied to the insertion site if desired, followed by a sterile gauze or transparent semipermeable membrane dressing. All edges of the dressing should be securely taped. Roller bandages obstruct visualization of the IV site and may impair circulatory flow. They are not recommended on an extremity where an IV cannula is placed. An armboard or handboard may be used if the cannula is placed close to an area of flexion.

A 3- to 6-inch portion of tubing is looped and taped at the insertion site. (The loop allows some slack to prevent dislodgement of the catheter caused by tension on the line.) Flow rate is adjusted, and all pertinent information is recorded.

Frequent monitoring of patients receiving IV therapy minimizes the risk of potential complications. Monitoring should include observation of the insertion site, flow rate, clinical data, and patient response to the prescribed therapy.

IV therapy can be discontinued on the order of a physician, on completion of therapy, for needle or catheter changes, or when infection or infiltration is suspected. The patient and/or a legally authorized representative also has the right to request discontinuation of treatment.

To remove a peripheral line, first the tubing is clamped, the tape is then removed from the skin, and the needle or catheter is withdrawn slowly and smoothly. Pressure should be maintained with a gauze pad at the insertion site until bleeding stops. When bleeding stops, the site should be cleansed with an antiseptic and a dry, sterile bandage should be applied.

Complications

IV therapy is an invasive procedure that is not without risks. Because the IV system provides direct access into the vascular system, stringent infection-control measures must be applied.

If an IV-related infection is suspected, the cannula, any purulent drainage, and the infusate should be cultured to identify the responsible microorganism. Blood cultures may be considered to determine the extent of the infection.

Other potential local, systemic, and mechanical complications associated with IV therapy include the following:

1. **Infiltration/extravasation;** the inadvertent administration of a solution/medication into surrounding tissue with escape of fluid from its physiologic space.
2. **Hematoma;** a swelling of tissue caused by a break in a blood vessel.
3. **Phlebitis;** (inflammation of a vein), marked by infiltration of vein and thrombus formation.
4. **Pyrogenic reactions;** including septicemia (blood poisoning) and bacteremia (presence of bacteria in the blood).
5. **Air embolism;** obstruction of a blood vessel caused by an air bubble.
6. **Catheter embolism;** or catheter fragments in the vascular system
7. **Pulmonary edema;** a potentially life-threatening accumulation of fluid in the lungs
8. **Speed shock/overload;** a systemic reaction that occurs when a foreign substance is introduced too rapidly into the circulation

These complications are listed in Table 21.1, with respective causes, signs and symptoms, and appropriate interventions.

Dosage calculations

The rate of flow of IV fluids can be affected by many factors, such as height of the fluid container, bent or kinked tubing, use of filters, medication additions, needle or catheter size, needle or catheter position, needle or catheter occlusion, or infiltration of IV fluid to the surrounding tissue. Patient movement or manipulation of the clamp may also be a factor. IV flow rate can be monitored by using a time tape, which indicates the prescribed solution level at hourly intervals.

The rules of ratio and proportion are used to calculate the rate of flow of IV fluids. It is important to check the rate of flow at least every 15 minutes for infants and children and at least every 30 minutes for adults if infusion pumps are not used. Every time the rate is checked, it is necessary to determine how much fluid is left to refigure the rate of flow needed and in what period of time it is to be administered.

Calculated infusion flow rates are only guidelines. Maintaining the calculated rate of flow does not relieve nurses of the responsibility to observe the patient for signs that the infusion is too rapid or too slow. Observation of

Table 21-1. Potential complications of intravenous therapy

Complication	Possible cause	Signs and symptoms	Intervention
Infiltration	Puncture of the vein wall or needle or cannula slipping out of the vein	Edema, pain, and burning at the venipuncture site	Discontinue infusion; remove cannula; restart at a different, more proximal location; elevate the affected part; apply cold compresses for the first 24 hrs, followed by warm, moist compresses
Hematoma	Unsuccessful attempt at venipuncture or infiltration of a blood transfusion	Painful, raised area, with blue or purplish patches	Remove needle or cannula; apply pressure and cold compresses
Phlebitis with or without clot formation	Vein irritation and inflammation; may occur postinfusion	Edema along the affected vein; sore, hard, cordlike, and warm vein	Discontinue infusion; remove cannula; apply warm, moist compresses; notify physician
Pyrogenic reactions	Contaminated equipment or solutions	Fever, chills, nausea and vomiting, backache, malaise	Discontinue infusion; culture cannula and solution and record lot number of solution; notify physician
Air embolism	Air in tubing; loose connections allowing air to enter tubing	Hypotension; cyanosis; heart murmur; tachycardia; syncope; vascular collapse; and loss of consciousness	Turn the patient on his or her left side with the head down; notify physician; check the system for leaks
Catheter embolism	Portion of a plastic cannula breaks off and flows into the vascular system; attempting to rethread the catheter with a needle; unsecured catheter	Vein discomfort; cyanosis; decreased blood pressure; weak, rapid pulse; loss of consciousness	Discontinue infusion; apply tourniquet above insertion site; notify physician; x-ray film taken to locate fragment
Pulmonary edema	Circulatory overload; excessive infusion flow rate	Headache; venous dilation; hypertension; coughing; dyspnea; tachycardia	Slow infusion to a keep-open rate; elevate the head of the bed and raise the patient's knees; notify physician
Speed shock	Too-rapid administration of solutions and medications	Shock; syncope; and cardiac arrest	Slow infusion to keep-open rate; resuscitate; notify physician

Modified from Hamilton H, ed: *Procedures,* Nurse's Reference Library, Springhouse, Pa, 1983, Intermed Communications patients for indications of too-rapid infusion is imperative. Pumps and controllers that automatically regulate the flow at a set rate should be used for infants, small children and older adults to prevent fluid overload. Smaller volume administration containers are also recommended for these groups.

Patient education

The establishment of rapport and an effective system of communication between the nurse and the patient is of utmost concern. It is important to explain the procedure to ensure cooperation and reduce anxiety, which can cause a vasomotor response resulting in venous constriction. IV therapy can be initiated only after the patient has exhibited signs of understanding and acceptance.

Before starting a continuous infusion, patient education needs to cover patient mobility, the importance of avoiding pressure to the IV site, keeping the site dry, and the fluid container at an appropriate height. Patients should be given an estimate of the approximate duration of therapy, warned not to adjust the flow rate and be advised to notify the nurse if they experience pain or other complications. Patient education and understanding requires documentation in the medical record directed by standards, policies and procedures utilized by the facility.

Documentation

Documentation of IV therapy should be legible and accessible to all healthcare professionals involved in the patient's care. Distinctive labeling should provide pertinent and easily identified information relative to the cannula, dressing, solution, medication, and administration set.

Documentation of any venipuncture should include the date and time of initiation, the amount and type of solution used, the type of needle or catheter and its gauge, the venipuncture site, and the rate of flow. The rate of flow should be recorded in ml/hr. Rates of flow in drops per minute are misleading, because drop factors vary from based on the tubing used. Any complications, anxiety, or untoward reactions on the part of the patient should be included in the record, along with nursing interventions taken.

INTRAVENOUS MEDICATION ADMINISTRATION

IV administration of medications has a number of advantages. Some drugs, including antibiotics, are frequently given intravascularly to provoke a quick, continuous therapeutic response. Other drugs may be given by the IV route because they are ineffective or dangerous by other routes. Some drugs are contraindicated for IV administration, including certain nonaqueous or suspension medications, because they obstruct blood flow.

Techniques and routes of administration

IV medications must have a physician's written order. Before medication administration, the nurse must assess; (a) the appropriateness of the prescribed therapy; (b) the patient's age and condition; (c) any medication allergies; and (d) the dose, route, and rate of the medication ordered. The nurse should be aware of the medication's indications, actions, and side effects, and appropriate nursing interventions in the event of adverse reactions. Before administering any medication it is important to verify the patient's identity and to check the label on the medication against the order on the patient's medication record and against the physician's order. Any discrepancies or concerns need to be brought to the physician's attention for clarification.

Before adding any drug to an IV solution it is also necessary to establish that the drug is compatible with the solution. Mixing of drugs in a continuous infusion should be done only after consultation with incompatibility lists and with the pharmacist. Aseptic technique should be used for admixing. The expiration date of solutions/medications must be ascertained. In addition, the physical and chemical compatibility of the delivery systems used must be confirmed. Incompatibilities can cause leakage, air embolism, occlusion, infection, and other undesirable effects. The addition of a drug to blood transfusions complicates identification of the source of adverse reactions, if any, and therefore should not be done.

Various methods can be used for IV drug administration, including the addition of drugs to the IV solution (continuous infusion); infusion through a secondary line (piggyback or add-a-line method); use of an intermittent infusion injection device (saline lock); and IV push injections.

1. Continuous infusions are diluted in a large quantity of fluid, from 250 to 1000 ml, and delivered over a 2- to 24-hour period. The medication is typically added to the infusion container by using a needle and syringe. After injecting the drug it is important to rotate the bottle or squeeze the bag to mix the solution thoroughly, observing the solution after the addition for any precipitation, discoloration, or cloudiness. After adding the medication, a label noting that medication has been added must be placed on the IV container. IV medications are often mixed in the pharmacy.

2. Implementing the piggyback method, a moderate quantity of fluid (usually 50 to 100 ml) is administered over a 5-minute to 2-hour period, using a separate small-volume IV fluid container that is attached either through the top of the drip chamber for the primary container or through a Y-connector on the tubing of the main line. This secondary container must be elevated above the level of the main line IV container. If the drug to be added through the piggyback set is incompatible with the primary IV solution, the line must be flushed with 0.9% sodium chloride before starting the drug infusion.

Intermittent infusion sets (saline or heparin locks) may be used for patients who are receiving IV medications regularly, either by the push method or intermittently, but who do not require continuous infusion of fluids. After insertion, saline is injected every 6 to 12 hours to maintain the patency of the infusion set. If the medication to be administered is compatible with heparin, the medication is injected in the time recommended, followed by an injection of heparinized saline to flush the medication and refill the catheter. If heparin is incompatible with the administered medications/solutions, the saline, administration, saline, heparin (SASH) procedure should be used. In this procedure, saline is used before and after administration of the medication and is followed by a final flush of heparinized saline.

IV push (bolus) medications may or may not be diluted in 0.25 to 50 ml of fluid. They are administered over a 5 second to 5 minute period, either by direct venipuncture or using in-progress infusion setups. If administered through an in-progress setup, the IV tubing above the injection site should be pinched during injection so the medication does not flow up to the bottle. The IV fluid should be permitted to flow rapidly for 30 to 60 seconds after injection to move the medication through the tubing.

The IV push method is often used in endoscopic procedures. It may be used to give conscious sedation, to provide an immediate drug effect in an emergency, to achieve peak drug levels in the bloodstream, or to deliver drugs that cannot be diluted or administered intramuscularly.

Indications for intravenous medication in gastroenterology

IV medications may be administered to gastroenterology patients for the following purposes:

(a) conscious sedation and/or analgesia; (e.g. use of diazepam (Valium), meperidine (Demerol), midazolam (Versed), or fentanyl (Sublimaze));

(b) control of variceal hemorrhage; for example, use of vasopressin (Pitressin) or octreotide (Sandostatin);

(c) treatment of narcotic-induced respiratory depression with naloxone (Narcan);

(d) treatment of bradycardia; for example, use of atropine; and

(e) reducing peristalsis or intestinal spasms; for example, use of glucagons.

In addition, IV antibiotics are given for prophylaxis in gastroenterology patients who are at risk for bacterial endocarditis or for patients with abdominal abscess, cholangitis, diverticulitis, or ulcerative colitis. Whenever prophylactic antibiotics are given, it is important to weigh the risks of infection against potential side effects of the medications.

Adverse reactions

After administering any drug it is important to observe the patient for signs of drug sensitivity or intolerance. If adverse effects occur, the medication should be discontinued and the physician should be notified.

Appropriate steps should be taken to reduce the risk of infection, as detailed above. To reduce vein irritation, the following steps may be taken:

1. Use the smallest gauge needle possible for IV push medications.
2. Use 3 to 10 ml saline following a 50- to 100-ml dose of antibiotic to prevent thrombus formation and vein irritation at the injection site.
3. Use intermittent, rather than continuous, infusions.

4. When possible, use normal saline as the IV fluid or diluent.
5. Use at least 50 to 100 ml of diluent with all antibiotics.
6. For IV therapy extending beyond 72 hours, rotate injection sites.

Medications should be timed as they are administered; exceedingly rapid administration can produce speed shock.

Certain complications of IV drug administration are specific to the method of administration.

1. Excessively high drug concentrations in the IV solution can cause complications, such as sclerosis, thrombosis (clot formation), hemolysis, or phlebitis.
2. With piggyback infusions, side effects and reactions to the infused drug can occur. Repeated punctures of the secondary injection port can cause an imperfect seal, with possible leakage or contamination.
3. Infiltration and a specific reaction to the infused drug are the most common complications of intermittent infusion devices.
4. With IV push injections, effects are often immediate, and signs of an acute allergic reaction or anaphylaxis can develop rapidly. If signs of anaphylaxis occur (i.e., dyspnea, cyanosis, convulsions, or increasing respiratory distress), the physician should be notified immediately and emergency measures should be instituted as necessary.

Infiltration is the leakage of infused solution from a vein into surrounding tissue, resulting from a needle puncturing a vascular wall or leakage around the venipuncture site. It causes local pain and itching, edema, blanching, and decreased skin temperature in the affected extremity. Infiltration of some drugs can severely damage tissue through irritative, sclerotic, vesicant, corrosive, or vasoconstrictive actions. Treatment of infiltrations of IV solutions and nonirritating drugs involves routine comfort measures, such as application of warm soaks. Infiltrations of corrosive drugs require emergency treatment to prevent tissue necrosis. If signs of infiltration occur, such as swelling, the absence of blood backflow, and/or a sluggish flow rate, the injection should be stopped, the amount of infiltration estimated, and the physician notified.

Documentation

Documentation requirements for IV medication infusions are similar to those that apply when administering fluids and electrolytes. In addition, it is important to document any medications added, the drip rate, and by whom they were added. For patients who arrive in an endoscopy unit with a line in place, the condition of the IV should be documented. The patient's response to IV medications should also be recorded. All unusual occurrences should be reported to the physician immediately. Written reports of adverse effects should include all signs, symptoms, treatment, and outcome. Encourage the physician to examine the patient and to draw a diagram on the chart indicating the location of pain or complications.

In the case of infiltration, record the site of the infiltration, the patient's symptoms, the estimated amount of infiltrated solution, the nursing treatment, the time, and the name of the physician notified. Continue to document the appearance of the infiltrated site and any associated symptoms.

BLOOD AND BLOOD COMPONENTS

The United States (U.S.) blood supply is among the safest in the world. The improvement of processing methods for blood products has reduced the number of infections resulting from these products. Each year, more than 11 million patients in the U.S. will receive blood therapy. Of those, approximately 1 in 10,000 - 20,000 may experience a mild febrile reaction. The frequency of blood transfusion complication related deaths are reported at 1 in 1,000,000 - 6,000,000 annually.

Federal, state and facility regulations require registered nurses to be trained before administering blood therapy. Blood therapy includes obtaining blood samples for type and crossmatching, ordering blood, checking blood supply with patient identification before administration, regulating blood infusing rate, observing the patient for adverse reactions, discontinuing blood, and documenting the therapy provided.

Techniques of blood administration

The trend in blood therapy is to administer fractionated blood components, as opposed to **whole blood,** to avoid circulatory overload. Whole blood can be fractionated into red blood cells **(erythrocytes);** platelet suspensions and concentrates; white blood cells **(leukocytes);** fresh plasma; frozen and stored plasma; cryoprecipitates or factor VIII concentrates; fibrinogen; factors II, VII, IX, and X concentrates (prothrombin complex); albumin; and gammaglobulin.

1. Whole blood contains red and white blood cells, serum, platelets, proteins (albumin, globulin, and fibrinogen), and other intravascular nutrients and substances. It is the best substance to transfuse in massive GI bleeding, because it replaces both blood volume and oxygen-carrying capacity. Whole blood transfusions carry the highest risk of complications.

2. Packed red blood cells (RBCs) raise the hemoglobin and hematocrit faster than whole blood, with less risk of circulatory overload. Packed RBCs are used in severe anemia, in patients whose bleeding has ceased and whose vascular volume has been replenished with saline or lactated Ringer's solution, and cautiously in patients with underlying cardiac disease or renal failure. RBCs may be frozen and then thawed for autologous transfusions.

3. Leukocyte-poor blood is produced by removing leukocytes and platelets from whole blood. It is administered to patients who are candidates for transplants, because it prevents sensitization to tissue antigens.

4. **Platelets** are administered to patients with thrombocytopenia (a decreased number of platelets), marked splenomegaly (enlargement of the spleen), or chronic depletion of platelets. In septic and/or febrile patients, platelet infusion should be doubled to achieve an increase in platelet count. Most patients require four or

more units of platelets to prevent or control bleeding.

5. **Plasma** is the fluid portion of blood that remains after centrifuging whole blood to remove the red blood cells. It contains most clotting factors but no platelets. The plasma may be prepared as a liquid or it may be frozen or dried. It is used to treat clotting factor deficiencies when specific concentrates are not available or when the precise factor deficiency has not been determined.

6. Fresh frozen plasma is used when there is little or no actual blood loss, such as in burns and in crush injuries. In emergencies, fresh frozen plasma may be used as a volume expander in hypovolemic bleeding until fresh whole blood is available. It is not required in most patients unless there is a clinically important disturbance in coagulation. Because a deficiency of coagulation factors is a preexisting phenomenon in many patients with cirrhosis, consideration should be given to providing these patients with fresh frozen plasma after every second or third unit of packed RBCs.

7. **Cryoprecipitates** are **serum** proteins, including factors VIII and XIII and fibrinogen, that settle out of solution at temperatures below 20° C. Cryoprecipitates are administered to patients with hemophilia A and von Willebrand's disease.

8. **Prothrombin** complex, which comprises factors II, VII, IX, and X, may be administered to treat hemophilia B, severe liver disease, and deficiencies of these specific factors. It carries a relatively high risk of transmitting hepatitis.

9. Volume expanders include 25% normal serum albumin; Plasmanate (a commercially prepared hypertonic solution of alpha and beta globulins, human albumin, sodium, and chloride), which is used in burn cases, hypovolemic shock, or hypoproteinemia; and the plasma substitutes dextran-40 or dextran-70, which have a molecular weight higher than that of blood and therefore cause osmotic diuresis and a resulting increase in blood volume when introduced into the vascular system.

10. Gammaglobulin is transfused to prevent infectious hepatitis, rubeola, mumps, pertussis, tetanus, and hypogammaglobulinemia and agammaglobulinemia.

The equipment required for transfusing blood and blood products includes: whole blood or components; a straight or Y-type blood administration set with a regular or microaggregate filter; infusion equipment including a 19- or 21-gauge needle or catheter; and a portable infusion standard. Both whole blood and packed cells contain cellular debris, necessitating in-line filtration during administration.

Nursing responsibilities in the administration of blood and blood components include but are not limited to the following:

(a) blood product inspection;

(b) verification of product expiration date;

(c) confirmation of compatibility between recipient and donor;

(d) confirmation of informed patient consent;

(e) patient education;

(f) Monitoring the patient at least 5 minutes post-administration, as per institution protocol;

(g) identification of immediate and delayed reactions;

(h) intervention in the case of adverse reactions;

(i) written documentation;

(j) communication with other healthcare providers; and

(k) adherence to aseptic technique.

All blood to be used for transfusion must be crossmatched with a sample of the patient's blood. Institutional protocols should be followed to ensure that the blood to be transfused is identified and double-checked with the patient's name, assigned hospital number, the number on the unit of blood, and the date of collection and crossmatching. It is vital that this identifying information be absolutely accurate: *Transfusing the wrong blood to a patient can be fatal!* It is advisable that two parties, registered nurses or physicians, check the blood before transfusion and report any discrepancies to the blood bank before administration.

After verifying the identifying information, the blood bag should be gently rotated to distribute the blood cells. The tubing, drip chamber, and filter(s) should be primed and flushed with 30 to 60 ml of sterile normal saline, which is accomplished by connecting an infusion container of saline to the tubing and filter. After flushing at a keep-open rate (about 10 drops per minute), the saline container is disconnected and the blood bag is connected to the tubing.

The blood is administered at a keep-open rate (25 to 30 drops per minute) for the first 30 minutes, while observing the patient for adverse reactions. After that, the flow should be adjusted to the prescribed rate, checking every 30 to 60 minutes for rate of flow, infiltration, and side effects. When the transfusion is complete, the blood bag, used tubing, and tag should be disconnected and returned to the blood bank.

To preserve blood and prevent contamination, it should be refrigerated at 40° C. If hanging of blood is delayed more than 30 minutes from the time it is received from the blood bank, it should be returned to the bank for refrigeration. Rapid transfusion of cold blood can lead to hypothermia. When multiple units of blood are required, portable or stationary blood warmers may be used to keep the blood at a constant temperature of 98.6° F.

If an infusion is to be administered following the transfusion, the tubing should be changed, the filter removed, and the needle or cannula flushed with 10 to 20 ml normal saline before reconnecting the infusion.

Whole blood and RBCs should not be used after 21 days. Frozen blood should be used within 24 hours after thawing and cannot be refrozen. Fresh frozen plasma should be used within 4 hours of thawing, because it does not contain preservatives. Blood may be heparinized to prevent clotting. Citrate is added to stored whole blood to prevent coagulation. If the blood is administered slowly, the patient's liver can remove citrate.

In autotransfusion, the patient's own blood may be salvaged after a traumatic injury or during an operative procedure and reinfused into a vein after it is filtered and treated with an anticlotting agent. Alternatively, the patient may donate his or her own blood before elective surgery. Potential complications of autotransfusion include blood clotting, hemolysis, coagulopathies, thrombocytopenia, particulate and air emboli, sepsis, and citrate toxicity.

Indications and contraindications

The primary purpose of blood transfusions is to improve tissue oxygenation (with RBCs) and/or to improve coagulation (with plasma and platelets). Other indications may include improving hemoglobin/hematocrit levels; increasing intravascular volume; or replacing certain substances, such as protein, platelets, or clotting factors.

Transfusions may be indicated for treatment of massive GI bleeding if the patient continues to bleed despite therapy, is in shock, has a very low hematocrit, or has symptoms related to poor tissue oxygenation. Treatment for massive bleeding is aimed at preventing hypovolemic shock, preventing dehydration and electrolyte imbalance, stopping the bleeding, and providing rest. Transfusions may also be given to increase the blood volume and help correct anoxia resulting from decreased RBCs. Infusion of crystalloids may dilute the red cell count. Stabilization of blood values may take 6 to 8 hours after volume replacement.

Exchange blood transfusions may be used in the treatment of hepatic coma. Fresh blood is used to replace the blood volume. This may be repeated in 12, 24, and 48 hours. Cross-circulation of blood between a donor and the patient may be done without the need for a large volume of typed and crossmatched blood. Either procedure gives the patient's liver cells time to regenerate and provides fresh blood or enables the donor to correct some of the patient's metabolic and electrolyte disturbances. In advanced cirrhosis when there is irreversible damage, these methods are of little benefit.

Patients should receive blood until their vital signs are stable, bleeding ceases, and enough RBCs are circulating to provide adequate oxygenation. A hematocrit of 30% is a reasonable goal in most patients.

Adverse reactions

Any nurse who administers blood must be able to recognize the signs and symptoms of adverse reactions. Potential adverse reactions to blood and blood component therapy include the following:

1. Circulatory overload, which occurs when too much fluid or too rapid an infusion is administered to patients with underlying cardiac, renal, liver, pulmonary, or hematological disease. Signs and symptoms include cough, chest pain, dyspnea, tachycardia, and cyanosis.

2. Bacterial reaction to the transfusion, which is characterized by the development of a fever, chills, abdominal and extremity pain, vomiting, hypotension, and bloody diarrhea. Bacteremic shock and death may follow the administration of as little as 25 ml of contaminated blood.

3. Allergic reactions, which may occur when the donor has

ingested substances to which the recipient is allergic. They may be manifested in mild cases by a mild urticaria, pruritus, and nasal congestion or in severe cases by bronchospasm, severe dyspnea, laryngeal edema, and circulatory collapse. Allergic reactions are usually treated with antihistamines.

4. Hemolytic reactions, which usually occur within the first 30 minutes of the transfusion and are caused by incompatibility between the transfusing blood and the patient's blood. Signs and symptoms in the initial phase include anxiety, headache, flushing, chest pain, shortness of breath, tachycardia, and low back pain or pains of the long bones. The reaction may progress to fever, nausea, vomiting, cyanosis, oliguria, anuria, uremia with shock, jaundice, and vascular collapse.

5. Hepatitis B, which may develop as long as 6 months after the use of contaminated blood, needles, catheters, tubing, or other equipment. Signs and symptoms include anorexia, jaundice, dyspepsia, abdominal pain, malaise, and weakness, often with hepatomegaly and splenomegaly.

6. Other transfusion related infectious agents (viral, bacterial, parasites) have been reported.

7. Massive transfusions of 8 to 10 or more units of blood may result in over transfusion reactions (uncontrollable hemorrhage), citrate intoxication (convulsions, impaired clotting, hyperkalemia, and ammonia intoxication), acid-base imbalances, or rapid pressure reactions. Other complications that can occur are hypothermia, decreases in serum calcium, magnesium and dilution thrombocytopenia.

If an adverse reaction occurs, the nurse should immediately stop the transfusion, save the substance being transfused, and keep the vein open with normal saline. The patient's vital signs should be assessed, and a urine specimen should be collected and sent to the laboratory immediately. The physician and the blood bank should be notified of a possible transfusion reaction. The labels of all blood containers should be compared to corresponding patient identification forms. Blood samples, all transfusion containers, and the administration set should be sent immediately to the blood bank.

The patient should be treated symptomatically and supportively. If ordered, oxygen, epinephrine, or other drugs should be administered. An alcohol bath or a hypothermia blanket may be used to reduce fever. The patient should be made as comfortable as possible, and reassurance should be provided as necessary. In the case of an anaphylactic reaction, emergency resuscitative measures must be instituted immediately.

Patient education

Blood transfusions always require a signed consent form from the patient.

To prevent recurrence of a transfusion reaction, patients who experience hypersensitivity reactions should be educated as to the cause and encouraged to carry this information in their wallets.

Documentation

After the transfusion is complete, it is important to record the time, date, and duration of transfusion; the type and amount of transfused blood or blood components; baseline vital signs; and the check of all identifying data.

In the case of a transfusion reaction, the nurse should record the time and date of the reaction, the type and amount of transfused blood or blood products, the clinical signs of the transfusion reaction in order of occurrence, the patient's vital signs, any specimens that were sent to the laboratory, any treatment, and the patient's response to treatment. Some institutions require completion of a transfusion reaction form.

In autologus, the nurse should record the duration of collection, suction pressure, type and amount of anticoagulant, the duration of transfusion, the use of a blood filter or washed cells, the amount and characteristics of drainage, and any complications.

CASE SITUATION

Davy Simms, the 6-month-old infant with a patent ductus described in Chapter 21, is scheduled for an esophagoscopy under general anesthesia. He is to receive ampicillin and gentamicin intravenously during the procedure.

Points to think about

1. How will the nurse assist the pharmacist in calculating the antibiotic doses for Davy?
2. Which antibiotic should be given first?
3. What type of IV catheter would be recommended for Davy?
4. With what solution should the ampicillin be diluted?
5. How might the potential adverse reactions to ampicillin be described?
6. What is the reason for giving Davy prophylactic ampicillin?

Suggested responses

1. The pharmacist will need an accurate height and weight to calculate the appropriate ampicillin and gentamicin doses for Davy.
2. Gentamicin should be given first, because the ratio of infusion is longer and the peak and half-life are longer than for ampicillin.
3. Davy will require multiple medications for his endoscopy procedure. It is therefore recommended that an angio-catheter be placed for stability and multiple injections. A 24-gauge angiocatheter can usually be placed in a 6 month old of average height and weight.
4. Ampicillin sodium can be diluted with either sterile distilled water or sterile normal saline. In this instance, the diluent used depends on the fluid used to keep the vein open. The fluid will probably be D5W, so the ampicillin would be diluted with sterile distilled water.

5. Potential adverse reactions to ampicillin include the following:
   (a) GI reactions, such as nausea, vomiting, or diarrhea; and
   (b) hypersensitivity reactions, such as urticaria, fever, laryngeal edema, and anaphylaxis (Skin rashes occur more frequently with ampicillin than with other penicillins.).

   With a patient this age, it is imperative that precise intake and output records be kept.

6. Davy is on prophylactic ampicillin to prevent bacterial endocarditis or great vessel arteritis while the physician evaluates the possibility of surgically closing the patent ductus. Ampicillin is the drug of choice in non-penicillin-allergic persons to prevent throat and ear infections caused by beta-hemolytic *Streptococcus,* which is the organism most commonly implicated in these problems in endemic areas of the country.

REVIEW TERMS

cannula, catheters, colloids, cryoprecipitates, crystalloids, D5W, electrolytes, erythrocytes, hemolysis, hypertonic, hypotonic, infiltration, isotonic, leukocytes, needles, normal saline, osmosis, phlebitis, plasma, plasmolysis, platelets, prothrombin, Ringer's solution, serum, tonicity, whole blood

REVIEW QUESTIONS

1. Salts that dissociate in solution into positive and negative ions are called:
   (a) Anions.
   (b) Cations.
   (c) Electrolytes.
   (d) Colloids.

2. The preferred instrument for delivering long-term, routine IV therapy is a(n):
   (a) Stainless-steel needle.
   (b) Over-the-needle catheter.
   (c) In-the-needle catheter.
   (d) Cannula.

3. A peripheral IV cannula would most likely be inserted in the:
   (a) Cephalic vein.
   (b) Femoral vein.
   (c) Superior vena cava.
   (d) Radial artery.

4. Elevation of the affected part and application of cold compresses for the first 24 hours, followed by warm, moist compresses, is the appropriate treatment for what complication of IV therapy?
   (a) Hematoma.
   (b) Infiltration.
   (c) Air embolism.
   (d) Catheter embolism.

5. Drugs should never be added to blood transfusions because:
   (a) They are incompatible.
   (b) It complicates determination of the source of any adverse reaction.
   (c) Drugs can cause clotting.
   (d) The rate of infusion is too slow.

6. Central venous catheters are used for long-term IV therapy or for repeated venous access and:
   (a) Are inserted into large veins.
   (b) Are threaded into the right atrium.
   (c) Can be used for medication administration.
   (d) All of the above.

7. When administering IV medications, vein irritation can be minimized by:
   (a) Using continuous, rather than intermittent, infusions.
   (b) Using the same injection site continuously.
   (c) Using 50 to 100 ml of diluent with antibiotics.
   (d) Avoiding the use of normal saline as the diluent.

8. What is the best substance to transfuse in patients with massive GI bleeding?
   (a) Whole blood.
   (b) Packed RBCs.
   (c) Platelets.
   (d) Plasma.

9. If the patient experiences an adverse reaction to a blood transfusion, the first thing the nurse should do is:
   (a) Assess the patient's vital signs.
   (b) Stop the transfusion.
   (c) Compare labels on blood containers with the patient's identification forms.
   (d) Return the blood to the blood bank.

10. Hemolytic reactions to blood transfusions usually occur:
    (a) Immediately.
    (b) Within the first 30 minutes of the transfusion.
    (c) Within 24 hours.
    (d) As long as 6 months after the transfusion.

BIBLIOGRAPHY

American Medical Association, Department of Drugs, Division of Drugs and Toxicology (1991). Drug evaluations annual. Chicago: American Medical Association.

Berstein, D.I. (2002, August 1). Management of natural rubber latex allergy. *J Allergy Clin Immunol 100(2Suppl),* S111-6. Journal of Allergy and Clinical Immunology.

Blume, D. (1980): *Dosages and solutions* (3rd ed.). Philadelphia: F.A. Davis.

Campbell, T. & Lunn, D. (1997). Intravenous therapy: current practice and nursing concerns. *Brit J Nurs 6,21, 1218-1228.* British Journal of Nursing.

Center for Disease Control (2003, February 14). *Safety of blood supply in the United States.* [On-line.] Available: www.CDC.org.

Coco, C. (1980). *Intravenous therapy: a handbook for practice.* St. Louis, MO: Mosby.

Crass, R. & Vanderveen, T. (1988). IV pumps and controllers: new technology stimulates increased sophistication. *J Healthcare Materials Management 6,* 51-61.

Damsgard, C. (1985). *GIA certification review manual.* Rochester, NY: Society of Gastrointestinal Assistants.

Dougherty, L. (2000). Drug administration. In Mammett, J. & Dougherty, L. (Eds.), *Royal Marsden Manuel of Clinical Nursing Procedures* (5th ed.). Oxford: Blackwell Science.

Given, B. & Simmons, S. (1984). *Gastroenterology in clinical nursing* (4th ed.). St. Louis, MO: Mosby.

Hamilton, H. (Ed.) (1983). *Procedures, Nurse's Reference Library.* Springhouse, PA: Intermed Communications.

Intravenous Nurses Society (1990). Intravenous nursing standards of practice. *J Intraven Nurs Suppl,* S1-S98. Journal of Intravenous Nursing Supplement.

Jagger, J. & Bentley, M. (DATE). Injuries from vascular access devices high risk preventable. *J Intrav Nurs 20, 65,* 533-37. Journal of Intravenous Nursing.

Kneedler, J. & Dodge, G. (1987). *Perioperative patient care: the nursing perspective* (2nd ed.). Boston: Blackwell Scientific.

Langfitt, D. (1984). *Critical care: certification preparation and review.* Bowie, MD: Brady Communications.

Medical Devices Agency (1996). *Latex Sensitization in the health care setting: use of latex gloves.* London: HMS.

Medical Devices Agency (1998). *Latex Medical Gloves (Surgeons) and Examination Powered Latex Medical Gloves.* London: HMS.

Needlestick Safety and Prevention Act, HR5178, Law 106 430 (2000, November 6). Available: http://www.thomas.loc.gov.

Perry, A.G. & Potter, P.A. (1994). *Clinical nursing skills and techniques* (3rd ed.). St. Louis, MO: Mosby.

Poley, G. & Slater, J. (2000, September). Current reviews of allergy and clinical immunology. *J Allergy Clin Immunology 106(3),* 585-90. Journal of Allergy and Clinical Immunology.

Sleisenger, M. & Fordtran, J. (Eds.) (2002). *Gastrointestinal disease: pathophysiology, diagnosis, management* (7th ed.). Philadelphia: W.B. Saunders.

Society of Gastroenterology Nurses and Associates (1997). Guidelines for nursing care of the patient receiving sedation and analgesia in the gastrointestinal endoscopy setting. *Gastroenterol Nurs 20,* pp. 1-13.

Springhouse Corporation (1999). *Handbook of Infusion Therapy.* Philadelphia: Springhouse.

Thompson, G. (1997). *Ways of avoiding latex allergy.* Community Nurse 3, 2, 33-4.

Wiggins, M. & Sesin, P. (1990). Guidelines for administering IV drugs, *Nursing 90(20),* 145-52.

Weinstein, S. (2001). *Plumers Principles and Practice of Intravenous Therapy* (7th ed.). Philadelphia: Lippincott, Williams & Wilkins.

Chapter 22

NUTRITIONAL THERAPY

This chapter will acquaint the gastroenterology nurse with the basic principles of nutrition and nutritional therapy. These principles are followed by detailed discussions of special diets in the practice of gastroenterology and the care of patients who are receiving enteral or parenteral nutrition.

Learning objectives

After reviewing the content of this chapter, the gastroenterology nurse should be able to:

1. Outline the basic principles of good nutrition, nutritional assessment, and nutritional therapy.
2. Describe a number of special diets that may be prescribed for patients with GI disorders.
3. Discuss the techniques used in the administration of enteral and parenteral nutrition, as well as factors to be considered in the care of patients receiving this type of therapy.

BASIC PRINCIPLES

A patient's nutritional status depends on the balance between the nutrient intake and energy expenditures. This balance may be affected by internal factors, such as age and physical condition, or by external factors, such as the quantity and quality of food available.

In patients with GI disorders, nutritional status may also be affected by the following:

(a) factors that interfere with food consumption such as impaired appetite, disease, or a special diet;

(b) factors that increase tissue destruction such as cancer, ulceration, or necrosis;

(c) factors that interfere with the patient's ability to absorb nutrients including absence of normal digestive secretions, intestinal hypermotility, or decreased absorptive surface;

(d) factors that interfere with nutrient utilization or storage such as impaired liver function, neoplasms, or pan-

creatitis;

(e) factors that increase nutrient excretion or loss including hemorrhage, abscess or fistula formation, nausea and vomiting, surgery, or diarrhea; and

(f) factors that increase nutritional requirements including fever, chronic infection, and malignancy.

For any patient, **nutrition** is an integral part of the total plan of care. A poor nutritional state can affect recovery, contribute to complications, and cause increased morbidity and mortality.

There are six general classes of essential nutrients, including carbohydrates, lipids, proteins, vitamins, minerals, and water.

Carbohydrates

Carbohydrates, which are composed of starches and/or sugars, are found in grains, vegetables, fruits, syrups, and sugars. They are all sources of glucose, which is needed for energy metabolism. It is recommended that both children and adults consume 130 grams of carbohydrates each day.

Ptyalin, an α-amylase secreted by acinar cells of the salivary glands, hydrolyzes about 40% of ingested starches into **disaccharides** in the mouth and stomach. In the duodenum, pancreatic amylase hydrolyzes the remaining 60% of ingested starch. In the jejunum, these newly formed disaccharides and ingested disaccharides are split into **monosaccharides** and are then absorbed with ingested monosaccharides. Any condition that compromises the duodenum or jejunum inhibits carbohydrate absorption.

The end product of carbohydrate **catabolism** is **glucose,** a monosaccharide that is the chief source of energy for all living organisms. Glucose is taken up by all of the cells of the body and burned for immediate energy. Excess glucose can be converted to **glycogen,** a long-chain polymer that is stored mainly in the liver and muscles. When necessary, liver glycogen can be converted to glucose for systemic distribution, but muscle glycogen is used primarily by the muscle itself. Excess dietary carbohydrates are also converted to triglycerides for storage in adipose tissue.

Lipids

Lipids consist of fats, oils, waxes, and related compounds. They provide a concentrated stored energy source, cushion vital organs, and insulate the body to help maintain a constant body temperature. The primary sources of lipids are oils, dairy products, egg yolks, meats, and nuts and seeds.

Ingested lipids are hydrolyzed and passed into the small bowel, where they form **triglycerides.** Short-chain triglycerides are broken down by gastric lipase and pancreatic lipase. Long-chain triglycerides are emulsified by bile, which allows pancreatic lipase to cleave them into **monoglycerides,** end-stage **fatty acids,** and **glycerol.** In the jejunum, these products form micelles, which allow fat to be absorbed. Both bile and lipase disorders and jejunal or ileal disease can cause fat malabsorption.

Proteins

Proteins are made up of various combinations of **amino acids.** Nine of the 22 recognized amino acids are considered essential for adequate nutrition. The chief dietary sources of protein are meats, dairy products, and starches. Ingested proteins may either be used to synthesize the proteins needed to build new tissue or may be catabolized for energy. Ingested protein must supply all of the amino acids needed for internal protein synthesis. The recommended levels of protein intake for adults is 0.8 grams per kilogram of body weight.

Nitrogen balance is an indication of the effect of diet on the body's protein supply. Depending on the patient's condition, nitrogen balance may be neutral, positive, or negative.

1. In a healthy adult, protein synthesis is equal to protein degradation, and the individual is said to be in nitrogen balance.
2. Positive nitrogen balance occurs when protein synthesis exceeds protein degradation. This state is normal and to be expected in children, who are building new tissue. In adults it may signify a rebuilding of wasted tissue.
3. Negative nitrogen balance occurs when protein losses are greater than protein intake; that is, protein breakdown exceeds protein synthesis.

Metabolism of ingested protein begins in the stomach, where pepsin, in the presence of hydrochloric acid, hydrolyzes proteins into amino acids and polypeptides of varying lengths. Then, in the duodenum and jejunum, pancreatic enzymes reduce these products to their basic peptides and amino acids. In the lower jejunum and ileum, the remaining peptides are hydrolyzed into amino acids and are absorbed. Protein absorption may be reduced by disorders that reduce gastric hydrochloric acid secretion or impair production of proteolytic enzymes, by duodenal or jejunal inflammation or infection, or by gastric or intestinal resection.

Vitamins

Vitamins are organic compounds that are essential in minute quantities for specific cellular metabolic reactions and for normal growth and health. They are classified as either fat-soluble or water-soluble.

1. Vitamins A, D, E, and K are fat soluble. They are absorbed with dietary fats and tend to be stored in the body in moderate amounts.
2. All other vitamins are soluble in water. They are excreted in urine and are not stored in the body in appreciable amounts.

The general functions of vitamins are to regulate metabolism, convert fats and carbohydrates to energy, and aid bone and tissue formation.

Minerals

Minerals are inorganic nutrients. They include major minerals, trace minerals, and trace elements. Major minerals include calcium, chloride, sodium, magnesium, potassium, sulfur, and phosphorus. These essential mineral nutrients are found in the human body in amounts in excess of 5 g. Trace minerals include chromium, cobalt, copper, fluorine, iodine, iron, manganese, and zinc. These essential mineral nutrients are found in the human body in amounts of less than 5 g.

Among other things, minerals serve to regulate enzyme metabolism, maintain nerve and muscle integrity, and facilitate membrane transfer of essential compounds.

Water

Water acts as an intracellular and extracellular solvent and provides a medium for transportation of nutrients and metabolic waste products. It also lubricates the tissues and helps maintain body temperature.

NUTRITIONAL ASSESSMENT

A thorough assessment of a patient's nutritional status includes the following:

1. Completion of a health and dietary history, including reports of any recent weight gain or loss; recurrent nausea, vomiting, or diarrhea; any chronic illness; and dietary habits.
2. Completion of a physical examination to obtain data: height, weight, weight-to-height ratio, body frame size, mid-arm circumference, and skin fold thickness. Note signs of nutritional deficiency, such as edema, loss of subcutaneous fat, and muscle wasting. In the case of a pediatric patient, correctly plot the child's height, weight, and head circumference on a growth grid.
3. Completion of a record of growth patterns and velocity of growth, which are very important in assessment of pediatric patients. Prior growth parameters help to define growth patterns and velocity.
4. Completion of diagnostic studies, including laboratory tests for serum proteins, total lymphocyte count, nitrogen balance calculations, hemoglobin and hematocrit, serum iron, and serum albumin.

For patients with recognized nutritional deficits, the physician may order oral, enteral, or parenteral nutritional therapy. Oral intake is the preferred means of administering a special diet, but it requires the patient to have an appetite, functioning GI tract and be able to ingest foods. Enteral (tube) feedings are used when patients are unable or unwilling to use the normal oral route, such as when a patient is unable to swallow, has altered central nervous system function, or has severe anorexia secondary to the primary underlying illness. Parenteral feeding (IV hyperalimentation) is provided through an IV line for patients without a functional GI tract or for whom a period of bowel rest is indicated.

SPECIAL ORAL DIETS

Many diets used in the treatment of GI illnesses involve restriction of a particular dietary component, such as fats or protein. Others alter the consistency of the diet or the amount of dietary fiber. When prescribing a special diet it is important to remember that dietary habits or customs are difficult to change. As allowed, when designing a special diet, consider the patient's cultural, socioeconomic, and religious background.

High-fiber diets

Dietary fiber is made up of complex polysaccharides and other polymers that are not digested in the bowel; they include cellulose, hemicelluloses, gums, mucilages, pectins, and lignins. Fiber acts to increase stool bulk and weight and also increases bowel transit time. The high-fiber diet is recommended as an aid in the prevention of constipation and diverticulosis and in individual cases for irritable bowel syndrome and diarrhea.

Approximately 25 grams for women and 38 grams for men of total fiber is recommended. Total fiber means dietary fiber and functional fiber. This additional fiber can either be supplied in the diet, with emphasis on whole-grain breads and cereals, fresh fruits, and fresh vegetables, or can be consumed in the form of psyllium seed, which is a rich source of hemicellulose, or bran, which provides both cellulose and hemicellulose. Bran has the highest fiber content of any food. If the additional fiber is to be supplied by diet alone, it is important to recognize that the fiber content in unprocessed foods may be altered significantly by processes that remove the fiber, such as eating fruits without the skins.

Low-fiber diets

The primary indication for a low-fiber diet is acute diarrhea. A low-fiber diet is also recommended in children who have active inflammatory bowel disease. Preparation for certain GI procedures, including air-contrast barium enema, colonoscopy, and intestinal surgery, also requires adherence to a very low-fiber diet, or even enteral nutrition for a few days. Partial low-fiber diets may be necessary to avoid recurrence of gastric phytobezoars or for patients with a very narrow ileal segment as a result of Crohn's disease.

Typically, a low-fiber diet used for chronic problems involves a reduction in the quantity of grains, fruits, and vegetables and limiting the intake of fats and proteins. The major drawback of a low-fiber diet is that it may provide an inadequate amount of calories and is deficient in many vitamins and minerals. If the patient's nutrition is marginal, the diet can be supplemented by enteral feedings.

Gluten-free diets

Gluten is a protein found in wheat, oats, rye, and barley. A lifelong gluten-free diet is used in the treatment of celiac sprue, a disease characterized by malabsorption of nutrients, and the absence of normal intestinal villi on the small bowel mucosa. Only the gliadin fraction of gluten protein is implicated in mucosal damage. To remove all cereal grains containing gliadin (i.e., wheat, barley, rye, and, in a few patients, oats), it is necessary for patients with celiac sprue to avoid the following:

(a) obvious sources of gluten, including baked goods, dry cereals containing wheat and/or oats, and pastas;
(b) less obvious sources of gluten, including wheat that has been used as an extender in processed foods and beverages, such as ice cream, salad dressings, canned foods, catsup, mustard, candy bars, and instant coffee. Even postage stamps and envelopes may contain gliadin; and
(c) foods with ingredients such as modified food starch, hydrolyzed vegetable protein, and malt.

Many sources of gliadin are not readily apparent to the consumer; it is very important that patients on gluten-free diets read all labels and carefully study the ingredients of all processed foods. Rice, soybean, corn, buckwheat, potato, and tapioca flours are appropriate substitutes or alternatives for gluten-sensitive patients.

Healthcare providers must remember that lifelong adherence to a gluten-free diet is a big commitment and may represent a significant social liability, especially for children and teenagers. Studies show that only 30% to 70% of celiac patients comply with their gluten-free diet. Patient education regarding the importance of compliance for continued good health is essential. Patients should be informed that failure to comply with a gluten-free diet results in lower stature and weight in young adults. Closely monitored follow-up and continued counseling are recommended. The Celiac Foundation offers excellent educational materials, cookbooks, and support for the celiac patient.

Within a week of removal of gluten from the diet, patients may experience a decrease in diarrhea, improved appetite, and an overall improvement in attitude and behavior. In other patients, clinical improvement may take several months.

The most common cause of failure to respond to a gluten-free diet is incomplete removal of gluten. Sometimes it may be necessary to hospitalize the patient for supervision by a knowledgeable dietitian to be certain that no glutens are consumed.

Some patients with celiac sprue may develop other nutritional deficiencies secondary to their gluten intolerance. If a secondary lactase deficiency develops, milk and milk products should be limited initially. In young children, initial dietary management also may require adequate calories and protein to sustain catch-up growth, multivitamin supplements, and iron and folic acid supplementation if the child is anemic. Most patients develop an increased tolerance to lactose and decrease their need for supplementation after gluten withdrawal as their intestinal structure and function begin to return to normal.

Lactose-free diets

A low-lactose diet is indicated for patients with symptoms of lactose intolerance, which is evidenced by a history of abdominal pain, diarrhea, bloating, and gas following ingestion of lactose and/or a positive lactose tolerance or hydrogen breath test.

Lactose intolerance may be the result of a lactase deficiency secondary to disease process, such as celiac sprue or Crohn's disease. Lactase deficiency may also occur in the absence of disease. Lactose intolerance may also result from decreased time of exposure to the intestinal mucosa, such as in short bowel syndrome or dumping syndrome. A low-lactose diet may be used in the treatment of patients with irritable bowel syndrome (IBS) or during the acute phase of a diarrheal illness in which intestinal transit is rapid or lactase deficiency is transient, as in acute gastroenteritis, ulcerative colitis, or Crohn's disease. A low-lactose diet may also be helpful in the initial phase of therapy for celiac sprue.

Patients with lactose intolerance should avoid milk and milk products, including ice cream, cheeses, and butter. Lactose-intolerant patients should also be alert to processed foods containing milk solids, whey, lactose, milk sugar, galactose, or skim milk powder. Yogurt containing active cultures may be well tolerated by lactose-intolerant individuals, because fermentation continues in the intestinal lumen.

Most lactose-intolerant patients can tolerate up to 3 g of lactose per day. More severe restrictions may be necessary in certain patients, such as patients with galactosemia. Dairy products typically provide a significant percentage of dietary calcium; thus calcium supplements may be necessary for patients on low-lactose diets, particularly for postmenopausal women. As well, many foods and other fluids such as juices are now fortified in calcium.

Cow's milk substitutes containing corn syrup solids and sodium caseinate may be used by patients on low-lactose diets. Also available are yeast preparations that may be added to milk to hydrolyze the lactose, and prehydrolyzed milk. Patients with a limited tolerance of lactose can use this milk in cooking or on cereal. In addition, tablets that contain lactase can be swallowed with meals to improve lactose tolerance.

The object of a low-lactose diet is relief of symptoms. After a period of time, small amounts of lactose can be carefully reintroduced into the diet, as long as the patient remains asymptomatic.

Low-protein diets

Restriction of dietary protein is indicated in patients who have symptoms of chronic renal insufficiency and in patients with severe liver disease who are at risk for portosystemic encephalopathy. Severe dietary restriction of protein requires restricting intake of milk, cheese, meat, fish, poultry, and eggs and limiting amounts of breads, cereals, and some vegetables.

To avoid a negative nitrogen balance and further deterioration of liver function, special mixtures of orally or intravenously administered amino acids may be prescribed. Supplementation with iron, calcium, B-complex vitamins, and calories may be required.

Some infants are intolerant to the protein constituents of cow's milk. A variety of substitute formulas that are prepared from hydrolyzed casein, vegetable proteins, or a meat base are available. Food labels must be checked for ingredients such as butter, cream cheese, any form of milk, casein, curds, whey, beef, and veal. After the infant has been symptom-free for 3 to 4 months, small amounts of milk may be reintroduced carefully and, if tolerated, may be slowly increased.

Low-fat diets

Low-fat diets are used to control symptoms of GI disease, particularly steatorrhea or diarrhea. They are indicated in all acute and chronic diseases in which the functions of lipolysis, micellar solubilization, mucosal absorption, transport out of the absorptive cell, or transport in the lymphatic system is impaired. A short-term low-fat diet may also be helpful in patients with acute gastroenteritis.

Because small amounts of cooking fats provide a large percentage of dietary fat, all foods prepared on a low-fat diet must be broiled, boiled, or baked. Skinless chicken and turkey are the staples of a low-fat diet. If red meat is eaten, all fat must be trimmed. Fish should be served without sauces. Consumption of breads, cereals, vegetables, and fruits should be emphasized. Dairy products made with whole or 2% milk should be avoided, as well as most desserts, cheeses, nuts, olives, bacon, mayonnaise, salad dressings, and cream sauces or gravies.

If table foods must be severely restricted to control fat intake, low-fat dietary supplements may be required to deliver adequate calories. Supplements containing preparations of vitamins A, D, E, and K may be necessary. Medium-chain triglycerides are available in oil and dry powder preparations that supply minerals, carbohydrates, and fat-soluble vitamins.

Low-sodium diets

The restriction of dietary sodium is indicated for gastroenterology patients with ascites and edema caused by severe liver disease. A combination of sodium restriction and diuretic administration is the mainstay of treatment for ascites. Sodium restriction prevents further expansion of the extracellular fluid volume and may be used alone for outpatients with minimal ascites. Once diuretic therapy has mobilized the ascites, patients may be maintained on a low-sodium diet without diuretics.

Patients on low-sodium diets should not add salt to their food, nor should they use salt in food preparation. Water that has been treated with sodium-containing water-softening compounds should be avoided, along with over-the-counter medications that contain sodium. Foods that are particularly high in sodium should be eliminated, including tomato juice, organ meats, smoked meats, shellfish, cheese, dry cereals, commercial mixes, commercially prepared desserts, spices, and commercially prepared soups. Supplementation with iron and B-vitamin preparations that do not contain sodium may be necessary.

ENTERAL NUTRITION

Enteral nutrition refers to the administration of a prescribed diet by means of a flexible tube inserted into the stomach or small bowel either transnasally, surgically, or endoscopically.

Indications and contraindications

Enteral nutrition is indicated for maintenance of nutritional status in patients who have a functioning GI tract but cannot ingest sufficient food and nutrients to meet energy requirements. Examples of conditions for which enteral nutrition may be indicated are anorexia, malabsorption syndromes, chronic malnutrition, infants with failure to thrive, major burns, severe trauma, hepatic or renal failure, and dysphagia resulting from AIDS, cerebrovascular accident, or esophageal tumor. It is contraindicated in patients with bowel obstruction, ileus, or severe diarrhea and should not be used immediately following a massive small bowel resection.

For patients in whom the GI tract is functional but oral feeding is not possible, enteral nutritional support is preferred over **total parenteral nutrition (TPN).** Compared to TPN, enteral nutrition is safer, is less expensive, and makes reintroduction of table foods easier. The use of a transnasal tube is 1/10th to 1/20th less expensive thancomparable parenteral nutrition, and significant complications are less frequent. In addition, enteral nutrition is just as effective as TPN in reversing malnutrition and restoring positive nitrogen balance.

Administration of enteral nutrition

Enteral nutrition is administered through a tube that may be inserted transnasally, surgically, radiographically, or endoscopically.

Transnasal insertion of a feeding tube involves the use of a nasogastric, nasoduodenal, or nasojejunal tube. Nasogastric tubes are indicated when pharyngeal reflexes are intact and there is little risk of aspiration. Nasojejunal or nasoduodenal intubation is indicated when the potential for aspiration is high or when a simple formula is required to assist nutrient breakdown in an impaired gut. However, it may be difficult to place a tube in the duodenum and maintain it there for any length of time. In addition, duodenal and jejunal tubes tend to be smaller in diameter and easily become obstructed. Discomfort and esophagitis as a result of lumen size or reflux may occur with any transnasal tube.

Tubes made of silicone or polyurethane plastics are thinner and more flexible than older tubes made of polyvinyl plastic. In addition, they do not stiffen or become brittle in the GI tract. Nasoenteral tubes come in a variety of lengths and diameters. Tubes for gastric feeding measure approximately 76 cm, whereas the longer tubes used for intestinal feeding are up to 120 cm. Some tubes are weighted at the distal end with tungsten; mercury is no longer used to weight these tubes because of complicated disposal issues. Nasoduodenal tube feedings are currently preferred for enteral nutrition because they offer less potential for aspiration than nasogastric tubes.

For patients who require long-term enteral nutrition, the feeding tube may be inserted by gastrostomy or jejunostomy. Intermittent bolus feeding through a gastrostomy tube (G-tube) is most suitable for the ambulatory patient who does not wish to be confined by a continuous infusion. G-tubes do not have most of the problems associated with nasogastric intubation but carry their own potential complications, such as drainage, infection, or formation of granulation tissue at the site. Both nasogastric tubes and G-tubes have a risk of aspiration of gastric contents.

Jejunostomy tubes (J-tubes) are most useful for patients who will undergo surgery for esophageal, gastric, pancreatic, or biliary disease.

Feeding tubes may also be inserted transnasally, orally, or endoscopically, such as in PEG or PEJ. Once the tube is in place, enteral feedings may be administered in the form of intermittent gravity drips or continuous drip infusion. With continuous drip infusion, a defined amount is given continuously with the use of an infusion pump. This method minimizes the risk of aspiration, abdominal distention, and diarrhea. Intermittent "bolus" infusions are more convenient but may not be tolerated as well by the patient.

It is important to check for proper tube placement before each intermittent feeding and at least once a shift during continuous feedings. Checking nasogastric placement by pH of stomach aspirate has shown to be a reliable method. Radiographic verification of tube placement may be needed before tube feedings are begun and after any event that may predispose a patient to tube dislocation.

The patient's head and thorax should be elevated at least 30 degrees. To minimize diarrhea, the solution should be diluted as ordered by the physician.

To allow the patient to adjust to tube feeding, the rate of administration of the solution should be increased gradually. For most patients, a 1 kcal/ml formula is used, beginning with 50 ml/hr and increasing the rate each day by 25 ml/hr intervals until a rate of 100 to 125 ml/hr is reached. For pediatric patients, hourly infusion rates and total volumes are calculated based on the child's size and individual nutritional needs. Once the prescribed rate is reached, the strength of the formula may be increased according to the patient's nutritional needs. Water supplements should be given as ordered.

The tube should be irrigated before and after each feeding

and every 3 to 4 hours when the patient is not receiving a continuous drip. It should be irrigated every 6 hours when the patient is receiving a continuous drip. To maintain optimum patency, the tube should be considered for replacement every 4 weeks.

Enteral diets

There are three basic types of enteral diets. The type of diet used depends on the status of the patient's GI tract and on his or her caloric and nutrient requirements.

1. Elemental diets are predigested, nutritionally complete powdered mixtures of basic nutrients that are reconstituted with water. Such diets are low-residue and lactose-free. They require little lipolytic or proteolytic activity and are relatively nonstimulating to pancreatic, biliary, and GI secretions. Elemental diets are used for patients with definite evidence of maldigestion and malabsorption. Disease-specific elemental diets are available for patients with renal failure, respiratory insufficiency, or hepatic encephalopathy.

2. Formulas with intact nutrients include blenderized meat-based meals; lactose-free feedings containing polymeric mixtures of proteins, fats, and carbohydrates in high-molecular weight forms; and nutrient-dense feedings that provide 1.5 to 2 kcal/ml compared with the 1 kcal/ml in blenderized or lactose-free feedings. Polymeric formulas are used when lipolytic and proteolytic GI function are almost normal.

3. Modular preparations contain only one nutrient group (fats, proteins, or carbohydrates). Modular preparations may be added to formula diets to increase specific components or to increase calories for patients on fluid restrictions.

Enteral calorie requirements may be calculated by using the Harris-Benedict equation for basal energy expenditures (BEE), where W is the patient's actual or usual weight in kilograms; H is the height in centimeters; and A is the age in years.

Women:

$$BEE = 655 + (9.6 \times W) + (1.8 \times H) - (4.7 \times A)$$

Men:

$$BEE = 66 + (13.7 \times W) + (5 \times H) - (6.8 \times A)$$

The enteral maintenance requirement is $1.2 \times BEE$; the enteral anabolic requirement is $1.5 \times BEE$.

Potential complications

Less than 1% of patients receiving enteral nutrition experience serious complications. The most common complication is aspiration. Aspiration may be minimized by placing nasojejunal or jejunostomy tubes well beyond the ligament of Treitz, by keeping gastric volumes less than 100 ml, and by elevating the patient's head and shoulders.

Other potential complications of enteral feedings include the following:

(a) tube obstruction;
(b) pharyngeal discomfort;
(c) nausea, vomiting, or cramping;
(d) diarrhea;
(e) dumping syndrome;
(f) hyperglycemia;
(g) excessive carbon dioxide production;
(h) hyponatremia and/or hypokalemia;
(i) constipation; and
(j) nasal or pharyngeal irritation or necrosis.

To avoid nausea, vomiting, or abdominal cramping, a slow rate of administration through a tube placed well into the stomach is best, with the patient in a sitting or low Fowler's position. Diarrhea can result from too-rapid infusion, infusion of hyperosmolar solutions, use of concomitant antibiotic, or fat malabsorption.

Nursing care

To avoid complications, patients on tube feedings should be monitored continuously to assess patient position, tube position and patency, and gastric residuals. For intermittent feedings, the position of the tube should be checked before each feeding. Adult patients should be given at least 50 ml of water before and after each intermittent feeding. In addition, fluid intake and output and weight gain or loss should be checked frequently. The effectiveness of enteral support should be assessed periodically by testing for metabolic imbalances and repeating nutritional assessments.

Patients who are receiving enteral feedings also need psychological support. Ambulation should be encouraged if possible, and both patient and family should be reassured that these feedings are necessary and that normal eating will be resumed as soon as possible.

Patients who are receiving enteral nutrition at home must be instructed in techniques of administration, record keeping of intake and output, and what physical symptoms to report to the physician.

TOTAL PARENTERAL NUTRITION

Total parenteral nutrition (TPN), or hyperalimentation, is the IV infusion of protein (amino acids), carbohydrates (dextrose), fat (lipid), and additives (vitamins, minerals, electrolytes, trace elements). It can be delivered through central or peripheral veins.

Indications and contraindications

Parenteral nutrition is indicated for patients who are moderately to severely malnourished or for those who are in negative nitrogen balance and are not expected to meet their nutritional requirements orally within a short period of time.

Parenteral nutrition may be ordered in the following situations: (a) for patients with GI disease such as inflammatory bowel disease, radiation enteritis, acute pancreatitis, and short-bowel syndrome; (b) for preoperative preparation of malnourished patients; (c) for patients with postoperative surgical complications, particularly fistulas; (d) for postoperative care of neonates; (e) for infants with intractable diarrhea; and (f) for patients with extensive burns or trauma, anorexia nervosa, liver disease, and renal failure.

Parenteral nutrition is usually not be used if oral or enteral nutrition is possible. Note peripheral parenteral nutrition as outlined below.

Administration of parenteral nutrition

To be practiced safely and successfully, parenteral nutrition should be administered by a trained TPN team consisting of a physician, nutritionist, pharmacist, and nurse. Most often, parenteral feedings are administered through an indwelling subclavian vein catheter via the superior vena cava. A Broviac or Hickman catheter may be used to permit capping of the catheter between infusions. For pediatric patients, a Broviac catheter with an inner diameter of 0.12 mm is available, compared to the regular size of 0.20 mm. In some cases the catheter is inserted via the femoral vein or antecubital vein to the subclavian vein (peripherally inserted central catheter [PICC]).

For some patients, **peripheral parenteral nutrition (PPN)** may be administered through a peripheral, rather than central, vein. PPN may be ordered for a patient who cannot ingest food orally for 2 or 3 days but who has adequate fat stores; for patients in whom a central line is precluded; and for patients who are eating but are not getting sufficient calories. PPN is also appropriate for low-birth-weight infants and for infants and children who need parenteral supplementation. PPN solutions contain a mixture of **dextrose** and amino acids. The concentration of dextrose should not be greater than 10%, however, because more concentrated solutions may be associated with vein sclerosing, the preservation of vein access and the development of thrombosis. Lipids may be given with peripheral alimentation to further dilute the dextrose concentration. Because of the limitations on dextrose content, the number of calories that can be given with PPN may be inadequate for long-term **anabolism.**

The initial infusion should be administered gradually, beginning with a rate of approximately 1 L in the first 24 hours. The concentration of the solution is increased slowly until the desired number of calories is delivered.

Parenteral diets

Parenteral formulas are concentrated liquids that usually provide 1 kcal/ml and about 42 g/L protein. Typically, parenteral formulas contain protein, carbohydrates, electrolytes, vitamins, trace minerals, and water.

In addition, lipid emulsions are often administered to meet essential fatty acid requirements. Fat should provide 30% or more of total calories.

In most hospitals, TPN solutions are ordered by the physician on a daily solution order form. Formulation of a parenteral solution must be carefully calculated so that it meets the complete needs of the patient in terms of calories, nitrogen, fatty acids, vitamins, trace elements, and water. Dextrose solutions and lipid emulsions are the main sources of energy in patients who are fed by central catheter.

The minimal amount of energy (calories) required to prevent weight loss or catabolism is 1.5 × BEE (the parenteral maintenance requirement). To achieve anabolism and positive nitrogen balance, the parenteral anabolic requirement is 1.8 × BEE.

Protein requirements are usually supplied by crystalline amino acids. The amount of protein needed is calculated according to the following formula:

Protein (g) = 6.25 × Energy requirements/day ÷ 150

Daily fluid requirements are calculated according to the following formula:

1000 ml for the first 10 kg body weight (100 ml/kg)
500 ml for the next 10 kg (50 ml/kg)
+ 20 ml for each kg of body weight thereafter

Daily fluid requirements

The maximum daily fat allowance is 2.5 g/kg. Not more than 60% to 70% of the total calories per day should be from fat. Usually, a lipid solution is added to the carbohydrate and protein solutions, and the combined mixture is administered to the patient. Some patients receive lipid solution only one or two times per week to prevent fatty acid depletion.

Vitamins and trace minerals are provided in parenteral alimentation solutions in amounts designed to meet daily requirements of patients with disease.

Potential complications of total parenteral nutrition

Serious complications occur in 5% to 10% of patients receiving TPN. The most common complication is catheter-related sepsis, which occurs in less than 5% of TPN patients. TPN-related infection may result from contamination of the catheter by skin flora, contamination of the TPN solution or tubing, or bacteremia originating from another source in the body. To avoid catheter infections, specific aseptic techniques must be followed in the care of the catheter and dressing. Fever in any patient with a central catheter should receive immediate attention, including blood culture and attempt to determine source of infection. If the patient has a positive blood culture, the catheter may need to be removed and replaced after treatment with antibiotics.

Potential mechanical complications of parenteral nutrition include thoracic injury during catheter insertion, such as subclavian artery puncture or myocardial perforation; air embolism from air entering the catheter during a line change; or venous thrombosis and thrombophlebitis. Metabolic imbalances may include hyperglycemia or hypoglycemia, electrolyte or mineral imbalances, and ketoacidosis. Hepatic complications may include hepatomegaly, fatty liver, enzyme elevations, and cholestasis.

Nursing care for patients receiving Parenteral Nutrition

Nursing goals in the administration of parenteral nutrition include prevention of infection, maintenance of the prescribed rate of flow, ongoing patient assessment, and the provision of patient/family education and support.

All aseptic precautions must be observed when preparing parenteral solutions and when caring for patients who are receiving parenteral nutrition. Careful aseptic insertion of the central venous catheter is the first step. Over the long term, care of the catheter dressing, the tubing, and the catheter itself must be meticulous. Hands should be washed with an antimicrobial solution before any contact with the TPN system or dressing. Most TPN teams have a nurse who changes dressings, otherwise a protocol is established for the floor nurses. Dressings are usually changed three times per week and more often if they become soiled, wet, or nonocclusive. Institutional policies and procedures for insertion-site care should be consulted, because they may vary.

Parenteral feeding solutions should be kept refrigerated until needed, then allowed to reach room temperature before infusion to prevent hypothermia. The solution should be administered at a steady rate. To prevent air embolism, the patient should bear down (Valsalva's maneuver) or be placed in the Trendelenburg position when the tubing is being changed.

The hospitalized patient on TPN should be monitored daily for fluid intake and output and weight gain or loss. Vital signs should be checked every 4 to 8 hours, and the urine should be checked for glucose every 4 to 6 hours. Regular laboratory tests should include creatinine and urea nitrogen, serum chemistries, electrolytes, magnesium, transferrin, triglycerides, complete blood count with differential, and platelet count. When parenteral nutrition is to be stopped, the glucose concentration should be decreased gradually.

For patients who continue to need parenteral nutrition but no longer require skilled nursing care, home parenteral nutrition can be safe and cost-effective. Home TPN with infusion done overnight permits the patient to return to a reasonably normal daytime routine and aids in social adjustment. Both the patient and his or her family members need to be trained before discharge regarding dressing changes, addition of fluids, record keeping of fluid intake and output, what symptoms to note, and how to contact a healthcare provider.

CASE SITUATION

Mrs. Ellen Marshall is a 60-year-old woman who is 5'6" and weighs 179 pounds. She has been diagnosed by endoscopy as suffering from reflux esophagitis. The gastroenterology nurse's initial assessment notes that Mrs. Marshall is overweight. Excessive weight gain can increase intraabdominal pressure and exacerbate reflux. Furthermore, eating the wrong foods can add calories, decrease lower esophageal sphincter tone, exacerbate pain, and increase the gastric acid secretion rate. One appropriate nursing diagnosis in Mrs. Marshall's case is "altered nutrition: more than body requirements, related to caloric intake exceeding metabolic need."

Points to think about

1. How might the gastroenterology nurse differentiate between the meanings of overweight and obesity?
2. What are the critical indicators (NANDA) in making a nursing diagnosis of "altered nutrition: more than body requirements, related to caloric intake exceeding metabolic need"?

3. How might the gastroenterology nurse describe the approach to obtaining these indicator data to confirm or refute such a nursing diagnosis?
4. What additional data are needed to complete a basic dietary assessment on Mrs. Marshall?
5. What nutritional advice might the nurse give Mrs. Marshall that might alleviate symptoms of esophageal reflux?

Suggested responses

1. The generally accepted definitions of overweight and obesity are as follows:
   (a) Overweight is any weight in excess of the ideal/desirable body weight for age, height, and body size. A person may be overweight but not obese because of muscle mass.
   (b) Obesity is an excess of body fat; that is, 20% or more above the ideal/desirable body weight.
2. The critical indicators for the nursing diagnosis "altered nutrition: more than body requirements, related to caloric intake exceeding metabolic need" are as follows:
   (a) body weight 10% to 30% over ideal weight for height and frame; and
   (b) in women, triceps skin fold greater than 25 mm (measures body fat).
3. To confirm or refute such a nursing diagnosis, it would be appropriate to do the following:
   (a) Obtain accurate weight, height, triceps skin fold, and wrist measurements.
   (b) Calculate body frame size as small, medium, or large (height in cm divided by wrist circumference in cm). For a woman: small = >11.0, medium = 10.1 to 11.0, large = <10.1.
   (c) Using derived frame size, use weight/height norms for age to arrive at ideal weight. (U.S. Public Health Service probability statistical norms are probably more accurate than insurance actuarial tables).
   (d) Calculate actual weight percentage over ideal weight. Note that there are other methods for calculating amount of body fat.
4. In addition to weight, height, and body frame, data needed to complete a dietary assessment on Mrs. Marshall might include the following:
   (a) usual food and fluid intake, including frequency of meals, snacks, method of food preparation, portion size, and types of foods normally consumed;
   (b) elimination patterns;
   (c) activity and energy levels;
   (d) ethnic or cultural background; and
   (e) conditions surrounding food consumption.
5. Nutritional advice that the nurse could give Mrs. Marshall to alleviate symptoms of esophageal reflux might include the following:
   (a) Avoid large meals and refrain from snacking before going to bed to keep gastric volume at a minimum.
   (b) Keep dietary fat to a minimum, because fat slows gastric emptying and decreases lower esophageal sphincter pressure.

(c) Minimize dietary intake of chocolate, alcohol, and coffee, which also reduce basal lower esophageal sphincter pressure.

(d) Avoid carminative substances, such as spearmint and peppermint, because they impair lower esophageal sphincter function.

(e) Avoid citrus juices, tomato products, and coffee, which are direct esophageal irritants.

(f) Encourage other dietary modifications to promote weight loss.

REVIEW TERMS

amino acids, anabolism, anorexia, carbohydrates, catabolism, dextrose, disaccharides, enteral nutrition, fatty acids, glucose, glycerol, glycogen, lipids, minerals, monoglycerides, monosaccharides, nitrogen balance, nutrition, percutaneous endoscopic gastrostomy (PEG), percutaneous endoscopic jejunostomy (PEJ), peripheral parenteral nutrition (PPN), proteins, total parenteral nutrition (TPN), triglycerides, vitamins

REVIEW QUESTIONS

1. Excess glucose is stored in the liver and in the muscles in the form of:
   (a) Adipose tissue.
   (b) Glycogen.
   (c) Disaccharides.
   (d) Triglycerides.

2. If a patient is in negative nitrogen balance, that means he or she is:
   (a) Building new tissue.
   (b) Ingesting the proper amount of protein.
   (c) Eating too much protein.
   (d) Not getting enough carbohydrates and lipids to meet energy requirements and using protein as an energy source.

3. Patients with celiac sprue must avoid eating:
   (a) Gluten.
   (b) Fiber.
   (c) Sodium.
   (d) Protein.

4. Low-fat diets are usually used to control:
   (a) Steatorrhea and diarrhea.
   (b) Intestinal gas and bloating.
   (c) Ascites.
   (d) Constipation.

5. The primary disadvantage of using a nasogastric feeding tube is:
   (a) Risk of aspiration.
   (b) Patient discomfort.
   (c) Risk of infection.
   (d) High cost.

6. Diarrhea may be avoided in patients receiving enteral nutritional support by:

(a) Placing the patient in a sitting or low Fowler's position.
(b) Slowing the rate of infusion.
(c) Increasing the strength of the formula.
(d) Using aseptic technique.

7. Peripheral parenteral nutrition is most appropriate for:
   (a) Patients who need long-term hyperalimentation.
   (b) Patients with inadequate fat stores.
   (c) Patients who require concentrated feeding solutions.
   (d) Infants with low birth weights.

8. To prevent an air embolism when central lines are being changed, the nurse should:
   (a) Place the patient in an upright position.
   (b) Use sterile technique.
   (c) Have the patient perform Valsalva's maneuver.
   (d) Flush the tubing with water.

9. The most common complication in patients receiving TPN is:
   (a) Thoracic injury.
   (b) Air embolism.
   (c) Metabolic imbalance.
   (d) Catheter-related sepsis.

BIBLIOGRAPHY

Beck, M. (1989). Percutaneous endoscopic gastrostomy. *Nursing 89 19*, 76-7.

Beck, M. (1986). Reflux esophagitis. *SGA J 9*, 77-8.

Chobanian, S. & Van Ness, M. (Eds.) (1988). *Manual of clinical problems in gastroenterology*. Boston: Little, Brown.

Dietitics.com.(2002, Fall). Dietary reference intakes released for carbohydrates, fats, protein, fiber, and physical activity. *Dietitics in Practice 2*(2).

Eastwood, G. & Avunduk, C. (1988). *Manual of gastroenterology: diagnosis and therapy.* Boston: Little, Brown.

Fullenkamp, P. (1990). Gluten-sensitive enteropathy, Part II; Dietary treatment of celiac disease. In Trivits, S. (Ed.), *Journal Reprints II*. Rochester, NY: Society of Gastroenterology Nurses and Associates.

Given, B. & Simmons, S. (1984). *Gastroenterology in clinical nursing* (4th ed.). St. Louis, MO: Mosby.

Goldberg, K. (Ed.) (1986). *Gastrointestinal problems, Nurse Review Series*. Springhouse, PA: Springhouse.

Jackson, B. (1989). Care of patients after percutaneous endoscopic gastrostomy (PEG) tube placement. *Gastroenterol Nurs 12*, 131.

Kundtz, J. (1988). PEG/PEJ: implications for nursing care. In Trivits, S. (Ed.), *SGA Journal Reprints*, Rochester NY: Society of Gastrointestinal Assistants.

Messner, R. (1988). Infection control in total parenteral nutrition. In Trivits, S. (Ed.), *SGA Journal Reprints*, Rochester NY: Society of Gastrointestinal Assistants.

Rodwell-Williams, S. &Schlenker, E. (2002). *Essentials of nutrition and diet therapy* (8th ed.). St. Louis, MO: Mosby.

Society of Gastroenterology Nurses and Associates, Inc. (2003). *Manual of gastrointestinal procedures* (5th ed.). Chicago: Society of Gastroenterology Nurses and Associates, Inc.

Short, N. (1990). Gastrointestinal intubations: nursing considerations. In Trivits, S. (Ed.), *Journal Reprints II*. Rochester, NY: Society of Gastroenterology Nurses and Associates.

Silverman, A. & Roy, C. (1983). *Pediatric clinical gastroenterology* (3rd ed.). St. Louis, MO: Mosby.

Sleisenger, M. & Fordtran, J. (Eds.) (2002). *Gastrointestinal disease: pathophysiology, diagnosis, management* (7th ed.). Philadelphia: W.B. Saunders.

Walker, A. Durie, P.R.,Hamilton, J.R.,Watkins, J.B., and Walker-Smith. (2000). *Pediatric gastrointestinal and liver disease* (3rd ed.). Ontario, Canada: Decker.

Waye, J. Geenen, J.E., Fleischer,D. (1987). *Techniques in therapeutic endoscopy*. Philadelphia: W.B. Saunders. [On-line.] Available: www.niddk.nik.gov/health/digest/pubs/celiac.

DIAGNOSTIC PROCEDURES AND TESTS

Chapter 23

ENDOSCOPY

This chapter will acquaint the gastroenterology nurse with endoscopic techniques that are used to diagnose disorders of both the upper and lower GI tract. Therapeutic endoscopy is discussed in subsequent chapters.

Learning objectives

After reviewing the content of this chapter, the gastroenterology nurse should be able to:

1. Describe the different types of endoscopes used in GI procedures and their main components.
2. Discuss the responsibilities of the gastroenterology nurse with respect to IV sedation and analgesia of gastroenterology patients.
3. Explain the indications, contraindications, techniques for, and potential complications of endoscopic investigations of the upper and lower GI tract, including esophagogastroduodenoscopy (EGD), endoscopic retrograde cholangiopancreatography (ERCP), colonoscopy, and flexible and rigid sigmoidoscopy.
4. Discuss nursing considerations involved in each of these procedures.
5. Describe several recent advances in endoscopic diagnosis, including small bowel enteroscopy, capsule endoscopy, endoscopic ultrasonography, and videoendoscopy.

TYPES OF ENDOSCOPES

GI **endoscopy** is the direct visual examination of the lumen of the GI tract. It is a safe, effective way of evaluating the appearance and integrity of the GI mucosa, detecting lesions, and providing access for therapeutic procedures.

The first endoscopes were rigid, metal instruments. Most have now been replaced by flexible fiberoptic or video scopes, which increase visibility and promote patient safety and comfort. Depending on the section of the GI tract that is to be explored, the endoscopist may use one of the following:

(a) flexible end-viewing or side-viewing (oblique) endoscopes, which are used to visualize the esophagus, stomach, and proximal duodenum, or to cannulate the biliary tract in ERCP;

(b) an anoscope, which is a rigid plastic or metal speculum that is used to inspect the anal canal;

(c) a proctosigmoidoscope or rectosigmoidoscope, which is a 15- or 25-cm rigid endoscope that is used to examine the rectum and the sigmoid colon; and

(d) a flexible sigmoidoscope, which may be up to 65 cm in length and is used for examining the rectum and the sigmoid and descending colon.

A colonoscope, which is a 120- to 180-cm flexible endoscope used to visualize the entire lower GI tract from the rectum to the ileocecal valve. In pediatric patients, many colonoscopies are done to rule out or monitor inflammatory bowel disease, so the usual goal endpoint is the terminal ileum. Although they are designed for specific uses, all endoscopes have certain common parts, which include the following:

1. A flexible insertion tube that is usually 8 to 12 mm in diameter. The insertion tube contains air/water and biopsy channels, fiber bundles, and cables. It extends from the distal end to the control head.
2. An umbilical cord that extends from the control head and inserts into the light source.
3. An optic system, which consists of **fiberoptic bundles** that conduct light through the shaft and transmit the image to the eye, used with a lens system that focuses the image at the eyepiece. In a video endoscope, the optic system consists of a one-piece, solid-state video camera (including the camera head, coupler, and focusable optics), which transmits the image to a television screen without the need for fiber optics.
4. A control head that houses the lenses; controls for maneuvering the tip up and down and left and right; and

valves that regulate irrigation, air or carbon dioxide insufflation, and suction.

5. Cables that extend the length of the insertion tube and serve to control the movement of the flexible tip.

6. Channels for air and water flow.

7. A suction/biopsy channel that also allows the passage of accessories, such as biopsy forceps, cytology brushes, polypectomy snares, laser fibers, electrocautery devices, or prostheses (stents). The suction channel also allows for suctioning fluid that obstructs the endoscopist's vision.

8. Optional cameras that can be attached to the endoscope to allow the taking of still 35-mm or instant photographs or video recordings.

Taken together, the various types of endoscopes and their accessories provide a powerful armamentarium for the diagnosis and treatment of GI disease.

SEDATION AND ANALGESIA

Many diagnostic and therapeutic procedures in the endoscopy unit, including EGD, ERCP, and colonoscopy, are performed using moderate sedation and analgesia. The American Society of Anesthesiologists (ASA) provides "Practice Guidelines for Sedation and Analgesia by Non-Anesthesiologist" which are utilized as guidelines in the endoscopy setting. The ASA defines four levels of continuum of sedation depth in the amended 2001document.

1. **Minimal Sedation or Anxiolysis** is a drug-induced state during which patients respond normally to verbal commands. Although cognitive function and coordination may be impaired, ventilatory and cardiovascular functions are unaffected.

2. **Moderate Sedation/Analgesia** ("Conscious Sedation") is a drug-induced depression of consciousness during which patients respond purposefully to verbal commands, either alone or accompanied by light tactile stimulation. No interventions are required to maintain a patent airway, and spontaneous ventilation is adequate. Cardiovascular function is usually maintained.

3. **Deep Sedation/Analgesia** is a drug-induced depression of consciousness during which patients cannot be easily aroused but respond purposefully following repeated or painful stimulation. The ability to independently maintain ventilatory function may be impaired. Patients may require assistance in maintaining a patent airway, and spontaneous ventilation may be inadequate. Cardiovascular function is usually maintained.

4. **General Anesthesia** is a drug-induced loss of consciousness during which patients are not arousable, even by painful stimulation. The ability to independently maintain ventilatory function is often impaired. Patients often require assistance in maintaining a patent airway, and positive pressure ventilation may be required because of depressed spontaneous ventilation or drug-induced depression of neuromuscular function. Cardiovascular function may be impaired.

Because sedation is a continuum, it is not always possible to predict how an individual patient will respond. Practitioners intending to produce a given level of sedation should be able to rescue patients whose level of sedation becomes deeper than initially intended (ASA, 2001).

For endoscopy procedures, the **Moderate Sedation/Analgesia ("Conscious Sedation")** level is approved by the ASA for the non-anesthesiology practitioner for best practice and positive patient outcomes. These guidelines are intended to ensure the performance of safe and effective diagnostic and therapeutic procedures. The goals of Moderate Sedation/Analgesia ("Conscious Sedation") include the following:

(a) maintain intact protective reflexes;

(b) allow relaxation to allay anxiety and fear;

(c) minimize changes in vital signs;

(d) diminished verbal communication;

(e) ensure cooperation;

(f) decreased pain perception;

(g) ensure easy arousal from sleep;

(h) maintain patient ability to respond to commands; and

(i) provide some degree of retrograde amnesia.

In endoscopy settings, Moderate Sedation/Analgesia ("Conscious Sedation") is most often induced by the IV administration of the benzodiazepines diazepam (Valium) or midazolam (Versed). These agents may be administered in combination with atropine and narcotic analgesics, such as meperidine (Demerol), morphine, and fentanyl. Titration of IV sedation/anlagesia medications to achieve the desired effect improves clinical efficacy and reduces adverse outcomes.

It is the responsibility of the conscious-sedation trained registered nurse to administer the sedation and analgesia during endoscopic procedures, in the presence of, and by the order of, a physician. In procedures that are complicated by the severity of the patient's illness, age, and/or complex technical requirements of the procedure, a second nurse may be needed to assist the physician while the first nurse assesses and monitors the patient throughout the entire process. It may be necessary to have the anesthesia department assess and monitor pediatric or high-risk patients as determined by the physician, or this may be standard practice in some institutions. Patients who need special consideration for increased risk include those who are over age 60; are unable to cooperate; or have a history of severe cardiac, pulmonary, hepatic, renal, or CNS disease, morbid obesity, sleep apnea, drug or alcohol abuse, pregnancy, metabolic imbalance, or airway difficulties. Emergency procedures performed on patients who have not been properly prepared for the procedure also represent additional risk.

Before the administration of sedation and analgesia, it is important that the registered gastroenterology nurse assess the patient for communication barriers or developmental stage factors; age and weight; vital signs and ECG; skin, drug, and latex allergies; current medications and medication history; use of substance history; relevant medical-surgical history; level of comfort; level of consciousness; mobility and associated safety measures; NPO status; type of bowel preparation and results if indicated; and laboratory results if indicated. Other preprocedure responsibilities include verification of signed informed consent; verification of transportation with a responsible adult for outpatients; establishment of venous access; and patient education, including what to expect during all phases of the procedure, as well as discharge instructions.

Before administration of sedation and analgesia, the patient should be kept NPO to reduce the risk of aspiration. Children under 6 months of age should not be allowed solids or full liquids for 4 hours before sedation but may be allowed clear liquids up until 2 to 3 hours before sedation. Children 6 to 36 months of age should not be allowed solids or full liquids for 6 hours before sedation but may be allowed clear liquids up until 2 to 3 hours before sedation. Children over 36 months of age and adults should not be allowed solids or full liquids for 8 hours before sedation but may be allowed clear liquids up until 2 to 3 hours before sedation (ASA, 1996). Patients who have delayed gastric emptying may require longer fasting times.

Both diazepam and midazolam must be slowly titrated in small incremental doses until the desired endpoint is reached, usually exhibited by onset of slurred speech and decreased responsiveness. Respiratory depression may be potentiated by the additional use of an analgesic, emphasizing the need to reduce the amount of incremental doses and closely assess and monitor the level of consciousness and respiratory function. Individual response varies with age, physical status, and current medications. Particular care must be taken with pediatric, elderly, and debilitated patients.

During any procedures performed under sedation and analgesia, it is the nurse's responsibility to monitor the patient's vital signs and response to both sedation and the procedure. Minimal monitoring for patients of all ages includes observation of oxygen saturation, blood pressure, pulse, respiratory rate and effort, level of consciousness (i.e., response to verbal and/or tactile stimuli and purposeful communication), warmth and dryness of skin, and pain tolerance. Physiological data from continuous monitoring should be documented at least every 5 minutes during medication titration and at least every 15 minutes thereafter until the patient meets pre-established discharge criteria. These intervals should be shortened with changes in the patient's status, need for additional medication, and increased complexity of the procedure. Continuous ECG and intermittent mechanical blood pressure monitoring are also useful but not required. Although automatic monitoring devices may enhance the nurse's ability to assess the patient accurately, they are no substitute for watchful, educated assessment.

It is important to document the diagnostic or therapeutic technique(s) used; any unusual events, including intervention and subsequent patient response; the status of the patient after completion of the procedure. The nurse must also document the name; dose/amount; route; time given; and patient response to all drugs, fluids, and blood products administered. Potential adverse reactions to sedation and analgesia include anaphylaxis, respiratory distress, tachycar-

dia, bradycardia, and seizures. Some patients may have a paradoxical reaction to sedation and analgesia, becoming incoherent, uncontrollable, and inconsolable. Caregivers should be educated regarding this possible response before the procedure. Because of increased potential adverse reactions, it is important that pediatric patients undergoing sedation and analgesia be monitored by individuals who are familiar with normal pediatric vital signs and are trained in pediatric basic life support and the use of respiratory emergency equipment. It is recommended that an individual trained in adult or pediatric advanced life support is immediately available in each setting. The emergency cart must be stocked with equipment and medications appropriate for the age and size of patients receiving sedation and analgesia.

After the procedure is complete, it is important that the nurse monitor the patient's vital signs and level of consciousness; observe and document any further unusual events or postprocedural complications and their nature; and review verbally the written postprocedure instructions that address diet, medications, safety-focused activity restrictions according to age or level of mobility, follow-up care, and course of action if a complication develops. At discharge, the nurse must ensure that institutional discharge criteria are met. These usually include return to presedation and analgesia oxygen saturation, vital signs, and level of consciousness; no nausea/vomiting; no abdominal pain; and steady ambulation.

The safe administration and maintenance of sedation and analgesia by order of the physician is one of the most important responsibilities of the registered nurse working in the GI endoscopy setting. The nurse must be trained and educated in endoscopy; must possess knowledge of medications used and the skills to assess, diagnose, and intervene in the event of complications; and may be given the responsibility for the administration of reversal agents prescribed by the physician, such as flumazenil (Romazicon) or naloxone (Narcan). Whether the registered nurse actually administers the medications, he or she is responsible for monitoring and assessing the patient receiving sedation and analgesia throughout diagnostic and therapeutic GI procedures. It is imperative that the registered nurse follows his or her state's nurse practice act and his or her institutional policy and procedures regarding sedation and discharge.

ESOPHAGOGASTRODUODENOSCOPY

In **esophagogastroduodenoscopy (EGD),** a flexible endoscope less than 10 mm in diameter is passed into the upper GI tract. The entire esophagus and stomach and the proximal duodenum are easily visualized. Smaller pediatric endoscopes may be used for younger patients or for patients with strictures. Larger-diameter gastroscopes with a larger suction channel or two suction channels may be used for therapeutic procedures.

EGD allows the physician to diagnose and document GI abnormalities through the use of direct vision and still and video photography. Diagnostic EGD may be indicated for patients with any of the following:

(a) dysphagia or odynophagia;

(b) dyspepsia (selected patients);

(c) esophageal reflux that persists despite appropriate therapy;

(d) persistent, unexplained vomiting;

(e) upper GI x-ray films showing lesions that require biopsy;

(f) acute or chronic upper GI bleeding (hematemesis or melena);

(g) suspected esophageal or gastric varices;

(h) suspected esophageal stenosis, esophagitis, hiatal hernia, gastritis, obstructive lesions, and gastric or peptic ulcers;

(i) chronic abdominal pain;

(j) suspected polyps or cancer;

(k) follow-up of patients with Barrett's esophagus; large, indeterminate ulcers; or previous gastric or duodenal surgery;

(l) removal of ingested foreign bodies;

(m) caustic ingestion; or

(n) oral aversion.

Diagnostic EGD may be contraindicated in uncooperative patients and inpatients with any of the following:

(a) suspected perforated viscus;

(b) shock;

(c) seizures;

(d) recent myocardial infarction;

(e) severe cardiac decompensation;

(f) large aortic aneurysm;

(g) respiratory compromise;

(h) severe cervical arthritis;

(i) acute oral or oropharyngeal inflammation;

(j) acute abdomen; or

(k) known Zenker's diverticulum (Mosby, 2002).

To decrease the risk of aspiration the patient undergoing EGD must be NPO before the procedure. Guidelines for fasting before sedation may be followed. A thorough medical and drug history and physical examination are important, with special attention given to any history of drug reactions; bleeding disorders; or associated cardiac, pulmonary, renal, hepatic, or central nervous system (CNS) disease. The mouth should be inspected for loose teeth and orthodontic appliances that could become dislodged. If ordered, a topical anesthetic may be applied to the oral pharynx to suppress the gag reflex.

Before insertion, the endoscope should be lubricated with a water-soluble lubricant. The patient should be placed in the left lateral position. The chin should be tilted toward the chest, keeping the head in the midline. The endoscope is passed in stages, examining each structure as the scope advances. To obtain the best possible view, mucus or other secretions are suctioned and air is instilled to distend structures.

As the endoscope passes through the pylorus, the patient may experience some abdominal discomfort or may retch. At this time, it may help to have the patient breathe deeply and slowly to help relax the abdominal muscles. The patient may also experience a feeling of fullness or an urge to defecate as air passes into the stomach and duodenum. It is important to reassure the patient and hold his or her head and shoulders to help maintain the proper position, keeping the chin tilted toward the table to allow secretions to drain.

Occasionally, duodenal spasm makes visualization of this structure difficult. Administration of a smooth-muscle relaxant, such as glucagon, decreases contractions so the mucosa and contour of the duodenum can be examined thoroughly.

Because of the narrow and collapsible airway in infants and small children, introduction of the endoscope may result in respiratory distress, such as stridor, apnea, or oxygen desaturation. A simple jaw-lift maneuver applied by the nurse is likely to reduce compression of the trachea and result in resolution of these symptoms. To apply a jaw lift, the nurse's fingers are gently placed along the lower jawbone and used to guide the jaw forward. An additional threat to the child's respiratory status is the increased potential for overinflation of the stomach (especially in infants), which decreases chest expansion. Symptoms may include abdominal distention, growing tachypnea, and oxygen desaturation; symptoms are usually relieved by removal of the air.

During EGD it is important to maintain the patient's oral airway, suctioning secretions and regurgitated material when necessary from the pharynx. Nasal oxygen should be used to treat hypoxia, and resuscitation equipment should be immediately available in the event of adverse cardiopulmonary reactions.

After the procedure the patient should remain NPO until the gag reflex returns, which may take 1 to 2 hours. After the gag reflex returns, any residual sore throat or hoarseness may be relieved by drinking liquids, using a normal saline gargle, or using anesthetic throat lozenges. Because of the risk of aspiration, throat lozenges cannot be given to patients who are still mildly sedated, nor should they be given to small children.

The nurse should monitor the patient's oxygen saturation and vital signs regularly and observe the patient for signs of bleeding, vomiting, change in vital signs, pain, and abdominal distention. The patient should be instructed to report any hematemesis, pain, or difficulty breathing, because these are symptoms of complications.

EGD is generally regarded as safe, but adverse events can occur, including the following:

(a) respiratory depression or arrest;

(b) perforation of the esophagus, stomach, or duodenum;

(c) hemorrhage related to trauma or perforation;

(d) pulmonary aspiration of blood, secretions, or regurgitated gastric contents;

(e) infection;

(f) cardiac arrhythmia or arrest;

(g) localized phlebitis related to IV diazepam (Valium); this reaction is seen less often now that midazolam (Versed) is in widespread use;

(h) vasovagal response; or

(i) allergic reaction to the topical anesthetic or IV medications.

The rate of complications increases when therapeutic maneuvers are performed. Patients at the highest risk are the elderly and those with advanced cardiac, pulmonary, hepatic, or CNS disease.

ENDOSCOPIC RETROGRADE CHOLANGIOPANCREATOGRAPHY

Endoscopic retrograde cholangiopancreatography (ERCP) uses a combination of endoscopic and radiological techniques to visualize the biliary and pancreatic ducts. ERCP is indicated for the following:

(a) evaluation of signs or symptoms suggesting pancreatic malignancy when results of ultrasonography and/or CT scan are normal or equivocal;

(b) evaluation of acute, recurrent, or chronic pancreatitis of unknown etiology;

(c) before therapeutic endoscopy of the biliary tree; for example, removal of retained common bile duct stones, endoscopic sphincterotomy, balloon dilatation of strictures, or placement of a stent or biliary drain;

(d) unexplained chronic abdominal pain of suspected biliary or pancreatic origin;

(e) evaluation of jaundiced patients suspected of having treatable biliary obstruction;

(f) evaluation of patients without jaundice whose clinical presentation suggests bile duct disease;

(g) preoperative or postoperative evaluation to detect common duct stones in patients who undergo laparoscopic cholecystectomy; or

(h) manometric evaluation of the ampulla and common bile duct.

The use of ERCP in pediatric patients is limited to rare cases of obstructive jaundice without dilated biliary ducts (such as in sclerosing cholangitis or congenital stricture of common hepatic duct), relapsing pancreatitis of unknown cause, and preparation of patients for pancreatic surgery when knowledge of the ductal anatomy is important.

ERCP is contraindicated in uncooperative patients and in patients who are physically unable to tolerate the procedure. It is also contraindicated inpatients with recent myocardial infarction, severe pulmonary disease, coagulopathy, or pregnancy. The physician should be notified if the patient has a known allergy to contrast media, and any necessary precautions should be taken. ERCP may be contraindicated in patients with acute pancreatitis, unless the clinical situation necessitates the procedure.

Before ERCP, patients should fast for 6 hours. Barium studies should not be conducted within 72 hours preceding ERCP, because the residual barium can obstruct the view of the contrast medium in the ducts. ERCP usually takes longer than routine EGD, and therefore IV sedation and analgesia is likely to be heavier.

Before the procedure, all equipment should be set up and tested in a radiographic examination room. The patient should be in either the prone or left lateral position. A side-viewing duodenoscope is passed into the second part of the duodenum. Glucagon may be injected intravenously to suppress duodenal peristalsis and enhance visualization.

When the endoscope is in the proper position to view the ampulla of Vater, the patient is moved to the prone position. The endoscopist then passes a plastic cannula through the endoscope and maneuvers it into the orifice of the ampulla. Further adjustment of the cannula using the endoscope's elevator control allows it to enter the pancreatic duct or the common bile duct.

Radiocontrast material is injected through the cannula. To be certain that the contrast medium is free of air bubbles, the cannula must be primed with contrast before being inserted into the endoscope. When the contrast medium is injected, the amount injected should be stated verbally. Contrast should be injected slowly to avoid overfilling the duct. X-ray films are then taken to identify the configuration of the appropriate ductal system. The patient should be observed for any allergic reactions to the radiocontrast dye. Before the scope is withdrawn, a biopsy examination or cytological brushing may also be done.

After the procedure is completed, delayed x-ray films may be ordered to determine the time and amount of drainage of the ducts. It is the responsibility of the nurse to perform the following procedures:

1. Assess, monitor, and document oxygen saturation and vital signs.

2. Observe the patient for abdominal distention and signs of pancreatitis, including chills, low-grade fever, pain, vomiting, and tachycardia.

3. Maintain NPO status until the patient's gag reflex returns or further orders are written.

4. Administer antibiotics as ordered.

The patient's temperature should be checked every 4 hours for 48 hours. In 2 to 4 hours a light meal may be served. the day after the procedure, a full diet may be resumed.

The most significant complications associated with ERCP are pancreatitis and sepsis. Injury to the pancreas can be the result of mechanical, chemical, enzymatic, microbiological, thermal, or hydrostatic factors. If pancreatitis does result, it usually occurs within 2 to 4 hours after the procedure.

Another frequent complication of ERCP is biliary sepsis, especially in patients with partial obstruction of either the pancreatic or common bile ducts. The introduction of infection into a stagnant duct system can result in cholangitis, pancreatitis and septicemia. The utilization of a reprocessed water bottle should be used for each ERCP. If a pseudocyst is present, ERCP should be used only as an immediate preoperative procedure under antibiotic prophylaxis. Parenteral antibiotics, usually gentamicin (Garamycin) and/or ampicillin, should be given immediately to anyone diagnosed by ERCP as having biliary or pancreatic stasis.

In many patients an asymptomatic rise in serum amylase is noted following ERCP. Unless accompanied by abdominal pain, this rise in amylase is usually insignificant and subsides shortly. Additional potential complications include aspiration, bleeding, perforation, respiratory depression or arrest, and cardiac arrhythmia or arrest. Patients may experience a rise in temperature, chills, nausea, vomiting, abdominal pain, or ascending cholangitis.

ANOSCOPY

An anoscope is a clear plastic or metal speculum designed for examining the anus and lower rectum. One type is cylindrical, with one side that is incomplete or slotted. The mucosa to be evaluated protrudes through this slot. By withdrawing and reinserting the anoscope in multiple orientations, excellent visualization of the entire circumference of the anal canal is possible.

The most common causes of bright red rectal bleeding in adults and children are hemorrhoids and fissures although hemorrhoids are not common in children. Protein allergy is the most common cause of rectal bleeding in neonates. **Anoscopy** is indicated for identification of these disorders. It may also be used before sigmoidoscopy or colonoscopy.

For anoscopy, the patient is positioned in Sims' left lateral position or the knee-chest position, which allows the sigmoid colon to straighten, thus promoting better visualization. Special proctological tilt tables (breakaway tables) are available that permit the patient to be placed in an inverted position with the head down, against a headrest. To minimize embarrassment, the patient is draped, exposing only the lower buttocks area.

A thorough visual and digital rectal examination is performed first, using a gloved, well-lubricated index finger (the little finger is used for infants under 2 years of age). At this time the examiner looks for anal anomalies, sphincter tone, polyps or adenomas, rectal prolapse, extracolonic masses, and hemorrhoids. Any stool remaining on the examining finger may be checked for blood.

Severe spasm induced by digital examination usually signifies low-lying inflammatory bowel disease, such as proctitis or ulcerative colitis (UC).

A warm, well-lubricated anoscope is inserted slowly, with the beveled surface of the tip facing laterally. The general appearance of the mucosa is noted, and the area is examined for fissures, abscesses, or signs of anal papillitis or cryptitis. Biopsies may be necessary to determine if abnormal mucosa is present.

PROCTOSIGMOIDOSCOPY

Proctosigmoidoscopy, also known as **rectosigmoidoscopy,** is an examination of the rectum and the sigmoid colon using a rigid proctosigmoidoscope. The proctosigmoidoscope is a small, hollow, stainless steel or plastic disposable tube that is 25 to 30 cm long and approximately 1.5 cm in diameter. A smaller **proctoscope** may be used with newborns or infants or for patients with strictures. A light source is attached to the end of the scope.

Indications for proctosigmoidoscopy may include the following:

(a) melena or bleeding from the anorectal area;
(b) persistent diarrhea;
(c) change in bowel habits;
(d) passage of pus and mucus;
(e) suspected chronic inflammatory bowel disease;
(f) bacteriology and histological studies;
(g) surveillance of known rectal disease;
(h) rectal pain;
(i) screening for suspected polyps or tumors;
(j) foreign body removal;
(k) as an adjunct to a barium enema; and
(l) surveillance following rectal surgery.

Contraindications include severe necrotizing enterocolitis, toxic megacolon, painful anal lesions, severe cardiac arrhythmia, and uncooperative patients.

Most patients should be given a hypertonic phosphate or saline enema the morning of the examination. Patients who have UC or acute diarrhea can be examined without the use of cleansing enemas or laxatives. Medication is rarely needed for adult or adolescent patients. Young children may require sedation and analgesia; infants under 3 months of age usually tolerate the procedure well without sedation.

With the patient in either a knee-chest or Sims' left lateral position, a thorough visual and digital rectal examination is conducted. The scope is warmed under running water and then gently pressed against the anal opening. While the patient is asked to bear down, the instrument is easily passed into the rectum, the obturator is removed, and the instrument is passed slowly into the colon. If spasm or difficulty is encountered, the scope should be withdrawn until the full lumen is seen and a second attempt should be made.

During insertion, the patient should breathe deeply with the mouth open, to keep the abdominal muscles relaxed. Cramping or a desire to defecate can be relieved by having the patient relax and take deep breaths or pant. If air is insufflated into the lumen to enhance visualization, the patient will normally experience some flatulence as the air moves down the bowel and escapes.

Once the desired depth is reached, the sigmoidoscope is gradually withdrawn, thus allowing examination of all sides of the bowel. A large cotton swab or suction may be used to remove any fecal matter, blood, or mucus that is obscuring vision. The examiner will note the color and friability of the mucosa, bleeding sites, petechiae, and ulcers. (Mucosal friability is established if pinpoint bleeding is noted immediately after application of mechanical pressure with a cotton swab or cytology brush.) If a biopsy examination is indicated, the site of the lesion or specimen and its distance from the anus should be recorded.

Throughout the procedure, the nurse should monitor the patient for vital signs; abdominal distention; pain tolerance; and warmth, color, and dryness of the skin. Sudden changes in position during the procedure should be prevented. Thus infants and children may need to be swaddled or held.

After the procedure is finished, the table should be returned to a low position and the patient should be brought slowly to a seated position before standing. The patient should be observed for signs of bleeding or perforation. Diet, fluids, and activity can return to normal following the procedure, unless complications occur.

Potential complications of rigid proctosigmoidoscopy

include perforation, minimal bleeding from lacerations, transient abdominal discomfort, and cardiac arrhythmias. If perforation is suspected and confirmed by clinical symptoms and roentgenographic examination, prompt surgical intervention is indicated. If there is excessive bleeding from a biopsy site, the patient's bleeding status should be checked and the biopsy site reexamined. Either silver nitrate or electrocautery of the bleeding area will usually stop the bleeding.

FLEXIBLE SIGMOIDOSCOPY

Sigmoidoscopy is the examination of the rectum and the sigmoid and descending colon using a flexible sigmoidoscope or colonoscope. In recent years, the flexible fiberoptic sigmoidoscope has largely replaced the standard 25-cm rigid sigmoidoscope for routine examination. The newer, flexible fiberoptic sigmoidoscopes, which measure up to 65 cm in length, have a much greater range than the older, rigid scopes. Flexible instruments are capable of reaching the descending colon in over 80% of patients, and it is possible to reach the splenic flexure. In addition, patients seem to tolerate flexible sigmoidoscopy better than rigid proctosigmoidoscopy.

Flexible sigmoidoscopy is indicated for the following:
(a) routine screening of adults over age 50;
(b) evaluation of suspected distal colonic disease when there is no indication for colonoscopy;
(c) inflammatory bowel disease;
(d) chronic diarrhea;
(e) pseudomembranous colitis;
(f) radiation colitis;
(g) sigmoid volvulus;
(h) foreign body removal;
(i) lower GI bleeding; and
(j) evaluation of the colon in conjunction with a barium enema.

Sigmoidoscopy is contraindicated in patients with fulminant colitis; toxic megacolon; severe, acute diverticulitis; peritonitis; or uncooperative patients.

Except in patients with watery diarrhea or suspected colitis, preparation for flexible sigmoidoscopy includes two warm tap-water or sodium biphosphate (Fleet) enemas 1 to 2 hours before the examination. In pediatric patients however, warm tap water enemas are not given due to the risk of electrolyte imbalances. A more thorough bowel preparation may be indicated by the patient's disease status. Compliance with the bowel preparation ordered by the physician should be verified. A medical history should be obtained, including medications, allergies, and any information pertaining to the current complaint. Antibiotic prophylaxis should be administered if ordered. Patients usually do not require sedation and analgesia.

After a thorough digital rectal examination, the patient is instructed to breathe slowly and deeply to relax the anal sphincters while the well-lubricated endoscope is inserted. While the endoscope is being advanced to the rectosigmoid junction, air is insufflated to facilitate passage into the sigmoid and descending colon. While the instrument is slowly withdrawn, the physician examines the sigmoid colon and then the rectal and anal mucosa. Suction may be used to remove residual matter, blood, or mucus that obscures vision.

During the procedure it is important for the nurse to monitor the patient's vital signs; color, warmth, and dryness of skin; abdominal distention; level of consciousness; pain tolerance; and vagal response. The physician should be notified if the abdomen is becoming excessively distended secondary to air insufflation. To help the patient cooperate, it may be helpful to offer back rubbing or instructions in breathing technique.

After the procedure is completed the patient may resume normal activity if no sedation has been administered. The patient should be observed for postbiopsy bleeding and persistent abdominal pain or distention.

Potential complications of flexible sigmoidoscopy include bleeding and perforation.

COLONOSCOPY

Colonoscopy involves direct visualization of the lower GI tract from the rectum to the ileocecal valve and even the distal ileum, using a long, flexible endoscope. Modern fiberoptic and video colonoscopes are similar in design to upper GI endoscopes but are longer, ranging in length from 120 to 180 cm. Suction removes liquid secretions that obscure vision, thereby permitting safe advancement of the instrument. Air and water controls help keep the lumen distended and the optics of the tip of the instrument clean.

An experienced endoscopist may view the entire colon and often the distal ileum, reaching the cecum in most patients.

Diagnostic colonoscopy is indicated for the following:
(a) evaluation of active or occult lower GI bleeding, such as hematochezia, melena with a negative upper GI investigation, unexplained fecal occult blood, and unexplained iron-deficiency anemia;
(b) evaluation of abnormalities found on radiographic examination;
(c) suspected cecal or ascending colonic disease;
(d) surveillance for colon neoplasia in patients who have had a previous colon cancer or previous colon polyps;
(e) screening in patients 50 years of age or older, in patients with a personal history of polyps or colorectal cancer, and in patients with a first-degree (parent or sibling) family history of colon cancer;
(f) surveillance in patients with chronic UC of several years' duration;
(g) diagnosis or management of chronic inflammatory bowel disease;
(h) chronic, unexplained abdominal pain; and
(i) confirmation of suspected polyps, rectal or colonic strictures, or cancer.

Colonoscopy is contraindicated in patients with fulminant UC; acute ischemic colitis; acute radiation colitis; suspected toxic megacolon; suspected perforation; acute, severe diverticulitis; the presence of barium; imperforate anus; massive colonic bleeding; shock; acute surgical abdomen or a fresh surgical anastomosis; or patients who are physically unable to tolerate the procedure. Relative contraindications include massive hematochezia, infectious bowel disease, pregnancy, coagulation abnormalities, unstable cardiovascular status, and uncooperative patients.

Standard bowel preparation for colonoscopy is to administer about 1 gallon of an isoosmolar electrolyte lavage solution. The solution may be consumed either orally or through a nasogastric tube over a 4-hour period, beginning 6 to 12 hours before the procedure. The only problem with this type of preparation is that some patients have difficulty consuming such a large quantity of fluid over a short period. A small-volume phospho-soda preparation has been more recently developed for use in healthy adults without cardiac, renal, or electrolyte problems. If rectal bleeding or severe abdominal pain occurs during bowel preparation, the physician should be notified immediately.

A variety of colonoscopy preparations are used for children. The child's age, size, and indication for the procedure must be considered before deciding what type of preparation will be used. Osmolar electrolyte solutions are often not well tolerated in the volume necessary for adequate bowel preparation, and they may be administered via nasogastric infusion. Current literature does not support the use of phospho-soda in children, although it is used by some institutions. Children may tolerate a regimen of clear liquid diet for 3 days before the procedure, in addition to enemas and cathartics, with good results.

The patient should be given an opportunity to urinate before the procedure. Because colonoscopy takes longer and is more uncomfortable than flexible sigmoidoscopy, it is customary to administer IV sedation and analgesia to promote relaxation and diminish discomfort. General anesthesia is used routinely in pediatric patients.

Colonoscopy is usually begun with the patient in the left lateral decubitus position. After a digital examination, the lubricated colonoscope is inserted into the rectum while the patient breathes slowly and deeply. Then the physician insufflates a small amount of air to help dilate the bowel lumen. When appropriate, the nurse should assist the physician in repositioning the patient smoothly to facilitate passage through the splenic flexure, the transverse colon, the hepatic flexure, the ascending colon, and the cecum. In addition, the nurse may apply pressure to areas of the abdomen as requested by the physician to assist with passage of the instrument.

Throughout the procedure it is important that the nurse monitor the patient for changes in oxygen saturation and vital signs; color, warmth, and dryness of the skin; abdominal distention; level of consciousness; vagal response; and pain tolerance. The physician should be notified if the abdomen becomes excessively distended because of air insufflation. To help the patient cooperate more readily, instructions in breathing technique may be offered.

During the procedure the physician may order the administration of atropine or glucagon in an attempt to decrease bowel spasms and/or motility. If either drug is used, the nurse should closely monitor the patient for hypotension and irregular or rapid pulse.

During insertion of the colonoscope, the objective is to reach the cecum as quickly and as safely as possible. During withdrawal, the objective is meticulous inspection. The mucosa is scanned by changing the position of the flexible tip while the instrument is slowly withdrawn. The bowel wall is examined for abnormalities, such as ulcerations, bleeding sites, polyps, inflammation, or tumors. Direct visualization allows for therapeutic procedures, such as polypectomy, dilatation, decompression, and fulguration of bleeding sites.

Following colonoscopy it is important for the nurse to monitor and document vital signs every 15 minutes until the patient is stable. The patient should be observed for signs of complications, such as bleeding, vomiting, a change in vital signs, severe or persistent abdominal pain and/or distention, and abdominal rigidity.

Major complications occur in less than 1% of patients undergoing colonoscopy. The two major complications, perforation and hemorrhage, are most likely to occur during or after polypectomy, which is discussed in Chapter 30. Other potential complications of colonoscopy include medication reactions, such as cardiac arrhythmias or arrest and respiratory depression or arrest; explosion of colonic gases; vasovagal reactions; and cardiac failure or hypotension, related to overhydration or underhydration of a susceptible patient during bowel preparation. Excessive bleeding from biopsy sites is rare unless the patient has a coagulation disorder or has been on products that contain aspirin. Unsuspected serosal tears and retroperitoneal emphysema have occasionally been found during laparotomy. Excessive use of air and advancement of the scope without a clear view of the lumen are most likely to cause these difficulties.

Colonoscopic complications may be minimized by advancing the colonoscope or sigmoidoscope with care and avoiding overdistention of the colon. Fluid and electrolyte status of elderly patients and those with renal and cardiac disease should be considered during bowel preparation. If soreness occurs at the IV injection site, it can be relieved with warm compresses.

ADDITIONAL TECHNIQUES

The technology available for endoscopic visualization of the GI tract continues to advance. Additional diagnostic techniques that are available to the endoscopist include small bowel enteroscopy, capsule endoscopy, endoscopy through an ostomy, videoendoscopy, and endoscopic ultrasonography.

Small bowel enteroscopy

Small bowel enteroscopy permits visualization of the small bowel beyond the ligament of Treitz. It is useful for patients with continued or intermittent blood loss in whom a GI bleeding site has not been found despite exhaustive testing. One technique uses a pediatric colonoscope as a push enteroscope to advance a long, thin, flexible endoscope into the small bowel. A balloon on the tip of the small bowel endoscope is inflated to hold it in place, and the push enteroscope is withdrawn. IV metoclopramide (Reglan) is administered, and the patient is sent to a recovery area for several hours while peristalsis advances the enteroscope through the small bowel. Once the enteroscope is positioned in the distal ileum, the small bowel is examined thoroughly while the enteroscope is slowly withdrawn. The complete procedure lasts 8 to 10 hours and enables visualization of all 20 feet of small bowel. A major disadvantage of this method is that because this scope does not accommodate accessories, no therapeutic interventions can be done.

A second technique uses a 210-cm push-type enteroscope similar to a standard GI endoscope, which accepts forceps and hemostasis devices in its biopsy channel. Because of the length of the endoscope, it is important to check length and compatibility of accessories before beginning a procedure. Patients are prepared as for EGD. Fluoroscopy and a compatible overtube may be used to facilitate passage of the endoscope, and IV glucagon may be used. The procedure can be completed much more quickly than the method described above, but it often takes longer than an EGD depending on ease of scope passage and number of therapeutic techniques used.

M2A™ Capsule Endoscopy

M2A™ Capsule Endoscopy is useful to help diagnose difficult and challenging small bowel cases where conventional methods have failed. Capsule enteroscopy is one of the newest diagnostic tools approved for the imaging of the small intestine. It is a non-invasive, diagnostic, easy-to-perform alternative technique that provides an improved level of visual imaging for diagnosis of diseases of the small bowel including obscure bleeding, irritable bowel syndrome, Crohn's disease, celiac disease, chronic diarrhea, malabsorption and small bowel cancer. The FDA has approved M2A™ Capsule Endoscopy as an adjunct tool for imaging of small intestine disorders and diseases. The capsule enteroscopy procedure is completely ambulatory. The patient does not need to be confined to a hospital or medical facility during the 8-hour process.

The complete system consists of four components.

1. A single use M2A™ Capsule endoscopy, which measures 11 mm X 26 mm, and contains four light emitting diodes (LEDs), a lens, color camera chip, two batteries, a radio frequency transmitter and an antenna. After the appropriate clearance and assessment, the capsule is activated and the patient swallows the capsule. Peristalsis moves the capsule through the gastrointestinal tract, allowing examination of the entire small bowel. The transmitter delivers over 50,000 images during the 8-hour procedure.
2. The 8-lead Sensor Array™ is a group of taped-on, latex-free sensors that are placed strategically around the abdomen to record signaled images from the capsule.
3. The DataRecorder™ is worn around the patient's waist on a supportive adjustable belt that stores the received images as the patient goes about their daily tasks.
4. On completion of the 8-hour procedure, the RAPID Workstation™ downloads the data for physician review.

Capsule endoscopy is contraindicated in patients with known or suspected gastrointestinal obstruction, strictures or fistulas, patients with known difficulty in swallowing, patients with cardiac pacemakers or automatic ventricular defibrillators, and patients under the age of 18.

Patient education is provided to explain the procedure, why it is being ordered and expectations during and after the procedure. Preprocedure patient preparation includes only that the patient has nothing by mouth for 6 hours prior to the scheduled procedure. At the scheduled procedure time the patient arrives, receives patient education and nursing assessment. The patient is than fitted with the sensor array which is attached to the data-recorder belt. The patient is now ready to ingest the M2A Capsule Endoscopy™ with a full glass of water. The patient is asked to remain NPO for the next 2-hours post-capsule ingestion and than free to take fluids. In 4 hours the patient may eat a light meal. Patients should be advised to avoid any contact with MRI while the capsule is in the body, and to contact the physician if any symptoms of nausea, vomiting, abdominal pain or discomfort should occur. Strenuous physical activity should be avoided for 8 hours after ingesting the capsule. The patient is instructed to return to the facility in 8 hours. When the patient returns, the sensors are removed and the data recorder downloads the collected images into the computer for physician review.

Capsule endoscopy holds some advantages over conventional small bowel imaging and diagnostic modalities:(a) the procedure is ambulatory and non-invasive, with no need for sedation; (b) no risks from exposure to x-ray; and (c) no infection control cross contamination issues. Patients return to their daily activities and with few restrictions, are easily compliant. A major disadvantage of this method is that the procedure facilitates diagnostic imaging only and does not allow for therapeutic intervention. Capsule endoscopy is FDA-approved for small intestine study. It does not replace EGD or colonoscopy.

Capsule endoscopy offers the patient and caregivers a major advance in gastrointestinal diagnoses. The imaging recorded data provides potential solutions in patient management for the unresolved diagnostic challenges of small bowel disease (Yu, 2002).

Endoscopy through an ostomy

Occasionally it may be necessary to directly visualize a segment of small or large intestine using a flexible endoscope that has been inserted through a stoma. This procedure is indicated for evaluation of an anastomotic site, identification of recurrent disease (e.g., Crohn's disease or cancer), or visualization and/or treatment of GI bleeding. It is contraindicated in patients with recent ostomy/bowel surgery, poor bowel preparation, suspected bowel perforation, presence of a large peristomal hernia, or massive lower GI bleeding.

Before the procedure it is necessary to examine the ostomy site to determine the size of the stoma, the type of effluent that can be expected during the procedure, and what ostomy appliance will be needed following the procedure. Compliance with bowel preparation orders should be confirmed and their effectiveness ascertained. The old ostomy appliance should be removed gently, working from the top downward, taking care to push the skin away from the appliance.

The patient should be in the supine position, with fluid-impervious towels draping the stoma. A large supply of sponges should be provided, especially for an ileostomy. The endoscope should be held at a right angle to the abdominal wall to facilitate entry through the ostomy. The patient's oxygen saturation and vital signs should be monitored throughout the procedure, as should the color, warmth, and dryness of the skin; abdominal distention; level of consciousness; and pain tolerance. The nurse should provide emotional support to the patient while also maintaining a tight seal around the endoscope as it enters the stoma so the physician is able to accomplish adequate insufflation.

After the procedure is completed it is important that the nurse monitor and document oxygen saturation and vital signs. The peristomal area should be cleaned carefully with a mild soap and water, and the skin should be thoroughly dried. An appropriate skin barrier and collecting pouch should be applied immediately. The patient should be observed for stomal bleeding, vomiting, a change in vital signs, severe or persistent abdominal pain, and abdominal rigidity.

Videoendoscopy

Video endoscopes have no coherent fiberoptic image bundle. Instead, a distal sensing device in the tip of the instrument electronically transmits an image to a video processor for display in color or black and white on a television monitor. Endoscopy is performed by reference to the monitor. An advantage of this technology is that all members of the endoscopy team are able to view the procedure, thus enhancing collaboration among team members.

A videotape deck may be added to the system for recording the procedure on videotape. The video processor has a freeze-frame function, and a character-generator keyboard is provided to make marginal notes on the video screen next to the endoscopic image. Individual photographs may be generated by adding a mavigraph to the system. New computer programs are continually being developed to enhance the capabilities of **videoendoscopy.** Now, patient data can be accessed for statistical purposes and reports of procedures can be generated by computer.

Controls for tip deflection are similar to those of conventional fiberoptic scopes, with two coaxial knobs for left, right, up, and down deflections. Valves are provided for air and water insufflation and for suction. An accessory/suction channel is also provided. Because of its high photosensitivity, the video endoscope requires less light and provides greater depth of visual field than fiberoptic endoscopes. However, because of the decreased light output, it is more difficult to transilluminate the right lower quadrant of the abdomen when the tip of the colonoscope is in the cecum.

The use of videoendoscopy or any form of photography is secondary to patient needs. It should be postponed if the safety of the patient is compromised in any way.

Endoscopic ultrasonography

New technology has combined the endoscope with ultrasonography to enhance visualization of the GI tract, which is obscured in conventional ultrasonographic examinations by intraabdominal gas and bony structures. With an oblique-viewing endoscope that has an ultrasonic transducer built into the tip, high-frequency, ultrasonic beams can be targeted in close proximity to existing lesions.

This procedure results in better-quality resolution, which enhances evaluation of the histological structure of targeted lesions. In addition, esophageal wall thickness may be evaluated and assessed. The walls of the esophagus, stomach, duodenum, and colon may be visualized, as well as the structure of several contiguous organs.

The act of scanning through the gastric wall, combined with changes in the patient's position, is sufficient for the study of the gastric wall itself, the gallbladder, pancreas, kidneys, left lobe of the liver, spleen, aorta, inferior vena cava, and various tributaries of the extrahepatic portal vein system.

An inflatable balloon covers the ultrasonic transducer and can be filled with water to compress the esophageal wall, eliminate the air space, and improve the quality of resolution, which enhances the evaluation of the targeted lesion. Endoscopic ultrasonography, as compared with radiographic and endoscopic examinations, has many advantages for detecting lesions in the wall of the GI tract.

CASE SITUATION

The nurse manager of a busy hospital endoscopy unit is adding a new nurse. Susie Jones has finished her hospital orientation and started in the unit. She is vaguely familiar with gastroenterology procedures but has no gastroenterology experience. The nurse manager needs to set up a training program for Susie.

Points to think about

1. The nurse manager begins by showing Susie the orientation manual. What should be included in this manual?
2. What other manuals and books should the manager make available to Susie to help her do her job?
3. It is Susie's third week, and she is beginning to learn how to assist with a colonoscopy. What has she probably learned so far?
4. The manager is now showing Susie how to assist with a colonoscopy. What types of things must she be taught?

Suggested responses

1. The orientation manual should include the following:
   (a) hospital and department philosophy statements and standards;
   (b) job descriptions and lists of essential duties;
   (c) an overview of the training period;
   (d) an outline of expected learning experiences with time frames for completion;
   (e) a tool for evaluating learning experience;
   (f) copies of policies specific to employee conduct (e.g., reporting on-the-job accidents, or infection control policies); and
   (g) policy and statements on patient rights.
2. Other manuals and books that the nurse manager might make available to Susie include the following:
   (a) hospital and department policy manuals;
   (b) hospital's fire and disaster manual;
   (c) hospital's manual on hazardous materials;
   (d) SGNA procedure manual;
   (e) SGNA core curriculum;
   (f) good GI anatomy and physiology book;
   (g) drug reference book;
   (h) other GI endoscopy books (see bibliography); and
   (i) recent volumes of *Gastroenterology Nursing*.
3. After her first 3 weeks, Susie has probably read the pertinent policy and procedure manuals and at least part of the core curriculum. In addition, she has probably learned the following:
   (a) how to handle the various forms and paperwork required in the department;
   (b) how to admit a patient to the unit and how to perform the nursing assessment and plan of care;
   (c) the necessary infection control techniques;
   (d) the different types of scopes and how to set up equipment for EGD and colon examination procedures;
   (e) how to assist with a simple EGD with minimal supervision; and
   (f) how to process biopsy and cytology specimens.
4. Before Susie assists with a colonoscopy, it is important that she know the following:
   (a) basic colon anatomy and physiology;
   (b) indications for colonoscopy;
   (c) techniques of preparing the colon for colonoscopy;
   (d) how to relate possible diagnosis with the equipment setup;
   (e) how the nurse can facilitate the passage of the scope by using gentle external hand pressure to prevent the scope from bowing in the sigmoid; how different patient positions can facilitate passage of the scope in difficult cases;
   (f) how to comfort the patient by talking gently and providing encouragement and praise, and that gently stroking the patient's back or forehead can be comforting and reduce the need for medication; and
   (g) pertinent information that should be provided to the patient before discharge.

Patients are usually receptive and supportive of a teaching situation if they feel that they will not be left alone in the care of a novice. The nurse manager should let the patient know that he or she will be teaching a new nurse but will be present throughout the procedure. The manager should leave technical discussions of any pathological conditions encountered and the treatment that will be used for them until after the procedure to avoid causing the patient any additional stress. When teaching, the nurse manager should always remember to support statements with a rationale.

REVIEW TERMS

anoscopy, capsule endoscopy, colonoscopy, endoscopic retrograde cholangiopancreatography (ERCP), endoscopy, esophagogastroduodenoscopy (EGD), fiberoptic bundles, proctoscope, proctosigmoidoscopy, rectosigmoidoscopy, sigmoidoscopy, small bowel enteroscopy, videoendoscopy

REVIEW QUESTIONS

1. The endoscopes used in EGD can visualize the upper GI tract as far as the:
   (a) Pylorus.
   (b) Ampulla of Vater.
   (c) Proximal duodenum.
   (d) Ileocecal valve.
2. Before EGD, the patient should be NPO for at least:
   (a) 2 hours.
   (b) 6 hours.
   (c) 12 hours.
   (d) 24 hours.
3. The major complication(s) associated with ERCP is (are):
   (a) Perforation.
   (b) Adverse effects of medication.
   (c) Hemorrhage.
   (d) Pancreatitis and sepsis.
4. The most common cause(s) of bright red rectal bleeding in adults and children is (are):
   (a) Inflammatory bowel disease.
   (b) Perforation.
   (c) Hemorrhoids and fissures.
   (d) Bleeding ulcers and varices.
5. One contraindication for rigid proctosigmoidoscopy is:
   (a) Severe cardiac arrhythmias.
   (b) Previous rectal surgery.
   (c) Rectal bleeding.
   (d) Rectal pain.
6. The usual bowel preparation for flexible sigmoidoscopy in adults is:
   (a) A single warm tap-water enema.
   (b) Two warm tap-water or Fleet enemas.
   (c) A 2-day liquid diet, followed by a strong laxative.
   (d) Electrolyte lavage.
7. For flexible sigmoidoscopy, the patient should be in the knee-chest or:

(a) Prone position.
(b) Supine position.
(c) Right lateral position.
(d) Left lateral position.

8. Patients who will undergo colonoscopy usually receive:
(a) Local anesthesia only.
(b) IV sedation and analgesia.
(c) General anesthesia.
(d) No sedation and analgesia or anesthesia.

9. Distention of the abdomen during colonoscopy is most likely caused by:
(a) Excessive insufflation of air.
(b) Excessive amounts of water used for irrigation.
(c) Perforation.
(d) Colonic obstruction.

10. Small bowel enteroscopy is indicated for patients with:
(a) Peptic ulcers.
(b) Inflammatory bowel disease.
(c) Persistent blood loss with no identifiable source.
(d) Intestinal polyps.

BIBLIOGRAPHY

American Society of Anesthesiologists (2002). Practice guidelines for sedation and analgesia by nonanesthesiologists. *Anesthesiology 96*, 1004-17.

Bertagnolli, M. (1990). Use of endoscopic ultrasound in patients with esophageal motility disorders. In Trivits, S. (Ed.), *Journal Reprints II*, Rochester, NY: Society of Gastroenterology Nurses and Associates.

Castell, D. (Ed.) (1999). *Endoscopy in The Esophagus*. Philadelphia, PA: Lippincott Williams & Wilkens.

Eastwood, G. & Avunduk, C. (1988). *Manual of gastroenterology: diagnosis and therapy*. Boston: Little, Brown.

Given, B. & Simmons, S. (1984). *Gastroenterology in clinical nursing* (4th ed.). St. Louis, MO: Mosby.

Hamilton, H. (Ed.) (1983). *Procedures, Nurse's Reference Library*. Springhouse, PA: Intermed Communications.

Keighley, M. & Williams, N. (1999). *Endoscopy, Surgery of the Anus, Rectum and Colon* (2nd ed.). London: W. B. Saunders.

Langmore, S. (2001). *Endoscopic Evaluation & treatment of Swallowing Disorders*. New York: Thieme Medical Publishers, Inc.

Lewis, B. & Czachor, K. (1990). Small bowel enteroscopy: the GIA's role. In Trivits, S. (Ed.), *Journal Reprints II*, Rochester, NY: Society of Gastroenterology Nurses and Associates.

Mathews, J., Maher, K. & Cattau, E. Jr (1990). The role of endoscopic retrograde cholangiopancreatography injection training sessions for the gastroenterology nurse and associate. In Trivits, S. (Ed.), *Journal Reprints II*, Rochester, NY: Society of Gastroenterology Nurses and Associates.

Ravenscroft, M. & Swan, C. (1984). *Gastrointestinal endoscopy and related procedures: a handbook for nurses and assistants*. Baltimore, MD: Williams & Wilkins.

Rayhorn, N. (Ed.) (1995). *Manual of gastrointestinal procedures: pediatric supplement*. Chicago: Society of Gastroenterology Nurses and Associates.

Saunderlin, G. (1996, May 20). *Small bowel enteroscopy*. Paper presented at the Twenty-Third Annual Course of the Society of Gastroenterology Nurses and Associates, Las Vegas, NV.

Silverman, A. & Roy, C. (1983). *Pediatric clinical gastroenterology* (3rd ed.). St. Louis, MO: Mosby.

Sivak, M. Jr. & Petrini, J. (Eds.) (1986). *Gastrointestinal endoscopy: old problems, new techniques: Gastrointestinal Series Volume 4*. New York: Praeger.

Society of Gastroenterology Nurses and Associates, Inc. (2003). *Manual of gastrointestinal procedures* (5th ed.). Chicago: Society of Gastroenterology Nurses and Associates, Inc.

Society of Gastroenterology Nurses and Associates, Inc (2002). Statement on reprocessing of water bottles used during endoscopy. *Gastroenterol Nurs 25*, 5.

Society of Gastroenterology Nurses and Associates, Inc. (2000). Guidelines for nursing care of the patient receiving sedation and analgesia in the gastrointestinal endoscopy setting. *Gastroenterol Nurs 23*, 6.

Squires, R.H. & Colleti, R.B. (1996). Indications for pediatric gastrointestinal endoscopy: A medical position statement of the North American Society for Pediatric Gastroenterology and Nutrition. *Journal of Pediatric Gastroenterology Nursing. 23*, 107 –10.

Thompson, J., McFarlane, G., Hirsh, J. & Tucker, S. (2002). *Diagnostic Procedures and Tests: Mosby's Clinical Nursing* (5th ed.). St. Louis MO: Mosby.

Watson, D. (1990). *Monitoring the patient receiving local anesthesia*. Denver, CO: Association of Operating Room Nurses.

Waye, J. (1989). Diagnostic and therapeutic endoscopy. In Sachar, D., Waye, J. & Lewis, B. (Eds.), *Gastroenterology for the house officer*. Baltimore, MD: Williams & Wilkins.

Waye, J. (1988). Light in the right lower quadrant during colonoscopy: a comparison of fiberoptic versus video colonoscopes. *SGA J 11*, 157-8. Society of Gastrointestinal Assistants.

Wiersema, M.J. (Ed.) (1997). Emerging technologies in gastrointestinal endoscopy. *Gastrointestinal Clinical of North America 7*, 191.

Yu, M. (2002). M2A TM Capsule Endoscopy: A breakthrough diagnostic tool for small intestine imaging. *Gastroenterology Nursing 25*, 1.

Zfass, A. & Brennan, P. (1988). Endoscopy of the bowel. In Gitnick, G. & Hollander, D. (Eds.), *Principles and practice of gastroenterology and hepatology*. New York: Elsevier.

Chapter 24

MANOMETRY

This chapter will acquaint the gastroenterology nurse with manometric procedures that are used in the diagnosis of GI disorders, focusing on manometry.

Learning objectives

After reviewing the content of this chapter, the gastroenterology nurse should be able to:
1. Describe the equipment and techniques typically used in manometric studies.
2. List the indications and contraindications for manometric procedures involving the esophagus, stomach, small bowel, sphincter of Oddi, and anorectum.
3. Discuss the types of manometric tracings that are observed in normal subjects and in patients with selected GI disorders.

BASIC PRINCIPLES

GI **manometry** is a diagnostic test that measures changes in intraluminal pressure and coordination of activity in the muscles of the GI tract. Although it is primarily used to measure esophageal motility, manometric techniques may also be used in the stomach, small bowel, sphincter of Oddi, and anorectum. The instrumentation used may vary, but virtually all manometric techniques involve a series of catheters and pressure transducers that measure GI motor activity and transform this activity into electrical signals that, in turn, produce graphical images on a physiograph or a computer.

ESOPHAGEAL MANOMETRY

Esophageal manometry is a highly technical evaluation of the regions of the esophagus, the upper esophageal sphincter (UES), the esophageal body, and the lower esophageal sphincter (LES). Disorders of the oropharyngeal region and the UES may be better diagnosed with radiography or by a simultaneous manometric and fluoroscopic study.

Indications and contraindications

Esophageal manometry is indicated to establish the diagnosis of suspected cases of achalasia, nutcracker esophagus, hypertensive LES, diffuse esophageal spasm, and nonspecific esophageal motility disorders. Because of the low incidence of diagnoses in patients with these disorders, more common esophageal disorders should be excluded with barium x-rays or endoscopy before manometric testing.

Esophageal motor problems associated with systemic disease (e.g., scleroderma, diabetes, collagen vascular diseases) should be evaluated using esophageal manometry if their detection would contribute to establishing a diagnosis or managing other aspects of patient care.

Esophageal manometry is indicated for placement of pH probes in adults, because position of the probe depends on the location of the LES. When a patient is being considered for antireflux surgery, manometry is possibly indicated for preoperative assessment of peristaltic function. Esophageal manometry in pediatric patients is less common, and other techniques are often used to place and confirm position of pH probes.

Esophageal manometry is not indicated for making the diagnosis of gastroesophageal reflux disease (GERD) and should not be the initial test for chest pain or other esophageal symptoms because of the low specificity of the findings.

Esophageal manometry is contraindicated in uncooperative patients; in patients with cardiac instability, recent gastric surgery, or severe esophageal ulcers; or in patients that have ingested, within the previous 24 hours, any medications that affect esophageal motor function. Complications of this procedure are rare.

Equipment

Manometry equipment consists of a **pressure sensor and**

transducer combination that detects the pressure in the esophagus and transduces it into an electrical signal and a recording device to amplify, record, and store that electrical signal. In esophageal manometry the only piece of equipment that enters the patient's esophagus is a long flexible tube: either a **water-perfused catheter,** in which the transducers are external, or a **solidstate probe,** in which the transducers are small and part of the probe itself. Each type has distinct advantages and disadvantages. The water-perfusion catheter uses an infusion pump powered by compressed nitrogen to perfuse distilled water through a multilumen catheter. The catheter has 3 to 8 lumens with side ports or openings in a set location, usually 1 to 5 cm apart. Each port is connected to a separate, external pressure transducer, which in turn is connected to the recording device.

Advantages of the water-perfusion system include a relatively low cost and external transducers, which can be easily replaced and can be assembled in a variety of configurations. The disadvantages of water-perfused systems include requirement for meticulous maintenance to achieve reliable test results and recording characteristics that are unsuitable for accurate pharyngeal studies.

Solidstate manometric probes contain transducers at fixed locations along the length. The probe plugs into a small electrical box, which is then connected to a recording device. The advantages of this system include suitability for recording any intraluminal pressure and its less cumbersome operation. The main disadvantage of the solidstate system is that the sometimes fragile probes are expensive (typically more than $1000 per channel) and cannot be modified.

Procedures

Before conducting an esophageal manometric study, it is important to verify the patient's NPO status, obtain the patient's medical history, and reassure the patient. In adult patients the procedure is performed while the patient is awake and without sedation, because premedication may interfere with swallowing and may have direct effects on motor events. In children, however, sedation may be required. Nitrates, calcium channel blockers, anticholinergics, promotility agents, and sedatives should be discontinued 24 to 48 hours before the study, because they can interfere with normal esophageal function. However, it is important to consult with the attending physician before discontinuing any medication.

The recording equipment must have the catheter attached, be filled with water, and be calibrated before insertion into the patient. The catheter should be initially calibrated at the level of the patient's esophagus. To avoid problems after actual tube insertion, patency of the catheter lumens should also be checked at this time. If one or more of the channels shows a straight line, the equipment may be malfunctioning or one of the catheter orifices may be blocked.

The catheter is traditionally inserted intranasally but may be inserted orally. The tube may be inserted with the patient in a sitting or a left lateral position. For comfort, the patient's nasal passage is anesthetized with a topical anesthetic such as lidocaine hydrochloride jelly applied with a cotton-tipped applicator. Cotton balls soaked in a solution of half tetracaine hydrochloride topical solution and half phenylephrine hydrochloride, then packed into the naris for 5 to 10 minutes before inserting the tube, also provide effective nasal anesthesia in adults. When the tip of the tube is in the back of the throat, the patient is instructed to tuck his or her chin down to the chest and swallow. It may be helpful to give the patient some water to drink through a straw to facilitate movement of the catheter through the esophagus and, finally, past the LES and into the stomach. Once the tube has been inserted into the stomach, the patient is helped into a supine or left lateral position.

Before beginning to withdraw the catheter, it is important to check catheter placement and function.

If all of the recording ports are in the patient's stomach, the physiograph should initially show a relatively flat, smooth tracing with a small pressure increase on inspiration or abdominal pressure. This pattern confirms placement in the stomach and is called the gastric baseline.

If one of the channels shows very rapid activity, this may be a result of cardiac interference. This type of pattern is most often seen during study of the esophageal body, when the recording orifice lies adjacent to the aortic arch.

Once it has been established that the recording equipment is working properly, the next step is to attach the equipment necessary to monitor the patient's swallows and respirations, if you desire these parameters.

Lower esophageal sphincter

The first step in a manometric study is to measure LES pressure (Table 24-1). The catheter may be moved steadily through the LES into the esophagus while the patient is not breathing or swallowing (rapid pull-through method) or may be withdrawn in a step-wise fashion while the patient breathes regularly and evenly (station pull-through). Under normal conditions, a **rapid pull-through** should show a rise in LES pressure, followed by a drop in pressure to below the gastric baseline as the recording ports enter the esophagus.

The **station pull-through** gives a more complete assessment of LES function. Using this method, the catheter is moved through the LES 1 cm at a time, with a pause at each point or station to observe LES pressure and relaxation. Relaxation of the sphincter is assessed by having the patient perform a series of controlled swallows, beginning with dry swallows and adding wet swallows. The swallow and accompanying relaxation of the LES should be reflected by a drop in pressure to about the level of the gastric baseline.

The point where the tracing goes down, rather than up, with an inspiration is called the *respiration inversion point* and represents the point where the recording port moves from the abdominal cavity into the thoracic cavity. If LES pressure is very weak, this inversion point may be the only way to locate the LES.

Table 24-1. Substances influencing LES pressure

Substance	Increase LES pressure	Decrease LES pressure
Hormones	Gastrin	Secretin
	Motilin	Cholecystokinin
	Substance P	Glucagon
		Somatostatin
		Gastric inhibitory polypeptide
		Vasoactive intestinal polypeptide
Neural agents	α-Adrenegic agonists	α-Adrenergic antagonists
	β-Adrenegic antagonists	β-Adrenergic antagonists
	Cholinergic agonists	Cholinergic antagonists
	No antagonists	No agonists
	Protein	Fat
Foods		Chocolate
		Ethanol
		Peppermint
Miscellaneous	Histamine	Theophylline
	Antacids	Prostaglandins
	Metaclopramide	E_2 and I_2
	Domperidone	Serotonin
	Prostaglandin $F_{2\alpha}$	Meperidine
		Morphine
		Dopamine
		Calcium channelblockers
		Diazepam
		Barbiturates

Esophageal body

The motility of the esophageal body is usually evaluated after anchoring the catheter at a point where the recording ports span the esophagus, usually at 3, 8, 13, and 18 cm above the LES. The recording ports may be located at different esophageal levels in children. Motility can be assessed by giving the patient about ten 3- to 5-ml swallows of water at 30 second intervals. The mean values for 10 wet swallows are analyzed, either manually or by computer. The precise steps to be followed in this procedure may vary according to the physician's preference. In some cases, food swallows may be given.

A normal tracing of a wet swallow should show an orderly progression of contractions from top to bottom, which is representative of normal esophageal peristalsis. Abnormal responses may include the following:

(a) simultaneous contractions, which occur at the same time throughout the esophageal body;

(b) retrograde contractions, which progress from the distal to the proximal esophagus;

(c) repetitive triple-peaked contractions; double contractions are considered a variant of normal contractions, whereas triple-peaked contractions are considered abnormal;

(d) nontransmitted contractions; and

(e) very strong or very weak contractions.

Upper esophageal sphincter

If assessment of the UES is desired, it is the final step in an esophageal motility study. For this process, each pressure port is pulled through the UES and relaxation of the sphincter with a swallow is assessed. Normally, a swallow causes a rapid decrease (or relaxation) in UES pressure, coordinated with pharyngeal activity and a resumption of resting UES pressure.

Cleaning

After the entire manometric study is completed, the water-infusion catheter lumens are flushed with detergent, followed by thorough rinsing and drying, and ethylene oxide gas sterilization. Solidstate manometry probes undergo high-level disinfection only.

PROVOCATIVE TESTING

Provocative testing is an optional technique designed to reproduce chest pain that may be esophageal in origin and is not generally not indicated/performed in children. It is imperative initially to exclude coronary disease, because of its more serious prognosis, as the cause of the patient's pain. In addition, an upper endoscopy or an upper GI series and gallbladder evaluation are usually performed to exclude other GI tract abnormalities.

Provocative testing is accomplished while the recording ports of the manometry catheter are located in the esophageal body. Interpretation is based on the patient's subjective pain and on manometric tracings.

Bernstein test

Noncardiac chest pain associated with acid reflux may be simulated by performing the **Bernstein test;** that is, alternating infusions of a placebo (normal saline) and 0.1N hydrochloric acid through one of the recording ports of a manometry catheter. The test is indicated in patients with atypical chest pain and is contraindicated in patients with an inability to tolerate intubation, with active or recent GI bleeding, or with known active ulcer disease (relative).

Before this test the patient should avoid ingesting antacids or coating agents, anesthetic gargle, or pain medication and should be NPO.

Because the patient's subjective pain is the diagnostic endpoint, the patient should be informed only that the test will attempt to determine the source of his or her chest pain. The two irrigating fluids should be out of the patient's visual field. With the patient in a sitting position, a nasogastric (NG) or motility tube is placed at midesophagus, and alternating solutions of normal saline and 0.1N hydrochloric acid are dripped through the tube in an attempt to reproduce the patient's symptoms. If the Bernstein test is performed following a manometric study, the manometry catheter may be used to instill saline and acid.

If discomfort occurs at any time, the patient should be instructed to point to the area and to describe the pain verbally, comparing it to previous symptoms (Fig. 24-1). A true

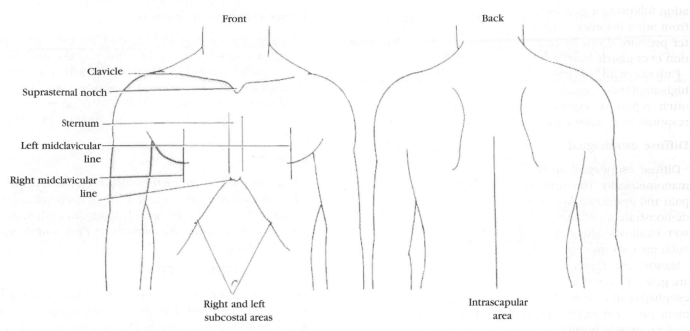

Fig. 24-1. Anatomical landmarks for differentiating discomfort evoked during intraesophageal acid drip test.

positive response to the Bernstein test requires that the symptoms be stimulated by acid infusion, lessened with saline infusion, and worsened with a subsequent acid infusion. If pain is related to gastric or duodenal lesions, it will not be relieved by the infusion of normal saline. Normal saline should be infused at the end of the test to flush hydrochloric acid from the esophagus.

Potential complications of the Bernstein test include aspiration and misplacement of the NG tube.

Edrophonium testing

The purpose of this edrophonium testing is to confirm the esophageal origin of noncardiac chest pain. It is indicated in patients with noncardiac chest pain and contraindicated in patients with an unstable cardiac history, atrial fibrillation, arrhythmias (or bundle branch block), severe asthma, bradycardia, or bronchial constrictive disease.

Before the test, any pain medications or any medications that could affect esophageal contractions should be withheld for 48 hours, as ordered by the patient's physician. Baseline esophageal manometry is conducted first. A motility catheter with at least four lumens should be positioned with the distal opening 3, 8, 13, and 18 cm above the LES. During edrophonium testing, the patient's subjective pain is the diagnostic endpoint, and the patient should not see the irrigating fluids administered. During continuous recording of esophageal pressures, a saline placebo is administered intravenously, after which the patient performs 10 wet swallows 30 seconds apart. Next, a bolus of the cholinesterase inhibitor edrophonium chloride (Tensilon) is administered rapidly in an IV bolus and the patient performs 10 wet swallows 30 seconds apart. The amplitude and duration of esophageal contractions should increase following edrophonium provocation. The test is complete after 5 minutes of

manometry tracings or 10 wet swallows. It is considered positive if typical chest pain is reproduced by edrophonium injection.

Adverse reactions to edrophonium may occur and are usually transient. They include tearing, dizziness, GI discomfort, and, less often, bradycardia, pupillary constriction, and laryngospasm. Atropine should be available as an antidote to bradycardia.

Disorders diagnosed using esophageal manometry

Esophageal manometry may be used in the diagnosis of both primary and secondary esophageal motility disorders.

Achalasia

Achalasia is characterized by long-standing, progressive dysphagia for both solids and liquids, often with weight loss, nocturnal regurgitation, and pulmonary symptoms. Definitive manometric findings include aperistalsis and incomplete LES relaxation (with or without an increase in resting sphincter pressure in 90% of patients). Patients with early achalasia may show complete LES relaxation, but of unusually short duration. In addition, LES pressure may be elevated, the length of the high-pressure zone may be increased, and intraesophageal pressures may be elevated relative to gastric pressure, a condition that is opposite to the normal relationship.

When assessing patients with suspected achalasia, it is important to advance the manometry catheter through the LES even though it may be difficult, because LES characteristics are important for manometric diagnosis. Fluoroscopy is often needed to confirm the location of the catheter and to aid in passage into the stomach. LES relaxation should be assessed with wet swallows, using a station pull-through technique. Demonstration of incomplete sphincter relaxation following a swallow is needed to distinguish achalasia from other disorders with aperistalsis. In most cases, sphincter pressure drops by only approximately 30% of its elevation over gastric baseline.

Patients with so-called *vigorous* achalasia demonstrate high-amplitude (greater than 60 mm Hg), simultaneous, often repetitive contractions of the esophageal body in response to swallows, along with elevated LES pressure.

Diffuse esophageal spasm

Diffuse esophageal spasm (DES) may also be diagnosed manometrically. The primary symptoms of DES are chest pain and dysphagia. Manometrically, patients with DES must demonstrate simultaneous contractions in more than 10% of wet swallows, along with intermittent normal peristalsis. Such patients may also show repetitive contractions.

Manometric findings in patients with esophageal spasm are generally restricted to the smooth muscle portion of the esophagus and are most pronounced in the 5- to 10-cm segment proximal to the LES. They do not seem to affect the skeletal muscle portion of the esophagus.

Nutcracker esophagus

Nutcracker esophagus is an abnormality of contraction wave amplitude, typified by a mean contraction amplitude greater than 2 standard deviations above a well-documented normal range. Patients with this disorder complain of chest pain and/or dysphagia. The duration of contractions may be prolonged, but peristaltic progression is normal. A high percentage of these patients have a positive response to the edrophonium chloride test.

Hypertensive LES

A hypertensive LES is characterized by abnormally high resting LES pressure. LES relaxation is normal, as is peristaltic progression. Patients may complain of chest pain.

Nonspecific esophageal motility disorders

The term nonspecific esophageal motility disorder is used to describe any abnormal motility pattern that does not fall into one of the other categories. Such disorders include weak (low-amplitude) contractions (less than 30 mm Hg), peristaltic contractions of prolonged duration, triple-peaked contractions, nontransmitted contractions (more than 20% of wet swallows), and retrograde contractions.

Diabetes mellitus

Patients with diabetes mellitus often exhibit manometric abnormalities, possibly as a result of the degenerative effects of diabetes on the autonomic nervous system. Esophageal motility is abnormal in approximately 80% of patients with diabetic neuropathy. These abnormalities may include occasional nontransmitted swallows and spontaneous contractions or may resemble DES. In the majority of cases, esophageal dysfunction is asymptomatic. In symptomatic patients, complaints are mild, consisting of heartburn and, rarely, dysphagia.

Scleroderma

Scleroderma, which is a form of progressive systemic sclerosis, is a connective tissue disorder characterized by a progressive thickening and induration of the dermis. A majority of patients with typical skin manifestations have evidence of esophageal involvement at autopsy, characterized by muscle atrophy and fibrosis that affect predominantly the smooth muscle region of the esophagus. The end results are failure of muscle contraction in the distal esophagus and incompetency in the LES. Manometry in these patients shows reduced contraction, aperistalsis in the distal esophageal body, and low to absent LES pressure.

Primary chronic intestinal pseudo-obstruction

The term chronic intestinal pseudo-obstruction describes a syndrome that is characterized by intermittent signs and symptoms of bowel obstruction, in the absence of a demonstrable obstructing lesion. It most commonly affects the small bowel. Esophageal manometry is abnormal in more than 80% of cases. Typical findings include incomplete LES relaxation, abnormal esophageal contractions (simultaneous and repetitive), and absent peristalsis.

Esophageal reflux

Esophageal manometry has limited usefulness in the diagnosis of esophageal reflux. It may be indicated to confirm adequate peristalsis amplitude in patients who are being considered for antireflux surgery. The presence of a significant motility disorder may be a contraindication to surgery.

In general, patients with esophageal reflux tend to have decreased LES pressure and lower peristaltic amplitude in the esophageal body, but these findings may also be seen in normal subjects. The finding of a hypotensive LES supports the diagnosis of esophageal reflux, although only about 25% to 50% of patients with esophageal reflux have hypotensive resting LES pressure. About 50% of patients with moderate or severe esophageal reflux exhibit some degree of impaired esophageal peristalsis.

Ambulatory esophageal pH monitoring is useful to quantify the amount of esophageal reflux in patients with typical gastroesophageal reflux symptoms who are unresponsive to medical therapy, patients with atypical symptoms (asthma, cough, laryngitis, sore throat) possibly caused by gastroesophageal reflux, and patients with GERD being considered for antireflux surgery. Before placement of the pH probe, esophageal manometry may be employed to document the location of the LES; the pH probe is typically placed 5 cm above the manometrically determined LES. In children, the probe tip is typically placed at 87.5% of the distance to the LES. The proper position of the probe in children may be estimated by a calculation based upon the child's height. Once the probe is in place, a chest x-ray is usually done to confirm proper positioning. Alternatively, the LES can be identified during endoscopy or manometry, and the probe placed accordingly.

Anorexia nervosa

A recent study found abnormal esophageal motility in up to 50% of patients with primary anorexia nervosa. Many of these patients had previously undiagnosed achalasia. Following the manometric diagnosis, pneumatic dilatation resulted in weight gain. The authors of this study conclude that esophageal motility studies should be performed in every adult patient diagnosed with primary anorexia nervosa.

GASTRODUODENAL SMALL BOWEL MANOMETRY

Gastric manometry may be indicated in patients with symptoms of delayed gastric emptying or clinically evident gastric motility disorders. Clinical conditions that have been associated with gastric arrhythmias include idiopathic gastroparesis, gastroparesis secondary to diabetes mellitus or anorexia nervosa, gastric ulcer disease, or gastric adenocarcinoma. Gastric arrhythmias have also been associated with the effects of certain drugs and hormones, including anticholinergics, metenkephalin, β-endorphin, epinephrine, glucagon, prostaglandin E_2, secretin, and insulin. Transient abnormal rhythms have also been observed postoperatively in otherwise normal individuals. Clinical signs of these disorders include severe gastric retention, nausea, vomiting, and weight loss.

Impaired gastric motor activity in patients with diabetic neuropathy may cause symptoms ranging from vague postprandial abdominal discomfort to invariable postprandial nausea and vomiting. Gastric stasis may also cause more serious problems, such as weight loss, poor diabetic control, and bezoars. The most commonly seen gastric motor abnormality in these patients is absence of the antral component of the interdigestive motor complex, which is normally responsible for clearance of indigestible solids. These patients may be helped by prescriptions of metoclopramide (Reglan) before meals and at bedtime.

Gastroduodenal small bowel motility studies include recording both fasting and fed patterns of phasic pressure activity in the antrum and upper small bowel, as well as responses to provocative testing. Both catheter perfusion techniques and transducer-containing probes are available. Perfusion catheters are inexpensive and easy to build or buy, but they are thicker than most transducer tubes.

The transducer tube is passed over a guidewire, and its location is confirmed fluoroscopically. Transducers are arranged spatially to sense the antrum, duodenum, and small bowel and are encased in a flexible polyurethane sheath that can be tolerated for long periods of time. Measurements can be made for up to 24 hours to sample a number of interdigestive, migrating motor complexes and to provide more opportunity to observe a disturbed or disrupted complex. These studies usually evaluate the liquid phase and solid phase of gastric emptying, with radionuclide and small bowel manometry studies performed simultaneously.

SPHINCTER OF ODDI PANCREATIC MANOMETRY

The sphincter of Oddi is a circular smooth muscle that surrounds the ampulla of Vater, the distal common bile duct, and the pancreatic duct (Fig. 24-2). During fasting, it exhibits peristaltic-like contractions that propel bile into the duodenum and prevent reflux of duodenal contents. Food causes the release of cholecystokinin from the duodenum, which inhibits contraction of the sphincter of Oddi and lowers the basal pressure.

Sphincter of Oddi manometry is indicated for diagnosis of papillary stenosis and for motility disorders of the sphincter of Oddi, which may be associated with choledocholithiasis,

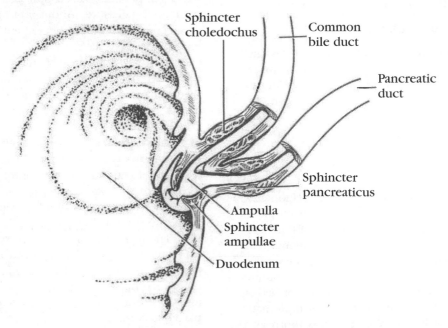

Fig. 24-2. Sphincter of Oddi anatomy.

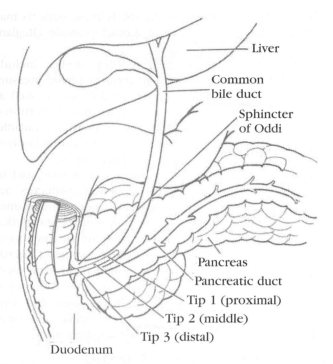

Liver

Common
bile duct

Sphincter
of Oddi

Pancreas

Pancreatic duct

Tip 1 (proximal)

Tip 2 (middle)

Tip 3 (distal)

Duodenum

Fig. 24-3. Placement of pressure catheter in sphincter of Oddi.

biliary pain, abdominal pain, or pancreatitis. Possible factors causing obstruction of bile flow include spasm of the sphincter of Oddi or retrograde contractions.

Sphincter of Oddi manometry is usually obtained during endoscopic retrograde cholangiopancreatography (ERCP) (Fig. 24-3). Like ERCP, sphincter of Oddi manometry is contraindicated in the following:

(a) uncooperative patients;
(b) recent myocardial infarction;
(c) acute pancreatitis;
(d) coagulopathy;
(e) barium in the GI tract;
(f) pregnancy; and
(g) severe pulmonary disease.

Before beginning sphincter of Oddi manometry, it is important to verify informed consent and NPO status, obtain the patient's medical history and laboratory results, establish a patent IV line, remove dentures, administer antibiotic prophylaxis as ordered, and record baseline vital signs.

The patient should be mildly sedated Anticholinergic drugs and opiates are not used before manometry, because they can alter sphincter pressures). A triple-lumen catheter is inserted through the biopsy channel of a side-viewing duodenoscope.

The duodenoscope is inserted orally. The ampulla of Vater is identified and cannulated with the triple-lumen manometry catheter, which is passed through the sphincter of Oddi into the common bile duct. This catheter is attached to a capillary infusion system, and three external transducers transmit the pressures to a physiograph. As the catheter is withdrawn slowly at 1-mm increments, a normal tracing shows basal pressures of less than 30 mm Hg, with peristaltic-like phasic waves. If a motility disorder is confirmed,

the physician may choose to perform an endoscopic sphincterotomy.

After the procedure is completed, it is important to monitor and document the patient's vital signs, observe for abdominal distention and signs of pancreatitis, maintain NPO status until the gag reflex returns, administer antibiotics as ordered, remove the IV line, provide written discharge instructions, and ensure that outpatients have someone to drive them home.

The most common complication of sphincter of Oddi manometry is pancreatitis, which may present as mild to incapacitating pain, beginning in the midepigastrium and radiating to the patient's back; nausea and vomiting; fever; distended abdomen; and decreased bowel sounds. Less likely complications are perforation, which may present with abdominal rigidity, rebound tenderness, an increase in pulse rate, and shallow and rapid respirations; or bleeding, which may present as a decrease in blood pressure and increased pulse rate.

ANORECTAL MANOMETRY

Anorectal manometry is indicated in patients with chronic constipation and/or fecal incontinence, after construction of a rectal pouch, before and after rectal surgery, in suspected scleroderma and dermatomyositis, and to rule out Hirschsprung's or Chagas' disease. It may be useful as a screening procedure in newborns with the meconium plug syndrome or with difficulty in passing stools. Anorectal manometry is also used as an operant conditioning technique to improve bowel control in patients with incontinence secondary to previous anorectal surgery, obstetrical trauma, spinal injury, irritable bowel syndrome, diabetic neuropathy, rectal prolapse, multiple sclerosis, scleroderma, or stroke.

Anorectal manometry is contraindicated in patients suffering from any severe or unstable medical or psychological condition, infectious diarrhea, or anal or rectal disease.

Anal manometry in infants and older children who are able to understand the procedure and cooperate can usually be performed without sedation. Toddlers and other children who are highly anxious or fearful will likely need sedation to accomplish the procedure and obtain interpretable data.

Before the procedure, it is important to verify informed consent and to review the patient's medical and surgical history and results of the physician's physical examination. The patient should be encouraged to have a bowel movement before the procedure; a Fleet enema may be administered if necessary.

The equipment used for anorectal manometry consists of pressure transducers and a balloon catheter.

(a) A distal sensor is positioned at the internal anal sphincter.
(b) A proximal sensor is placed at the external sphincter.

The test procedure consists of recording the reflex response of the two anorectal sphincters to transient distention of the rectal balloon. In most individuals, distention of the rectal balloon causes the internal sphincter to relax, while the external sphincter contracts to prevent defecation.

Anorectal manometry may also be used for biofeedback therapy in patients with fecal incontinence. Such patients should be shown their baseline manometric tracings of external sphincter pressure and then should be instructed in the maneuver necessary to produce a rise in pressure on the tracing. Following this instruction, the patient should be asked to contract the external sphincter briefly whenever he or she perceives an increase in the distending volume in the rectal balloon. As appropriate responses are made, the distending volume in the rectal balloon should be decreased progressively, out of sight of the patient, until the patient responds appropriately to smaller volumes. After the initial instruction period the patient should be asked to apply the learned techniques consciously for 2 weeks whenever the sensation of fecal distention is felt. In addition, the patient should practice sphincter contractions 30 to 50 times a day for the first few weeks.

Potential complications of anorectal manometry include hemorrhage, perforation, and sepsis.

PATIENT EDUCATION

Before any manometric procedure, it is important that the patient be fully informed. Patients should be advised of the following:

(a) purpose of the test;
(b) positioning that will be used;
(c) effective relaxation methods;
(d) techniques to be used;
(e) approximate length of the procedure;
(f) sensations the patient is likely to experience;
(g) risks of the procedure; and
(h) importance of patient cooperation.

Patient education and comprehension should be documented. After the procedure, the physician may want to discuss the results of the test with the patient. The nurse should discuss and document postprocedural instructions and recommendations for follow-up care.

CASE SITUATION

We met Doris Johnson in Chapter 13. She has suffered significantly with chest discomfort. She has had heartburn; reflux of sour, bitter-tasting liquid up into her mouth; and several chest colds that her physician said were caused by the acid getting into her lungs at night. On upper endoscopy, she was found to have esophagitis. Mrs. Johnson says she has had trouble adhering to her antireflux regimen. She does not have the head of her bed up on blocks yet, but she has been sleeping on several pillows. She thought the pillows would be sufficient, but she admits that when she wakes up in the morning she has invariably rolled off the pillows. She is in the endoscopy department now for esophageal manometry.

Points to think about

1. The gastroenterology nurse has set Mrs. Johnson up for her motility study. The equipment is all ready and the nurse is prepared to place the tube into her esophagus. Mrs. Johnson jumps up in alarm and says, "You mean you aren't going to put me to sleep like the last time?" How should the nurse respond?

2. What techniques might help the nurse pass the manometry tube successfully?

3. The nurse would expect that Mrs. Johnson has a hypotensive LES, which allows reflux of gastric material into the esophagus. What else might be seen on the tracing?

4. There are two types of esophageal motility disorders: primary and secondary. What does that mean?

Suggested responses

1. When Mrs. Johnson expresses surprise that she will not be sedated, the nurse might respond as follows:

   (a) Explain that this is not the same procedure she had before.

   (b) Explain that this test will determine how the muscles in her esophagus contract and that the sedating medication could affect the test by artificially relaxing those muscles.

   (c) Reassure Mrs. Johnson that the tube to be inserted through her nose is much smaller than an ordinary NG tube and that everything possible will be done to make her comfortable.

2. To help pass the manometry tube successfully, the nurse might:

   (a) Measure the tube to know how far to insert it. The manometry tube must pass through the esophagogastric junction into the stomach, with all of the lower side openings positioned below the diaphragm.

   (b) Have the patient remove her dentures, if any.

   (c) If the physician allows, anesthetize the inner nares.

   (d) Ask Mrs. Johnson if she breathes better through one side of the nose. If so, that side should be tried first.

   (e) Listen to Mrs. Johnson if she says she has had problems in the past with NG tube insertion. Even if the nurse is an expert at passing tubes, listening and being compassionate foster trust and confidence.

   (f) Advance the tube slowly and carefully around the back of the nose and into the back of the throat. The nurse must never push against an obstruction, and if one naris is obstructed, the other side should be tried. After some experience the nurse will know how to maneuver the tube from one side to the other, or up or down, or curl the tip to get around the back of the nose and throat.

   (g) When ready to enter the esophagus, the nurse should have the patient bend her head forward and swallow. This causes the epiglottis to open the esophagus and close the trachea. Unless there is suspicion of achalasia or other obstruction, it is usually permissible for the patient to take a few sips of water.

(h) Once the patient is able to swallow, the tube usually passes easily into the stomach. If any obstructions are met, the nurse should stop and check tube placement on the manometry machine. If the tube is pushed against a lower esophageal obstruction, it will curl back on itself.

(i) If the patient gags inordinately, it may be a good idea to have another nurse sit by the patient to calm her and coach her while the tube goes down.

3. In addition to a hypotensive LES, the nurse might expect to see a secondary spasm of the esophagus. Reflux of gastric contents into the esophagus is usually caustic to the esophageal mucosa, causing esophagitis. In turn, esophagitis can cause secondary spasm of the esophagus, which can be painful. On manometry, DES may show normal peristalsis interspersed with simultaneous contractions, often of high amplitude and prolonged duration. These contractions may be repetitive, and there is usually an incomplete relaxation of the LES.

4. Primary motility disorders are those that involve only the esophagus, such as achalasia, DES, nutcracker esophagus, hypertensive LES, and nonspecific esophageal motility disorders. Secondary motility disorders occur when the esophagus is affected as part of a more generalized disease process, such as diabetes mellitus, scleroderma, or chronic idiopathic pseudo-obstruction.

REVIEW TERMS

Bernstein test, manometry, pressure sensor and transducer, rapid pull-through, solidstate probe, station pull-through, water-perfused catheter

REVIEW QUESTIONS

1. The function of a pressure transducer is to:
   (a) Convert electrical signals to pressure readings.
   (b) Convert pressure changes to electrical signals.
   (c) Record ink tracings that represent GI motility.
   (d) Apply pressure to the GI tract.
2. Esophageal manometry is contraindicated in patients with:
   (a) Dysphagia.
   (b) Recent gastric or esophageal surgery.
   (c) Diabetes mellitus.
   (d) Noncardiac chest pain.
3. Compared to water-perfused systems, the transducers used in solid-state manometry probes are:
   (a) Larger.
   (b) Less expensive.
   (c) More difficult to repair.
   (d) More reliable.
4. If one of the recording channels shows unusually rapid activity during an esophageal motility study, this is most likely a result of:
   (a) Esophageal spasm.
   (b) Too-rapid pull-through.

(c) A malfunctioning transducer.
(d) Cardiac interference.

5. Motility of the esophageal body is best assessed while the patient:
   (a) Performs a series of wet swallows.
   (b) Performs a series of dry swallows.
   (c) Takes a series of deep breaths.
   (d) Holds his or her breath and does not swallow.
6. The Bernstein test is used to:
   (a) Stimulate esophageal peristalsis.
   (b) Calibrate the pressure transducers.
   (c) Reproduce chest pain that may be a result of acid reflux in the esophagus.
   (d) Reproduce chest pain that may be a result of esophageal spasm.
7. Aperistalsis of the esophageal body and incomplete relaxation of the LES are manometric symptoms associated with:
   (a) Achalasia.
   (b) Diffuse esophageal spasm.
   (c) Nutcracker esophagus.
   (d) Nonspecific esophageal motility disorders.
8. Manometric manifestations of advanced scleroderma include:
   (a) Simultaneous and repetitive esophageal contractions.
   (b) Aperistalsis in the distal esophageal body and low to absent LES pressure.
   (c) Abnormally high resting LES pressure.
   (d) A mean contraction amplitude at least two standard deviations above normal.
9. Anticholinergic drugs and opiates are not used before manometric procedures primarily because they can:
   (a) Make the patient nauseous.
   (b) Sedate the patient.
   (c) Change the patient's breathing pattern.
   (d) Alter GI motility.
10. In anorectal manometric studies of normal subjects, distention of the rectal balloon causes the external anal sphincter to:
    (a) Spasm.
    (b) Relax.
    (c) Contract.
    (d) Exhibit no change in sphincter pressure.

BIBLIOGRAPHY

Arndorfer, R. (1988). Techniques of esophageal manometry. In Trivits, S. (Ed.), *SGA Journal Reprints*, Rochester, NY: Society of Gastrointestinal Assistants.

Carlson, L. & Anderson, B. (1988). Sphincter of Oddi dysfunction: a cause of biliary obstruction. In Trivits, S. (Ed.), *SGA Journal Reprints*, Rochester, NY: Society of Gastrointestinal Assistants

Castell, D., Richter, J. & Dalton, C., (Eds.) (1987). *Esophageal motility testing*. New York: Elsevier.

Chobanian, S. & Van Ness, M. (Eds.) (1988). *Manual of clinical problems in gastroenterology*. Boston: Little, Brown.

Chopra, S. & May, R. (Eds.) (1989). *Pathophysiology of gastrointestinal diseases*. Boston: Little, Brown.

Dalton, C., Richter, J. & Castell, D. (1990). Esophageal manometry. In Trivits, S. (Ed.), *Journal Reprints II*, Rochester, NY: Society of Gastroenterology Nurses and Associates.

Kahrilas, P., Clouse, R. & Hogan, W. (1994). An American Gastroenterological Association medical position statement on the clinical use of esophageal manometry. *Gastroenterology 107*, 1865-84.

Sachar, D., Waye, J. & Lewis, B. (Eds.) (1989). *Gastroenterology for the house officer*. Baltimore, MD: Williams & Wilkins.

Silverman, A. & Roy, C. (1983). *Pediatric clinical gastroenterology* (3rd ed.). St. Louis, MO: Mosby.

Sleisenger, M. & Fordtran, J. (Eds.) (2002). *Gastrointestinal disease: pathophysiology, diagnosis, management* (7th ed.). Philadelphia: W.B. Saunders.

Society of Gastroenterology Nurses and Associates, Inc. (2003). *Manual of gastrointestinal procedures* (5th ed.). Chicago: Society of Gastroenterology Nurses and Associates, Inc.

Society of Gastroenterology Nurses and Associates, Inc. (1994). *Manual of gastrointestinal procedures* (3rd ed.). Baltimore, MD: Williams & Wilkins.

Stachner, G., Kiss, A. & Wiesnagrotzki, S. (1986). Oesophageal and gastric motility disorders in patients categorized as having primary anorexia nervosa, *Gut 27*, 1120-6.

Chapter 25

BIOPSY AND CYTOLOGY

This chapter will acquaint the gastroenterology nurse with the techniques used to obtain biopsy samples, cell cultures, and cytology specimens for the diagnosis of GI disease. Endoscopic methods used to obtain biopsy specimens from the esophagus, stomach, small bowel, and colorectum are detailed. Procedures for percutaneous liver biopsy and pancreatic fine-needle aspiration are outlined, in addition to techniques for suction biopsies of the small bowel and rectum. Methods employed in the collection of tissue specimens for cell culture and cytological analysis are also explored.

Learning objectives

After reviewing the content of this chapter, the gastroenterology nurse should be able to:

1. Describe the techniques used for endoscopic biopsy of the esophagus, stomach, small bowel, and colorectum, including indications, contraindications, potential complications, and patient care and patient education considerations.
2. Explain the techniques that are used for percutaneous liver biopsy, fine-needle aspiration of the pancreas, and suction biopsy of the small bowel and rectum.
3. Discuss the methods used in gastroenterology for the collection of specimens for cell culture and cytology.

BASIC PRINCIPLES

Biopsy and **cytology** both allow direct sampling of GI tissue for diagnostic purposes. Biopsy involves excision of pieces of living tissue from a suspected pathological site, with subsequent **histopathological analysis** in the laboratory. Specimens may be obtained either by using biopsy forceps that are passed through the biopsy channel of an endoscope or by using a suction method (e.g., small bowel or rectal suction biopsy) or a needle that is inserted percutaneously (e.g., percutaneous liver or pancreatic fine-needle

aspiration). Liver biopsy specimens may also be obtained surgically or laparoscopically.

Specimens for cell culture or cytological analysis may be obtained either endoscopically, by using brushings, or by using **washing** and/or **aspiration** techniques.

ENDOSCOPIC BIOPSY

Endoscopic biopsy is indicated when there is a suspicion of abnormal mucosal tissue or for confirmation of normal tissue in any portion of the GI tract. It is contraindicated in patients with severe coagulopathy or active bleeding. A bleeding profile should be obtained, if clinically indicated. Caution must be exercised in patients who are currently using anticoagulants or who have recently ingested nonsteroidal antiinflammatory drugs (NSAIDs) or medications containing acetylsalicylic acid (ASA), unless bleeding time is verified as normal. Ideally, patients should discontinue ingestion of aspirin and NSAIDs for 1 week before endoscopic biopsy.

To obtain an endoscopic biopsy specimen, an endoscope is inserted into the esophagus, stomach, small bowel, or colon, as described in Chapter 23. Once the endoscope is in place, biopsy forceps are passed down the biopsy channel.

A whole range of **biopsy forceps** is available, with different-shaped jaws and sometimes a central spike or bayonet. The most common biopsy forceps are simple cupped forceps, but elongated or even fenestrated types, with smooth or dentate edges, are available. Forceps with a central spike can be especially helpful to hold the tissue in place and prevent the forceps from slipping so an accurate biopsy specimen can be taken. Jumbo forceps can be used with large-channel scopes to obtain larger pieces of tissue.

Electrocoagulating, or **"hot" biopsy forceps** are used to coagulate tissue when the patient is at an increased risk of bleeding. Hot forceps are insulated by a nonconducting sheath. An active cord connects the handle of the forceps to the cautery unit. Regular forceps are sometimes coated for passage. Because of the thin wall of the right colon and the greater risk of perforation, care should be taken when using hot biopsy forceps in this location.

Once the forceps are in place, the nurse opens and closes the forceps, in response to the physician's request. The act of closing the forceps and pulling on the tissue tears off a specimen of the target tissue. The specimen is then retrieved by bringing the biopsy forceps out through the channel of the endoscope. As the forceps are withdrawn, the shaft should be wiped with a gauze sponge to remove secretions.

In most cases the accuracy of histopathological interpretation of endoscopic biopsy specimens can be improved by obtaining multiple specimens of the suspicious area. Specimens should be prepared according to institutional policy, and the container should be labeled with patient information and the site of the biopsy.

If immediate denial or confirmation of malignancy is required, the endoscopic biopsy specimen, in the form of a **frozen section,** may be sent to the laboratory for immediate microscopic examination by a pathologist. No fixative of any kind is used for frozen sections. Instead, the specimen is placed on mounting material, labeled, and immediately taken to the laboratory.

After use, reusable forceps should be cleaned and steam-sterilized, in accordance with SGNA infection-control guidelines. Disposable biopsy forceps are also available.

Excessive bleeding and perforation are the most likely complications of endoscopic biopsy. After the procedure is completed, the patient should be instructed to notify the physician of signs and symptoms of bleeding or perforation which would include fever or pain.

Endoscopic esophageal biopsy

Endoscopic biopsy of the esophagus is indicated for the diagnosis of mucosal abnormalities in the esophagus, such as a radiologically demonstrated stricture or suspected carcinoma. It may be used to look for evidence of Barrett's esophagus in patients with esophageal reflux or, in children, to verify esophagitis.

When radiological interpretation identifies a stricture as benign, endoscopy with multiple biopsies and brush cytology are also recommended to rule out any possibility of malignancy.

To correctly diagnose esophageal cancer, it is important to dilate any strictured lesion sufficiently to allow passage of the endoscope down to its distal margin. Numerous biopsy specimens should be obtained from tissue that is clearly abnormal but not necrotic. Brush cytology can also be helpful in some cases. Specimens for cytology may be obtained by using a sheathed disposable brush that is inserted through the endoscope.

Esophageal biopsy specimens from patients with chronic esophageal reflux often show thickening of the esophageal squamous epithelium. Findings of polymorphonuclear leukocytes, eosinophils and ulceration in esophageal biopsy specimens also provide strong support for a diagnosis of active esophagitis. Additionally, biopsy of ulcer margins may enhance detection of viral infection such as HSV.

Endoscopic gastric biopsy

Endoscopic biopsy is indicated in the diagnosis of gastric mucosal abnormalities associated with active and chronic gastritis, gastric polyps, carcinoma, or gastric ulcers. In addition, biopsy specimens may be used for the diagnosis of *Helicobacter pylori* (H. pylori) infections.

All polyps of the stomach should be examined by endoscopic biopsy. The biopsy technique used depends on the type and size of the protruding lesion. If possible, polyps should be removed endoscopically. If polyps cannot be removed, biopsies should be performed. Adenomatous polyps, large hyperplastic polyps, and any polyp with a stalk should be removed by using an endoscopic snare technique, as described in Chapter 30.

Endoscopic visualization is not sufficient for a definitive diagnosis of gastric cancer; a biopsy should be performed in all suspect cases. Most neoplasms of the stomach are adenocarcinomas. For patients with suspected gastric adenocarcinoma, the appearance of the lesion is assessed, a biopsy of the lesion is performed, and the lesion is brushed for cytology. It is possible to detect lesions as small as 2 to 3 mm in diameter and to obtain a histological diagnosis.

For submucosal tumors, the mucosa overlying the tumor can be lifted off with biopsy forceps, but this will not always provide a positive diagnosis of the tumor itself. To obtain submucosal tissue, a large-particle biopsy, hot biopsy, or a lift-and-cut biopsy employing a snare may be used. Needle biopsy may also be used to aspirate tissue from submucosal nodules.

The benign appearance of a gastric ulcer should always be confirmed by multiple biopsies and **exfoliative brush cytology** (Fig. 25-1). Biopsies of the ulcer edges are necessary to be certain whether or not the lesion is malignant. When endoscopy is performed, six to ten biopsy specimens should be obtained in a circumferential pattern from the ulcer margin.

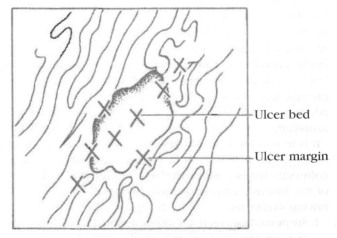

Fig. 25-1. Recommended ulcer biopsy sites.

In patients with suspected *H. pylori* infections, the specimen may be obtained by using standard biopsy forceps from the dependent portion of the antrum, along the greater curvature. The sample can then be inserted into an agar gel test kit that contains urea, a pH indicator, buffers, and a bacteriostatic agent. A rapid color change indicates the presence of the urease enzyme typically produced by *H. pylori*. Tissue may also be sent to the pathology lab and stained for *H. Pylori*. The gastroenterology nurse should request appropriate laboratory stain as per institution protocol.

After an endoscopic gastric biopsy, the patient should be observed for signs and symptoms of complications such as bleeding and perforation, including abdominal pain, tenderness, distention, nausea, vomiting, chills, hypotension, or temperature elevation.

Endoscopic small bowel biopsy

Small bowel biopsy is a simple technique that provides important diagnostic information. The direct visualization that is permitted by endoscopic biopsy is advantageous in patients with focal disease.

Small bowel biopsy is indicated for the differential diagnosis of malabsorption syndromes and other entities that are responsible for chronic diarrhea or weight loss. A diagnosis of celiac sprue, for instance, should never be made without a biopsy. Diseases such as intestinal lymphangiectasia, agammaglobulinemia, and Whipple's disease also give rise to highly specific lesions. Small bowel biopsy is also useful for obtaining tissue to check for *Giardia*.

Requirements for small bowel biopsies to be of maximum diagnostic value include the following:

(a) precise localization of the biopsy site;

(b) proper orientation and prompt fixation of biopsy specimens;

(c) careful study of serial sections of the central half or two thirds of each biopsy specimen; and

(d) obtaining the specimen from the region of the duodenal-jejunal junction, in the area of the ligament of Treitz.

Endoscopic colorectal biopsy

Although colonoscopy permits visualization of the entire inner surface of the colon, mucosal biopsy is often necessary to arrive at a specific diagnosis. Colonic biopsies of the mucosa and colonic lesions are obtained routinely for diagnostic purposes. The main advantages of taking biopsy specimens through an endoscope are the ability to sample the entire colon and to precisely target the area of interest. In addition, multiple specimens are easily obtained endoscopically.

It is important to note that significant and potentially diagnostic abnormalities may be present in tissue obtained by colorectal biopsy, despite a normal endoscopic appearance of the mucosa. Colorectal biopsies are indicated in the following situations:

1. Suspected collagenous or microscopic colitis in middle-age women with unexplained, chronic nonbloody diarrhea and grossly normal colonic mucosa.

2. Suspected neoplastic lesions of the rectum and colon.

3. Suspected Crohn's disease, in which the typical mucosal biopsy shows a focal ulcerative and inflammatory process, rather than the diffuse abnormality seen with ulcerative colitis. Histological documentation of granulomatous inflammation of bowel mucosa argues strongly for a diagnosis of Crohn's disease, particularly when discrete noncaseating granulomas are found and other causes of granulomatous disease have been excluded.

4. Suspected ulcerative colitis, which is characterized by inflammation of the colonic mucosa, with changes ranging from mild degrees of inflammation to microscopic erosions of the epithelium and crypt abscesses. A complete colonoscopy with biopsy is especially useful when prior sigmoidoscopic findings are equivocal.

5. As an adjunct to cultures and smears of rectal mucosa for detecting an infectious process in men and women who engage in anal intercourse and may be at risk for acquiring HIV infection. Mucosal biopsy in such patients may demonstrate focal crypt epithelial cell degeneration, which has been described as a characteristic pathological feature in AIDS. When performing a culture for AIDS-related diseases, the tissue should be examined for cytomegalovirus (CMV), herpes (HSV), cryptosporidium, *Micrococcus,* and amoeba.

6. Diagnosis of a suspected neural lipidoses and patients with unexplained signs of a degenerative nervous system disorder. Morphological and histochemical staining characteristics of the biopsy specimen can help diagnose certain neural diseases, including Niemann-Pick disease, amaurotic idiocies such as Tay-Sachs disease, and Hurler's syndrome.

7. Schistosomiasis, in which the eggs of the parasite can be identified in a squash preparation of the mucosal specimen.

8. Amebiasis, in which volcano-like lesions are seen; the center of the volcano may have organisms.

9. Assessment of progress in patients who are undergoing therapy.

Rectal suction biopsy

Most intraluminal biopsies of the GI tract go no deeper than the muscularis mucosa, which is adequate for most diagnoses. Suction biopsy more consistently penetrates into the submucosa. There are two disorders in which submucosal tissue assists in the diagnosis. The first disorder is Hirschsprung's disease, in which evidence of the myenteric ganglia is sought within the submucosa. The second disorder is systemic amyloidosis, a disorder in which amyloid accumulates between muscle layers of the intestine. The diagnosis is often obtained in both of these disorders by rectal suction biopsy.

The capsule of the biopsy tool is placed within the rectum and held against the rectal wall. Using a manometer to measure suction pressure, the tissue is suctioned into the capsule's side hole. When the suction is maintained, the trigger is fired and the tissue is cut in a guillotine fashion. The specimen is sent to pathology in the usual manner. Biopsy should be below the peritoneal reflection (within 7 to 10 cm of the anal verge in adults) to reduce the chance of perforation.

To provide useful diagnostic information from a colorectal biopsy specimen, the following activities should be performed:

1. The intestinal location of the biopsy specimens must be clearly defined by anatomical area (e.g., rectum, descending colon, splenic flexure). Centimeter designation is not usually accurate, especially if that number is used to find the location a second time.
2. Labeled, separate containers must be used for tissue specimens from different biopsy sites.
3. Multiple sections should be made of all specimens and thoroughly examined.

Rectal Culture

A rectal culture is a very simple and easy test to perform by the healthcare provider. A cotton swab is gently inserted into the rectum and rotated completely, then removed. This is quick and normally painless to the patient. A smear from the swab is placed in culture media in an effort to grow microorganisms for evaluation. As growth occurs, organisms can be identified.

Rectal culture is used to isolate and identify organisms that can cause symptoms or disease in the lower gastrointestinal (GI) tract. There are organisms that are normally present in this area of the GI tract but some are disease-causing pathogens. Rectal culture is indicated when GI distress is present and an infection is suspected as the cause. It may be performed initially or when a stool sample is difficult to obtain. The main pathogens that are isolated are: bacterial or parasitic enterocolitis, gonorrhea infection, and vancomycin-resistant Enterococcus.

Small Bowel Suction Biopsy

Suction biopsy has been proven safe, provided there is no tendency to bleed. In addition, the tube can be positioned rapidly and is easily visualized fluoroscopically. Compared to endoscopic biopsies, suction biopsies of the small bowel can be larger, easier to orient, and less traumatizing. In addition, suction biopsies can avoid the more proximal duodenum, where Brunner's glands and lymphoid follicles are abundant and potentially complicate histological interpretation. The procedure can be performed on an outpatient basis and is particularly valuable in the evaluation of patients with malabsorption syndromes.

Small bowel biopsy is diagnostic in Whipple's disease, agammaglobulinemia and severe hypogammaglobulinemia, and abetalipoproteinemia.

Small bowel biopsy *may* be diagnostic in the following:
 (a) intestinal lymphoma;
 (b) intestinal lymphangiectasia;
   eEosinophilic enteritis;
 (c) mastocytosis;
 (d) amyloidosis;
 (e) Crohn's disease;

 (f) giardiasis;
 (g) coccidiosis; and
 (h) CMV gastroenteritis.

Small bowel biopsy is abnormal, but not always diagnostic, in the following:
 (a) celiac sprue, unclassified sprue, and tropical sprue;
 (b) viral gastroenteritis;
 (c) intraluminal bacterial overgrowth;
 (d) folate and/or B_{12} deficiency; and
 (e) acute radiation enteritis.

Small bowel biopsy is contraindicated in patients with coagulopathy, in uncooperative patients, and in patients who are not NPO.

Platelet count or platelet smear, prothrombin time, partial thromboplastin time, and bleeding times should be obtained before suction biopsy if clinically indicated. Aspirin-containing products, anticoagulants, and NSAIDs should be avoided for 2 weeks before biopsy. The patient should fast for 4 to 8 hours, depending on age. The posterior part of the pharynx may be anesthetized with a topical anesthetic; infants and uncooperative younger children may be sedated.

Before beginning the procedure, it is important to complete the following activities:

1. Verify a written informed consent and the length of the patient's NPO status.
2. Obtain laboratory results, medical history, and baseline vital signs.
3. Notify the physician if the patient is currently on anticoagulant therapy, ASA, or NSAIDs; if laboratory results are abnormal; or if the patient's history indicates a need for prophylactic antibiotics (e.g., prosthetic heart valve).
4. Inform the patient of the purpose of the test, the techniques to be used, and the sensations he or she is likely to experience.

A number of instruments of various designs can be used for small bowel biopsy, including a **Carey capsule** or **Crosby capsule**. Capsule biopsy allows collection of a larger tissue sample and is able to reach areas of the small bowel not accessible to an endoscope.

A dissection microscope or a hand lens permits a reasonably good assessment of villous morphology and often leads to an immediate diagnosis of the atrophy that is typical of celiac disease. In addition to histological examination, biopsy samples may be useful for enzymatic, metabolic, immunological, and other microscopic studies. Tissue for morphology is placed in formalin, while the portion for intestinal enzymology is immediately quick-frozen at −40° C on a piece of aluminum foil lying on dry ice. Enzymatic studies include the determination of enzyme activity in tissue homogenates from patients with suspected isolated lactase deficiency, congenital sucrase-isomaltase deficiency, or a general decrease of disaccharidase activity associated with various mucosal disorders.

In addition, a small portion of the tissue sample can be placed in glutaraldehyde for electron microscopy. Another portion can be quick-frozen in isopentane, to be evaluated later by immunofluorescent studies designed to confirm the presence of immunity defects or to identify bacteria, viruses, or parasites.

Intestinal mucosa specimens may also be incubated with a radioactive substrate placed in an incubation medium to help characterize inborn errors of intestinal transport, such as cystinuria and glucose-galactose malabsorption.

Complications of small bowel biopsy are rare but may include perforation, hemorrhage, or entrapment of the capsule in the duodenum. The patient's hematocrit should be checked 4 to 6 hours after completion of the biopsy. Risk of perforation is greatest in severely hypoproteinemic, edematous patients.

FINE-NEEDLE ASPIRATION OF THE PANCREAS

Pancreatic abnormalities may be diagnosed by direct percutaneous **fine-needle aspiration** of the pancreas using ultrasonography or computed tomography (CT) guidance. Pancreatic aspiration appears to be a highly successful method of obtaining a cytohistological diagnosis of pancreatic cancer, with reported diagnostic accuracy rates of 80% to 90%. False-positive biopsy results are unlikely, but the absence of malignant cells in an aspirated biopsy does not definitively exclude pancreatic cancer.

Fine-needle aspiration is indicated in patients with large pancreatic masses that have been identified by noninvasive imaging studies. Cytological examination of biopsy specimens can provide tissue diagnosis and differentiation of lymphoma or endocrine tumors from adenocarcinoma without surgery, which is especially useful in elderly patients in whom the morbidity and mortality from laparotomy is high. For patients with small focal mass lesions, diffuse enlargement of the pancreas with calcification, or equivocal findings on ultrasonogram or CT scan, endoscopic retrograde cholangiopancreatography (ERCP) should be performed first, as described in Chapter 23.

In performing a fine-needle aspiration, either ultrasonography or CT guidance is used to pass a needle directly into the mass lesion. The aspirated material is then used for cytological examination. Several attempts at aspiration may be needed to obtain an adequate number of cells for cytological examination. Accuracy may be improved by the presence of a cytologist in the examining room to immediately prepare the cytology slides for assessment of specimen adequacy. Complications of fine-needle aspiration are infrequent, but there has been at least one report of seeding of malignant cells along the needle tract after aspiration. Accuracy depends greatly on the skill of the operator and the experience of the cytologist.

ENDOSCOPIC ULTRASOUND-GUIDED FINE NEEDLE ASPIRATION

Endoscopic ultrasound (EUS) is the most sensitive modality in the detection of pancreatic tumors. EUS is additionally utilized in the staging of esophageal, gastric, and rectal cancers. For endoscopists, EUS's limitations arise from the fact that the EUS is strictly an imaging modality. With the introduction of an echoendoscope with a sector scanner (Pentax/Hitachi) the technique of EUS-guided fine-needle aspiration (FNA) biopsy was developed. The pie-shaped image (sector) seen on the ultrasound screen enables the needle to be seen as it is advanced through the tissues, thus directing the needle to a targeted area for cell aspiration.

A specially designed needle, stylet, and handle have been developed for endoscopic use. The need for protecting the endoscopic channel, as well as allowing for flexibility during tip deflection of the endoscope, dictated the design of the needle. The needle, within an outer sheath, passes through the biopsy channel and exits above the optic lens. The needle can be seen both endoscopically and with ultrasound as it is advanced from the sheath. If used, the balloon is deflated to avoid puncture.

The performance of EUS-guided FNA is similar to other aspiration techniques. After both endoscopic and EUS evaluation the needle may be passed into the targeted tissue. In EUS/FNA, the assistant is often responsible for the aspiration of the cytological material. This is necessary because of the endoscopist's need to maintain the position of the endoscope with the transducer in contact with the GI wall during needle puncture. Under ultrasound guidance the needle punctures the targeted lesion, the stylet is removed, and suction is applied using a 10-ml syringe. While maintaining constant suction the needle is moved back and forth within the lesion. Suction is released while the needle is within the lesion to reduce the risk of aspiration of surrounding tissue. The entire needle assembly is removed from the endoscope, and the cell material is smeared on a glass slide for staining and review by a histocytologist. One to five passes may be needed to obtain adequate specimens for diagnosis. The presence of a histocytologist greatly improves the accuracy of diagnosis.

EUS/FNA is indicated in patients with pancreatic lesions, especially those that are difficult to locate with the more common procedure of percutaneous CT-guided FNA. Of most importance is the use of EUS/FNA in the staging of lymph node involvement of GI, pancreatic, and pulmonary cancers. This is an important addition to the care of cancer patients and may assist in directing chemotherapy and radiation therapy, and it may preclude unnecessary surgery for some.

Complications of EUS/FNA are similar to those of any endoscopic procedure. Although bleeding is a concern, as with any biopsy, the addition of Doppler ultrasound enables the endoscopist to distinguish vascular and solid structures. Most procedures are performed on outpatients; however, medication, IV fluids, and monitoring should be prudently adjusted, because EUS/FNA usually requires additional procedure time.

PERCUTANEOUS LIVER BIOPSY

In most cases, liver biopsy is performed percutaneously, but it can also be done under direct vision via laparoscopy or surgery. **Percutaneous liver biopsy** is a relatively low-cost bedside procedure.

Percutaneous liver biopsy is indicated for the evaluation of the following:

1. Acute and chronic cholestatic jaundice, after extrahepatic bile duct obstruction has been ruled out.
2. Acute viral hepatitis, pathological features of which include diffuse spotty parenchymal infiltration of hepatic lobules by lymphocytes and occasional plasma cells and neutrophils; ballooning degeneration and necrosis of hepatocytes; acidophilic body formation; swollen Kupffer cells; cholestasis; and inflammation of the portal tracts.
3. Alcoholic hepatitis, histological features of which include Mallory bodies, scattered fat, hepatocyte swelling, neutrophilic inflammation, and varying degrees of fibrosis, progressing to cirrhosis.
4. Documentation of cirrhosis and provision of information about the etiological agent. In suspected alcoholic cirrhosis, liver biopsy is used to confirm the stage of hepatic fibrosis and to exclude the presence of non-alcohol-related liver disease. In primary biliary cirrhosis, liver biopsy shows four progressive histological stages: florid duct lesions, followed by bile ductule proliferation, scarring, and micronodular cirrhosis. Percutaneous liver biopsy is complicated in cirrhotic patients, because penetration into the liver is made more difficult by subcapsular fibrosis and bile duct proliferation. In some patients, diagnostic laparotomy may be more productive because it helps to eliminate sampling errors.
5. α_1-Antitrypsin deficiency. In α_1-antitrypsin deficiency, liver biopsy shows globules in the cytoplasm of liver cells that stain positively with periodic acid-Schiff stain and resist digestion with diastase.
6. Unexplained hepatomegaly or liver abnormalities, as identified by ultrasonography, CT, or radionuclide scanning.
7. Space-occupying lesions or infiltrative neoplastic disease. Biopsy will indicate malignancy in patients with hepatocarcinoma only if the specimen is obtained from the site of the malignant lesion. Blind percutaneous needle biopsy with cytology is positive in 75% of patients with metastatic liver disease. CT-guided and peritoneoscopic needle biopsies may have higher diagnostic yields.
8. Assessment of a patient's response to therapy.
9. Lipid or glycogen storage diseases.
10. Drug related liver disease.
11. Wilson's disease. In the absence of Kayser-Fleischer rings, a liver biopsy for quantitative copper determination is essential in patients with suspected Wilson's disease. It is important in these patients that the biopsy needle and container be free from copper contamination.
12. Hemochromatosis, a genetic disorder of iron absorption. Liver biopsy permits estimation of tissue iron stores by histochemical staining, measurement of hepatic iron concentration by dry weight by chemical analysis (analysis for hemochromatosis-related genetic mutations may be performed on fixed tissue), and histological assessment of liver damage.
13. Screening of relatives of patients with familial liver disease.
14. Staging of malignant lymphoma.

Percutaneous liver biopsy is contraindicated in uncooperative or confused patients and in patients with any of the following:

1. Significant coagulopathy (although, if necessary, such patients may be prepared with infusions of fresh-frozen plasma and platelets).
2. Severe anemia.
3. Extrahepatic obstructive jaundice.
4. Inadequate movement of the right diaphragm secondary to right pleural effusion, right lower lung pneumonia, or fibrosis.
5. Moderate to large amounts of ascites.
6. Severe uremia, unless bleeding time is normal.
7. Excessive obesity.
8. Local skin infections involving the planned biopsy site.
9. Peritonitis.
10. Suspected hemangioma or hepatoma.
11. Suspected hepatic vein thrombosis.
12. Amyloidosis (relative), because of the possible risk of liver rupture.

Before performing percutaneous liver biopsy, it is important that laboratory studies (hemoglobin, hematocrit, white blood cell count, platelet count, prothrombin time, and partial thromboplastin time) be done to establish proper clotting factors, adequate blood volumes, and absence of infection. Other preliminary procedures may include obtaining baseline vital signs, blood typing and crossmatching, prophylactic vitamin K, chest and abdominal radiographs and scans, and a history of drug allergies. Foods and fluids should be withheld for at least 6 hours and NPO status verified.

Written informed consent must be obtained and the patient's medical history verified, including nonuse of anticoagulants, aspirin, or NSAIDs. The patient should be reassured, and the risks of the procedure and possible alternatives should be explained. An IV line may be started, if ordered. Because the patient will have to remain in bed for several hours after the biopsy, he or she should be encouraged to void before the procedure. The purpose of the test, techniques to be used, and sensations the patient is likely to experience should be explained. Breathing techniques that will be needed during the procedure should be explained and reinforced.

To minimize discomfort, the patient may be premedicated with sedatives, analgesics, mild narcotics, and/or barbiturates. The patient is placed in a supine position near the right side of the bed with a pillow under the right side; the right arm is placed under the head and the head is turned toward the left. Because pediatric patients cannot be expected to cooperate, they must be adequately sedated. Infants may be restrained on a circumcision board or held by assistants.

The biopsy site is chosen, and the surrounding skin is cleansed with acetone-alcohol and iodine solutions. Sterile drapes are arranged around the biopsy site (Fig. 25-2). The skin, subcutaneous tissues, and deeper intercostal muscles at

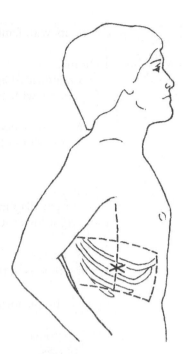

Fig. 25-2. Liver biopsy site.

the insertion site are infiltrated with a local anesthetic, such as procaine (Novocain) or lidocaine (Xylocaine), assuming that the patient has no known allergy to these substances.

A 4-mm skin incision is made at the biopsy site. A biopsy needle is attached to a syringe that contains a small amount of sterile saline. The type of needle used depends on the probable nature of the lesion. For example, a standard biopsy needle (Klatskin, Menghini, or similar) has the potential for causing a serious hemorrhage, but a fine needle may not obtain enough tissue for diagnosis. Tru-Cut disposable needles are commonly used, even for children.

After the needle is attached to the syringe, it is pushed through the skin incision and advanced into the intercostal muscles. The saline is injected to expel any tissue fragments from the needle. To prevent pleural cavity or diaphragm puncture, the patient holds his or her breath at full expiration while the biopsy needle is pushed into the liver. For pediatric patients, the biopsy should be timed to the respiratory cycle.

While constant aspiration is maintained, the needle is advanced 4 to 5 cm and then quickly withdrawn. Throughout the procedure, the needle is actually in the liver for only a fraction of a second. The patient resumes breathing 5 to 10 seconds after the specimen is obtained. A second biopsy through the same incision at a slightly different angle may be necessary.

The biopsy sample may be expelled from the needle temporarily into saline or directly into 10% formalin and then sent to the laboratory for analysis. If lymphoma is suspected, accurate diagnosis requires that a portion of the biopsy specimen be placed in saline, not formalin. The minimal amount of tissue necessary for evaluation by the pathologist is usually a core sample longer than 1 cm.

Potential Complications: percutaneous liver biopsy

Local pain and infection	Needle breakage
Hemorrhage into the peritoneum	Hemobilia
Bile peritonitis	Liver laceration
Perforated gallbladder	Pleurisya and peri-
Subcapsular or intrahepatic	hepatitis
hematoma	Shock
Pleural pain and pneumothorax	Hemothorax
Penetration of abdominal	Anesthetic reactions
viscera	Endotoxic shock
Capsular bleeding	Septicemia
Bacteremia	Tumor seeding
Arteriovenous fistulas	

If the apparent tumor is of a size or in a location unlikely to be reached with the standard blind-needle technique, sonography-guided or CT-guided biopsy may be more appropriate. Lesions that are more than 3 cm in diameter and peripherally located may be biopsied with sonographic guidance. CT guidance makes it easier to perform a biopsy of smaller, deeper lesions or those in relatively inaccessible locations. Angiographic techniques may be used to obtain liver tissue in patients with abnormal clotting parameters or massive ascites.

After the procedure is completed, an adhesive bandage is applied to the insertion site, and the patient is turned onto his or her right side against a firm support (e.g., bath blanket, sandbag, pillow). The patient maintains that position for the first 2 hours, with strict bed rest for the next 6 to 8 hours. If bleeding from the site persists, a pressure dressing may be needed. The insertion site must be observed closely for intraperitoneal hemorrhage or peritonitis. Vital signs should be taken regularly during this time. Patients may be allowed clear liquids shortly after biopsy. Solid food may be reintroduced after several hours if no serious complications have developed. If vital signs do not change, and hemoglobin and hematocrit are normal, outpatients may be discharged after 4 to 6 hours of observation, but they must remain on bed-rest for 8 to 12 hours.

The physician should be notified immediately in the following situations:

(a) the patient's pulse increases and systolic blood pressure decreases;

(b) the patient experiences prolonged pain that radiates to the back, abdomen, or shoulder;

(c) there is abdominal distention or obvious bleeding from the insertion site;

(d) the patient's temperature increases; and

(e) the patient's respiration changes.

Major complications have been reported in about 3 out of every 1000 biopsies, and deaths have been reported in about 1 out of every 1000. Potential complications of percutaneous liver biopsy are listed in the box above.

Complications can be minimized by using a needle that is 1.2 mm in diameter or less, avoiding biopsy in high-risk patients, and adhering strictly to protocol for obtaining the biopsy.

CELL CULTURE AND CYTOLOGY

When the presence of an infection is suspected, tissue specimens may be needed for the **culture** of bacteria, fungi, or other organisms. Specimens for culture may be obtained by using a cytology brush, by washing, or by aspiration. When whole cells are needed for microscopic examination, cytology specimens are collected, using either a cytology brush or a washing technique.

Indications for cytology

There are a number of different indications for obtaining endoscopic cytology specimens, including the following:
(a) suspected malignancy;
(b) suspected candidiasis;
(c) examination of duodenal aspirate for *Giardia,* secretory immunoglobulins, bile acid patterns, pancreatic amylase and trypsin levels, or evidence of strongyloidiasis; and
(d) pancreatic and bile ductal lesions.

Brush cytology

Information about the nature of some lesions can be obtained by **brush cytology,** using a tiny brush that is passed through the endoscope in much the same way as the biopsy forceps.

Sheathed disposable brushes are commercially available in various sizes and lengths. Appropriate selection depends on the location of the lesion, the endoscope length, and channel diameter being used. The brush is lined up with the suspicious area, extended beyond its plastic sheath, and rubbed across the mucosa. After harvesting cells from the suspect lesion, the head of the brush is withdrawn into the outer sheath before it is removed from the endoscope. Use of a sheathed brush minimizes the shedding of cells into the suction/biopsy channel.

After the brush is removed from the endoscope, thin smears of cells are made on clean microscope slides. The brush is gently rotated over the slide, brushing in one direction only. Specimens should be fixed with a cellular fixative, labeled, and sent to the laboratory as per institution protocol. The tips of disposable brushes may be cut off after the sample has been taken and sent intact to the laboratory, after moistening with 1 or 2 drops of sterile saline for culture, or in a container of 3 to 6 drops of sterile saline for cytological examination.

Obtaining specimens by washing

If a washing technique will be used to obtain specimens for culture or cytology, a specimen trap is attached to the endoscope suction port and the specimen is aspirated through the endoscope into the trap, injecting 20 to 30 ml of nonbacteriostatic saline through the biopsy channel to obtain the specimen. The trap is disconnected from the endoscope and sealed, and the endoscopic specimen is labeled and sent immediately to the laboratory.

Esophageal secretions may be obtained during esophagoscopy or by aspiration of iced saline that is injected through a nasogastric tube positioned at progressively higher positions in the esophagus.

For gastric cytology, vigorous gastric lavage is performed with a large volume of normal saline. This solution is aspirated and placed in an ice-water bath for later analysis. Then, a buffered solution of sodium acetate with chymotrypsin is instilled to promote exfoliation of malignant cells. Lavage is performed with the patient in different positions, and the solution is then aspirated, placed on ice, and taken to the laboratory for analysis.

For aspiration or lavage cytology of the pancreatic duct, pancreatic juice is collected into tubes containing a fixative. The tubes are centrifuged, and smears are made and fixed. For lavage cytology, small amounts of saline are injected into the main pancreatic duct and then aspirated with a syringe.

For colon cytology, the patient is prepared with a cathartic and with cleansing enemas. Warm saline, with or without chymotrypsin added, is instilled. After several minutes the solution is collected, placed on ice, and taken to the laboratory.

CASE SITUATION

This is the second hospital admission for Gary, age 28, who is diagnosed with AIDS. Initially, Gary was admitted for severe dysphagia (difficulty swallowing) and odynophagia (pain on swallowing). His upper endoscopy at that time revealed severe esophageal inflammation with whitish patches. Specimens taken at that time revealed candidiasis. Gary now has diarrhea and weight loss, in addition to some continuing odynophagia. He is scheduled for both upper and lower endoscopy, with biopsy and cytology.

Points to think about

1. Immunocompromised patients, especially those with AIDS, are susceptible to a host of GI problems. What are some of the normal defenses the gut has to prevent invasion by pathological organisms, and how are these defenses affected by HIV infection?
2. On upper endoscopy, Gary is found to have dense patches of creamy, waxy exudate; esophagitis; and two very large, deep ulcerations. His duodenum is normal, but there are two raised, dark red, 10-mm lesions in his stomach. What types of specimens will help diagnose the cause of these problems?
3. The gastroenterology nurse is now involved in much more specimen collection than in the past. Why is it important to develop a good working relationship with laboratory personnel?
4. Diarrhea can have many causes in the patient with AIDS, including amebiasis, shigellosis, gonorrhea, CMV, herpes

simplex, syphilis, lymphogranuloma venereum, cryptosporidiosis, and *Chlamydia.* What tests would help determine the cause of Gary's diarrhea?

5. In dealing with infectious specimens, what special practices should be employed?

Suggested responses

1. The normal defenses the GI tract has against pathological organisms include the bactericidal effect of gastric acid, intestinal motility, normal bowel flora, intact mucosa, humoral immunity, lymphocytes, macrophages, and neutrophils. In patients with HIV infection, deficiencies in the immune system (neutropenia and alterations in hormonal and cell-mediated immunity) affect the normal defense mechanisms of the GI tract. In addition, infections can disrupt intact mucosa, decrease motility, and overrun normal flora. Because of this, the gut is susceptible to local and systemic infections.

2. In AIDS patients, the esophagus is often involved with opportunistic infections such as *Candida,* herpes simplex, and CMV. Comprehensive testing is recommended, because having the scope in place allows for easy specimen acquisition. Specimens that will help diagnose the cause of Gary's symptoms include the following:

   (a) Brush cytology to test for *Candida.* Disposable brushes are packaged sterile and are inexpensive enough that nondisposable brushes should no longer be used for specimen acquisition. It is important to know the institution's routine for preparing specimens. Often, the brush may be delivered to the laboratory in its package with orders for fungal culture and stains, and the laboratory will prepare it. Although symptoms of *Candida* infections may improve or disappear with therapy, this does not always indicate disappearance of mucosal lesions. Follow-up endoscopies are often necessary.

   (b) Biopsy of the deep esophageal ulcerations. If the pathologist knows the suspected diagnosis, special stains can be applied to identify fungal, viral, or parasitic invasion.

   (c) Viral cultures. Special media are usually obtainable from the laboratory for viral cultures. They are kept refrigerated and have a relatively short outdate. A forceps biopsy specimen is placed in the viral culture medium and labeled.

   (d) Biopsy of the dark red lesions in the stomach. These lesions are most likely Kaposi's sarcoma. They can appear anywhere in the gut and vary in color from red to deep purple. Fifty percent of AIDS patients who present with Kaposi's skin lesions will also have GI tract lesions, which have a much poorer prognosis. In the gut, these lesions lie submucosally; standard forceps biopsy, which only penetrates mucosal tissue, may be negative. It would be helpful to use the largest forceps that will fit through the channel of your scope. This may be a time for the snare lift-and-cut

technique. Care should be taken in case there is excessive bleeding from these lesions at biopsy.

3. Laboratory personnel can be very helpful. Specimens must often be taken to different departments within the laboratory (e.g., pathology for biopsy and cytology, microbiology for cultures and staining). There are many different ways to order tests, and many specimens need special collection methods and media. Having this knowledge before the procedure can save time and can help avoid mistakes and loss of specimens.

4. Tests that can help specify the cause of Gary's diarrhea include the following:

   (a) Colonoscopy, to examine the whole large bowel and ascertain the extent of disease.

   (b) Flexible sigmoidoscopy for specimen collection.

   (c) Stool cultures and microscopic examinations. In the colon, it may be difficult to determine what agent is causing colitis. The list of possible agents is long. Many of these organisms may be present simultaneously, or they may not appear in every specimen. This means that stool cultures and microscopic examinations may need to be done on a serial basis and must often be repeated.

   (d) Specimens for Gram stain, bacterial culture, ova and parasites, viral cultures, and special staining techniques. Again, each institution uses different methods and media. It is important to be familiar with institutional procedures and to give the pathologist and laboratory personnel as much information as possible regarding the potential diagnosis.

   (e) Biopsy to help differentiate colitis from Crohn's disease or ulcerative colitis.

   (f) Biopsy of the characteristic red lesions of Kaposi's sarcoma.

5. It is unlikely that handling infectious specimens would cause infection in healthcare personnel unless they are immunocompromised. However, the contaminated hands or clothing of healthcare personnel may spread infections to other patients who might be immunocompromised. It is important to remember that AIDS patients are immunocompromised and therefore more susceptible to infection than most patients. Special practices to think about when dealing with infectious specimens include the following:

   (a) Wear gloves, protective gowns, masks, and protective eyewear when collecting specimens.

   (b) Wash hands thoroughly when gloves are removed and leaving protective clothing in the procedure room hamper.

   (c) Do not handle patient care equipment when exudative lesions or weeping dermatitis are present

   (d) Put all specimens in well-constructed containers with secure lids to prevent leaking during transport.

   (e) Collect each specimen carefully to avoid contaminating the outside of the container and the laboratory form accompanying the specimen.

   (f) Implement standard precautions for blood and body fluids for *all* patients; this eliminates the need for special warning labels on specimens, because all specimens should be considered infective.

(g) Subject endoscopes used on HIV-positive patients to the same scrupulous cleaning and disinfecting regimen given to all endoscopes.

(h) Use biopsy forceps that are sterile, because they are designed to break the mucosal barrier; they may be disposable and packaged sterile, or they may be reusable and sterilized after use by ultrasonic cleaning and steam under pressure.

(i) Use disposable cytology brushes.

REVIEW TERMS

aspiration, biopsy, biopsy forceps, brush cytology, Carey capsule, Crosby capsule, culture, cytology, exfoliative brush cytology, fine-needle aspiration, frozen section, histopathological analysis, hot biopsy forceps, percutaneous liver biopsy, suction biopsy, washing

REVIEW QUESTIONS

1. Endoscopic biopsy is contraindicated in patients with:
   (a) Carcinoma.
   (b) Severe coagulopathy.
   (c) Inflammatory bowel disease.
   (d) GI polyps.

2. Frozen sections are used when:
   (a) The biopsy specimen will be preserved for a long period of time.
   (b) A fixative is needed to preserve the specimen.
   (c) Immediate denial/confirmation of malignancy is required.
   (d) A pathologist is not immediately available.

3. The most likely complication of endoscopic biopsy is:
   (a) Excessive bleeding.
   (b) Infection.
   (c) Tumor seeding.
   (d) Nausea and vomiting.

4. Suspect esophageal tissue is most often sampled using what technique?
   (a) Suction.
   (b) Needle aspiration.
   (c) Endoscopic biopsy.
   (d) Polypectomy.

5. Specimens for small bowel biopsy are usually taken from what general area?
   (a) The duodenum.
   (b) The jejunum.
   (c) The ileum.
   (d) The ligament of Treitz.

6. During EUS/FNA, aspiration of tissue is accomplished using suction applied with:
   (a) A 5-ml syringe.
   (b) A 10-ml syringe.
   (c) A 20-ml syringe.
   (d) A 60-ml syringe.

7. The length of time a patient should stay in bed under direct observation of a medical staff member after having a liver biopsy is:
   (a) 2 to 4 hours.
   (b) 4 to 6 hours.
   (c) 6 to 8 hours.
   (d) 8 to 12 hours.

8. To prevent pleural cavity or diaphragm puncture during the procedure, insertion of the needle for percutaneous liver biopsy in pediatric patients should be:
   (a) Timed to the patient's respiratory cycle.
   (b) Done while the patient holds his or her breath on expiration.
   (c) Done slowly.
   (d) Done under ultrasonography or CT guidance.

9. If disposable cytology brushes are sent intact to the laboratory, they should be moistened with:
   (a) Nonbacteriostatic saline.
   (b) Glutaraldehyde.
   (c) Isopentane.
   (d) Cellular fixative.

10. A solution that may be instilled in the GI tract to promote exfoliation of malignant cells is:
   (a) Normal saline.
   (b) Secretin-cholecystokinin.
   (c) Chymotrypsin.
   (d) Formalin.

BIBLIOGRAPHY

Bowlus, B. (Ed.) (1998). *Gastroenterology Nursing: a core curriculum* (2nd edition), St. Louis, MO: Mosby.

Branski, D., Faber, J. & Shiner, M. (1996). A comparison of small-intestinal mucosal biopsies in children obtained by blind suction capsule with those obtained by endoscopy. *J Pediatr Gastroenterol Nutr* 22, 194-6. Journal of Pediatric Gastroenterology and Nutrition.

Chang, K.J. & Wiersema, M.J. (1997). Endoscopic ultrasound-guided fine-needle aspiration biopsy and interventional endoscopic ultrasonography. *Gastrointest Endosc Clin North Am* 7(2), 221-35.

Chobanian, S. Van Ness, M. (Eds.) (1994). *Manual of clinical problems in gastroenterology* (2nd ed.). Boston: Little, Brown.

Eastwood, G. & Avunduk, C. (1994). *Manual of gastroenterology: diagnosis and therapy* (2nd ed.). Boston: Little, Brown.

Friesen, C. (1995). Grasp biopsy, suction biopsy, and clinical history in the evaluation of esophagitis in infants 0-6 months of age. *J Pediatr Gastroenterol Nutr 20*, 300-4. Journal of Pediatric Gastroenterology and Nutrition.

Geramizadeh, B. (2002). Brush cytology of gastric malignancies. *Acad Cytol 46*(4), 693-6.

Howden, C. & Hunt, R. (1998). Guidelines for the management of helicobacter pylori infection. *Amer J. Gastroent 93*(12), 2330-8. American Journal of Gastroenterology.

Johns Hopkins Pathology (2003). *Pancreas cancer fine needle aspiration.* Baltimore, MD: Johns Hopkins Hospital.

Kotton, C., (2002). *MEDLINE plus Medical Encyclopedia: Rectal Culture, VeriMed HealthCare Network.*: A.D.A.M., Inc.

Misiewicz, J. J., Bartram, C.I., Cotton, P.B. (1994). *Atlas of clinical gastroenterology* (2nd ed.). London: Gower Medical.

O'Donoghue, J. (1995). Adjunctive endoscopic brush cytology in the detection of upper gastrointestinal malignancy. *Int Acad Cytol 39*(1), 28-34. International Academy of Cytology.

Pennazio, M. (1995). Clinical evaluation of push-type enteroscopy. *Endoscopy 27*, 164-70.

Society of Gastroenterology Nurses and Associates, Inc. (2003). *Manual of gastrointestinal procedures* (5th ed.). Chicago: Society of Gastroenterology Nurses and Associates, Inc.

Shah, J. (2002). *MEDLINEplus Medical Encyclopedia: Liver biopsy, VeriMEd Healthcare Network*.: A.D.A.A., Inc.

Shah, J. (DATE). *Updater MEDLINEplus Medical Encyclopedia: Small bowel biopsy, VeriMed Healthcare Network*.: A.D.A.M., Inc.

Silverman, A. & Roy, C. (1991). *Pediatric clinical gastroenterology* (4th ed..). St. Louis, MO: Mosby.

Sivak, M. (2000). *Gastrointestinal Endoscopy, Volume 1 and 2* (2nd ed.). Philadelphia, Pennsylvania: W.B. Saunders.

Sleisenger, M. & Fordtran, J. (Eds.) (1988). *Gastrointestinal disease: pathophysiology, diagnosis, management* (6th ed.). Philadelphia: W.B. Saunders.

Thampanitchawong, P. & Piratvisuth, T. (1995). *Liver biopsy: complications and risk factors*. World J. *Gastroenterology 5*(4), 301-4. World Journal of Gastroenterology.

Vilmann, P. (1995). Endoscopic ultrasonography-guided fine-needle aspiration biopsy of lesions in the upper gastrointestinal tract. *Gastrointest Endosc 41*(3), 230-5. Gastrointestinal Endoscopy.

Wiersema, M. (1994). Combined endosonography and fine-needle aspiration cytology in the evaluation of gastrointestinal lesions, *Gastrointest Endosc 40*(2), 199-206. Gastrointestinal Endoscopy.

Yamada, T. Laine, L., Alpers, D.H. (1999). *The textbook of gastroenterology* (3rd ed.). Philadelphia: J.B. Lippincott.

All techniques in this chapter, except fine-needle aspiration of the pancreas, are also discussed in:

Society of Gastroenterology Nurses and Associates, Inc. (2003). *Manual of gastrointestinal procedures* (5th ed.). Chicago: Society of Gastroenterology Nurses and Associates, Inc.

Chapter 26

OTHER PROCEDURES AND TESTS

This chapter will acquaint the gastroenterology nurse with nonendoscopic diagnostic tests and procedures that are used in the practice of gastroenterology. Radiographic and nonradiographic imaging techniques are discussed, including plain and contrast radiography, ultrasonography, and computed tomography. Studies involving the analysis of GI secretions are described and laboratory tests involving the analysis of blood, urine, and fecal samples are reviewed.

Learning objectives

After reviewing the content of this chapter, the gastroenterology nurse should be able to:
1. Describe radiographic and nonradiographic imaging studies performed on gastroenterology patients, including indications, contraindications, and patient care instructions.
2. Discuss a variety of diagnostic tests and procedures used to analyze GI secretions.
3. Briefly explain the diagnostic tests that are used most frequently to analyze the blood, urine, or feces of gastroenterology patients.

BASIC PRINCIPLES

In addition to the diagnostic techniques discussed in the preceding chapters, gastroenterology patients are often required to undergo a variety of other laboratory tests and procedures.

The importance of discussing these tests with the patient cannot be overemphasized. To educate and prepare patients for such tests, it is important that the nurse understand the role of these tests in the diagnostic process and communicates this information to the patient. Complete instructions and explanations help ensure the patient's compliance and also allay any feelings of anxiety. Most patients do better during a test when they have received information about the procedure they will undergo and the sensations they are likely to experience. It may be helpful to provide patient instruction when a member of the patient's family is there to offer support and to reinforce the teaching. After completion, patient education and comprehension should be documented.

It is also important to review the patient's history before any diagnostic testing is conducted and to verify compliance with any necessary preparations, such as length of NPO status, withholding of certain medications, or preliminary blood work. During the procedure the nurse may be responsible for patient positioning, handling specimens or test samples, gathering instruments and supplies, and calibrating any recording devices.

After the procedure is completed, the patient should be monitored for adverse effects, provided with discharge instructions, instructed how to obtain test results, and what follow-up is recommended.

RADIOGRAPHIC AND NONRADIOGRAPHIC IMAGING

Radiographic studies of the GI tract help detect abnormalities such as obstructions, strictures, ulcers, or structural changes. Flat and upright plain x-ray films of the abdomen and upright chest x-ray films are often the first tests performed on patients with acute abdominal symptoms. In most cases, other tests are also required.

Generally speaking, radiology is easier for the patient than endoscopy and has fewer complications; however, endoscopy has greater diagnostic potential. The local availability of radiological and endoscopic expertise may also influence the physician's choice of diagnostic method.

Administration of a contrast medium before or during radiographic studies accentuates differences in the densities of abdominal regions and structures, thus facilitating interpretation of the radiographs. Most radiographic tests for GI disorders use **barium sulfate** as the contrast medium. Barium is a chalky, radiopaque, inert, nonallergenic substance that enables **fluoroscopic examination** and **x-ray (roentgenographic) examination** of the esophagus, stomach, and small and large intestines. It may be administered orally, rectally, or via intestinal stoma. Any routine x-ray examinations, lower GI studies, or oral cholecystograms should be done *before* barium studies because the ingested barium may obscure other films. Barium studies are contraindicated in patients with digestive tract obstruction or perforation.

Patients who undergo barium studies must be cautioned to report failure to pass the barium within 2 to 3 days so cathartics or enemas may be prescribed to avoid constipation or obstruction. In some institutions, an enema or a laxative is given routinely after barium studies. Patients may also be advised to increase their intake of fluids. They should be told to expect stools to be chalky and light-colored for 24 to 72 hours after the barium.

Iodine-based contrast media are administered intravenously for radiographs of the gallbladder, pancreas, spleen, and the various ducts. Radiographic studies with iodine-based contrast media require careful review of the patient's history of allergies to iodine, seafood, or iodine-based contrast agents. They also require careful patient preparation before the test and close observation afterward for delayed hypersensitivity reactions.

Barium swallow

A **barium swallow** permits radiographic examination of the esophagus after ingestion of a thick barium solution. This test can reveal the presence or absence of foreign bodies, diverticula, ulcerations, varices, polyps, tumors, a hiatal hernia, or motility disorders. It may discover, but is not sensitive for, esophagitis or Barrett's esophagus. A barium swallow is contraindicated in patients with intestinal obstructions. For patients with suspected perforations, Gastrografin is the preferred contrast medium.

Patients scheduled for a barium swallow should:

(a) fast for a given period of time before the examination; and

(b) consult their physicians to determine if it is appropriate to take oral medications prior to the procedure.

During the test, the patient swallows a barium mixture while in a supine position. The Trendelenburg position may be used to detect gastric reflux or a sliding hiatal hernia. For patients with dysphagia, a barium tablet or food/marshmallow bolus should be used in addition to the liquid barium, so that strictures can be better identified.

Upper gastrointestinal series

In an **upper gastrointestinal (UGI) series** with small bowel follow-through, the esophagus, stomach, and small intestine are all examined following ingestion of a barium solution. An UGI series can be used for diagnosis of hiatal hernia, diverticula, varices, strictures, ulcers, tumors, Crohn's disease, malabsorption syndromes, or motility disorders. Gastric x-ray films may show masses or ulcers. Films of the small intestine may indicate obstruction, regional ileitis, or diverticula.

Patients scheduled for a UGI should remain NPO after midnight. Some institutions also recommend that patients:

- follow a low-residue diet for 2 to 3 days;
- avoid anticholinergic or narcotic medications for 24 hours;
- refrain from smoking after midnight; and
- avoid antacids for several hours before the test.

After swallowing the barium, the patient assumes various positions on the x-ray examination table so the barium will outline all parts of the gastric wall. In addition, the abdomen may be palpated or compressed. Air may be introduced into the abdomen to improve visualization of small lesions that can be missed when using barium alone. This is called a double-contrast and the patient will be asked to swallow a gas-producing substance in the form of a powder, pills, or carbonated beverage.

Enteroclysis

When small bowel follow-through fails to provide a satisfactory study, **enteroclysis** may be used to detect subtle small bowel disease.

Patients scheduled for an enteroclysis should (a) receive a bowel prep (enemas are not recommended since some fluid may be retained in the small bowel); and (b) have someone with them to drive home if sedation is needed.

This test is invasive, requiring intubation of the patient either intranasally or orally with a flexible feeding tube. The tip of the tube is positioned in the duodenum, and barium is injected through the tube into the small bowel under fluoroscopic guidance. The barium is then followed by an injection of water and/or methylcellulose solution to give a **double-contrast effect.** Multiple spot films of the various segments of the small bowel are obtained, including the ileocecal valve. Enteroclysis is able to show small polyps, mass lesions, and subtle mucosal involvement of inflammatory bowel disease more clearly than conventional small bowel follow-through. Sedation may be necessary to ensure patient comfort during the examination.

Barium enema

The **barium enema** is a common and valuable diagnostic test for patients with colon disorders. Both single-contrast and double-contrast barium enemas are safe and well tolerated without premedication, although double-contrast enemas are generally the method of choice. In double-contrast studies, a thicker barium solution is used. After rotation to cover the bowel wall, air is introduced into the bowel so that smaller lesions can be seen.

A barium enema is indicated for the evaluation of the large intestine, evaluation of inflammatory disease and to detect polyps, masses, diverticula, and structural changes. The procedure is contraindicated in patients with fulminant ulcerative colitis associated with systemic toxicity, toxic megacolon, or suspected perforation or obstruction.

Patients scheduled for a barium enema should:

(a) be well educated about the procedure, since full cooperation is essential for a successful exam;

(b) receive a bowel-cleansing regimen to allow for adequate examination of the bowel; and

(c) follow a clear liquid diet for 1 to 2 days.

A conventional cathartic and an enema preparation or a balanced electrolyte lavage solution is given after the procedure. Defecation of barium should be monitored and laxatives given if not passed within 2 to 3 days.

"Unprepped" barium enema examination is indicated for children when Hirschsprung's disease is suspected. The barium is administered as an enema, and the patient is encouraged to retain the barium, despite any cramping or urge to defecate. In some cases the barium is administered through a Foley type of catheter, and the balloon is inflated slightly to prevent the patient from expelling the solution. The use of a catheter may increase the urge to defecate and exacerbate patient discomfort. The patient is instructed to move about to allow the barium to spread throughout the colon. In some cases a tilt table may be used to achieve a semi-erect or Trendelenburg position that will allow the barium to cover all areas of the colon.

Capsule Endoscopy

Capsule endoscopy is a new technique that employs a disposable video capsule swallowed by the patient allowing visualization of much of the small bowel not within reach of standard upper and lower endoscopy. The U.S. Food and Drug Administration (FDA) approved this procedure on August 1, 2001.

Indications include:

(a) to aid in the diagnosis of GI bleeding especially when upper endoscopy and colonoscopy are negative; and

(b) to evaluate conditions of the small bowel that cause diarrhea, pain or weight loss (ie. Crohn's Disease).

Patients swallow a plastic capsule with a sip of water. The capsule is approximately the size of a large vitamin and contains a disposable, miniature camera in order to visualize the digestive system. Images captured by the camera are transmitted to a number of sensors attached to the patient's torso and recorded digitally on a recording device, similar to a Walkman, worn around the patient's waist. After approximately 8 hours (the life of the battery) the capsule has progressed through the small intestine. At this time the recorder and the sensors are removed from the patient. The system acquires about 50,000 images of the small intestine. The data is then downloaded to a workstation, and software processes the images to produce a video of the small intestine for interpretation by the physician.

Patients scheduled for capsule endoscopy should follow these instructions:

1. Take no iron tablets for 7 days.

2. No bowel prep is required.

3. Remain NPO after midnight.

4. The sensors will be applied to the abdomen with adhesive pads and will be connected to the recorder that will be worn in a belt around the patient's waist. Some patients may have to shave their abdomens 6 inches above and below the navel the night before the procedure to assure that the sensors will stay attached.

5. Sign informed consent.

6. Some physicians give simethicone prior to capsule endoscopy to decrease gas bubbles and increase visualization.

7. After ingesting the capsule, patients will be NPO for at least 2 hours. After 4 hours they may have a light lunch. After completion of the study (8 hours), they may return to their normal diet.

8. Patients should contact the hospital immediately if they have any abdominal pain, nausea or vomiting anytime after ingesting the capsule.

9. Some images may be lost due to radio interference (e.g. from amateur radio transmitter, MRI, etc). On rare occasions this may result in the need to repeat the capsule procedure. In such a case, the patient will be advised to stay within the premises of the clinic for the duration of the capsule procedure to prevent this problem from recurring.

10. The data-gathering period lasts 8 hours and during this time, patients should avoid any strenuous physical activity, Bending, or stooping. The belt should remain secure throughout the procedure. The recorder is actually a small computer and should be treated with care.

11. Periodically during the data-gathering period, the patient will need to verify that the small light on top of the recorder is blinking. If blinking stops, patient should record the time and contact the hospital. The patient should also record the nature of any event such as eating, drinking and unusual sensations. These notes are given to the caregivers at the time the equipment is returned.

12. At the end of 8 hours, the patient must return to the hospital for the Data Recorder, and sensors to be removed. Pulling the wires of the sensors or attempting to remove any part of the apparatus by the patient should be avoided. The data recorder holds the images of the examination. The data recorder, recorder belt, sensors and recorder battery pack must be handled carefully.

13. If patients cannot positively verify the excretion of the capsule, or they develop unexplained abdominal pain, vomiting or other symptoms of obstruction, the physician must be contacted to evaluate the patient and possibly order an abdominal X-ray.

14. Undergoing an MRI while the capsule is inside the patient may result in serious damage to their intestinal tract or abdominal cavity. If positive verification of the excretion of the capsule from your body can't be done the physician may order an abdominal x-ray before undergoing an MRI examination.

15. The capsule is disposable and will be excreted naturally in a bowel movement. In the rare case that it will not be excreted naturally, it will have to be removed endoscopicaly or surgically.

16. The examination may be incomplete due to technical difficulties, poor preparation, or slow bowel function. (No test, including capsule endoscopy, can offer 100% accuracy for diagnosis.)

Magnetic Resonance Cholangiopancreatography

Magnetic Resonance Cholangiopancreatography (MRCP) is a new application of MRI. With this technique, a patient's hepato-biliary and pancreatic systems are imaged using MRI imaging with special software. This type of imaging can reproduce images similar to those obtained from the more invasive approach with ERCP without the added risk of pancreatitis, sedation, or perforation. There is no patient preparation, or radiation exposure. The patient is injected with Gadolinium intravenously with 1 cc for every 10 pounds of body weight. It is currently the most benign dye used for radiological procedures. The patients feel no flushing, nausea, or vomiting, and Gladolinium can be administered to patients with a known IV contrast allergy. It has been shown to be effective in detecting gallstones and visualizing the biliary and pancreatic ducts. Currently the major shortcoming lies in the experience of the interpreting physician, and the fact that the procedure does not allow for therapeutic interventions. If an intervention is needed the patient would require an Endoscopic Retrograde Cholangiopancreotography.

Percutaneous transhepatic cholangiography

Percutaneous transhepatic cholangiography (PTC) is used to visualize the biliary ductal system. It may be used to distinguish between obstructive and nonobstructive jaundice or to determine the location, extent, and cause of mechanical bile duct obstruction, which may be caused by stones, tumors, inflammation, stenosis, or stricture. PTC is often used to place a drainage catheter for the treatment of obstructive jaundice. PTC is contraindicated in patients with cholangitis, massive ascites, allergies to iodine, or uncorrectable coagulopathy.

Under fluoroscopic visualization, a Chiba needle (a "skinny" needle) is introduced into the liver, through the locally anesthetized seventh or eighth intercostal space, parallel to the plane of the table. The needle is slowly withdrawn until a green fluid is aspirated, indicating that a bile duct has been entered. A radiopaque iodine dye is then injected, and radiographs are taken to define the site, cause, and extent of bile duct obstruction.

Patients scheduled for a PTC should:

(a) receive antibiotics (these may be given for 2 days before and 3 days after the procedure);

(b) be carefully observed after completion of procedure (The patient's vital signs should be checked regularly and be observed for 24 hours for signs of hemorrhage from the site, including a decrease in blood pressure, an increase in pulse rate and respirations, restlessness, pallor, or diaphoresis. Bleeding may result from PTC and can be massive.);

(c) remain in bed for the first 6 hours, lying on the right side; and

(d) be monitored for pain, temperature elevation, chills, abdominal distention, peritonitis, bile leakage, or septicemia.

Cholangiography can also be performed intraoperatively and postoperatively via a T-tube or cholecystectomy tube that is placed in the cystic duct.

Abdominal ultrasonography

Ultrasonography is indicated to show the size and configuration of organs. It identifies abnormalities of the structures and spaces within the abdomen or pelvis through the transmission of sound waves. Sound waves are used to create images of organs.

Ultrasonography is the best noninvasive test for the detection of gallstones, because it does not involve patient preparation or radiation and is simple to perform and interpret. It is also indicated in screening for biliary dilatation. It may be useful in detecting changes caused by appendicitis, such as a dilated appendix, thickened wall, or paraappendiceal fluid accumulation. Ultrasonography is also sensitive for acute cholecystitis.

The skin over the area to be studied is exposed and lubricated to seal out air pockets and keeps the transducer from rubbing the patient's skin. While the patient lies still, a microphone transducer is slowly rubbed over the skin surface for approximately 20 to 30 minutes. An image of the structures within the target area is produced on a screen throughout the test.

Oral cholecystography

Although ultrasonography is the initial diagnostic procedure of choice for the detection of gallstones, **oral cholecystography** is an acceptable alternative when ultrasonography is unavailable, or not diagnostic, or when the cholecystogram will be performed in conjunction with a UGI series. Oral cholecystography may be superior to ultrasonography for demonstrating the patency of the cystic duct, assessing gallbladder function, or showing the apparent density of stones. It is also necessary before oral dissolution therapy of gallstones to be certain the cystic duct is open.

Patients scheduled for oral cholecystography should know that:

(a) it will involves oral administration of pills containing iodinated radiocontrast material;

(b) films are taken 10 to 14 hours later;

(c) fat may be ingested following the initial gallbladder films to cause contraction of the gallbladder, filling the common bile duct;

(d) radiography takes 30 to 45 minutes; and

(e) they may resume a normal diet and continue with their prescribed medications.

Oral cholecystography is contraindicated in patients with severe renal or hepatic damage or in patients with a known allergy to iodine. This test may prove unsuccessful when patients have elevated bilirubin, do not take the pills correctly, or cannot tolerate them.

Arteriography

Arteriography, which is also called **angiography,** involves the catheterization of selected arteries, followed by injection of an iodinated dye via the catheter. Subsequent x-ray films can help to locate the source of GI bleeding, evaluate cirrhosis and portal hypertension, or determine the extent of vascular damage to the liver and spleen after abdominal trauma. Vascular tumors may be located by selective celiac and superior mesenteric arteriograms. Selective arteriography can also be therapeutic. Autologous clots or vasopressin (Pitressin) can be injected into appropriate vessels to control bleeding, or chemotherapeutic agents can be delivered directly to the tumor. Arteriography is contraindicated in patients who are allergic to iodine.

Computed tomography

Computed tomography (CT) is a noninvasive, radiological scanning technique that relies on differences in tissue density to reflect organ configurations. Because it gathers information in all three dimensions, CT provides a more detailed and more precise view of the area being scanned than does abdominal ultrasonography. However, CT scanning also requires more personnel and expensive equipment to operate than does ultrasonography, and it does use ionizing radiation. The diagnostic accuracy of CT scanning can be enhanced by IV injection of contrast material to visualize the biliary system or by oral ingestion of a contrast agent to delineate the GI system.

CT scanning is indicated for evaluation of gallbladder carcinoma, common bile duct stones, liver masses, pancreatic adenocarcinoma, intraabdominal abscess, and complications of acute pancreatitis.

Scintigraphy

Scintigraphy relies on the use of radioactive isotopes, such as technetium (^{99m}Tc), iodine (^{131}I), or indium (^{111}In), to reveal displaced anatomical structures, changes in organ size, and the presence of neoplasms or other focal lesions, such as cysts or subphrenic and subhepatic abscesses. New pharmaceuticals being introduced will be organ specific for making diagnoses.

Hepatic Scintigraphy

Hepatic scintigraphy with ^{99m}Tc-labeled sulfur colloid is widely used for noninvasive evaluation of the liver. The most common use is for diagnosing and following the progression of metastatic disease. In addition, its sensitivity for hepatocellular dysfunction or diffuse infiltrating diseases such as alcoholic liver disease, cirrhosis, lymphoma, amyloidosis, or infiltrating metastatic disease may be higher than other imaging methods.

The Kupffer cells and other phagocytic cells in the liver and spleen absorb the radiolabeled chemical. Because most intrahepatic masses do not contain these phagocytes, such masses appear as "cold" spots on the hepatic scintigram.

Biliary scintigraphy

For biliary scintigraphy, the patient must be NPO after midnight. A ^{99m}Tc-labeled iminodiacetic acid derivative is administered intravenously. In normal subjects, this labeled compound is taken up by the hepatocytes and excreted into bile. Scans are obtained 5 to 60 minutes or longer after radionuclide injection to outline the bile ducts, gallbladder, and proximal small bowel.

If the ducts are visible but the gallbladder is not, acute cholecystitis is suggested but not proven. In patients with nonacute gallstone disease, gallbladder filling may be delayed by up to 3 hours. False positive scans may occur in patients with acute pancreatitis, chronic cholecystitis, alcoholism, neoplasms of the gallbladder and liver, and patients receiving total parenteral nutrition. False negative scans may occur in patients with acute acalculous cholecystitis.

Radionuclide evaluation of gastric emptying

For evaluation of gastric emptying, radionuclide testing is preferred over intubation methods. The ability of radionuclides to tag a solid test meal offers quantitative results that are not possible with barium radiography.

The radionuclide technique is useful for evaluation of any functional cause of delayed gastric emptying, but its most common clinical use is in the diagnosis of diabetic gastroparesis. It is also of value in evaluating rapid emptying, particularly the "dumping syndrome" that may be noted after gastric surgery.

The liquid component of the meal is labeled with ^{111}In. Either egg salad or chicken liver is labeled with ^{99m}Tc, which serves as a marker of the solid component of the meal. Following ingestion of the radiolabeled solid and liquid meal, the patient reclines under a scintiscanner that measures the initial level of intragastric radioactivity and the rate of passage of radioactivity out of the stomach (i.e., gastric emptying). In this manner, differential rates of solid and liquid emptying can be detected.

Gastric emptying studies may also be done without radionuclides.

Scintigraphic scanning

GI bleeding may be diagnosed through the use of one of two scintigraphic techniques. One technique uses ^{99m}Tc-labeled sulfur colloid; the other uses ^{99m}Tc-labeled red blood cells using the patient's own blood. Using the labeled red blood cell technique, a sample of the patient's blood is drawn and red blood cells are separated from other blood components before the addition of technetium. After injection with the labeled substance, the patient is placed in a supine position and gamma camera views of the abdomen are obtained at intermittent intervals. When the labeled substance enters the bleeding site, its location is identified through nuclear scanning. This procedure is less invasive than arteriography and has been shown to be more sensitive in series of adult patients with GI bleeding. The test is only reliable if the patient is experiencing active bleeding at the time of the procedure.

Inflammatory foci may be identified using ^{99m}Tc-labeled white blood cells, employing a similar technique as that of labeled red blood cell studies. The patient's white blood cells are isolated, and technetium is added before the substance is administered intravenously. Nuclear scanning techniques allow for identification of inflammatory foci (as seen in inflammatory bowel disease) in areas where the labeled white blood cells cluster.

Transjugular intrahepatic portosystemic shunts

Transjugular intrahepatic portosystemic shunt (TIPS) is an invasive radiological procedure. The two main indications for employing the TIPS procedure are: (a) acute variceal bleeding uncontrolled by medical or endoscopic management, and (b) recurrent variceal bleeding in patients who are refractory or intolerant to conventional management.

The procedure is performed under fluoroscopic guidance and conscious sedation is used. After explaining the procedure to the patient and obtaining informed consent, the nurse or physician preps and drapes the right side of the neck. A wire is introduced into the right hepatic vein via the right internal jugular vein. A sheath through which contrast is injected to confirm entry into the portal vein replaces the catheter. The parenchymal tract is dilated with an angioplasty balloon. The balloon is deflated, and a wall stent catheter is advanced over a wire across the hepatic vein to the portal vein. The metallic stent is left in place. Venography is performed and shows hepatopedal flow to the inferior vena cava with collapse of the varices. Doppler ultrasound is used to monitor shunt patency approximately every 3 months.

TIPS are effective in lowering portal pressure and controlling acute variceal bleeding. The long-term effectiveness of TIPS in preventing recurrent bleeding has not been established. Unproven indications are initial therapy of acute variceal hemorrhage, prophylactic therapy to prevent variceal hemorrhage, refractory ascites, Budd-Chiari syndrome, and to reduce intraoperative morbidity during liver transplant surgery.

The patient must be monitored for possible complications following the procedure. Such complications include inadvertent puncture of the gallbladder, colon, or other abdominal organ; blood loss; and infection. There is a high occlusion rate from thrombosis or stenosis. Stenosed stents can usually be revised. The main symptom is worsening hepatic encephalopathy.

Contraindications include heart failure, polycystic liver disease, infection, severe hepatic encephalopathy, and fulminant liver failure.

SECRETORY STUDIES

Secretory studies evaluate the secretion of bile and various GI enzymes, with or without external stimulation.

Biliary drainage

For biliary drainage procedures, a duodenal tube is passed to the second portion of the duodenum, and the gallbladder is stimulated by instillation of magnesium sulfate or IV administration of sincalide (Kinevac). Specimens of bile are obtained and examined microscopically for cells, crystals, and parasites.

Although biliary drainage is no longer a major diagnostic aid, it may be helpful in special cases. It may be indicated in the following situations:

(a) for patients with absent or poor gallbladder function and a clinical picture of cholelithiasis;

(b) for patients with deep jaundice or sensitivity to the iodine in the contrast medium;

(c) when there is a probability of common duct stones in a postcholecystectomy patient;

(d) in patients with suspected cholesterolosis, where cholesterol crystals are imbedded in the submucosa of the gallbladder; and

(e) whendiagnosing giardiasis or bacterial overgrowth.

It is contraindicated in uncooperative patients, including patients with strong gag reflex, and in patients with vomiting and/or pyloric obstruction.

Successful intubation depends on the nurse's ability to achieve good rapport with the patient and inspire confidence.

Patients scheduled for biliary drainage procedures should:

(a) receive thorough teaching that may include use of an anatomy chart or diagram;

(b) remain NPO for at least 6 hours before the test, avoiding even oral medications;

(c) Have allergies reviewed for magnesium or kinevac hypersensitivity;

(d) remove dentures, unless they are tight fitting upper dentures, which may help the patient swallow more normally; and

(e) receive topical spray to anesthetize the posterior pharynx if they retch or gag excessively; however, pharyngeal anesthesia increases the risk of aspiration and should be avoided if possible.

A lubricated double-lumen nasogastric or intestinal tube is inserted into the duodenum, with the patient sitting upright. A triple-lumen tube, which allows isolation of the second and third portions of the duodenum between two inflatable balloons, may be used for pediatric patients. Oral passage of the duodenal tube to the stomach can be facilitated if the patient is able to relax. To prevent gagging after the initial insertion, it is best to keep the tube on the side of the mouth between the cheek and teeth.

To avoid contamination of the duodenal drainage by stomach contents, gastric contents should be aspirated as the tube passes through the stomach. The gastric aspirate is placed in a container marked "gastric residual."

With the patient in the right lateral position, the tube is then passed slowly (about 1 inch every 4 or 5 minutes) into the duodenum, until the tip of the tube is near the ampulla of Vater. To increase gastric activity and help the tube to be carried more rapidly through the pylorus, it may be helpful to suggest relaxation techniques or to ask the patient to pretend to eat a favorite meal or to walk around the room.

During intubation the tube should be allowed to drain freely by gravity drainage into a specimen container. When the tip of the tube passes through the pylorus, the drainage should change from the cloudy, colorless, or bile-tinged acid secretions of the stomach to the clear, yellow, alkaline secretions of the duodenum. The drainage should be tested for pH intermittently to determine when the tube enters the duodenum. If duodenal intubation is difficult, the physician may order metoclopramide (Reglan) to increase peristalsis.

Correct positioning of the duodenal tube is of primary importance if good specimens are to be obtained. Fluoroscopic guidance may be used to confirm correct placement. The tube should lie along the greater curvature of the stomach and should not coil in the stomach.

Once correct placement of the tube has been confirmed fluoroscopically or by the color and alkalinity of the drainage, bile originating in the common bile duct (A bile) should be collected for 15 to 20 minutes. Then the patient may be tested for sensitivity to the stimulant drug(s). In accordance with the physician's order, sincalide (Kinevac) may be administered intravenously to contract the gallbladder, or 30 ml of 25% magnesium sulfate may be instilled through the duodenal tube to relax the sphincter of Oddi and allow bile to flow into the duodenum.

If magnesium sulfate is used for gallbladder stimulation, the tube should be clamped for 5 minutes following instillation, then reopened, and the solution permitted to run out. If Kinevac is used, the collection of A bile should be continued by gravity drainage. When the color of the bile drainage becomes dark green, the specimen collection container should be changed, and this gallbladder bile (B bile) should be collected for approximately 20 to 30 minutes. Failure to collect B bile is frequently caused by gallbladder disease with loss of the concentrating function, or cholelithiasis, which causes cystic duct obstruction. If the patient has had a cholecystectomy, of course, there will be no B bile.

When the bile drainage color becomes light yellow, this liver bile (C bile) should be collected until it almost stops, approximately 20 to 30 minutes. Finally, 30 ml of air should be injected to clear the tube, and the tube should be clamped and removed. All specimens should be labeled and delivered to the laboratory, where they will be examined microscopically for cells, crystals, and parasites. Parasites are easily identified in a fresh specimen. The laboratory may also identify cells that could be indicative of an inflamed gallbladder or biliary tract, or crystals that are diagnostic for cholelithiasis, common duct stones, or cholesterolosis.

If a topical anesthetic was used, the patient should remain NPO until the gag reflex returns. The patient should be offered mouthwash to remove the bitter taste of bile from his or her mouth.

Duodenal drainage specimens may also be collected during esophagogastroduodenoscopy (EGD). Kinevac is administered intravenously and, after 5 to 10 minutes, bile is suctioned through the biopsy channel into a specimen trap. If dark green bile is not obtained, a second Kinevac stimulation may be ordered.

Another alternative is to insert a nasobiliary catheter endoscopically and leave it in the duodenum for use in collecting bile specimens following stimulation.

Potential complications of biliary drainage include entrapment of the tube in the duodenum.

Pancreatic stimulation

Diagnosis of pancreatic disease often depends on tests that indicate alterations in pancreatic enzyme levels or pancreatic function. Pancreatic stimulation involves the determination of the volume, bicarbonate content, and pancreatic enzyme concentration in the duodenal juice before and after direct IV stimulation of the pancreas with the hormones secretin and/or cholecystokinin. An orally passed radiopaque duodenal tube is guided under fluoroscopic control through the duodenum to the ligament of Treitz. Secretin is administered intravenously over a 1-minute period, and samples of duodenal fluid are collected in ice-cooled flasks for a total of approximately 50 minutes. Each specimen is examined for volume, bicarbonate concentration, pH, and the enzymes trypsin, chymotrypsin, lipase, and amylase.

Results are approximate, because the duodenal aspirates consist of pancreatic and duodenal juices and bile. In addition, not all of the secreted juice will be aspirated. A finding of less than 90 mEq/L of bicarbonate is 74% to 90% sensitive and 80% to 90% specific for chronic pancreatitis. Increases in duodenal secretion (volume and/or bicarbonate level) may occur with chronic alcoholism, hepatic or biliary cirrhosis, gastrinomas, or hemochromatosis. Decreases in secretions are associated with pancreatic carcinoma, collagen disease, diabetes mellitus, and Billroth I and II surgeries. Patients with cystic fibrosis have a substantial reduction in volume and bicarbonate and an 80% to 90% reduction in or absence of enzymes. Normal to slightly reduced volume, reduced bicarbonate concentration, and greatly reduced enzyme secretions are found in patients with pancreatic exocrine insufficiency that is not caused by cystic fibrosis.

Gastric analysis

The purpose of gastric analysis is the objective measurement of gastric acid secretions. It is indicated in patients with intractable ulcer symptoms, suspected Zollinger-Ellison syndrome (hypersecretory disease), or achlorhydria. It may be indicated to assess the efficacy of treatment regimens in peptic ulcer disease. For patients with suspected achlorhydria or gastric hypersecretory states, it may also be helpful to obtain a serum gastrin level, as discussed in the section on blood tests.

Gastric analysis is contraindicated in patients with gastric outlet obstruction, recent UGI bleeding, inability to freely pass a nasogastric tube, an allergy to the stimulating agent, or when food particles or fresh blood are present in the gastric aspirate.

Patient preparation includes the following requirements:

(a) remaining NPO for 12 hours

(b) withholding of histamine$_2$ (H$_2$) receptor antagonists,

proton pump inhibitors, anticholinergics, tricyclic antidepressants, sucralfate (Carafate), and antacids for 48 hours before testing.
(c) withholding of proton pump inhibitors for a minimum of 72 hours before testing.

If the test is being done to check the effectiveness of the medications, then the medications should be continued up until 12 hours prior to the test.

After lubricating the tube, a radiopaque polyethylene nasogastric tube is passed, fluoroscopy may be used if needed, and so the tip lies in the most dependent part of the stomach and along the greater curvature. Proper placement is confirmed by instillation of 30 ml of water with immediate recovery of at least 80%.

With the patient lying on the left side, suction is used to aspirate the stomach contents as completely as possible, and the aspirate is discarded. Four 15-minute basal acid output samples are then obtained separately. Pentagastrin (Peptavlon) is injected subcutaneously, and four 15-minute maximal acid output samples of gastric secretions are again collected. Each sample is analyzed for volume, pH, free acid, color, consistency, and occult blood. Although less invasive and less time-consuming methods are available for obtaining this data, there are isolated cases in which gastric analysis may be indicated.

Complications of gastric analysis are rare but may include nosebleeds, tube misplacement, or an adverse reaction to the gastric stimulant. The patient's nose and throat may feel irritated so gargling with warm salt water or sucking on throat lozenges may help.

Twenty-four-hour pH monitoring

Measuring the pH will show the degree of acidity or alkalinity of the gastric secretions. Prolonged esophageal pH monitoring is the most sensitive method of directly detecting esophageal reflux, quantifying it, and correlating symptoms with reflux events. **Ambulatory pH monitoring** is also indicated in patients with suspected pulmonary complications of esophageal reflux; other atypical presentations of esophageal reflux, such as nonulcer dyspepsia, wheezing, and hoarseness; typical presentation of esophageal reflux with a negative workup; and follow-up for esophageal reflux patients after medical or surgical therapy. pH monitoring may also be used to determine if episodes of apnea or bradycardia are associated with reflux in infants. Adults with chest pain may undergo pH monitoring to determine a noncardiac source for pain. Ambulatory pH monitoring may be performed in patients before proposed antireflux surgery, to prevent unnecessary surgery in patients with atypical symptoms who do not, in fact, have esophageal reflux. It is contraindicated for patients with any esophageal condition that would prevent correct placement of the probe.
Patient preparation includes:
(a) Remaining NPO after midnight or at least 6 hours;
(b) Discontinuing H_2 blockers for 24 hours;
(c) Discontinuing proton pump inhibitors for at least 72 hours before the procedure; and

(d) In children, fasting for 2 to 4 hours before the procedure.

Sometimes pH monitoring is done to assess the adequacy of acid suppression and these patients should not discontinue medication before the procedure. The pH probe and equipment must be calibrated for each patient. For the test, a pH probe is inserted through the patient's nostril to a position 5 cm above the lower esophageal sphincter (LES). The patient may be asked to take a few sips of water to help advance the probe. The LES is located by esophageal manometry, fluoroscopic placement, endoscopic visualization, or by measuring the pH in the stomach and withdrawing the probe until it enters the esophagus, where the pH is higher. In children, the proper location is in the distal esophagus, at a distance that is 13% above the LES. Proper placement of the probe may need to be confirmed by radiographic examination. The tube is then taped securely to the nose and side of the face. Some types of pH monitoring equipment require the use of an external reference electrode, which is secured to a flat area of skin surface (usually the chest or back). The area may need to be shaved before the electrode is applied, to allow optimal conduction.

The probe is connected to an external recording device. The patient proceeds with his or her daily routine while wearing the device for 24 hours. Symptoms (i.e. chest pain, heartburn, or coughing) and activities are recorded in a diary and also a button is pressed and the event is marked on the recording device. Children may need to be hospitalized overnight if the parent or guardian is unable to record events accurately. Baths, showers, and strenuous activities must be avoided because of the possibility of damaging the monitor, dislodging the probe or disrupting the recording. At the completion of the monitoring period, the stored data are downloaded into a computer that analyzes the information and prints a graphical display of esophageal pH over the recording period, along with a summary of these values. Normal pH in the esophagus ranges between 6.5 and 7.0. Acid reflux is defined as a fall in intraesophageal pH below 4.0.

BLOOD TESTS

Blood tests are frequently ordered for gastroenterology patients to test for coagulopathy, to reveal alterations in basic metabolic functions, and/or to indicate the severity of a disorder.

Table 26-1 shows the reference range for some of the more commonly used blood tests. It is important to note that reference ranges are determined by testing a large group of healthy individuals and then taking as the normal range the values that fall within 2 standard deviations of the mean, thus encompassing 95% of the sample studied. The range established by this method is dependent on two important factors: the method used, including reagents and instrumentation; and the geographical location of the population tested. It may be necessary to establish more than one reference interval for any given test (e.g., for different age-groups or for males and females).

Table 26-1. Normal adult values for selected blood tests

Diagnostic test	Low range	High range
Hematocrit (%)	38-F	47-F
	40-M	54-M
Hemoglobin (g/dl)	12-F	16-F
	13.5-M	18-M
Prothrombin time (seconds)*	11-14	
Activated partial thromboplastin time (seconds)*	32.0-47.0	
Platelets (mm³)	150,000	450,000
Albumin (g/dl)	3.6	5.1
Globulin (g/dl)	2.1	3.8
Albumin/globulin ratio	1.0	2.0
Total protein (g/dl)	6.4	8.3
Glucose (mg/dl)	65	115
Cholesterol (mg/dl)	150	240
Triglycerides (mg/dl)	30	170
AST/SGOT (mU/ml)	6	41
(IU/1)	10	40
ALT/SGPT (mU/ml)	8	50
(IU/1)	5	35
Alkaline Phosphatase		
0-15 yr (IU/ml)	50	300
Adult (IU/ml)	30	115
Total bilirubim (mg/dl)	0.10	1.3
Indirect bilirubin (mg/dl)	0.0	0.4

Not all values that fall outside the reference range are clinically significant. A clinically significant change in a test result is a numerical change that also reflects a change in the individual's condition.

Hemoglobin and hematocrit

Hemoglobin is the oxygen-carrying pigment of the red blood cells. It is formed by the developing red blood cell in bone marrow. **Hematocrit or Packed Cell Volume (PCV)** refers to the volume percentage of erythrocytes in whole blood. Both hemoglobin and hematocrit levels are decreased when the patient is anemic and increased when the patient is dehydrated, as a result of concentration of cells proportionate to fluid volume.

Prothrombin level

Prothrombin is a glycoprotein in the plasma that is normally converted to thrombin upon activation. A deficiency in this factor leads to hypoprothrombinemia. Decreased prothrombin levels may be associated with impaired absorption of vitamin K from the intestine. It may also be related to decreased availability of vitamin K, resulting from absence of bile salts or decreased intestinal flora caused by antibiotic suppression. Low levels of prothrombin are seen in infectious hepatitis, cirrhosis, biliary tract obstructions, and small bowel disorders.

Prothrombin time

Prothrombin time (PT) measures the rapidity of blood clotting through examination of factors I, II, V, VII, and X. Prolonged PTs are seen in patients with poor nutrition, vitamin K deficiency from decreased absorption, liver disease leading to decreased synthesis of clotting factors, warfarin sodium (Coumadin) therapy, and inherited blood disorders.

Activated partial thromboplastin time

Activated partial thromboplastin time (APTT) also measures the rapidity of blood clotting. It reflects clotting time by examining factors I, II, V, VIII, IX, X, XI, and XII. A prolonged APTT is observed in patients who are taking heparin, in those with liver disease, and in those with inherited coagulopathies.

International Normalized Ratio (INR)

The INR is the ratio of the patient's PT compared to the mean PT for a group of individuals. Use of the INR allows physicians to determine the level of anticoagulation in a patient independent of the laboratory reagents used.

BLEEDING TIME

If the platelet count is extremely low, clotting mechanisms may be impaired. To assess platelet function, bleeding time is measured by making small cuts in the patient's arm and monitoring the time until bleeding stops. Aspirin products and nonsteroidal anti-inflammatory drugs (NSAIDs) such as ibuprofen (Motrin) can prolong bleeding time for up to 14 days after ingestion.

PLATELET COUNT

Platelets play an important role in blood clotting. A platelet count measures the number of platelets present in the blood. A decrease in platelets is seen in bone marrow depression, lupus, severe hemorrhage, or intravascular coagulation. An increase in platelets may occur with blood vessel injury or cancer.

Serum albumin-globulin ratio

Serum albumin and globulin occur in inverse proportion to one another (i.e., as one increases, the other decreases proportionately). Decreased albumin is associated with cirrhosis, chronic hepatitis, temperature elevations, far-advanced carcinoma, malabsorption, fasting, and malnutrition; very low levels are often associated with edema and ascites. The highest levels of globulin occur in post hepatic cirrhosis and active chronic hepatitis.

Protein loss

An abnormal loss of proteins into the GI tract may be associated with a variety of disorders. In patients with unexplained edema and hypoalbuminemia, an enteric loss of albumin should be considered, such as protein-losing enteropathy, a decreased rate of albumin synthesis, or an increased rate of albumin catabolism. Protein-losing enteropathy can be identified by examining serum and fecal

α_1-antitrypsin levels. ^{131}I-labeled albumin may be used to evaluate the albumin pool and the rate of degradation of albumin. Albumin tagged with 51-chromium (^{51}Cr) is used to measure enteric albumin loss. For patients in whom the cause of hypoalbuminemia is unclear, the combined use of ^{131}I-albumin and ^{51}Cr may be needed.

In another test of excessive protein loss, ^{131}I-labeled polyvinylpyrrolidone (povidone) is injected intravenously, and blood specimens are collected after 2, 4, 6, and 24 hours.

Galactose tolerance

In the galactose tolerance test, IV galactose is administered, and blood is drawn at half-hour intervals for 2 hours. The presence of large amounts of galactose in the serum after this period of time is indicative of liver disease (failure of the liver to convert galactose to glycogen).

Glucose tolerance

In the glucose tolerance test, oral glucose is given to a fasting patient, and blood samples and urine specimens are taken at intervals of 30, 60, 120, and 180 minutes. Failure of the glucose level to return to normal in 1 to 2 hours is indicative of impairment of glucose utilization by the body tissues. In some patients it may be more appropriate to use an IV glucose test, which measures the ability of the liver to maintain glucose levels in the blood.

Disaccharide tolerance

Disaccharide intolerance may be measured by administering an oral loading dose of the suspect disaccharide after an 8-hour fast. A fasting serum glucose sample is obtained, the loading dose is given, and serum glucose is measured at 30, 60, 90, and 120 minutes after the loading dose is administered. A careful record is kept of the number, character, pH, and Clinitest results (presence of reducing substances) for all stools passed during the test and for 8 hours after the test is completed. In most individuals, serum glucose rises more than 30 mg/dl over the fasting level during the test period. In patients with disaccharide intolerance, the increase in serum glucose is usually less than 20 mg/dl.

Serum d-xylose

This test measures the intestines ability to absorb D-xylose, a simple sugar, as an indication of whether nutrients are being properly absorbed. Disease processes that alter or compromise the mucosa of the upper small bowel result in decreased absorption and excretion of xylose. A delay in gastric emptying time is a major reason for falsely low serum and urine levels of xylose. This test is useful in evaluating the integrity of the upper intestinal mucosa in celiac disease, idiopathic steatorrhea, regional enteritis involving the upper small bowel, starvation, short bowel syndrome, blind loop syndrome, and milk-protein sensitivity. In celiac disease, with clinical improvement and restoration of the normal mucosa while the patient is on a gluten-free diet, the serum and urine values of xylose approach and ultimately reach normal levels. Renal failure will give falsely low urine xylose levels.

To measure xylose absorption, d-xylose is given orally after an overnight fast, and serum and urine xylose are measured 1 or 2 hours later.

SERUM CHOLESTEROL

Cholesterol is an important normal body constituent, used in the structure of cell membranes, synthesis of bile acids, and synthesis of steroid hormones. Elevated cholesterol levels may be caused by biliary cirrhosis, familial hyperlipidemia, high cholesterol diet, nephritic syndrome and diabetes. Low cholesterol levels may be caused by liver disease, malabsorption, malnutrition, pernicious anemia and hyperthyroidism. In 2001, guidelines from the National Cholesterol Education Panel recommended that all lipid tests should be performed after fasting for 9-12 hours. The test consists of four parts:

1. Total cholesterol, the sum of LDL, HDL and VLDL. The normal range is less than 200 mg/dl.
2. LDL- Low Density Lipoproteins. The normal range includes the following ranges: Optimal, less than 100 mg/dl; Borderline High, 100-159 mg/dl; and High, 160 mg/dl and above.
3. HDL- High Density Lipoproteins. Also known as the "good cholesterol" because it functions to take excess cholesterol to the liver for excretion in the bile. The normal range is greater than 37 mg/dl in men, and greater than 47 mg/dl in women.
4. Triglycerides are compounds used by the body to move fatty acids through the blood. The normal range is anything less than 150 mg/dl.

Serum AST and ALT

The extent of liver disease may be determined by measuring aspartate aminotransferase (AST) and alanine aminotransferase (ALT). These cytoplasmic enzymes are released into the blood following disruption of cell membranes. Normal values are less than 40 international units (IU).

ALT is a cytosolic enzyme. Very high levels of this enzyme (i.e., as much as 100 times normal) indicate viral or drug-induced hepatitis with extensive cirrhosis. ALT levels in the thousands may indicate "shock liver," which is related to prolonged hypotension. Moderate to high ALT levels (i.e., less than 10 times normal) are suggestive of other forms of liver disease, such as biliary obstruction. Slight to moderate levels of ALT indicate hepatocellular injury. ALT may be used to differentiate between alcoholic and viral hepatitis, with alcoholic hepatitis having a lower elevation of ALT.

AST is a microsomal enzyme. It is not as specific to liver damage as ALT and must be used in conjunction with other liver tests. Increases in AST reflect cell permeability and cellular response to injury.

Serum bilirubin

A total serum bilirubin test measures both the secretory and excretory functions of the liver. Abnormal elevations of total bilirubin indicate hepatocellular disease, biliary tract disease, or overproduction of bilirubin at a rate beyond the liver's capacity to metabolize it. It is not a sensitive indication of biliary obstruction or liver cell injury.

Unconjugated (indirect) bilirubin measures the secretory function of the liver. Conjugated (direct) bilirubin measures excretory function. Elevations in this value usually indicate hemolysis or decreased cell permeability. Elevated direct bilirubin is indicative of hepatobiliary disease, hemolysis, liver cell damage, and obstructed bile flow in the common bile duct. Direct bilirubin may also be elevated in various genetic disorders of bilirubin metabolism, such as Dubin-Johnson syndrome or Gilbert's syndrome.

Serum alkaline phosphatase

Increased alkaline phosphatase levels may reflect post-hepatic obstructive jaundice, hepatic metastasis, or fatty infiltration. Marked elevations usually indicate cholestatic processes, such as mechanical biliary obstruction or drug-induced secretory failure. Serum alkaline phosphatase may also rise after administration of vitamin D, albumin, or drugs such as barbiturates, oral contraceptives, or phenothiazides. Levels of alkaline phosphatase are also elevated in osteoblastic diseases, Paget's disease, and hyperparathyroidism, and normally during pregnancy and growth. If there is complete obstruction of the common bile duct, both alkaline phosphatase and bilirubin are usually elevated. If a single hepatic duct is obstructed, only alkaline phosphatase is elevated.

γ-Glutamyl transferase

If γ-glutamyl transferase (GGT) is normal in conjunction with alkaline phosphatase elevation, the source of alkaline phosphatase elevation is probably bone. If GGT is elevated, it pinpoints the liver as the source of alkaline phosphatase elevation.

Serum amylase

The amount of amylase activity in serum may be altered in patients with penetrating or perforated peptic ulcer, peritonitis, bowel obstruction, biliary tract disease, liver disease, pelvic inflammatory disease, diabetic ketoacidosis, acute pancreatitis, parotid or other salivary gland disease, or ischemic bowel. In patients with pancreatic pseudocysts, serum amylase is elevated. Amylase levels may be elevated as early as 6 hours after the onset of acute pancreatitis, remain high for 3 to 5 days, and drop to normal in about 7 days.

Serum lipase

Lipase is produced in the pancreas and secreted into the duodenum, where it converts triglycerides and other fats into fatty acids and glycerol. Elevation is most common in acute pancreatitis but may also occur in perforated peptic ulcer, intestinal obstruction, acute cholecystitis, infectious hepatitis, cirrhosis, or jaundice. In patients with pancreatitis, it is not uncommon for serum lipase levels to reach 100 times the normal level. Lipase increases later and remains elevated longer than amylase, usually decreasing after 7 to 10 days.

Serum gastrin

Gastrin is a hormone that is secreted in the pyloricantral mucosa of the stomach. It stimulates secretion of hydrochloric acid by the parietal cells of the gastric glands. The gastrin stimulation test is indicated in patients with severe or unusual gastric or duodenal ulcerations, suspected Zollinger-Ellison syndrome, and suspected gastric hypersecretion. In this test, timed serum gastrin levels are drawn after stimulation with IV secretin. Patients must fast for 12 hours before the test, and H_2 antagonists and anticholinergics should be withheld for 24 hours. Proton-pump inhibitors should be withheld for at least 72 hours.

A large-bore IV needle is inserted to secure adequate blood samples. Blood specimens are drawn 10 minutes before, immediately before, and 1, 2, 5, 10, and 30 minutes after injection of secretin. For each sample, 5 ml of blood is withdrawn and discarded, followed by collection of a 10-ml specimen for testing. Serum gastrin levels are calculated for all seven samples.

Potential complications include infiltration of the IV fluid, inability to withdraw the correct amount of blood for the sample, and a local or systemic allergic reaction to administration of secretin.

Hepatitis antigens and antibodies

Hepatitis B surface antigen (HBsAg) is a measure of hepatitis B infection. Testing is positive in carriers and in those with acute and chronic infections. Hepatitis B surface antibody (HBsAb) is seen in patients who have recovered from hepatitis B and/or have formed antibodies by other means. HBsAb titers may be valuable in confirming immunity after immunization with the hepatitis B vaccine series.

Hepatitis B core antibody (HBcAb) is present in both acute and recovered disease states; immunoglobulins must be assessed to make a differential diagnosis. If immunoglobulin M (IgM) is positive, the patient's disease is active and infectious; if immunoglobulin G (IgG) is positive, the patient has developed the antibody and is no longer infective.

Hepatitis B e antigen (HBeAg) is indicative of a highly infectious state. Patients with hepatitis B e antibody (HBeAb) are no longer infectious.

If hepatitis A antibody (HAVAb) is negative, there is no history of or currently active hepatitis A virus. HAVAb is positive in both acute infections and in those who have recovered from infection. Patients with acute infectious hepatitis A are IgM positive. Patients who have recovered from hepatitis A are IgG positive.

The diagnosis of hepatitis C virus (HCV) infection in patients with chronic hepatitis (defined as infection persisting for more than 6 months) entails the detection of anti-HCV in serum, confirmed with a positive recombinant immunoblot assay (RIBA-2). The diagnosis of acute HCV infection is more problematic, because anti-HCV may not appear in serum for 2 to 6 months. In addition, immunocompromised patients may not mount an anti-HCV response.

Because hepatitis D virus (HDV) occurs only in patients

infected with hepatitis B virus (HBV), the initial step in diagnosis of HDV is confirmation that the patient is seropositive for HBsAg. Anti-HDV IgG or IgM is found in the acute and chronic phases of HDV infection, respectively.

Carcinoembryonic antigen

Carcinoembryonic antigen (CEA) is a glycoprotein that is associated with fetal growth. In adults, however, plasma CEA levels are elevated with endodermal tumors or neoplasia involving the lung, breast, ovary, bladder, testes, brain, or reticuloendothelial system, in addition to a wide range of benign inflammatory disorders. It has been studied as a possible prognosticator in colorectal cancer; elevated preoperative levels should be followed postoperatively and if there is a rise after an initial fall, it may be indicative of a recurrence.

CA-19-9

This is a commercially available monoclonal antibody to a tissue glycoprotein that also recognizes a mucin-type glycoprotein in serum. This is sensitive for gastric, pancreatic, and hepatobiliary tumors. This test is not a useful screening method and needs further study.

Serum antibodies

Antibodies sometimes develop to cytoplasmic constituents, including antimitochondrial antibodies and antismooth muscle antibodies. Indirect immunofluorescence is used to demonstrate the presence of these antibodies. They seem to have no etiological significance but are useful markers for a limited range of conditions of probable immune etiology, nearly all of which involve the liver. Antibody to smooth muscle occurs in 90% or more of patients with chronic active hepatitis. Antimitochondrial antibody, usually in high titers, is found in 90% or more of patients with biliary cirrhosis. Neither antibody, however, is specific for the single disease.

Celiac screening panel

Individuals with untreated celiac disease may have abnormally elevated antiendomyseal, antireticulin, and IgA antigliaden antibodies. Although detection of these antibodies has a valuable role in initial screening, individuals with celiac disease may have no circulating antiendomyseal antibodies, and such antibodies may occur in other enteropathies. As a result, small bowel biopsy is necessary to confirm the diagnosis. These antibodies disappear with mucosal healing on a gluten-free diet, and they may be used to monitor patient compliance with the dietary regimen.

URINALYSIS

In gastroenterology patients, urine samples may be analyzed to determine levels of bilirubin or urobilinogen, vitamin B_{12} absorption, or the extent of biliary obstruction. Most urinalysis is semiquantitative in nature and is done on random clean-catch samples.

Urine bilirubin

Only direct bilirubin can be measured in the urine. Significant amounts of bilirubin in the urine are indicative of hepatic disease or biliary obstruction. The urine specimen for a bilirubin test must be collected in a dark bottle and immediately taken to the laboratory, because light decreases the bilirubin level. Alternatively, the specimen may be shaken at bedside; brown urine with yellow foam is a positive result.

Urine urobilinogen

Elevated levels of urobilinogen indicate failure of the liver cells to reabsorb the urobilinogen that is broken down in the intestine by the action of intestinal bacteria on bilirubin. Urine specimens that will be analyzed for urobilinogen levels should be put in a dark brown container and immediately taken to the laboratory.

Schilling test (vitamin B_{12} absorption)

The **Schilling test** is used to determine vitamin B_{12} (cyanocobalamin) malabsorption. In preparation for this test, the patient fasts from midnight the previous night until 2 hours after the oral administration of radioactive vitamin B_{12} capsules. The test is done in two stages: ^{58}Co-cyanocobalamin alone and ^{57}Co-cyanocobalamin combined with intrinsic factor. An IM injection of 1 mg of nonradioactive vitamin B_{12} is administered to the patient immediately or up to 2 hours after the administration of the radioactive capsules. All urine is collected for 24 hours after the administration of the radioactive capsules. The urinary excretion of each isotope is determined, and the ratio is calculated to provide information about the relative absorptions of the two isotopes and the site of the absorptive defect.

FECAL ANALYSIS

Stool specimens should be analyzed for patients with diarrhea, steatorrhea, constipation, bleeding, or persistent abdominal discomfort. Usually only a small amount of stool needs to be collected on a tongue blade and placed in a disposable container. If an enema is needed to obtain a specimen, only tap water or normal saline should be used.

The length of time it takes for stool passage can be determined by the administration of a carmine marker or charcoal marker when a meal is ingested. The color, form, odor, consistency, content, and pH of the stool may also be important. The nurse should explain to the patient the method to be used to collect the stool specimen, whether it should be delivered fresh, and the process whereby it should be stored. The patient should also be instructed to record the times of bowel movements and to note stool color, consistency, and any associated pain.

Fecal urobilinogen

Specimens collected for this test should be put in light-resistant containers and immediately sent to the laboratory. If possible, the specimen should be collected between noon and 4 p.m., because urobilinogen production peaks at that time. An increased amount of urobilinogen darkens the color of the stool, whereas a decreased amount causes clay-colored stools. Decreased amounts are usually the result of biliary obstruction.

Occult blood

Occult blood testing is most often used for cancer screening. It is not useful in patients with frank bleeding from the GI tract, actively bleeding hemorrhoids, or in women who are menstruating.

The most common test for the detection of occult blood in the feces is **Hemoccult,** which uses guaiac-impregnated paper slides or guaiac tape and a developing solution. It is readily available, convenient, and inexpensive. However, its effectiveness depends on the degree of fecal hydration, the amount of hemoglobin degradation, and the presence of interfering substances that enhance or inhibit oxidation of the indicator dye.

Before occult blood testing, the patient must:

(a) Adhere to a high-fiber diet for 48 hours, with no rare red meat;

(b) Avoid foods that are high in peroxidase, such as turnips, broccoli, or horseradish; and

(c) Avoid iron preparation, bromides, iodides, salicylates, NSAIDs, or high doses of ascorbic acid.

(d) Ideally, aspirin and NSAIDs should be avoided for 1 week before Hemoccult testing.

Three stools must be collected without being contaminated by urine or toilet tissue. The delay between collection and laboratory testing should not exceed 6 days, and the specimens should not be refrigerated. For analysis, a small piece of stool is placed on the slide or tape and is wetted with the appropriate developing solution. A blue color appears in 30 to 60 seconds if blood is present. Positive results indicate GI bleeding and may be important in the early detection of colorectal cancer. False positive results may be caused by patient noncompliance with dietary and/or medication restrictions. Vitamin C (ascorbic acid) can cause false negative results.

Fecal fat

Little if any dietary fat is unabsorbed when bile and pancreatic secretions are adequate. The presence of abnormal fecal fat content (steatorrhea) is significant in malabsorptive disorders such as Crohn's disease and blind loop syndrome. Typically, fatty stools are greasy, pale, frothy, floating, and foul-smelling.

For a qualitative test of fecal fat, a random sample of stool is examined for evidence of malabsorption and various fats. Neutral fat, which accounts for 20% to 30% of total stool fat in pancreatic insufficiency, stains red with Sudan and appears as globules, whereas fatty acids do not stain with Sudan and appear as fatty acid crystals.

Seventy-two-hour fecal fat collection is an accurate method of testing for fat malabsorption. The patient is kept on a high-fat diet, with no alcohol, throughout the stool collection period. A diet record is kept and analyzed for the amount of fat ingested during the collection period. Total amount of fat in the stool collection is measured and compared with the patient's intake. The test result demonstrates the amount of fat that was not absorbed. Some test centers require the administration of a nonabsorbable "marker" (e.g., charcoal) at the beginning and end of the collection period. Plastic wrap used inside the diaper helps to facilitate collection of stools in small children. Parents should be asked to refrain from using diaper creams or ointments during the specimen collection period.

Fecal chymotrypsin

Fecal chymotrypsin determination is a reliable, semiquantitative test for exocrine pancreatic insufficiency. It can be applied to the same 72-hour stool collection procedure used for quantitation of fecal fat. It is more suitable than biliary drainage for routine screening of malabsorption syndromes.

Stools are collected for 72 hours between two nonabsorbable markers, such as charcoal. Specimens are frozen as soon as possible after they are passed and are pooled in a preweighed container. Enzyme activity in the stool samples is measured titrimetrically or by using an ultraviolet spectrophotometer.

Protein loss

α_1-Antitrypsin is a natural plasma protein that resists proteolytic digestion. The purpose of measuring fecal α_1-antitrypsin is to detect protein loss. Its concentration in the stool can be measured simply and accurately by immunological methods. In addition, measurement of α_1-antitrypsin does not require the use of radioisotopes.

Another way of detecting excessive protein loss is to inject ^{131}I-labeled polyvinylpyrrolidone (povidone) intravenously and collect stool samples over a 72-hour period. A patient with a disease that involves protein loss will excrete large amounts of polyvinylpyrrolidone in the stool.

Alternatively, ^{61}Cr-albumin may be injected intravenously, and all stools collected for a 96-hour period, taking care not to contaminate the stool specimens with urine. Normal subjects excrete less than 1% of the administered dose of tagged albumin. In patients with protein-losing enteropathy, between 4% and 20% and as much as 40% of the administered dose is recovered in the stool.

Fecal organisms

Stool may be collected and examined for organisms by following the instructions provided by the laboratory designated to perform the test. Testing for bacterial infection (e.g., *Salmonella, Shigella, Campylobacter, Escherichia coli*) usually involves collecting fresh stool and placing it into culture media immediately. Parasites (e.g., *Giardia, Cryptosporidium*) may require placement of the specimen into media designed to preserve both the ova and parasites, such as formalin. Specimens for *Clostridium difficile* may need to be collected fresh and either frozen or kept in a container on ice and delivered to the laboratory immediately.

Patient education regarding specimen collection techniques is vital to ensuring a reliable test result.

HYDROGEN BREATH TEST

Breath tests commonly involve the ingestion of a radioactive substance and the measurement of certain exhaled gases after a given time period. Usually the patient is asked to exhale through a solution containing specific chemicals that change color in the presence of certain concentrations of the gas. **Hydrogen breath tests** are used in the diagnosis of bacterial overgrowth of the intestine, short bowel syndrome, sugar intolerance, and tests of fat absorption.

At present the hydrogen test for malabsorption of lactose and other carbohydrates is the most widely used breath test. Hydrogen is produced in the body by bacterial fermentation of carbohydrates. Under normal circumstances, lactose is broken down into glucose and galactose and is absorbed in the small intestine, which has virtually no anaerobic bacteria. In patients who are deficient in lactase or who have delayed transit times, mucosal damage, or colonic flora in the UGI tract, lactose will come into contact with the fermenting bacteria in the colon and hydrogen gas will evolve.

The objective of hydrogen breath testing is to measure the volume of hydrogen that is produced in the colon, absorbed from the colon into the blood, and expelled in the breath. Hydrogen breath testing is indicated in patients with suspected carbohydrate malabsorption, abnormal GI time, or bacterial overgrowth of the small intestine. It is contraindicated in uncooperative patients. Patients must fast for 12 hours before the test and must refrain from smoking after midnight the previous night. Antibiotics and bowel cleansers should not be given within a week before the test.

End-expired tidal air is collected twice before and every 30 minutes for 3 hours after ingestion of a carbohydrate drink. Hydrogen gas concentration is determined by gas-liquid chromatography. Normal individuals expire less than 20-ppm hydrogen, whereas persons with malabsorption syndromes expire greater than 80 ppm.

To avoid the problem of false positive results, a positive lactose test may be followed by a glucose breath test to differentiate between true lactose intolerance and bacterial overgrowth. At least 10% of the population lacks hydrogen-producing bacteria in the colon. To avoid false negative results, a negative lactose test may be followed by a lactulose test to confirm the presence of hydrogen-producing colonic bacteria.

HELICOBACTOR PYLORI TESTS:

H. pylori is diagnosed through blood, breath, stool, and/or gastrointestinal biopsy tests. Blood and breath tests are most common because they are least invasive. The Urea breath test, carbon-13 blood test and H. pylori stool antigen tests are used to detect *H. pylori*:

1. **Urea Breath Test.** This test is usually used in combination with the blood test for diagnosing *H. pylori*, or after treatment to determine the effectiveness of that treatment. The patient drinks a urea solution that contains a special carbon atom. If *H. pylori* is present, it breaks down the urea, releasing the carbon. The blood carries the carbon to the lung, where the patient exhales it. The breath test is 96-98% accurate. Patient must be NPO for at least 4 hours and not be taking any antibiotics, proton pump inhibitors (PPIs), or Bismuth compounds for one month.

2. **Carbon- 13 Blood Test.** This is a simple blood test that detects antibodies to the H. Pylori bacterium. The accuracy of antibody detection is variable ranging from 85-95%.

3. **H. Pylori Stool Antigen (HpSA) Test.** This Stool test may be used to detect h. pylori infection in the patient's fecal matter. Patient must be NPO for 4 hours and off all antibiotics, PPIs and Bismuth compounds for one month.

CASE SITUATION

Jennifer Roth, a 28-year-old female, is scheduled for a gastroscopy on Tuesday. She is being treated for alcoholism and has GI bleeding and acute pain.

Points to think about

1. What tests would most commonly be ordered before a procedure for this patient?
2. What laboratory tests might be increased or decreased, and why?

Suggested responses

Abnormal test result	Possible cause
ALT	Cirrhosis or hepatitis, depending on the degree of alcoholism
AST	
Lactic dehydrogenase (LDH)	
Red blood count	GI bleeding resulting in iron deficiency
Hemoglobin	
Hematocrit	
Red cell indexes/morphology	
Platelet count	Impaired platelet production because of toxic effects of alcohol on the bone marrow
PT	Liver disease impairs production of protein synthesis
APTT	
Urinary bilirubin	Normal to elevated, depening to the degree of bleeding and the stage of liver disease (The liver converts the hemoglobin from the red cells to bilirubin)
Occult blood	GI bleeding

1. The following tests would probably be ordered for this patient:
   (a) Liver profile, including ALT, AST;
   (b) Complete blood count, including hematocrit, hemo-

globin, white cell count, the proportions of the different white cells, red blood cell indexes and morphology, and platelet count;

(c) PT, PTT, INR;

(d) Urinalysis, including bilirubin and urobilinogen; and

(e) Occult blood.

REVIEW TERMS

activated partial thromboplastin time (APTT), ambulatory pH monitoring, angiography, arteriography, barium enema, barium sulfate, barium swallow, capsule endoscopy, cholangiography, computed tomography (CT), double-contrast effect, enteroclysis, fluoroscopic examination, hematocrit, Hemoccult, hemoglobin, hydrogen breath tests, magnetic resonance cholangiopancreatography (MRCP), occult blood, oral cholecystography, percutaneous transhepatic cholangiography (PTC), prothrombin time (PT), radiographic studies, Schilling test, scintigraphy, ultrasonography, upper gastrointestinal (UGI) series, x-ray (roentgenographic) examination

REVIEW QUESTIONS

1. The usual position of the patient during a barium swallow is the:
   (a) Standing position.
   (b) Sitting position.
   (c) Prone position.
   (d) Supine position.

2. In a double-contrast barium enema, visualization is improved by the introduction of:
   (a) Air.
   (b) An inert dye.
   (c) Radioactive isotopes.
   (d) Methylcellulose.

3. Patient teaching prior to capsule endoscopy should include which of the following:
   (a) NPO after midnight.
   (b) Iron tablets should be avoided one week prior to test.
   (c) MRIs must be avoided until confirmed excretion of the capsule.
   (d) Abdominal pain , nausea, or vomiting require calling their physician.
   (e) All of the above.

4. The three-dimensional image produced by CT is based on:
   (a) Differences in tissue density.
   (b) The differential transmission of sound waves by different tissues.
   (c) The differential uptake of radioactive isotopes.
   (d) Visualization of radiopaque structures.

5. Which of the following is true about Magnetic Resonance Cholangiography?
   (a) There is more radiation exposure than chest x-ray.
   (b) The major shortcoming is the lack of ability to perform therapeutic interventions.
   (c) The dye (gadolinium) used causes severe nausea.
   (d) The patient must remain NPO after midnight.

6. For gastric analysis, gastric acid secretions are stimulated by the injection of:
   (a) Secretin.
   (b) Metoclopramide (Reglan).
   (c) Glucose.
   (d) Pentagastrin (Peptavlon).

7. An increase in platelet levels could indicate:
   (a) Cancer.
   (b) SLE.
   (c) Cirrhosis.
   (d) Crohn's disease.

8. Extremely high levels of ALT are indicative of:
   (a) Viral or alcohol-induced hepatitis.
   (b) Biliary obstruction.
   (c) Hepatocellular injury.
   (d) Hepatic metastasis.

9. The Schilling test is used to evaluate:
   (a) Disaccharide tolerance.
   (b) Vitamin B_{12} absorption.
   (c) Immunity to hepatitis.
   (d) Bilirubin levels.

10. In patients with lactose intolerance, most of the excess hydrogen that is detected in a hydrogen breath test is produced:
    (a) In the small intestine.
    (b) By aerobic bacteria.
    (c) In the colon.
    (d) In the lungs.

BIBLIOGRAPHY

Ballinger, P. (1995). *Merrill's Atlas of Radiographic Positions and Radiologic Procedures Vol. 2* (8th ed.). St. Louis, MO: Mosby.

Ballinger, P. (1995). *Merrill's Atlas of Radiographic Positions and Radiologic Procedures, Vol. 3* (8th ed.) St. Louis, MO: Mosby.

Chait, P. (1996). Interventional gastrointestinal radiology. In Walker, W. Durie, P.R., Hamilton, J.R., Watkins, J.B., and Walker-Smith. (Eds.), *Pediatric gastrointestinal disease* (2nd ed.). St. Louis, MO: Mosby.

Cotton, P. & Williams, C. (1990). *Practical gastrointestinal endoscopy* (3rd ed.). Oxford: Blackwell Scientific.

Emslie, J. (1996). Technetium-99m-labeled red blood cell scans in the investigation of gastrointestinal bleeding. *Dis Colon Rectum 39*(7), 750-4.

Gainey, M. (1996). Radionucleotide diagnosis. In Walker, W. Durie, P.R., Hamilton, J.R., Watkins, J.B., and Walker-Smith. (Eds.), *Pediatric gastrointestinal disease* (2nd ed.). St. Louis, MO: Mosby.

Henry, J. (1996). *Clinical diagnosis and management by laboratory methods* (19th ed.). Philadelphia: W.B. Saunders.

Johnson, L.R. (Ed.) (1994). *Physiology of the gastrointestinal tract* (3rd ed.). Philadelphia: Lippincott-Raven.

Johns Hopkins Medical Laboratories (2000). *Department of Pathology Alphabetical Test Listings*. Baltimore, MD.

Ogilvie, J. Norwitz, L., Kalloo, A.N., Kallo, A.N. (2002). *Johns Hopkins Manual for Gastrointestinal Endoscopy Nursing*. Thorofare, NJ: Slack Inc.

Society of Gastroenterology Nurses and Associates, Inc. (2003). *Manual of gastrointestinal procedures* (5th ed.). Chicago.

Walker-Smith, J. (1996). Celiac disease. In Walker, W. Durie, P.R., Hamilton, J.R., Watkins, J.B., and Walker-Smith. (Eds.), *Pediatric gastrointestinal disease* (2nd ed.). St. Louis, MO: Mosby.

Yamada, T. Laine, L., Alpers, D.H. (1999). *Textbook of Gastroenterology Vol. 2* (3rd ed.). Philadelphia: Lippincott.

THERAPEUTIC PROCEDURES

Chapter 27

DILATATION

This chapter will acquaint the gastroenterology nurse with the procedures used for endoscopic dilatation of GI strictures.

Learning objectives

After reviewing the content of this chapter, the gastroenterology nurse should be able to:

1. Describe the indications, contraindications, techniques, and potential complications of using sheer force to dilate GI strictures, using rubber bougies or tapered polyvinyl chloride dilators.
2. Explain the indications, contraindications, techniques, and potential complications of using hydrostatic or pneumatic balloons for GI dilatation.
3. Discuss nursing considerations pertinent to each of these techniques.

BASIC PRINCIPLES

There are two basic types of GI dilatation; a sheer-force method, which involves forcing a dilator through a narrowed area, using axial force to enlarge the lumen; and hydrostatic or pneumatic balloon dilatation, which involves inflating a balloon within the lumen, thereby providing a radial force that accomplishes the dilatation. Obstructing tumors may also be ablated by using a laser or bipolar tumor probe, as discussed in Chapter 28.

There are two different types of sheer-force dilators:

(a) mercury or tungsten weighted "bougies" (Hurst or Maloney type) made of rubber or silicone; and

(b) tapered polyvinyl chloride Savary-Gilliard or American dilators (these have replaced the early Eder Puestow and Celestin dilators).

The sizes of esophageal dilators are expressed in terms of their diameter in millimeters (mm) or in French units (Fr), which are based on the circumference of the instrument (i.e., the diameter in millimeters multiplied by pi). For con-

venience, a factor of 3 rather than 3.14 may be used for pi when converting from millimeters to French units.

PROCEDURE

Dilatation procedures are contraindicated in uncooperative patients and in patients with significant coagulopathy, esophageal impaction, recent myocardial infarction, active ulcers, recent biopsy examination, or severe cervical arthritis.

Before upper GI dilatation, the patient should be NPO for at least 6 hours. Verify signed informed consent. Obtain medical history including allergies, current medications and any other information pertinent to current complaint. Dentures should be removed, and a topical anesthetic or gargle may be used. Establish a patent IV line and obtain baseline vital signs. Notify physician if the patient is currently on anticoagulant, ASA or NSAID therapy or if labs are abnormal.

The patient is positioned in a sitting, standing, or left lateral position. It is the nurses responsibility to ensure that the correct position is maintained throughout the procedure. If the dilators deviate from the midline during the procedure, perforation of the pharynx, esophagus, or stomach could occur.

Bougienage with Hurst or Maloney dilators alone is usually performed without premedication in adults. Children typically require sedation. Other forms of dilatation are performed using sedation and endoscopy. Some dilatation procedures are performed with fluoroscopic guidance, particularly when carcinomas or long strictures are being dilated. The distal 5 to 6 inches of the dilator should be lubricated with a water-soluble lubricant.

The nurse should assemble the dilators and monitor the patient's response to the procedure, providing nursing intervention (such as suction) as indicated. The nurse also assists the physician. When a guidewire is used, it is the nurse's responsibility to pass the guidewire to the physician, ensuring that there are no kinks or bends. The spring tip is inserted first, while the nurse controls the loose end. Then, the lubricated dilator is fed onto the correctly placed guidewire. The nurse must stabilize the guidewire to maintain the correct position during advancement and withdrawal of the dilator. Guidewire markings should be used to confirm the correct placement. The physician should be notified if there is any blood on the used dilator or in the patient's secretions. The sizes of the dilators should be documented.

It is best to begin dilatation procedures with a dilator that is one or two sizes smaller than the diameter of the stricture. Dilatation can be repeated daily, every other day, or several times per week, depending on the patient's response, the severity of the stricture, and the sense of resistance that is felt. On subsequent sessions, the physician may begin with a dilator that is one size smaller than the largest dilator passed at the previous session. As a general rule, not more than three increasing French sizes should be used in any one session.

The esophagus is the most common target of GI dilatation. The primary goal of esophageal dilatation is to restore the patient's ability to eat and drink normally. In most cases, dysphagia in response to solid food will not be completely relieved until a minimal luminal diameter equivalent to 38 or 40 Fr (14 mm diameter) is achieved. If the esophageal lumen can be fully dilated to 52 Fr (17 mm diameter), the patient should be able to eat a normal diet. Patients with a lumen less than 39 Fr will require a modified diet.

After any upper GI dilatation procedure, the patient should remain NPO until the gag reflex returns if local anesthesia is used. Vital signs and patient condition should be monitored and documented. The patient should be instructed to notify the physician immediately in the event of chest pain, fever, regurgitation of blood, pain on swallowing, back pain, shoulder pain, abdominal pain, abdominal distention, rectal bleeding, chills, black stools, or nausea.

Potential complications of dilatation include hemorrhage, perforation, aspiration, and bacteremia. The most common site of perforation is the area immediately proximal to a stricture. With dilators that use guidewires, the risk of perforation is more likely related to the guidewire than to the dilator. Fluoroscopy is generally advised to be sure that the guidewire does not bend to form a sharp point or loop and to verify correct placement of the dilator at the stricture. Perforation may also occur if the guidewire is misplaced or damaged. In patients who have undergone previous surgery, the use of guidewires is riskier and more complicated, because the anatomy may be distorted.

It is critically important that perforation be identified as soon as possible. Cervical perforation is usually obvious. It is associated with fever, chest pain, leukocytosis, pain on swallowing, change in the quality of the voice, and air in the subcutaneous tissues of the neck (i.e., subcutaneous emphysema). Radiographic examination usually reveals air in the retroesophageal space. The most common symptom of esophageal perforation is persistent pain, even if it is mild, after dilatation.

When perforation is suspected, it is important to obtain upright and lateral x-ray films of the chest to serve as a baseline and to search for free air under the diaphragm, pneumothorax, or pleural effusion. In addition, an x-ray examination should be performed, using a water-soluble contrast medium. Use caution, because aspiration of contrast media can cause pulmonary toxicity. Many times, perforation can be managed conservatively by administering antibiotics, providing suction, and keeping the patient NPO. At other times, surgery may be necessary.

Bleeding is a rare complication of dilatation for the management of benign lesions. When bleeding occurs, it is usually minor and transfusions are seldom needed. Bacteremia has developed after dilatation procedures, but it is a serious problem only in immunocompromised patients and in patients with prosthetic valves or a history of endocarditis. The bacteria in the blood may originate from either the dilator or the oropharynx. For this reason, it is important to clean and disinfect dilators adequately after each use according to manufacturers' directions.

If blood and/or mucus are present on the dilator on removal from the affected site, this observation should be documented. If there is a question about the malignancy of the stricture, any blood or mucus that is present may be rinsed into a bottle with cytological fixative and submitted for cytological examination.

Different types of dilators are used in different situations. Indications for the use of several different types of dilators are discussed, along with techniques for insertion and specific risks associated with each technique.

Bougienage

Bougienage is the dilatation of the esophagus by using mercury-filled, soft-rubber, or tungsten-filled silicone dilators (**bougies**) of graduated sizes, ranging from 18 to 60 Fr. Dilators less than 32 Fr are so flexible that little effective pressure can be applied from above without bending them.

The mercury or tungsten provides the proper combination of rigidity and flexibility, so the bougies can be swallowed. The force applied to the shaft of the dilator can be transmitted to the stricture. There are two types of bougies: tapered **Maloney dilators** and blunt or rounded **Hurst dilators**. The Maloney dilator, with its tapered end, seems to be easier for patients to swallow. The tapered tip of the Maloney dilator is more likely to enter a small-diameter stricture but is also more likely to bend, causing the dilator to be misdirected.

Indications for bougienage include the following:

1. Esophageal strictures, including peptic, postsurgical, postradiation, or malignant strictures.
2. Chemically induced strictures caused by lye ingestion or a sclerosing agent. Esophageal injury associated with a gray-white exudate, ulcers, and hemorrhage can have nonforceful dilatation 3 to 7 days after injury. Esophageal injury that is associated with extensive ulceration, gray-black exudate, mucosal sloughing, and a dilated and atonic lumen without peristalsis should not

be dilated until mucosal healing is noted endoscopically.

3. Esophageal rings or webs. In bougienage for lower esophageal rings, it is best to use one pass of a large dilator, such as a 50 Fr. If this treatment is not successful, it may be preferable to use a pneumatic dilator similar to that used in patients with achalasia.

4. Diffuse esophageal spasm, with a normal lower esophageal sphincter (LES).

5. Scleroderma.

Before the procedure a topical anesthetic may be applied to the patient's throat. The patient is usually placed in an upright sitting position, but a left lateral position may be used to avoid aspiration, to facilitate endoscopic examination preceding dilatation, or if fluoroscopy is to be used.

Maloney or Hurst dilators are passed into the hypopharynx and esophagus in much the same way as a flexible endoscope. Before use, the distal end of the bougie is well lubricated. The physician introduces the bougie into the mouth and uses a forefinger to direct it into the pharynx. A swallowing motion allows gentle passage into the upper esophagus. An experienced operator can feel when the dilator engages the stricture. When it does engage a stricture, the dilator is held lightly between the thumb and fingers, and gentle force is applied to dilate the stricture.

Aspiration of oral secretions is usually necessary during the procedure. The physician should be notified of any blood on the used dilator or in the patient's secretions. The size of the dilators used should be documented.

Care and maintenance of rubber bougies are not difficult. Before each use, the bougies should be inspected carefully. Most bougies are stamped with an expiration date from the manufacturer: usually about 5 years. If the rubber cracks, splits, or has expired, it should be replaced. Most manufacturers have a trade-in policy, and the mercury can be recycled.

After use, bougies should be cleaned of all patient debris with an enzymatic cleaner and then disinfected according to the manufacturer's directions. Rubber dilators should be removed from the disinfecting solution promptly. Prolonged soaking will cause deterioration of the rubber. After disinfection, bougies should be thoroughly rinsed and dried. They should be stored horizontally, as straight as possible, in a closed, clean, and dry area.

Care and maintenance of silicone bougies requires inspection of each dilator before each use. After the procedure, wash the dilator with mild soap and water; enzymatic cleaner or alcohol-based solvents may adversely affect the silicone. Refer to the manufacturer's instructions.

The problem with all bougienage techniques is that they are dependent on an externally applied axial force. If the stricture is too tight, the axial force applied may cause the pusher to bend laterally and rupture the esophagus, rather than push the dilator through the stricture. Bougies are of little benefit when the stricture is unyielding, is angulated, or causes severe luminal narrowing.

POLYVINYL CHLORIDE DILATORS

Strictures may also be dilated by inserting a guidewire past the affected area and introducing a semiflexible, tapered, polyvinyl chloride dilator over the wire. Guidewires should be introduced via the biopsy channel of the endoscope with the endoscopist observing the route of the wire. The scope is then removed, leaving the wire in place. The dilators are then inserted over the guidewire with or without fluoroscopic guidance. The polyvinyl chloride dilators should never be used as a bougie or without the use of the guidewire.

Savary-Gilliard dilators consist of a series of semiflexible, tapered, polyvinyl dilators that have a lumen for the guidewire in the center. They range in size from 5 to 20 mm (15 to 60 Fr). The dilators fit over a stainless-steel guidewire that is 1 82 cm long and 0.8 mm in diameter. The wire has a graduated, flexible spring tip that reduces the risk of retroflexing on itself or lumenal perforation. A radiopaque marker is incorporated into the dilator to aid in fluoroscopic monitoring.

The **American dilator** system is an adaptation of the Savary-Gilliard dilators. The distal tapered end of the dilator shaft is shorter, and they are completely radiopaque. Dilators in the American system range in size from 5 to 18 mm (15 to 54 Fr).

Polyvinyl chloride dilators are easily passed through the mouth, and the flexible tip readily traverses the pharynx. They are used for esophageal strictures with the following indications:

(a) dilatation of peptic, malignant, postsurgical, or postradiation strictures;

(b) dilatation of obstructing tumors to permit passage of an endoscope through which laser therapy can begin at the distal tumor margin;

(c) placement of a stent;

(d) patients with esophageal webs or rings, diffuse esophageal spasm, chemically induced strictures, or scleroderma; and

(e) pediatric patients who may have the above-mentioned indications.

Potential complications of dilatation utilizing this method include perforation, bleeding, aspiration, and bacteremia.

Hydrostatic Balloons

The technique of luminal dilatation by using a balloon was initially performed for occlusive vascular disorders. Today, balloon dilatation has become an integral part of therapeutic endoscopy. **Hydrostatic balloons** are made of a specially treated polyethylene, which is altered to greatly increase strength and minimize stretching. A pressure gauge keeps the applied pressure within recommended limits. The balloon is filled with fluid (e.g., water or dilute radiopaque dye). (Full-strength contrast material crystallizes easily and occludes the lumen of the dilator, thereby rendering it useless.)

There are two types of balloon dilators: through-the-scope (TTS) balloons and over-the-guidewire balloons. Both are inflated using the appropriate manufacturer's device.

1. TTS balloons have an inflated diameter of 4 to 25 mm. They are passed through the biopsy channel of the endoscope, and dilatation is accomplished under direct vision.

2. Over-the-guidewire balloons have an inflated diameter of 4 to 40 mm. A guidewire is passed, the scope is removed, and the dilators are passed. Fluoroscopy may be used.

Hydrostatic balloons are used for the following:

(a) filatation of benign or malignant esophageal, pyloric, duodenal, rectal, or left-colon strictures;

(b) temporarily opening the rectosigmoid luminal pathway when it is obstructed by a tumor, before endoscopic laser therapy (For rectal cancers, it may be easier to use a rigid proctoscope and hand-held laser fiber.);

(c) pyloric stenosis (not congenital pyloric stenosis seen in infants);

(d) biliary tract strictures; and

(e) food impactions above an esophageal stricture.

Esophageal strictures that lend themselves to conventional bougienage should be treated in the traditional manner because it is less complicated, less time consuming, and less expensive than balloon dilatation.

In patients with food impactions above an esophageal stricture, the bolus is dislodged and the guidewire is passed through the stricture. The dilator is passed and inflated, and the bolus is then pushed into the stomach. This procedure avoids the potentially greater complications of aspiration secondary to removal of the foreign object. Throughout the procedure the nurse should assist the physician with guidewire control.

Before any balloon dilatation procedure it is important to inflate the balloon with water to check for leakage. Spraying the balloon with silicone may assist passage through the scope.

After the balloon is in place, a syringe pressure gauge assembly should be used to inflate it to a fixed pressure according to the manufacturer's recommendations or as directed by the physician. X-ray contrast material may be used and followed by fluoroscopy to ensure placement and dilatation. The balloon is then left inflated for a short period of time, as determined by the physician. After the appropriate time has elapsed, the balloon is deflated. Once it is removed it should be checked for signs of bleeding. Patient discomfort may serve as a guide to the number of dilatations attempted during a single session. With the use of three progressively larger inflatable balloons, esophageal peptic strictures can be dilated dramatically in one session. The schedule for subsequent dilatation sessions is based on the type of stricture, its response to initial and subsequent dilatation, and the patient's tolerance of the procedure. Each stricture requires an individually tailored approach.

After use, balloon dilators should be reprocessed and stored according to the manufacturer's guidelines. If contrast material was used to inflate the balloon, it must be rinsed out completely before reprocessing. If it is not

removed the balloon walls may adhere and destroy the balloon. Hydrostatic balloons can withstand temperatures up to 65° C, which allows for sterilization with ethylene oxide.

Potential complications of dilatation by using a hydrostatic dilator are the same as those for other dilatation procedures.

HYDROSTATIC DILATATION IN PYLORIC STENOSIS

In patients with pyloric stenosis, a TTS or over-the-guidewire technique may be used to insert a hydrostatic balloon. In the TTS technique, a well-lubricated balloon is passed through the biopsy channel of an endoscope and into the stricture. The balloon is inflated to maximum pressure with water or dilute contrast medium, using a pressure gauge. Dilatation is repeated three or four times, maintaining maximum inflation for at least 1 minute during each dilatation. After dilatation is complete, the balloon is withdrawn, and the endoscope is passed through the pyloric ring for inspection of the duodenum.

For over-the-guidewire balloon dilatation of the pylorus, a heavy-gauge guidewire with a spring tip is passed through the stricture and advanced far enough to serve as an anchor. Dilatation may be carried out with fluoroscopic guidance, filling the balloon with dilute radiographic contrast material. Following dilatation, endoscopy is used to evaluate the pyloric ring and duodenal bulb.

BALLOON DILATATION OF BILIARY TRACT STRICTURES

Bile duct strictures may be dilated with balloon catheters during endoscopic retrograde cholangiopancreatography (ERCP) or percutaneous transhepatic cholangiography (PTC). After dilatation, a biliary stent may be placed through the stricture either endoscopically or percutaneously during PTC. Indications for balloon dilatations of the biliary tract include the following:

(a) inflammatory strictures;

(b) postoperative strictures, especially after liver transplantation;

(c) benign or malignant strictures;

(d) stenoses at a choledochoenterostomy site;

(e) sclerosing cholangitis;

(f) sphincter of Oddi dysfunction and biliary dyskinesia; and

(g) before stent placement.

For dilatation of the biliary tract, a no-profile dilating balloon is selected by the physician. Choice of balloon is determined by the size and length of the strictured area. These balloons come in a variety of sizes measuring 2 to 4 cm in length, with a diameter of 4 to 10 mm. The guidewire that is used in conjunction with a stent or nasobiliary tube is used to achieve correct placement of the balloon.

Before dilatation, a diagnostic ERCP is performed to determine the size, location, and anatomy of the stricture. The ERCP cannulating device should then be flushed with saline to clear the contrast media. A guidewire that is compatible with the inner diameter of the cannulating device is placed into the cannulating device and advanced into the common bile duct. The cannulating device is then removed, leaving the guidewire in place.

With the guidewire in place, the dilating balloon is sprayed with silicone and then fed over the guidewire, through the biopsy channel of the scope, and into the common bile duct. The nurse should keep tension on the guidewire to make passage easier. The physician will position the balloon over the center of the strictured area.

A pressure gauge should be attached to the Luer-lok end of the balloon. These gauges typically show pressures from 0 to 300 pounds per square inch (psi) or 0 to 20 atmospheres (atm). The maximum amount of pressure for each balloon should be noted on the balloon or the package, and this maximum pressure should not be exceeded during the dilatation. Using a syringe with dilute contrast medium, inflate the balloon to the correct pressure and hold for 1 minute. When fully inflated, the balloon may show a waist at the site of the stricture. Balloon size, maximum inflation pressure, and length of inflation time should be documented at the end of the procedure.

Following dilatation, the balloon is deflated and withdrawn from the scope and discarded. Repeated dilatations with increasingly larger balloons may be necessary to achieve the desired patient outcome. In patients with common bile duct strictures, a stent may be placed across the stricture for up to 3 months to promote reepithelialization of the duct lumen and prevent restricturing.

Following balloon dilatation, a clinical improvement in jaundice and a drop in serum bilirubin should be observed, in addition to a decrease in the incidence of cholangitis. Use of dilating balloons for temporary dilatation and the placement of a long-term stent produces the best patient outcomes. Studies have shown a technical success rate of 70% to 75% and symptomatic improvement in two thirds to three quarters of patients. Eighty-three percent of patients followed up to 42 months postprocedure have shown good to excellent results.

Complications occur in approximately 7% of patients, including pancreatitis and injury to the bile duct. Most cases of pancreatitis respond to conservative treatment. Laceration of the bile duct often resolves spontaneously when the lacerated area is bridged by a stent.

Pneumatic Balloons

Pneumatic balloons are used for forceful stretching of the LES in patients with achalasia. Forceful dilatation to a diameter of approximately 3 cm is necessary to tear the circular muscle and produce a lasting reduction in LES pressure. The success rate in treatment of achalasia with pneumatic dilators is 80% to 85% with a 0.2% mortality rate and 2.6% perforation rate.

Pneumatic dilatation may also be used in cases of diffuse esophageal spasm with a hypertensive LES. The object of this procedure is to decrease the resistance at the LES to allow the esophagus to empty. It may also be used for dilatation of lower esophageal rings, if bougienage is unsuccessful.

One successful dilatation should cure this condition permanently. Although the ring may still be visible on radiographic examination, the patient's dysphagia should not recur.

Many types of balloon dilators have been used for pneumatic dilatation. Balloons are available in various lengths and diameters. Most popular are the Rigiflex dilators, available in 3-, 3.5-, and 4-cm sizes. Although manufacturers recommend inflation to a fixed pressure, many experts dilate by feeling the esophagus.

The patient may be hospitalized, and a liquid diet should be instituted the day before dilatation. Before the procedure the patient should be warned that moderate to severe discomfort will be experienced. The patient should be assured that additional pain medication will be administered if necessary. The procedure is done under local anesthesia, with meperidine (Demerol) or fentanyl given preoperatively to reduce discomfort. Atropine may be given intravenously to reduce oral secretions, and diazepam (Valium) or Versed may be administered for sedation, but it is preferred that the patient remain alert and cooperative. It is important to lavage and empty the esophagus of retained material, if present, and to set the pressure gauge according to the manufacturers specifications.

The collapsed pneumatic balloon should always be introduced over a guidewire, and the procedure should be performed under fluoroscopic control. When the center of the balloon is positioned at the level of the LES, the bag is inflated rapidly with air, fluid, or dilute contrast medium to a preset pressure (at least 6 lbs/sq in) for 15 to 60 seconds. After the length of time determined by the physician, the balloon should be deflated and removed.

During the procedure the patient should be observed for severe chest pain and additional medication administered as ordered.

After the procedure the head of the patient's bed should be elevated. The dilator should be checked for evidence of blood. The physician should be notified if the patient experiences chest pain, fever, regurgitation of blood, pain on swallowing, back pain, shortness of breath, shoulder pain, or chills. The patient should be instructed to notify the physician of continuing chest pain, back pain, or other pain.

Some endoscopists immediately follow dilatation with a radiographic contrast study to identify any distal esophageal leaks near the region of the esophagogastric junction. If no leak is seen, the patient is observed over the subsequent 6 hours, and the diet is gradually resumed.

Because of the importance of monitoring the patient for severity and character of chest pain, the physician may prefer inpatient observation for 24 hours. In addition, the physician may want the patient to remain on a clear liquid diet for 24 hours after the procedure.

Potential complications of pneumatic dilatation include perforation, bleeding, and aspiration. Risk of perforation is somewhat higher than in standard dilatation, occurring in 2% to 4% of patients. Patients with small perforations and contrast material extending beyond the normal esophageal lumen can be managed conservatively, with antibiotics and close observation for signs of worsening pain and fever. Clinical deterioration or the presence of free-flowing contrast material into the mediastinum mandates immediate thoracotomy and repair. If the tear is small, the repair and a Heller myotomy can be performed in the same operation.

CASE SITUATION

Mrs. Doris Johnson, whose case was presented in Chapters 13 and 24, suffers from esophageal reflux, which was diagnosed 2 years ago. Her husband died 18 months ago and she was unable to force herself to comply with her treatment regimen during the grieving period. Emotional recovery has been slow, and she has not returned to the prescribed therapy. Now she is experiencing dysphagia in reaction to solid food but not to liquids. She is to have an esophageal endoscopy and possible dilatation.

Points to think about

1. Given Mrs. Johnson's history and symptoms, what might the nurse expect to find on endoscopic examination?
2. Based on these expectations, what equipment should the nurse have ready?
3. The nurse discovers that Mrs. Johnson has a knowledge deficit in relation to her current diagnosis and treatment. What should the nurse review with her?
4. Mrs. Johnson might be considered noncompliant in relation to her esophageal reflux medical regimen. What are the ethical issues to be considered in labeling a patient noncompliant?
5. In the nursing diagnosis "noncompliance in relation to esophageal reflux medical recommendations," what one factor is inherent in the definition and must be known before an individual can be labeled as noncompliant?
6. What areas must be assessed before a nurse can assist Mrs. Johnson in overcoming noncompliance?
7. What might the nurse tell Mrs. Johnson regarding postdilatation follow-up?

Suggested responses

1. The endoscopic findings demonstrate a stricture of the distal esophagus. This type of stricture may or may not permit passage of the endoscope.
2. The equipment that the nurse should have available for the procedure to be performed on Mrs. Johnson would include:
   (a) Biopsy forceps and cytology brush. All strictures should be diagnosed histologically to rule out a malignancy or Barrett's esophagus (the presence of gastric mucosa above the squamocolumnar junction).
   (b) Dilators. Depending on the type of stricture and/or physician preference, the nurse may need balloon (TTS) dilators, polyvinyl (Savary-Gilliard) dilators, and/or mercury-weighted or tungsten-weighted bougies (Maloney dilators).

3. Information the nurse should discuss with Mrs. Johnson would include the following:
   (a) The current diagnosis and ways the problem can be alleviated, so that the nurse can ascertain Mrs. Johnson's recall of what her physician has told her. In addition, the nurse should answer questions or refer them to the physician.
   (b) The physiological process of reflux and ways to manage it, such as not eating late at night, not lying down after meals, not wearing constricting clothing, and elevating the head of the bed on 6-inch blocks.
   (c) The need to reduce weight, which will help with managing reflux and hypertension. The nurse should refer Mrs. Johnson for counseling in this area.
   (d) Dietary and medication restrictions, such as eliminating caffeine, alcohol, acetylsalicylic acid, and nonsteroidal antiinflammatory drugs.
   (e) The label noncompliant can carry a judgmental connotation and place blame on the patient for failing to comply with a therapeutic recommendation. Healthcare providers must be able to identify all of the variables or factors that contribute to or interfere with a persons ability to comply with recommendations before labeling a patient as noncompliant. Some nursing authorities believe that such a label inflicts unnecessary discomfort or pain on patients by professionals presumably dedicated to 'do no harm.'

The definition of noncompliance involves the expressed desire and intent not to adhere to therapeutic recommendations. Without this expression, a nurse cannot apply this type of label. It is important to identify not only the variables for nonadherence but also the degree to which compliant behavior has occurred.

Before attempting to assist Mrs. Johnson in overcoming noncompliance, the nurse should assess the following:
   (a) Defining characteristics of noncompliance, such as observation of noncompliant behavior or results of objective measures that reveal noncompliant behavior (e.g., physiological measures, development of complications, or increase in symptoms).
   (b) Personal factors, which include values and beliefs about health, illness, threat, and the prescribed therapy.
   (c) Interpersonal factors, such as support from others and satisfaction gained from it.
   (d) Environmental factors, including barriers to compliance in the environment in which the patient must exist (e.g., economic difficulties).
4. Instructions for follow-up after esophageal dilatation might include:
   (a) Symptoms of complications, such as increased chest pain, vomiting of blood, difficulty breathing, scapular pain, and fever.
   (b) Dietary modifications needed (e.g., eat slowly and chew food well).
   (c) Prescribed medications.
   (d) Required follow-up visits.

REVIEW TERMS

American dilator, bougienage, bougies, dilators, French units, Hurst dilators, hydrostatic balloons, Maloney dilators, pneumatic balloons, Savary-Gilliard dilators

REVIEW QUESTIONS

1. The primary goal of most esophageal dilatation procedures is to:
   - (a) Permit passage of the endoscope.
   - (b) Allow the patient to eat and drink normally.
   - (c) Treat achalasia.
   - (d) Cure esophageal cancer.

2. Before the patient can resume a normal diet, the esophageal lumen must be dilated to a diameter equivalent to at least:
   - (a) 20 Fr.
   - (b) 30 Fr.
   - (c) 40 Fr.
   - (d) 50 Fr.

3. A mercury-filled, rubber bougie with a tapered tip is called a:
   - (a) Maloney dilator.
   - (b) Hurst dilator.
   - (c) Balloon dilator.
   - (d) Savary dilator.

4. After bougienage with local anesthesia, the patient should remain NPO:
   - (a) For 2 hours.
   - (b) Until the gag reflex returns.
   - (c) Until the possibility of perforation has been ruled out.
   - (d) For 8 hours.

5. One advantage of polyvinyl chloride dilators over the rubber bougies is that:
   - (a) There is no risk of perforation.
   - (b) Fewer passes through the pharynx are needed.
   - (c) The placement of the guidewire through the narrow area makes dilatation of tortuous strictures easier and safer.
   - (d) The endoscopist can see the dilatation through the scope.

6. The method used most often for dilatation of pyloric or colonic stenosis is:
   - (a) A polyvinyl chloride dilator.
   - (b) A pneumatic balloon.
   - (c) A hydrostatic balloon.
   - (d) A rubber bougie.

7. A hydrostatic dilating balloon is filled with dilute contrast media because:
   - (a) Full-strength contrast medium could crystallize, damaging the balloon.
   - (b) Full-strength contrast medium may cause an allergic reaction.
   - (c) It helps stimulate peristalsis, thus aiding passage of the balloon through the upper GI tract.
   - (d) It exerts more pressure than water or saline.

8. The primary use of hydrostatic balloons of the biliary tract may be able to:
   - (a) Permanently treat biliary strictures.
   - (b) Dilate the duct before long-term stent placement.
   - (c) Treat sphincter of Oddi dysfunction.
   - (d) Remove common bile duct stones.

9. In pneumatic dilatation, the balloon remains inflated:
   - (a) For up to 1 minute.
   - (b) For up to 10 minutes.
   - (c) Until the patient experiences chest pain.
   - (d) Until the preset pressure is obtained.

BIBLIOGRAPHY

Abele, J.E. (1992). The physics of esophageal dilatation. *J-Iepalo Gastroenterol 39*, 486-9.

Dalzell, A.M. (1992). Esophageal stricture in children: fiber-optic endoscopy and dilatation under fluoroscopic control. *J Pediatr Gastroenterol Nutr 15*, 426-30. Journal of Pediatric Gasterology and Nutrition.

Fleischer, D.E. (1989). A marked guidewire facilitates esophageal dilatation. *Am J Gastroenterol 84*, 359-61. American Journal of Gastroenterology.

Kozarek, R. (1995). Gastrointestinal dilation. In Yamada, T. (Ed.), *Textbook of gastroenterology* (2nd ed.). Philadelphia: Lippincott, Williams & Wilkins.

Microvasive Product Information. Natick: MA.

Nostrant, T.T. (1995). Esophageal dilatation. *Digest Dis 13*, 337-55.

Richter, J.E. (1995). Motility disorders of the esophagus. In Yamada, T. (Ed.), *Textbook of gastroenterology* (2nd ed.). Philadelphia: JB Lippincott.

Society of Gastroenterology Nurses and Associates, Inc. (2003). *Manual of gastrointestinal procedures* (5th ed.). Chicago.

All techniques in this chapter are discussed in:
Society of Gastroenterology Nurses and Associates, Inc. (2003). *Manual of gastrointestinal procedures* (5th ed.). Chicago.

Chapter 28

HEMOSTASIS AND TUMOR ABLATION

This chapter will acquaint the gastroenterology nurse with endoscopic and other techniques that are used to stop GI bleeding. Indications, contraindications, techniques, and potential complications of monopolar and bipolar electrocoagulation, heater probes, laser photocoagulation, esophageal-gastric balloon tamponade, photodynamic therapy, injection sclerotherapy, and variceal ligation are all described in detail. Nursing considerations for managing these patients are outlined as they relate to the role of the gastroenterology nurse.

Learning objectives

After reviewing the content of this chapter, the gastroenterology nurse should be able to:

1. Discuss the general principles and the role of the gastroenterology nurse in thermal coagulation procedures and methods, including monopolar and bipolar electrocautery, heater probes, and laser photocoagulation.
2. Discuss indications, contraindications, and techniques for esophageal-gastric tamponade.
3. Explain the use of injection sclerotherapy, variceal ligation, and chemical injection therapy in the treatment of esophageal and gastric varices.

BASIC PRINCIPLES

In planning endoscopic therapy for GI bleeding, it is important first to confirm the location of the hemorrhage (upper or lower GI tract). Most of the causes of upper GI bleeding and some of the causes of lower GI bleeding are amenable to endoscopic therapy. Causes of upper GI bleeding include esophageal, gastric, and duodenal ulcers; erosive esophagitis, gastritis, and duodenitis; Mallory-Weiss tears; varices; tumors; and arteriovenous malformations (AVMs). Although approximately 70% to 80% of upper GI bleeding episodes are self-limited, the overall mortality rate for patients with upper GI bleeding remains at 6% to 7%. Factors that increase this risk include the severity of bleeding, significant coexisting medical illness, age above 60 years, need for surgery, and continued or recurrent bleeding. At the time of diagnostic endoscopy, the physician and nurse should be prepared to treat the bleeding site with injection therapy, photocoagulation, or electrocoagulation.

Several factors affect the timing of the endoscopic examination. The likelihood of finding the source of the bleeding is higher when the procedure is done within 24 hours of the bleed. Ongoing upper GI bleeding requires urgent endoscopy as soon as the patient is medically stable. For upper GI bleeding that is not thought to be active, endoscopy should be performed as soon as personnel and equipment become available. For active lower GI bleeding, colonoscopy should not be performed until the colon has been cleansed properly.

Causes of lower GI bleeding include hemorrhoids, diverticulosis, polyps, cancer, AVMs, colitis, colonic ischemia, post polypectomy, and hemorrhage from the upper intestinal tract (found in 10% of patients in whom the provisional diagnosis of upper GI bleed has been made). Of these, endoscopy management is most often used for bleeding cancers, AVMs, and polyps.

Premedication for endoscopic hemostasis is similar to that administered for diagnostic endoscopy. Avoid use of Demerol if AVMs are suspected. However, because patients with major blood loss may be hypotensive, the blood pressure-lowering effects of commonly used narcotics and sedatives must be considered. Antiperistaltic agents such as glucagon may be administered to diminish motility when searching for or treating nonbleeding angiodysplasia.

A number of endoscopic methods are available to control GI hemorrhage, including monopolar and bipolar electrocautery, heater probes, and laser therapy. Variceal bleeding may be treated with IV vasopressin (Pitressin), injection sclerotherapy, injection of hypertonic or epinephrine solutions, esophageal variceal ligation, or esophageal-gastric tamponade. Injection therapy is also used to treat bleeding ulcers.

ELECTROCAUTERY

Electrosurgery can be used to produce cutting and/or **coagulation (fulguration** and **desiccation)** effects. When both **cutting current** and **coagulating current** are applied, the resulting energy is referred to as a "blended" current.

Electrocoagulation (electrocautery) occurs when current flows through resistant tissue, thereby coagulating protein and producing hemostasis. It is used to treat active bleeding from a visible vessel, visible vessels without bleeding, or blood oozing from a clot in the base of an ulcer. It is also used in conjunction with the excision of polyps, large mucosal biopsies, and endoscopic retrograde sphincterotomy. Polypectomy and sphincterotomy are discussed in detail in Chapter 30.

In addition, electrocoagulation is used for treatment of hereditary hemorrhagic telangiectasias (Osler-Weber-Rendu syndrome) of the GI tract and for acquired vascular abnormalities of the stomach, duodenum, or cecal area (angiodysplasia). For AVMs in the stomach and duodenum, electrocoagulation is achieved by placing an electrode on the peripheral border of the malformation, applying moderate pressure, and moving circumferentially until the AVM has been completely encircled. If the center of an AVM is electrocoagulated before its periphery has been treated, torrential bleeding may occur.

Electrocautery is contraindicated in patients with excessive bleeding, esophageal varices, or coagulopathy. It can be performed safely with the majority of newer model pacemakers, but a case-by-case determination must be made before the procedure.

Electrosurgical units (ESUs) are all different; even those that are provided by the same manufacturer vary. Avoid twisting and wrapping cords as this causes increased resistance. It is important to thoroughly understand the tissue effects caused by the use of each unit.

All electrosurgical equipment should be inspected regularly for frayed or cracked cords, loose connections, or deterioration in the power cord and plug. A working backup for the ESU should be readily available. Unit functioning should be checked and documented before each use.

Before attempting electrocoagulation in the upper GI tract, the stomach must be free of blood, and the patient's condition must be stabilized. An oral bite block should be placed, and sedation and analgesia should be achieved as appropriate. Diagnostic esophagogastroduodenoscopy (EGD), using a therapeutic scope if available, should be performed to determine the cause of the bleeding.

Before electrocoagulation of the colon or rectum, it is important that the colon be well prepped to eliminate the risk of exploding the hydrogen and methane gases that are normally present in the stool. It is also important to remember that the colon wall is thinner than the upper GI tract and thus the risk of perforation is greater, particularly if the lumen is over distended.

Both before and during electrosurgical procedures, it is the nurse's responsibility to perform the following activities:

1. Inspect all equipment to make sure it works properly.
2. Verify settings with each use of the ESU.
3. Position the grounding pad on the patient (for monopolar electrocoagulation only) and document placement.
4. Turn on the power when the physician is ready to use the ESU and turn it off immediately after use.
5. Check the placement of the foot pedal.
6. Verbally confirm the physician's orders for mode of operation (coagulation, cutting, or blended current) and settings.
7. Reassure and encourage the patient to stay as still as possible.

After the procedure is completed, it is important to check for skin damage or burns near and under the grounding pad (when using the monopolar modality); monitor the patient's vital signs and document results; monitor the patient for abdominal pain and/or distention; and document power settings and status of grounding pad site.

Potential complications of electrocautery include thermal injury, hemorrhage, perforation, transmural burns, and explosion.

The following are two ways of applying electrocoagulation:

1. In the monopolar modality, electrical current flows from a small, active electrode that is in contact with the target tissue, through the patient, and toward a grounding pad that is attached to the patient's skin. The site chosen should be muscular, well vascularized, and not over bony prominences, joint prosthesis, or where circulation is likely to be impaired. The preferred site is the upper thigh. The high current density at the relatively small electrode site generates a significant amount of heat in the resistor (the target tissue), thereby causing coagulation. The current density at the grounding pad is lower, because the amount of tissue in contact with the grounding plate is much larger.
2. In the bipolar modality, the current flows between two small electrodes that are in contact with the tissue and are separated by a space of only a few millimeters. The localized current pathway between the two electrodes results in tissue heating. The bipolar modality therefore does not require a grounding pad.

Monopolar electrocoagulation

There are certain safety factors associated with the use of the grounding pad in **monopolar electrocoagulation.** Before the procedure the nurse should explain the purpose of the grounding pad to the patient. The patient should be instructed not to touch side rails, IV poles, or other metal objects during the procedure (Fig. 28-1).

A number of different types of grounding pads are available. Disposable pads with gel and adhesive edges are preferred, because they conform to patient contours and do not have to be repositioned if the patient's position is changed. The nurse should apply the grounding pad according to the

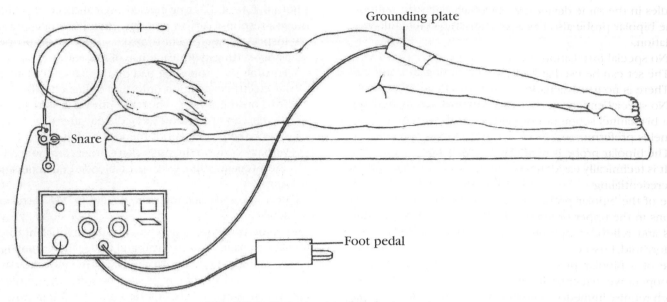

Fig. 28-1. Patient setup for electrocautery.

manufacturer's guidelines. The pad should have generous contact on healthy tissue, avoiding bony prominences and large scars that could decrease skin area contact. Excessive hair should be removed from the site of attachment.

Incorrect application of a grounding plate may result in "hot spots" where current density remains high because of limited skin contact. Spot burning can also occur. To avoid pacemaker malfunction and burns from internal metal prostheses, the grounding pad should be as far away as possible from any pacemaker, hip pin, or artificial joint, and as close as possible to the site of use.

With the use of high-frequency currents, current leakage can be a problem.

1. Current may pass through the accessory, leak through the endoscope, and pass back to the endoscopist, causing burns to the operator.
2. Current may pass through the accessory, leak through the scope, and pass to the patient at an internal point in which the patient is in contact with the scope, and then continue to the grounding pad, presenting the potential for a burn at a scope-patient contact point.
3. Current may also pass through the accessory, through the tissue at the site of electrosurgery, and through the patient's body to a part that is in contact with a grounded piece of metal (e.g., table edges, Mayo stands, IV poles).

It is important to remember that any personnel in contact with equipment or the patient during use of the generator can become part of the electrical circuit.

To avoid these problems, the gastroenterology nurse should take the following steps:

1. Securely attach the grounding pad to the patient.
2. Wear rubber gloves to decrease conduction and contact with the scope.
3. If a fiberoptic instrument is being used, ensure that a nonconductive material covers the eyepiece.
4. Avoid touching the patient during activation of the ESU.

5. Place metal objects far enough away from the x-ray table or examination table to prevent accidental patient contact.
6. Prevent patient contact with metal railings or edges of the litter.

Bipolar electrocoagulation

A bipolar electrode is a specialized, hemostatic probe that is inserted through an endoscope channel to control GI hemorrhage and bleeding. The **bipolar probe** does not require a grounding pad, because the current travels back through the bipolar electrode. Because there are two electrodes, coagulation takes place only between the two points. One point delivers the current and the other closes the circuit returning to the generator. Electrical energy is converted into thermal energy on contact with the tissue, thereby producing a more predictable depth of injury than with monopolar therapy. The tip of the bipolar probe consists of an array of longitudinal or circumferential microelectrodes. The probes are 7 and 10 Fr in size; the 10-Fr probe can only be used with a large-channel scope. Through a hole in the center of the tip, a powerful water jet can be delivered intermittently or constantly to irrigate the bleeding lesion and to increase the precision of targeting. Coagulation is possible with the top and sides of the probe tip.

Bipolar electrocoagulation has certain advantages over the monopolar modality. Depth of tissue penetration is limited, thus reducing the risk of perforation and avoiding full-thickness burns. There is a rapidly decreasing energy and heating effect at short distance from the electrodes. Two additional features of the bipolar probe are its ability to tamponade the vessel before delivering thermal energy and the fact that the thermal energy can be delivered from the sides of the probes. Studies have shown that although bipolar electrocoagulation is technically more difficult to use, it produces less mucosal injury and is equally effective as monopolar electrocoagulation. Bipolar products with injection needles in the same device are available.

The bipolar probe also has advantages over laser photocoagulation.

1. No special installation is necessary.
2. The set can be used at bedside.
3. There is no gas evacuation.
4. No special endoscopic adaptation is necessary, although a bi-channel scope or one with a large instrument channel is preferred.
5. The bipolar probe is relatively inexpensive.
6. It is technically easier to use and does not require special credentialing.

Use of the bipolar probe is indicated for actively bleeding lesions in the upper or lower GI tract, to destroy neoplastic cells and relieve symptoms of obstruction, and to destroy hemorrhoidal tissue.

Use of a bipolar probe is contraindicated in combative, uncooperative patients; in cases of massive hemorrhage, which require immediate surgery; where visualization of the bleeding site is inadequate; and where free peritoneal air is observed on x-ray films.

Potential complications of bipolar electrocoagulation include perforation, delayed hemorrhage, and deep ulcerations.

When setting up the bipolar unit, the water bottle is filled with sterile water and connected to the port on the machine. The probe and foot pedal are then connected to the unit, and the probe primed with water. By placing several drops of normal saline on a glass slide, putting the tip in the saline, and depressing the bipolar pedal the nurse will be able to test the probe and unit to assure proper function. If the probe is working properly, the saline will heat and bubbles will form. Following a successful test, the unit should be turned off until needed during the procedure. Lubricating the probe with silicone will facilitate smooth passage through the endoscope, as well as prevent tissue from adhering to the probe.

For application of a bipolar probe, the electrode is placed within 2 to 3 mm of the vessel and firm pressure is applied. The probe is activated in 1- to 2-second bursts until circumferential coagulation has occurred. During the procedure the nurse's responsibilities are to maintain the water level in the water bottle, set the energy levels and water pressure designated by the physician, wipe secretions from the probe with gauze as it is withdrawn from the endoscope, and clean the probe tip as needed during the procedure.

As in any endoscopic procedure that involves sedation and analgesia, the nurse should establish an IV line as ordered. This procedure does not usually require two nurses as the sedation nurse can start the IV. The nurse is responsible for monitoring the patient's vital signs, level of consciousness, and abdominal distention caused by the instillation of large amounts of air and water. After the procedure is completed, the nurse should continue to monitor the patient's vital signs, observing the patient for bleeding, vomiting, abdominal pain, and distention.

The bipolar cautery unit should be cleaned and disassembled, and the water completely flushed from the unit. The water bottle should be emptied and sterilized in accordance with institutional policy and probes maintained and processed according to the manufacturer's directions.

Bipolar ablation of obstructing gastrointestinal tumors

For palliative ablation of obstructing esophageal or rectal tumors, a specialized bipolar probe may be used to ablate the strictured area. The local delivery of heat to the site of the cancer may destroy neoplastic cells and relieve symptoms.

The standard bipolar tumor probe kit has five probes of different diameters. Each probe has four sections; a distal flexible, 'slinky'-like tip that is 6 cm in length; an electrically activated bipolar probe that is similar to the Eder-Puestow olives in shape and size; a flexible shaft that is 60 cm in length with markings at centimeter intervals; and the electrical connection, which attaches by a cord to a 50-watt bipolar electrocoagulating generator.

Preliminary screening tests are needed to confirm that the patient is a good candidate for the procedure. The tumor should be symmetrical, and there should be no contraindications to therapy. Screening tests for esophageal tumors include the following:

(a) a screening endoscopy to determine the location, size, and shape of the tumor;
(b) a contrast radiographic study of the esophagus to define the length, location, and shape of the tumor and to exclude the presence of a tracheo-esophageal fistula; and
(c) an imaging study to determine the extent of the disease, the thickness and symmetry of the esophageal wall at the tumor site, and the tumor's proximity to critical structures.

Before the procedure the patient may receive IV sedation and analgesia. An anticholinergic medication may also be used if the tumor is in the proximal esophagus.

A small-caliber endoscope is passed into the stomach, and a guidewire is inserted to the junction of the body and the antrum. Although fluoroscopic guidance is not absolutely necessary, it adds an extra measure of safety. The guidewire is then left in place while the endoscope is withdrawn. If the endoscope cannot advance beyond the proximal margin of the tumor, polyvinyl dilators are passed over the guidewire to dilate the tumor until the probe can be passed beyond the distal margin of the tumor. It is important not to "overdilate" the tumor, however, because good contact between the probe and the tumor is necessary. The nurse's role is to assist with the passage of guidewires, inflate dilators to the size and duration as directed, and monitor the patient's response to the procedure.

Thermal treatments are initiated distally and proceed stepwise proximally. Once the tumor probe reaches the proximal margin of the tumor and the last burn is delivered, the probe and guidewire are removed, and the treated area is evaluated endoscopically. If the burn has been delivered perfectly, a circumferential white burn should be seen. When the burn is incomplete, or if the probe pulls tissue with it as it advances, some areas will appear white and others will be friable and hemorrhagic.

After the procedure the tumor probe should be cleaned and processed according to the manufacturer's instructions. The patient should be NPO for at least 4 hours, and vital signs monitored for evidence of perforation or bleeding. If there is any concern that a perforation may have occurred, a chest x-ray may be done. If there are no complications, clear liquids may be given after 4 hours. In some institutions, patients remain NPO until the following morning, after a barium swallow has been performed.

Some dysphagia may be expected in the first 24 hours following the procedure. It is not uncommon for the patient to have a low-grade fever, mild leukocytosis, and chest pain. A second endoscopy is carried out 48 hours after the first to determine whether a second treatment is necessary, and once luminal patency has been achieved, monthly follow-up is often conducted.

HEATER PROBES

The **heater probe** is very similar in application to the bipolar probe. It consists of a hollow aluminum cylinder with an inner heat coil and an outer coating of Teflon. The aluminum has high thermal conductivity, which provides for a precise and uniform distribution of heat to tissue from its end or sides. A coaxial channel is provided to wash away blood and debris. Heater probes are available with diameters of 3.2 or 2.4 mm; the 3.2-mm size must be used with a large-channel endoscope.

The attributes of the heater probe are its portability, coaxial channel for application of a water jet, capability for controlling and presetting the rate of pulses, effectiveness, low cost, and capability for use at angles other than directly vertical. Like the bipolar probe, the heater probe also permits direct tamponade of bleeding sites. Moreover, the tip of the probe is covered with Teflon, which prevents sticking and frequent removal of the probe to wipe off adherent blood and tissue. In addition to controlling GI bleeding, heater probes have been used successfully to treat patients with hemorrhoids.

Steps in the application of the heater probe unit and bipolar unit are very similar with the exception of testing. By submerging the tip in water and depressing the Coag pedal the heater probe can be tested to determine if the unit is functioning properly. Should a malfunction occur an alarm will sound and a fault light will be activated.

The heater probe is applied directly to a vessel with firm pressure. Several brief applications of thermal energy may be required to produce hemostasis. A disadvantage of the heater is that delivery of the maximum amount of thermal energy requires up to 8 seconds, during which time the contact between the probe and the bleeding point must be maintained. Furthermore, the probe must be allowed to cool before it is withdrawn through the scope; if it is still hot, it can melt the channel lining.

LASER THERAPY

The word **laser** is an acronym for light amplification by stimulated emission of radiation. Because laser light is coherent and collimated it can be intensely focused, which allows it to be precisely aimed. To date, only argon and neodymium:yttrium-aluminum-garnet (**Nd:YAG**) lasers have been widely used in endoscopy. Carbon dioxide lasers are not adaptable to the current generation of flexible endoscopes.

In endoscopic applications, laser light energy is transmitted through a flexible quartz waveguide, which is usually protected by a plastic catheter passed through a flexible endoscope. Between the fiber and the catheter is free space, through which coaxial air, carbon dioxide, or helium flows, thus keeping the fiber and the surface of the treatment site clear of blood and other debris. Because this coaxial gas can lead to problems with overdistention, a two-channel endoscope is preferred so the gas can be exhausted through the suction channel. More than 95% of the lasers used for GI work are Nd:YAG lasers. Unlike the Nd:YAG laser, the argon laser is absorbed by hemoglobin and therefore will not penetrate clots. The depth of penetration of the **argon** laser is less than that of the Nd:YAG lasers (approximately 1 mm, compared with 4 mm). The argon laser beam is visible; the Nd:YAG beam is not visible and thus requires an additional xenon or helium-neon aiming beam. The Nd:YAG laser also carries the greater risk of potential damage to the eye of the examiner, observer, or patient.

Flexible endoscopes may be damaged if laser energy is reflected from the target surface to the tip of the endoscope. This can be avoided by the following preventive measures:

1. Use endoscopes that are designed for laser therapy and are manufactured with stainless-steel or white porcelain reflective tips rather than black tips.
2. Make sure that the laser fiber is well outside the endoscope channel and clearly visualized before activating the laser.
3. Do not work too closely to the target surface during extensive coagulation.

The temperature generated at the treatment site determines the effect of the laser on tissue. Generally speaking, protein coagulates at 60° C (photocoagulation), and tissue vaporizes at 100° C (photovaporization).

1. **Photocoagulation** creates a white, blanched appearance with edema. The coagulative effect of lasers allows them to be used to achieve hemostasis for acute GI bleeding and to treat GI lesions that are not actively bleeding (e.g., angiodysplasia or ulcers with visible vessels).
2. **Photovaporization** may cause a divot, charring of tissue, and smoke. The photovaporization effect of lasers allows them to destroy neoplastic tissue and to cut through normal tissue to achieve therapeutic goals.

Conventional laser therapy differs from heater probe and electrocoagulation treatment in that it is a noncontact method. The laser waveguide does not come into contact with the tissue. Newly developed sapphire endoprobes, however, permit the laser to be used as a contact device. These tips, which attach to the tip of the standard laser waveguide, serve as lenses to concentrate the energy at the tip of the waveguide, so much lower wattages are required.

Laser treatment may be used for hemorrhagic conditions of the GI tract, such as Mallory-Weiss tears, bleeding peptic ulcers, angiodysplasia, or Osler-Weber-Rendu syndrome. Patients with stigmata of recent hemorrhage, including active bleeding, a visible vessel, or a fresh clot, are ideal candidates for laser photocoagulation. In addition, laser photo-vaporization has been used for neoplastic disease, benign esophageal webs and anastomotic strictures, intrahepatic and extrahepatic biliary obstruction, and gallstones. In the colorectal area, the laser may be used for benign pedunculated polyps or sessile lesions, tumor vaporization, and photocoagulation of hemorrhoids.

Endoscopic laser therapy is contraindicated in uncooperative patients or in patients with coagulopathy, extremely large vessels in the field, or inaccessible lesions.

Before laser therapy the power emission from the laser probe must be checked. Patients usually receive IV sedation and analgesia and are placed in the left lateral decubitus position. Everyone in the room, including the patient, should wear safety glasses or goggles. Endoscopists may use goggles or, if using a fiberoptic endoscope, may rely on the protective ocular lens cover once the laser is inserted. Laser masks should be worn to protect personnel against smoke and possible aerosolization of tissue particles. The water-cooling system should be in operation. The power emission from the laser probe should be checked. "Laser in use" warning signs should be placed at all doors. A smoke evacuator may also be beneficial.

During the procedure it is the responsibility of one nurse to maintain the laser on standby mode when it is not in the firing position, to set power and duration as ordered by the physician, and to clean the tip of the fiber frequently with hydrogen peroxide and a soft-bristled brush. Removal of the fiber from the biopsy channel allows an excellent opportunity to remove excess smoke and debris. The nurse also assists the physician with use of biopsy forceps for possible debridement of the treatment site. The patient should be monitored during the procedure for abdominal distention and possible vasovagal reaction. Pain level should be observed so additional IV conscious sedation can be administered as necessary.

After the procedure is completed, the entire exterior of a reusable fiber, including the brass tip, is wiped with a gauze pad saturated with hydrogen peroxide. However, some laser equipment is disposable so it is important to refer to the manufacturers' instructions. The interior is cleaned by lavaging with hydrogen peroxide in a syringe without a needle, while a constant flow of carbon dioxide is maintained. The flow of carbon dioxide prevents the peroxide from traveling more than a few centimeters up the fiber. The peroxide can be removed by depressing the foot pedal, with the laser lamps off, to produce a burst of carbon dioxide gas.

Fibers should be reprocessed according to the manufacturer's instructions.

Following laser treatment, the patient is kept NPO until the physician's orders permit resumption of oral intake. Vital signs should be checked as per institution guidelines for care of patients receiving IV sedation and analgesia.

Swallowing is often worse immediately after laser therapy of the esophagus because of edema. If there is odynophagia, antacids may relieve symptoms. If ordered by the physician, a nasogastric tube may be inserted to relieve abdominal distention. Narcotic analgesics may be necessary to relieve chest pain. Chest x-ray films and/or abdominal films may be ordered to exclude the possibility of perforation. It is not uncommon for patients to experience a low-grade fever and mild leukocytosis 12 to 36 hours after laser therapy.

To obtain adequate patency of a tumor site with laser therapy, several treatments may be required. After the final treatment, a water-soluble x-ray contrast swallow may be obtained to rule out perforation and to document the effects of therapy. The first follow-up endoscopy is usually carried out in 3 to 4 weeks.

Potential complications of endoscopic laser treatments include hemorrhage, tissue slough, perforation, gaseous abdominal distention, ulceration, delayed healing, and fistula or stricture formation. If perforation and/or bleeding are suspected, they should be treated as described in Chapter 31. Complications from endoscopic laser therapy increase with the amount of energy delivered and the length of the procedure. Minor increases in bleeding during laser therapy are relatively common, but laser-induced massive GI bleeding is also possible and may require emergency surgical intervention.

Laser treatment of upper gastrointestinal bleeding

Before laser photocoagulation of upper GI bleeding, a large-bore tube is used for thorough lavage of the stomach. Vasopressin (Pitressin) should be available for IV use if uncontrollable bleeding occurs, and a snare or grasper should be available for transecting and removing large adherent clots. A syringe irrigator may be used to remove smaller clots. A blood pump is necessary to allow rapid blood infusion if needed.

For the treatment of bleeding ulcers, the laser fiber is held 1 to 2 cm from the target, and pulses of high power and short duration are used for coagulation. If a vessel is visible, the beam is aimed circumferentially around it. When visible edema develops, the vessel itself is treated.

Laser therapy for vascular abnormalities

Endoscopic obliteration and clinical benefit have been reported in patients with angiodysplasia after use of both the argon and the Nd:YAG laser. When the laser beam strikes a large, abnormal vessel, it may initially cause a dormant lesion to bleed, but further laser therapy can bring this hemorrhage under control. Although angiodysplastic lesions may be seen in both the stomach and intestines, gastric and proximal duodenal lesions are responsible for the majority of upper GI bleeding.

Angiodysplasia of the colon, particularly the cecum, has also been treated with argon and Nd:YAG laser therapy. Results are best when it has been established that the colonic lesion has bled and the lesion is not just an incidental finding. Risk of perforation is greater in the right colon, because it is thinner than other areas of the GI tract.

In patients with Osler-Weber-Rendu syndrome, laser therapy may reduce treatment time when many lesions are present. Laser treatment has also been shown to significantly reduce the potential for rebleeding and requirement for transfusions.

Laser coagulation of hemorrhoids

Nd:YAG laser photocoagulation and obliteration is a viable alternative to surgical removal of internal and external hemorrhoids. This technique delivers extensive heat therapy directly to the hemorrhoidal structures. It attempts to both fix the mucosa and remove some or all of the internal hemorrhoidal tissue. Compared with a surgical approach, laser therapy requires only local, rather than general, anesthesia; there is less trauma; and laser therapy causes less pain.

The infrared photocoagulator is another recent innovation for the treatment of hemorrhoids. This device is *not* a laser; it focuses infrared radiation on the tissue via a specially made polymer tip. The source is a low-voltage tungsten-halogen lamp. The light source is directed at the base of the hemorrhoid and is used to produce a visible eschar. It is generally painless for patients receiving treatment on an outpatient basis and is expected to have minimal long-term sequelae or serious complications.

Laser treatment of gastrointestinal tumors

Endoscopic laser treatment is also indicated for palliative or curative treatment of benign or malignant tumors of the esophagus, stomach, duodenum, ampulla, colon, or rectum. When palliative treatment is undertaken, the goal is usually to relieve obstruction or to reduce blood loss; attempts to relieve pain have generally not been successful. Blood loss may be reduced by coagulating tumor bleeding sites or by destroying the tumor vasculature. Palliation of bleeding and/or obstruction with laser photocoagulation appears to be a true alternative to bypass surgery. In some cases, intended curative treatment has been achieved.

The use of laser therapy may be indicated in the following situations and types of malignant and premalignant lesions:

(a) benign polyps and large villous adenomas that are sessile, at least 5 mm in transverse diameter, and not amenable to electrosurgical snaring;

(b) periodic removal of polyps to prevent development of rectal cancer in patients with Gardner's syndrome or familial polyposis who have had subtotal colectomies with ileorectal anastomoses;

(c) palliative treatment of malignancies in which there is widespread disease and no chance for surgical cure;

(d) to reestablish luminal patency and relieve dysphagia in patients with incurable esophageal cancer;

(e) to relieve gastric outlet obstruction, control chronic bleeding, or reduce tumor bulk in patients with gastric cancer; and

(f) to relieve obstruction, control bleeding, or reduce tumor bulk in patients with colorectal cancer who are not surgical candidates or who decline surgery.

To determine whether a patient with GI cancer is a candidate for laser therapy, the following three preliminary examinations are required:

(a) a barium swallow to define the location and extent of the tumor in the upper GI tract;

(b) diagnostic endoscopy to view the gross appearance of the tumor and to obtain biopsies and cytology; and

(c) a computed tomography (CT) or nuclear magnetic resonance (NMR) scan to define the extent of the disease.

If there is any possibility of a cure for GI cancer, and there are no medical contraindications, exploratory surgery may be performed. In patients whose functional status is so poor that even if the lumen were opened it would not greatly improve the quality of life, laser therapy should not be considered.

As in thermal treatment, it is preferable to begin at the distal margin of the tumor. If a two-channel endoscope cannot be advanced to the distal margin of the tumor, the esophagus may be dilated. Dilatation is usually sufficient to allow for treatment to begin at the distal tumor margin. If not even the smallest endoscope will pass beyond the obstruction, the endoscopist may begin treatment at the proximal tumor margin.

To begin laser therapy, the quartz wave-guide that carries the laser beam is passed through the biopsy channel and beyond the distal tip of the scope. The beam is aimed at the portion of the neoplastic tumor closest to the lumen, and treatment progresses in increasingly larger concentric circles toward, but not to, the wall of the target organ. Usually the tumor is destroyed by vaporization. Some endoscopists prefer to accomplish tumor destruction by coagulation because, although this is a slower process, less smoke is generated. At the end of treatment, the tissue is often edematous and charred black secondary to thermal damage. Major blood loss is not usually a problem.

It is uncommon for any patient with esophageal tumors to require more than three laser sessions. Patients are usually treated every other day until maximal luminal opening is achieved. The 48-hour period between treatments allows for maximal tissue necrosis and is well tolerated by most patients. In subsequent sessions, surveillance endoscopy is used to observe the effects of the last treatment. If necessary, necrotic tissue can be pushed distally into the stomach, and dilatation may be perfomed.

Patients with rectal tumors are generally more amenable to outpatient treatment than patients with esophageal cancer, who are often more debilitated. When the colonic lumen is almost completely obliterated by the tumor, a temporary opening may be provided by dilatation with a through-the-scope balloon dilator. For rectal cancers, a rigid proctoscope and hand-held laser fiber may be used. If the lesion has advanced to the anal verge, treatment with the Nd:YAG laser is painful and a saddle block may be required. If a rectal lesion is circumferential, treating only 270 degrees of the lesion can reduce the risk of rectal stenosis.

PHOTODYNAMIC THERAPY

A treatment called photodynamic therapy (PDT), has been used effectively to treat superficial esophageal cancers, high-grade dysplasia, Barrett's esophagus, and superficial adeno-carcinomas of the colon in the United States, Europe, and Japan. PDT drugs called *photosensitizers* are injected into the patient's body, where they collect naturally in cancerous and precancerous cells.

The dose of photosensitizer is calculated according to the patient's weight and is administered intravenously. Approximately 24 to 48 hours after injection, a red light laser is directed endoscopically at the tumor or lesion. The first observable changes are blanching of the tumor tissue and diffuse hemorrhage. Necrosis and eschar formation occur over a 2 to 3 week period, followed by healing after approximately 6 to 8 weeks. Patients may require one to three treatments.

The patient is instructed to avoid exposure to sunlight for a period of about 4-6 weeks. At the end of this time, the patient may gradually increase his or her exposure to sunlight as tolerated. The following side effects may occur after the PDT treatment: decrease in appetite, nausea, difficulty in swallowing, and pain in the middle chest. Intravenous fluids or nutritional therapy may be necessary during the first 1 to 2 weeks after the procedure.

As technology in this therapy improves and experience increases, researchers feel this treatment shows great promise as a minimally invasive technique.

When compared to surgical intervention, PDT is emerging as a promising treatment with outcomes including lower morbidity, mortality, and cost. The advantage of this treatment is that it does not involve the use of heat or the vaporization of tissue caused by conventional laser therapy.

INJECTION THERAPY

Endoscopic injection therapy was first used to stop variceal bleeding in 1939. After being supplanted temporarily by portacaval shunt techniques, it was reintroduced in 1974 and has become increasingly popular since then. This therapy method involves the injection of a chemical agent through a needle injector into or around a bleeding site to stop bleeding through variceal thrombosis or local edema.

Injection therapy is contraindicated in uncooperative patients or in patients with severe coagulopathy. The procedure is performed under direct endoscopic visualization, most often by using a flexible upper endoscope. A double-channel endoscope is helpful to permit additional suction when the patient is actively bleeding.

Injection-therapy needle assemblies are disposable. The greatest flexibility is obtained with a simple tubular system made of synthetic material, with a needle fixed to the distal tip. A second outer sheath is added, into which the needle may be withdrawn/retracted when not in use.

In addition to the choice of agent, the volume, rate of injection, and placement of injections are all important in determining the overall effect.

Before the procedure it is important to verify the patency of a large-bore IV line, to verify blood type and cross match, and to obtain the results of laboratory testing. The patient should be instructed to remain still and to refrain from coughing. IV sedation and analgesia should be administered to maximize patient cooperation and minimize patient movement. Because some of the agents used in this procedure can cause corneal ulcerations, the patient's eyes should be covered by a small towel during the procedure, and all personnel should wear protective eyewear, gloves, and masks.

A 5- or 10-ml syringe containing the chemical agent should be attached to the proximal end of the needle injector. The injector should be flushed with the agent to rid it of air and to check for patency and leaks. The needle injector should be checked to ensure that the needle properly protrudes from and retracts into the sheath.

A complete endoscopic examination of the esophagus, stomach, and duodenum is performed to locate the bleeding site or varices. The injector is passed through the biopsy port of the endoscope. A gauze sponge held around the injector-syringe connection will prevent leakage. With the patient in the left lateral position, the endoscope is positioned at the bleeding site. Air is insufflated to distend the esophageal lumen, thus enhancing visualization. The needle is advanced. Once the needle tip is visualized, it should be maneuvered into position, and the needle should be thrust directly into the desired site by rapidly advancing the injector and plunging the needle into the wall up to its junction with the sheath.

As soon as entry has been achieved, the nurse rapidly injects 0.5 to 3 ml of the chemical agent at the physician's direction, using slow, steady pressure. The nurse should verbally state the amount of injection in increments of 0.5 ml, and should say "stop" as soon as the injection has been completed.

Throughout the procedure the patient should be monitored for abdominal distention, and the number, type, and amount of injections should be documented. Following the injection, the needle should be withdrawn into the sheath. The entire assembly is then removed from the accessory channel and discarded in an appropriate sharps container. The stomach should be suctioned to decompress the gastric distention caused by continuous insufflation of air.

Nonvariceal injection therapy

Nonvariceal GI bleeding, such as with Mallory-Weiss tears, angiodysplasias, ulcers, and postpolypectomy bleeds, has been treated with a hypertonic saline-epinephrine solution. Injection of hypertonic saline-epinephrine is a relatively simple maneuver and has satisfactory hemostatic efficacy in the endoscopic treatment of nonvariceal GI bleeding caused by vasoconstriction and platelet aggregation effects.

A common sclerosing agent used for hemostatic control of bleeding ulcers is dehydrated (98%) ethanol (alcohol).

Alcohol works by dehydrating and fixating the exposed blood vessel and surrounding tissue. The resulting local vasoconstriction, vascular wall degeneration, and endothelial destruction lead to thrombosis.

Injection is often combined with thermal treatment to control bleeding. New products are available that allow for injection therapy and bipolar electrocoagulation in one device.

Variceal sclerotherapy

Injection **sclerotherapy** involves the injection of a sclerosing (hardening) agent into a blood vessel (Fig. 28-2). It is indicated for the following:

(a) temporary control of acute bleeding from esophageal varices pending shunt placement or in patients who are poor surgical risks;

(b) eradication of esophageal varices to prevent rebleeding;

(c) treatment of small hemorrhoids with bleeding; and

(d) temporary control of acute hemorrhage from gastric varices.

Gastric varices do not respond as well to sclerotherapy as do those in the esophagus. Needle puncture of a gastric varix may be associated with prolonged bleeding from the injection site that is difficult to tamponade.

Injection sclerotherapy is rarely used as a prophylactic measure for patients who have never bled from varices. In children who are awaiting liver transplantation, however, grade III or IV varices are injected prophylactically.

The physician chooses the sclerosing agent. Ideally, it should induce rapid thrombosis followed by intimal damage to the vein and ending in obliteration with minimal damage to the underlying esophageal musculature. It should be innocuous when it reaches the extraesophageal vascular system and other organs. The sclerosing agents used most commonly in the United States for control of variceal bleeding are morrhuate sodium (Scleromate), sodium tetradecyl sulfate (Sotradecol), and ethanolamine oleate (Ethamolin). Sodium tetradecyl sulfate may be less ulcerogenic than mor-rhuate sodium, and ethanolamine oleate may be the least ulcerogenic of the three. Allergic reactions have been reported with all three agents. If skin comes into contact with the sclerosant, it should be rinsed immediately with water.

Sclerotherapy is difficult if there is active hemorrhage, because blood must be cleared from the field to make precise injections. It is usually started 4 to 6 hours after relative hemodynamic stability has been achieved by transfusion, IV vasopressin, and/or **balloon tamponade.** The currently accepted practice is to control acute bleeding by IV vasopressin (Pitressin). This procedure usually relieves acute bleeding in 75% to 90% of cases and allows the patient to be stabilized.

As soon as the sclerosant is injected, the needle is withdrawn and rapidly reinserted into another site. The needle is fully withdrawn into the sheath after each injection. If undue pressure is needed to inject, it usually means that the needle is against the wall or that the varix has been injected previously. Forcing sclerosant into the wall of the esophagus will probably result in a superficial esophageal ulcer.

The endoscopist determines the number and pattern of injections which may be given intravariceally, paravariceally, or using a combination of both. Paravariceal (submucosal) injection can be recognized if the site blanches after injection; intravariceal injection results in ballooning of the blood vessel with a characteristic dark blue color within a few minutes of the injection.

In patients with active hemorrhage, when the bleeding point can be identified, the first injection should be made immediately above the bleeding point in the same column, and then to the right and left. As the flow subsides, an injection may be made distally to the bleeding point. Even if injection therapy is unsuccessful in stopping active bleeding, it is important to make an injection below the varix.

After each injection, there is frequently some back-bleeding. Oozing is possible and stops in 1 to 2 minutes. If a

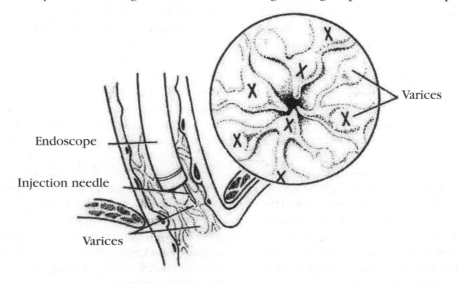

Fig. 28-2. Variceal sclerosing. Insert shows accepted sites for sclerosing.

stream of blood arises from a puncture site, the puncture pattern for active hemorrhage should be followed.

After the procedure an extended period of observation follows, in which the patient should be monitored for signs of GI blood loss and esophageal perforation. A patent IV line should be maintained until discharge. The patient may need additional pain medication, as ordered. After the procedure the physician may order laboratory work and antacids or sucralfate (Carafate) slurry.

Transient side effects of injection sclerotherapy include mild to severe chest pain, dysphagia, and fever. Chest pain usually subsides within 24 hours. Severe pain that lasts more than 24 hours may be indicative of perforation. A low-grade fever can be observed in about 28% of patients and usually subsides in 24 hours. Esophageal ulceration should also probably be considered a side effect of sclerotherapy, because up to 78% of these patients have some degree of ulceration. A long-term complication is esophageal stricture. Many of these patients suffer chronic dysphagia.

More serious potential complications of injection sclerotherapy include hemorrhage, aspiration, necrosis, mediastinitis, esophageal perforation, pleural effusion, sepsis, or portal vein thrombosis. Perforation is manifested by persistent chest pain, dysphagia, fever, and pleural effusion. Septicemia is rare, but prophylaxis is probably warranted for patients with clinically significant heart disease, prosthetic heart valves, or ascites. Pleural effusion seems to be related to the amount of sclerosant used and the amount of chest pain the patient experiences; it usually resolves without therapy.

Complete eradication of varices may require several endoscopic sessions or may occur early in the patient's course, with an average of five sessions for complete eradication of varices. Varices recur in 10% of these patients, even once they are varix-free. Annual checkups are recommended.

ENDOSCOPIC VARICEAL LIGATION (EVL)

A newer method for the treatment of bleeding varices is **endoscopic variceal ligation (EVL),** a technique that has also been used successfully for the eradication of hemorrhoids. With EVL, rubber bands or O-rings are applied around the varices. The tensile strength created by the bands is sufficient to eradicate the varices.

With one manufacturer's ligator, the outer cylinder of a friction-fit adaptor is carefully attached to the distal tip of the endoscope. A tripwire is inserted down the biopsy channel of the scope. The inner cylinder of the adaptor, with a latex O-ring attached, is attached to the tripwire and then to the outer cylinder.

With the overtube properly positioned, and the need for EVL confirmed, the preloaded ligator and endoscope are introduced. The varix is aspirated into the inner cylinder, and the tripwire is pulled to release the O-ring. Suction is released, and the endoscope is withdrawn. At the physician's discretion, serial ligations may be performed after removing the spent inner cylinder and reloading a new one. Disadvantages of this technique are poor visibility with profuse bleeding, reloading bands, and overtube trauma.

Compared to injection sclerotherapy, however, EVL seems to result in less substernal discomfort and stricture formation.

Multiple-band ligation is also used to treat esophageal varices. There are multiple products that range from 4- to 12-band placement per intubation. The setup includes a ligator unit, handle unit with tripwire and scope fastener, and irrigation device. Manufacturer information should be followed in setting up all devices. The handle unit controls the deployment of bands. The physician will identify the varix, make contact, suction, and then deploy one band by turning the handle unit. Varices should be ligated in a distal-to-proximal sequence to avoid obscuring the endoscopist's field of vision. Nurses need to be aware that the device decreases the ability to aspirate secretions and the patient could be at higher risk for aspiration.

Advantages of multiple-band ligation include the following:
(a) no overtube-associated complications, such as trauma and increased patient discomfort;
(b) no need for multiple intubations or removal of cassettes, which results in time savings and less exposure of staff to blood and body fluids; and
(c) usable on any size scope (except 160 scopes).

Although the advantages are numerous, it should be noted that it is considerably more expensive than the single-banding technique.

ESOPHAGEAL-GASTRIC TAMPONADE

Esophageal-gastric **tamponade** involves the insertion of specialized tubes to provide pressure on bleeding areas of the esophagus or esophagogastric junction. It is indicated in patients with acute upper GI bleeding from esophageal varices or tears at the esophagogastric junction. Because of the variety of potential complications and because it is more difficult to use than vasopressin (Pitressin), it is generally performed in patients with variceal bleeding after the administration of vasopressin, sclerotherapy, or EVL has failed. It is used rarely for Mallory-Weiss tears that are unresponsive to medical therapy.

Esophageal-gastric tamponade is contraindicated for patients with cardiopulmonary failure, recent surgical trauma to the esophagogastric junction, or when variceal bleeding has stopped. It should not be attempted when the source of upper GI bleeding cannot be identified. It is also contraindicated in patients who are surgical candidates and in whom prior tamponade has failed.

Before the procedure it is important to establish and confirm a patent oral airway, monitor vital signs, and establish one or two large-bore IV lines for fluid and blood replacement. Because patients with acute upper GI bleeding may become extremely agitated, it is important to explain the benefits of the procedure, assure the patient of constant nursing care and monitoring, and explain that some pressure will be felt when the tube balloons are inflated.

The following three different types of tubes may be used for this procedure:

1. The **Sengstaken-Blakemore tube** is a three-lumen tube with esophageal and gastric balloons. It provides a

gastric aspiration port to allow drainage from below the gastric balloon. Esophageal aspiration is accomplished by a secondary tube, such as a Levin or Salem sump tube that is inserted orally or nasally to rest above the esophageal balloon. A manometer is used to insufflate the balloons and to measure pressure.

2. The **Linton tube** is a three-lumen tube that uses a gastric balloon but no esophageal balloon and provides ports for both esophageal and gastric aspiration. Elimination of the esophageal balloon reduces the risk of esophageal necrosis. A manometer is used to measure pressures from the gastric inflation port.

3. The **Minnesota tube** is a rubber, radiopaque, 18-Fr, four-lumen, double-balloon tube. The four lumens are used for gastric lavage and aspiration, esophageal aspiration, esophageal tamponade, and gastric tamponade. Medications may be instilled through the gastric lavage port. Lavage and gastric and esophageal suction may be performed while the balloon is inflated.

Before insertion, all balloons should be inflated and examined for defects. They should be checked for air leaks by submerging in water. The patient should be placed in a semi-Fowler's or left lateral position. If a Sengstaken-Blakemore tube is used, a nasogastric tube should be inserted above the esophageal balloon to provide esophageal suction. Intermittent suction should be attached to the nasogastric tube.

The lubricated balloon tube should be inserted through the patient's mouth or nose, and the position of the tube should be confirmed by x-ray examination. Gastric contents should be aspirated, and the gastric balloon should be inflated in increments of 100 ml of air until the balloon is full (250 to 500 ml for a Sengstaken-Blakemore tube; 450 to 500 ml for a Minnesota tube; and 700 to 800 ml for a Linton tube). If the patient complains of sudden substernal pain or if insufflation of air is not audible over the epigastric area, inflation should be stopped immediately.

Once the gastric balloon is inflated, the tube should be pulled back gently until resistance is felt against the gastroesophageal junction. The balloon inlet should be clamped, and the tube should be secured with 1 to 2 pounds of traction. Traction may be initiated by the use of a nasal sponge guard, an over-the-bed traction set-up with 1 pound of weight, and a football helmet or catcher's mask. External traction may cause ulceration of the nasal mucosa and should not be used for prolonged periods.

Suction should be connected to the gastric and esophageal lumens, and drainage from each port should be observed.

If bleeding continues after the gastric balloon is inflated, the esophageal balloon should be attached to a manometer and inflated with air to 25 to 45 mm Hg. The esophageal balloon inlet should be clamped, and the nasogastric tube should be changed to constant suction. If bleeding is clearly from esophageal varices above the gastroesophageal junction, the esophageal balloon may be inflated simultaneously with the gastric balloon. If bleeding continues during esophageal tamponade, it may be from a gastric varix.

The procedure for insertion of a Linton tube is the same as for a Sengstaken-Blakemore tube, except there is no esophageal balloon, and the esophageal suction lumen obviates the need for a secondary nasogastric tube. The Minnesota tube also has an esophageal suction lumen.

Regardless of the type of tube used, scissors should be taped to the head of the bed so they are within easy reach in case transection and emergency removal of the tube becomes necessary.

While the tube is in place it is important to check the traction on the tube regularly, monitor vital signs, irrigate the gastric tube as ordered and assess fluid return, recheck and adjust the esophageal balloon pressure every 2 hours, provide good oral care, and keep the patient NPO.

After 24 hours, if bleeding is controlled, the esophageal balloon should be deflated. The nurse should check for rebleeding per the physician's orders. The gastric balloon should be deflated if no bleeding recurs over the next 6 to 12 hours. Frequent oral care should be provided, and frequent coughing and deep breathing should be encouraged.

Potential complications of esophageal-gastric tamponade include aspiration, rupture of the esophagus from pressure secondary to a misplaced gastric balloon, tissue necrosis from excessive pressure and/or prolonged inflation time, and airway obstruction secondary to dislodgement of the esophageal tube.

NURSING CONSIDERATIONS

Nursing considerations for patients with GI bleeding require special attention. GI bleeding is usually the result of another, less obvious problem.

A thorough nursing history is of paramount importance. It is necessary to obtain as much information as possible about the patient's current health problems. In addition, a family health history can help to determine whether there is any family history of alcohol abuse or other problems that can cause GI bleeding. The patient's past and current work environments should be assessed to determine if exposure to chemicals or inhalants of any type might be a causative factor.

A physical assessment including weight, skin quality, and muscle tone provides data specific to the general appearance of the patient. Any discoloration of the skin should be documented. Joint Commission requirements include nutritional assessment, information which may be related to other concurrent disease processes.

Once a total physical assessment is completed and documented, the gastroenterology nurse can formulate the nursing diagnosis. Nursing diagnoses that may apply to patients with GI bleeding include the following:

(a) anxiety, related to uncertainty of prognosis, multiple diagnostic procedures, and treatment regimen;

(b) ineffective breathing pattern, related to decreased lung expansion, decreased energy, and fatigue;

(c) potential for injury: bleeding, related to altered clotting mechanisms;

(d) chronic low self-esteem, related to unknown etiology; and

(e) knowledge deficit with respect to treatment regimen.

The gastroenterology nurse must work with the patient and family members to identify outcomes that will be realistic for the patient. The overall goal is to prevent further damage and to improve the patient's overall physical and mental condition. Examples of desired outcomes for patients with GI bleeding might include the following:

(a) patient is free of injuries and bleeding;

(b) skin integrity is good;

(c) patient has normal respiratory function;

(d) family demonstrates support for patient; and

(e) patient is free of infection.

Patient care must be planned specifically for the individual patient. For patients with bleeding problems, it is important to implement nursing care that assists in controlling hemorrhage. Patient comfort is maintained by assessing the need for pain medication. Fluid and electrolyte status is constantly assessed. The patient and family members and/or significant others must be taught appropriate self-care techniques. Potential problems and solutions are reviewed. The patient should be made aware of helpful community resources.

CASE SITUATION

Mr. Ben Harrison, age 54, was offered an executive physical when he was promoted. As a routine part of his physical, a stool test was done to check for blood, and a flexible sigmoidoscopy was performed. The stool was positive for occult blood and a small polyp was found at 30 cm from the anus on sigmoidoscopy. Mr. Harrison's internist knows that findings of stool positive for occult blood and a polyp in the sigmoid may indicate a synchronous lesion higher in the large bowel. For this reason, he refers Mr. Harrison to the gastroenterology department for a colonoscopy.

Points to think about

1. Mr. Harrison exhibits the following signs and symptoms:
   (a) increased heart and respiratory rates;
   (b) increased systolic blood pressure;
   (c) profuse palmar sweating;
   (d) increased muscular tension;
   (e) urinary frequency and urgency; and
   (f) anger concerning need for various diagnostic tests.
   To what nursing diagnosis do these data seem most applicable?

2. What interventions might the gastroenterology nurse use before and during the colonoscopy to reduce Mr. Harrison's anxiety?

3. The procedure has started, and the doctor has passed the first small polyp at 30 cm. The patient is tolerating the procedure very well. As the doctor advances to the ascending colon, he finds a larger, more vascular appearing polyp. He moves on to the cecum, which is normal, and comes back to the ascending colon to remove the polyp. What are the responsibilities of the nurse operating the ESU?

4. The body uses its own mechanisms to achieve hemostasis. Three of these mechanisms are local reactions, which would be a response to cell disruption, as in a cut. What are they?

5. By what mechanism does electrosurgery help to provide hemostasis?

6. The heat produced by a monopolar electrode is dependent on four factors. What are they?

7. When using an electrocautery device during a procedure, what should the nurse chart on the record specific to electrocautery?

8. Colonoscopy with polypectomy is a safe, outpatient procedure. Barring any complication, Mr. Harrison will go home when he has recovered from sedation. What instructions will the nurse give him?

Suggested responses

1. The most applicable nursing diagnosis is anxiety related to threat to bodily health and lack of control over events.

2. Appropriate anxiety-reducing interventions the nurse may take might include the following:
   (a) Provide a relaxing, reassuring, professional atmosphere.
   (b) Discuss with Mr. Harrison the types of feelings he may experience during the examination, such as slight crampy abdominal pain caused by air insufflation or stretching of the bowel by moving the colonoscope.
   (c) Tell the patient that he or she will be there throughout the procedure to take care of his needs.
   (d) Speak softly to the patient during the procedure and rubbing his back gently.

3. The nurse responsible for the ESU should:
   (a) Set up and check the unit before the procedure and establish that it is working correctly.
   (b) Place the grounding pad on the patient (because the nurse is using a monopolar unit); disconnect the heart monitor, because it can be an alternate pathway for current (this is debatable, but better to be safe than sorry); and move the patient's hands and legs away from the side rails.
   (c) Be sure that the unit is plugged in, that all connections are secure, and that all personnel are wearing gloves.
   (d) Hand the snare to the physician to feed through the scope, and open and close the snare per the physician's instructions.
   (e) Once the polyp is removed, turn the machine to stand by while removing the snare.
   (f) Document site of polypectomy, placement of grounding pad, and ESU type and number.

4. The body's own mechanisms for achieving hemostasis include the following:
   (a) Vessel spasm. Vessels contract in an effort to diminish blood loss; spasm lasts from a few seconds to 30 minutes, so suspected bleeding vessels must be watched.
   (b) Platelet aggregation. Circulating platelets have an affinity for the moist, irregular endothelium that is exposed in a broken vessel and will adhere there, thus forming a platelet plug.

(c) Clot formation. Within seconds or minutes after damage, platelet aggregates and altered blood structure release activator substances; this triggers formation of fibrin threads, thus forming a network in which plasma and red blood cells can coalesce into a clot.

5. Electrosurgery helps provide hemostasis by the following mechanism: kinetic energy relayed to the cells from the ESU excites the ions in the cells, and they collide with other cellular particles, thereby creating heat in the cell. The effect on tissue is thermal, not electrical.

6. The heat produced by a monopolar electrode depends on the following factors:

(a) The power setting.

(b) Tissue resistance. The heat in the tissue increases in relation to the resistance of the tissue. Tissue with a lot of water content has low resistance. Dry tissue has higher resistance. When heat dries out the tissue, it may take a higher setting to continue cutting.

(c) Current density. Heat varies according to current density. When the snare loop is closed, it increases the current density and raises the temperature to the adjacent tissue. In the monopolar modality, the current density diminishes as it spreads out to the larger surface area of the dispersive electrode (grounding pad). If the surface area is large enough, the return electrode disperses the current and the patient does not feel the heat. If the large electrode were to come loose at the edges and have only a small contact with skin, the current density going to that small spot could be great enough to cause a burn.

(d) Time. The longer the physician depresses the foot pedal, the greater the heating depth will be.

7. When using an electrocautery device, the following should be documented:

(a) The equipment and accessories used, including brand name and whether it was monopolar or bipolar;

(b) A description of the lesion and any tissue that was recovered and sent to pathology;

(c) Machine settings and number of applications;

(d) How the lesion looked after heat application; any bleeding that is present; and

(e) How the patient tolerated the procedure; any complications.

8. Instructions the nurse should give Mr. Harrison when he goes home include the following:

(a) Do not drink alcohol, drive a car, or operate machinery until the next day.

(b) Observe any dietary or medication restrictions the physician has ordered; for instance, the use of aspirin or NSAIDs may be restricted after polypectomy because it interferes with blood clotting.

(c) Some bloating is normal because of the air instilled during the procedure and that it will subside as air is expelled.

(d) Call the physician if any rectal bleeding occurs, or if there is severe abdominal pain or temperature elevation.

REVIEW TERMS

argon, balloon tamponade, bipolar electrocoagulation, bipolar probe, coagulating current, coagulation, cutting current, desiccation, electrocautery, electrocoagulation, electrosurgical unit (ESU), endoscopic variceal ligation (EVL), fulguration, heater probe, laser, Linton tube, Minnesota tube, monopolar electrocoagulation, Nd:YAG, photocoagulation, photovaporization, sclerotherapy, Sengstaken-Blakemore tube, tamponade

REVIEW QUESTIONS

1. Thermal coagulation of bleeding vessels is achieved in gastroenterology patients by using:

(a) Monopolar electrocautery.

(b) Bipolar electrocautery.

(c) Lasers.

(d) All of the above.

2. Leakage of current in monopolar electrocoagulation can cause burns to the:

(a) Endoscopist.

(b) Patient.

(c) Nurse/associate.

(d) All of the above.

3. When using bipolar electrocoagulation, all of the following are true *except:*

(a) There is less mucosal injury than monopolar.

(b) A grounding pad is needed.

(c) Silicone prevents tissue adherence.

(d) Perforation is a potential complication.

4. The type of laser used most often in endoscopic applications is:

(a) Carbon dioxide.

(b) Nd:YAG.

(c) Argon.

(d) KTP/532.

5. Laser fibers used in endoscopic applications are cleaned with:

(a) Alcohol.

(b) Glutaraldehyde.

(c) Hydrogen peroxide.

(d) Sterile water.

6. The specialized three-lumen tube with esophageal and gastric balloons that is used for esophageal-gastric tamponade is called a:

(a) Sengstaken-Blakemore tube.

(b) Linton tube.

(c) Minnesota tube.

(d) Salem sump tube.

7. In esophageal-gastric tamponade, the esophageal balloon should be inflated to what pressure?

(a) 2.5 to 4.5 mm Hg.

(b) 25 to 45 mm Hg.

(c) 125 to 145 mm Hg.

(d) 1 psi.

8. The first line of treatment in patients with actively bleeding esophageal varices is usually:

    (a) IV vasopressin (Pitressin).

    (b) Balloon tamponade.

    (c) Injection sclerotherapy.

    (d) Electrocoagulation.

9. Severe chest pain that persists for more than 24 hours in patients who have undergone sclerotherapy for esophageal varices is most likely a result of:

    (a) Myocardial infarction.

    (b) Residual effects of the sclerosing agent.

    (c) Aspiration pneumonia.

    (d) Perforation.

10. Which of the following statements is *false?*

    (a) Esophageal varices can be treated with sclerotherapy.

    (b) Multiple-band ligation is often complicated by overtube trauma.

    (c) Gastric varices do not respond well to invasive treatments.

    (d) Eradication of varices may require an average of 5 sessions.

BIBLIOGRAPHY

Chen, P., Wu, C. & Liaw, Y. (1986). Hemostatic effect of endoscopic local injection with hypertonic saline-epinephrine solution and pure ethanol for digestive tract bleeding. *Gastrointest Endosc 32*, 319-23. Gastrointestinal Endoscopy.

Dennison, A. (1989). The management of hemorrhoids. *Am J Gastroenterol 84*, 475-81. American Journal of Gastroenterology.

Fleischer, D. (1988). BICAP tumor probe therapy for esophageal cancer: a practical guide. *Endosc Rev 5*, 2-13. Endoscopy Review.

Fleischer, D. (1988). The therapeutic use of lasers in GI disease. In Trivits, S. (Ed.), *SGA Journal Reprints*. Rochester, NY: Society of Gastrointestinal Assistants.

Grossweiner, L.J. (1995). Photodynamic therapy. *J Laser Appl 7*, 51-7.

Gruber, M. & Camara, D. (1988). Injection sclerotherapy: seven years' experience. In Trivits, S. (Ed.), *SGA Journal Reprints*. Rochester, NY: Society of Gastrointestinal Assistants.

Heier, S.K. (1994). Photodynamic therapy for esophageal malignancies. In Barkin, J.S. (Ed.). *Advanced therapeutic endoscopy* (2nd ed.). Philadelphia: Lippincott-Raven.

Henderson, B.W. & Dougherty, T.J. (1992). How does photodynamic therapy work? *Photochem Photobiol 55*(1), 145-57.

Kirby, D. (1989). Management of esophageal varices: a review of treatment options and the role of the gastroenterology nurse and associate. *Gastroenterol Nurs 12*, 10-4. Gastroenterology Nursing.

Laine, L. & Peterson, W. (1994). Bleeding peptic ulcer. *Med Prog 331*, 717-27.

Lightdale, C. (1995). Photodynamic therapy with porfimer sodium versus thermal ablation therapy with Nd:YAG laser for palliation of esophageal cancer: a multicenter randomized trial. *Gastrointest Endosc 42*(6), 507-12. Gastrointestinal Endoscopy.

McFarland, P. & McFarlane, J. (1997). (Ed.), *Nursing diagnosis and intervention*. (3rd Edition) St. Louis, MO: Mosby.

Palmer, K.R. & Choudari, C.P. (1995). Endoscopic intervention in bleeding peptic ulcer. *Gut 37*, 161-4. Schapiro, M. (1989). The gastroenterologist and the treatment of hemorrhoids: is it about time? *Am J Gastroenterol 84*, 493-5. American Journal of Gastroenterology.

Sheck, P. (1988). GI assistant's role in laser therapy. In Trivits, S. (Ed.), *SGA Journal Reprints*. Rochester, NY: Society of Gastrointestinal Assistants.

Shields, N. (1988). The role of the GIA in electrosurgery. In Trivits, S. (Ed.), *SGA Journal Reprints*. Rochester, NY: Society of Gastrointestinal Assistants.

Short, N. (1989). Gastrointestinal intubations: nursing considerations. *Gastroenterol Nurs 12*, 43-9. Gastroenterology Nursing.

Silvis, S. (Ed.) (1985). *Therapeutic gastrointestinal endoscopy*. New York: Igaku-Shoin.

Sleisenger, M. & Fordtran, J. (Eds.) (2000). *Gastrointestinal disease: pathophysiology, diagnosis, management* (7th ed.). Philadelphia: W.B. Saunders.

Society of Gastroenterology Nurses and Associates, Inc. (2000). *Manual of Gastrointestinal Procedures* (4th ed.). Chicago, IL.

Swartz, M., Carey, K. & Danzi, J. (1989). Laser therapy of the gastric lesions of the Osler-Weber-Rendu syndrome, *SGA J 12*, 143-4. Society of Gastrointestinal Assistants.

Tytgat, G.N.J. & Classen, M. (Eds.) (1994). *The practice of therapeutic endoscopy*. New York: Churchill Livingstone.

Waye, J. Geenen, J.E., Fleischer, D. (1987). *Techniques in therapeutic endoscopy*. Philadelphia: W.B. Saunders.

Williams, S. & Westaby, D. (1995). Recent advances in the management of variceal bleeding. *Gut 36*, 647-8.

Zinberg, S. (1989). A personal experience in comparing three nonoperative techniques for treating internal hemorrhoids. *Am J Gastroenterol 84*, 488-92. American Journal of Gastroenterology.

All techniques in this chapter, except bipolar ablation of obstructing GI tumors, are also discussed in:

Society of Gastroenterology Nurses and Associates, Inc. (2003). *Manual of Gastrointestinal Procedures* (5th ed.). Chicago, IL.

Chapter 29

INTUBATION AND DRAINAGE

This chapter will acquaint the gastroenterology nurse with indications, contraindications, and techniques for GI intubation and drainage. A variety of intubation and drainage procedures are covered, including nasogastric intubation, gastric lavage, insertion of nasobiliary/nasopancreatic catheters, biliary and pancreatic duct stent placement, intestinal intubation, colon decompression, abdominal paracentesis, and endoscopic placement of self-expanding metal stents (SEMS).

Intubation for esophageal-gastric tamponade is discussed in Chapter 28. The use of feeding tubes and percutaneous endoscopic gastrostomy/jejunostomy (PEG/PEJ) devices for long-term enteral nutrition are discussed in Chapter 22.

Learning objectives

After reviewing the content of this chapter, the gastroenterology nurse should be able to:

1. Discuss techniques for the insertion of nasogastric and nasoenteric tubes.
2. Explain indications and techniques for the insertion of esophageal prostheses.
3. Describe the use of nasobiliary/nasopancreatic catheters and biliary/pancreatic stents.
4. Discuss procedures for gastric lavage, colonic decompression, and abdominal paracentesis.
5. Identify the indications for endoscopic metal stent placement and discuss special nursing care before, during, and after self-expanding metal stent placement.

NASOGASTRIC TUBE INSERTION

Nasogastric intubation is indicated for the following:
(a) treatment of gastric distention or gastric outlet obstruction;
(b) assessment and treatment of upper GI bleeding;
(c) certain gastric/esophageal tests;
(d) gastric lavage;

(e) aspiration of gastric secretions;
(f) administration of medications and feedings;
(g) prevention of vomiting by decompressing the stomach after major surgery; and
(h) emptying the upper GI tract before emergency surgery.

Insertion of a **nasogastric tube** must be performed cautiously in pregnant patients and in patients with an aortic aneurysm, recent myocardial infarction, gastric hemorrhage, or esophageal varices. It is contraindicated in patients with nasopharyngeal or esophageal obstruction, severe maxillofacial trauma, or severe uncontrolled coagulopathy.

The diameter of nasogastric tubes used for normal adults is usually 14 or 16 Fr and 55 to 66 cm in length. When choosing a nasogastric tube for a pediatric patient, consider the size of the child and the reason for the tube. Feedings of thick formulas require a larger tube than feedings of thin formulas. Nasogastric suction requires a larger tube, especially if blood or clots are present. A wide range of diameters is available (i.e., 3.5 Fr for neonates; 5, 8, 10, and 12 Fr for children of all age-groups). Smaller diameter tubes are appropriate (and more comfortable) for children who require long-term nasogastric intubation. The length of tubing needed to reach the stomach should be determined by placing the end of the tube at the tip of the patient's earlobe and extending it to the nose and down to the xiphoid process.

The most commonly used nasogastric tubes are the Levin tube, the Salem sump tube, and extended-use nasogastric feeding tubes.

1. The **Levin tube** has only one lumen. If a vacuum forms, causing the tube to adhere to the stomach lining, the gastric mucosa may be damaged. Intermittent low suction is recommended for the Levin tube.
2. The **Salem sump tube** has a primary suction-drainage lumen and a smaller vent lumen. Continuous airflow through the vent lumen prevents a vacuum from forming. When a Salem sump tube is used with suction, the

larger lumen is connected to the suction equipment. Intermittent high suction or continuous low suction may be used with the Salem sump tube.

3. **Extended-use nasogastric feeding tubes** are made of soft, flexible plastic material, with either a weighted or unweighted tip. They may require use of a guidewire to facilitate insertion. Some manufacturers state that the tube may be left in place for up to 30 days before requiring replacement.

4. The **Moss tube** is a double lumen tube with a gastric retention balloon, a port for distal duodenal feedings and several esophageal, gastric and proximal duodenal aspiration ports.

5. The **Compat tube** is a 9fr nasojejunal feeding tube combined with an 18fr gastric suction port lumen. The gastric port serves for decompression and drainage as well as providing a port to administer medications. Refer to manufacturer's instructions for placement options.

Before insertion of a nasogastric tube, the patient or caregiver should be questioned regarding any history of nasal surgery, fractures, or a deviated septum and to verify the length of the patient's NPO status. Small children may require bundling or being held for tube insertion. Children who are unable to cooperate by sitting up should be held supine.

To facilitate insertion, a limp rubber tube may be placed on ice for about 3 minutes, or a stiff plastic tube may be softened by immersion in warm water. The tube should be inserted in the nostril with the greatest airflow while the patient is in a high Fowler's or left lateral decubitus position. Before insertion the nostrils should be examined for any obvious obstruction. To determine which nostril has the greatest airflow, the nurse should perform the following activities:

1. Question the patient about any previous nasal surgery, trauma, or a deviated septum.

2. Inspect the nostrils with a penlight for any obvious obstruction.

3. Occlude one nostril at a time while the patient breathes through the nose.

A topical anesthetic should be applied if ordered. Dentures should be removed so they will not be dislocated if the patient gags. While wearing disposable gloves, the nurse should lubricate the nasogastric tube with a water-soluble lubricant. With the patient's head tilted slightly back, the tube should be inserted into the nostril and rotated gently toward the center. When the tube is in the back of the patient's throat, the chin should be tipped toward the chest to close the trachea and open the esophagus. If the patient's condition or test permits, the patient may sip water through a bendable straw while the tube is guided gently down the esophagus and into the antrum. The tube should then be taped to the nose. To confirm correct placement:

1. Ask the patient to talk. If the patient cannot talk, the tube may be coiled in the throat or may have passed through the vocal cords.

2. Use a tongue depressor and penlight to confirm that the tube is not curled in the mouth or throat, especially in unconscious patients.

3. Inject air through the tube and use a stethoscope to auscultate a "whooshing" sound just below the xiphoid process. If the patient belches, the tube may be in the esophagus.

4. Attempt to aspirate the stomach contents.

5. Perform an x-ray examination or fluoroscopy.

If the patient coughs frequently or experiences dyspnea during insertion, the tube should be removed immediately because it may be in the trachea or coiled in the pharynx.

Once proper placement is confirmed, the tube should be clamped or attached to intermittent suction or gravity drainage, or feeding as ordered by the physician. Do not tape until placement has been confirmed.

In some patients, such as those with a deviated septum, the tube can be placed orally. In such cases, the distal tip of the tube should be placed on the back of the patient's tongue. The patient should be asked to tip the chin toward the chest and swallow, keeping the upper and lower teeth slightly apart. If the patient is unconscious or cannot swallow for any reason, the tube should be advanced between respirations. It may be helpful to stroke the patient's neck to facilitate passage down the esophagus. Again, the tube should be inserted gently with each swallow.

After insertion the tube should be taped to the nose with adhesive tape. A pin or tape will support the weight of the tube on the patient's clothing. Adequate tubing should be used to allow the patient free movement and turning. Taping the tubing just below the naris (as opposed to in an upward direction) reduces friction and damage to the nose. Also, a manufactured tube holder may be used to secure the tube. Refer to the manufacturer's instructions for specific directions on application.

Patency of the tube should be confirmed periodically by irrigating with normal saline. The frequency of irrigation and the amount of solution should be specified by the physician. Fluid inserted during irrigation should be removed and measured.

The nares should be cleansed, and the tube should be retaped as necessary. Mouth care should be provided once a shift or as necessary. Depending on the patient's condition, lemon-glycerin swabs may be used to clean the teeth, or the patient may brush them. The lips should be coated with petroleum jelly to prevent dryness. The patient may be allowed to chew gum, suck on hard candy, or use throat lozenges to promote comfort, if indicated by patient condition and physician order.

When nasogastric suction is used, bowel sounds should be assessed regularly to check GI function. The color, consistency, and odor of gastric drainage should be observed. Normal gastric secretions are colorless or yellow-green from bile and have a mucoid consistency. Gastric drainage that has the color of coffee grounds may be an indication of bleeding and should be reported immediately. Nausea, vomiting, a feeling of fullness, epigastric discomfort, and distention may be indications that the tube is not patent. Patients should also be observed for fluid and electrolyte imbalances. In critically ill patients, periodically remove tape and rotate tube gently, then retape. This helps prevent serous mucosal breakdown. Repositioning the tip may lessen the chance of gastric bleeding due to chronic suction in one area.

If medications are to be instilled through the tube, it is important to irrigate the tube before and after instillation. Suction should be omitted for 30 to 45 minutes after instillation to permit absorption of the medication.

Before removing a nasogastric tube, it should be flushed with a small amount of air to clear the tube of stomach contents that would cause irritation during removal. The tube should be untaped from the patient's nose, and the patient should be instructed not to breathe to ensure closure of the epiglottis. The tube should be withdrawn gently and steadily until the distal end reaches the nasopharynx, when it can be pulled quickly. If possible, the tube should be quickly covered and removed. The patient should be assisted with mouth care, and tape residue should be cleaned from the nose with adhesive remover. If signs of GI dysfunction recur, reinsertion of the tube may be necessary.

Potential complications of nasogastric tube insertion include respiratory distress caused by incorrect tube placement, pulmonary aspiration, epistaxis (nosebleed), necrosis of the nasal mucous membrane caused by incorrect taping of the tube, skin erosion at the nostril, sinusitis, esophagitis, esophagotracheal fistula, gastric ulceration, pulmonary and oral infection, and esophageal or gastric hemorrhage or perforation. An additional complication of nasogastric intubation is otitis media caused by eustachian tube irritation. The use of suction can cause electrolyte imbalance and dehydration.

ESOPHAGEAL PROSTHESES

To provide a patent lumen for purposes of nourishment and oral secretions in patients with terminal, obstructive esophageal cancer, a prosthesis may be inserted endoscopically through the obstruction. For tracheal-esophageal fistula, a prosthetic may be inserted to cover the TE fistula and control aspiration of oral secretions into the lungs.

Until the early 1990s, esophageal prostheses were made of latex or silicone rubber, polyvinyl chloride or other plastics. With the advent of Self Expanding Metal Stents (SEMS), these are no longer used. The SEMS are much easier to insert and are far superior to the rigid tubes of the past.

Indications include circumferential stenosis resulting from malignant carcinoma of the lower two thirds of the esophagus when dysphagia becomes a problem, and esophageal-pulmonary fistulas or extrinsics compression of the esophagus.

Contraindications include the following:
(a) when another medical condition takes priority;
(b) for cancers that are less than 2 cm below the upper esophageal sphincter;
(c) if tumor invasion compresses the trachea and/or bronchus;
(d) if the stricture cannot be adequately dilated; and

(e) in uncooperative or unmotivated patients.

Before insertion, patient must be NPO for 2-8 hours. The nurse should assess the patient for any indication of cardiopulmonary compromise, establish a patent IV, administer antibiotics as ordered, and remove dentures. The patient should be informed that the stent will cause the feeling of pressure in the chest as it expands over a few days.

The patient should be placed in the left lateral position. The throat should be anesthetized as ordered. The G.I. nurse's responsibilities are to provide emotional support to the patient, maintain the oral airway and manage oral secretions, assist the physician, monitor vital signs, observe the color, warmth, and dryness of the patient's skin, and monitor the patients level of consciousness, pain and respiratory status. A GI technician or second nurse should provide careful assistance to the physician in prosthesis placement. The primary RN should monitor the patient as indicated.

The esophageal lumen should be dilated to accommodate the SEMS and will be specified in the instructions. The amount of dilitation is minimal in comparison to the amount required to insert the rigid plastic stents used in the past.

The area to be stented is identified and marked using an injection catheter and contrast. The distal margin and the proximal margin are injected. Measurements are taken and appropriate stent is chosen.

Stents are available in various lengths and are either coated or non-coated. Once the appropriate size is determined, the stent should be placed using the manufacturer's instructions.

Fluoroscopy is used to confirm the position of the stent and to rule out perforation. When the effects of sedation have worn off, contrast medium may be used to confirm that there is no perforation.

Post-procedure monitoring should include vital signs, symptoms of compromised respirations, respiratory depression, aspiration, bleeding, signs or symptoms of perforation. The patient should be NPO except for ice chips for several hours, after which liquids can be started. The following day the diet may be advanced to a soft diet. When the stent crosses the GE junction, the patient is treated with antacids and/or H_2 blocker or proton pump inhibitors and antireflux measures.

After discharge, the patient ingests a regular diet with proper dentition. They must chew well and drink liquids often during the meal.

Potential early complications of inserting an esophageal stent include perforation, necrosis, or bleeding retrosternal pain. Later complications may include food bolus obstruction secondary to tumor overgrowth, or esophagitis secondary to efflux if the prosthesis extends across the GE junction.

GASTRIC LAVAGE

Gastric **lavage** involves insertion of a gastric tube through the nose or mouth. It is indicated in patients with acute GI bleeding, when preparing the stomach for endoscopy after barium or food ingestion, and for evacuating the stomach after ingestion of toxic substances. In patients with acute GI bleeding, lavage gives a good indication of the rapidity of bleeding, cleanses the stomach before endoscopy, and, in patients with cirrhosis, removes blood to lessen the likelihood of hepatic encephalopathy. A smaller-diameter nasogastric tube is used to localize the bleeding. A large-bore (often in sizes 30 to 36 Fr) tube is placed orally for instillation of aliquots of fluid and removal of residual gastric contents.

Gastric lavage is contraindicated in patients with possible esophageal or gastric perforation, known esophageal obstruction, or maxillofacial trauma. It is also contraindicated after ingestion of corrosive substances, such as lye and some cleaning compounds, because the nasogastric tube may perforate the esophagus. When gastric lavage is performed in conjunction with an esophagogastroduodenoscopy (EGD), an overtube may be used to isolate the esophagus from the airway. This is particularly advisable if the patient is sedated, because it decreases the potential for aspiration of gastric contents or lavage solution.

The setup required for gastric lavage includes a container of irrigation solution to which is attached a piece of tubing ending in a Y-connector. One side of the Y-connector is attached to the patient's nasogastric or orogastric tube, and the other side is attached to another piece of tubing that is connected to a calibrated collection container.

A number of gastric tubes are available including:

1. The basic **double-lumen orogastric "stomach pump" tube** is indicated in situations where intermittent gastric lavage and evacuation are required. The larger lumen is used for evacuation of gastric contents, and the smaller lumen is used for instillation of an irrigant. It is especially suitable for emergency removal of toxic agents, overdose of oral medications, or ingestion of hazardous substances. Activated charcoal slurries may be administered through the large suction lumen. In situations where there is a high risk of aspiration, such as loss of consciousness, seizures, or delirium, a cuffed endotracheal tube should be inserted before insertion of the double-lumen tube.

2. The **single-lumen tube** with several openings at the distal end is usually passed orally, but it can be inserted nasally. Single-lumen tubes allow rapid lavage and evacuation of large volumes of fluid, but continuous irrigation is not possible because the same lumen must be used for both instillation and evacuation of fluid. During an emergency the single-lumen tube may be used to aspirate large amounts of gastric contents quickly.

Before inserting a gastric tube for lavage it is important to obtain baseline vital signs, ensure an adequate airway, and establish a large-bore IV line for volume replacement as ordered. Patients should be informed that the tube may cause some gagging, but they will be able to breathe. The importance of remaining on the left side should be emphasized.

The patient should be placed in the left lateral position. If a nasogastric tube is being used, the patient may be in Fowler's position. The nasogastric intubation procedure just described should be used for inserting a nasogastric tube. If the tube is inserted orally, the well-lubricated tube should be guided into the back of the mouth while the patient is encouraged to suck on the tube and swallow. To check tube placement, 20 to 40 ml of air (5 ml in children) should be injected, and the epigastric area should be auscultated with a stethoscope. Before instilling any irrigation solution, the stomach contents should be aspirated to ensure correct placement. If the patient begins to cough or experiences dyspnea, the tube may be in the trachea. The tube should be removed immediately and another insertion attempted. It is important to provide frequent patient reassurance and support during the procedure.

The irrigating solution container is hung from the highest level of an IV pole. The inflow tube is unclamped and 250 ml of irrigation is instilled gradually to evaluate the patient's tolerance and prevent vomiting. (Iced saline lavage is no longer recommended, because it has a tendency to lower the patient's core temperature.) After instillation, continuous negative pressure should be applied with a syringe or by removing the clamp on the outflow tube, thereby allowing the fluid to flow via gravity into a collection container that is lower than the patient's head. The procedure should be repeated, increasing the amount of irrigating solution to 500 ml, until the return is clear, or of acceptable clarity. In patients with upper GI bleeding, lavage should be continued until bleeding stops or until it becomes evident that other measures will be necessary. If the amount instilled is significantly greater than the amount recovered, the tube should be repositioned.

The patient should never be left alone during gastric lavage. He or she should be observed continuously for changes in level of consciousness, and vital signs should be monitored frequently. Throughout lavage, frequent suctioning of the oral cavity may be needed to prevent aspiration. When lavaging the stomach after ingestion of poisons or drugs, all return fluid should be saved for possible laboratory analysis.

When the return is of acceptable clarity, the tube should be withdrawn slowly, and aspiration of any fluid in the stomach or esophagus should be continued. The patient should exhale slowly as the tube is withdrawn.

Potential complications of gastric lavage include aspiration of gastric contents, which is most likely to occur in groggy patients; perforation; electrolyte imbalance from prolonged lavage; and hemorrhage. Bradyarrhythmias may also occur. If the gastric tube becomes clogged, unrelieved gastric distention may occur, thus leading to potentially fatal shock.

NASOBILIARY/NASOPANCREATIC CATHETERS

Nasobiliary catheters (NBCs) and **nasopancreatic catheters (NPCs)** are used for short-term decompression or perfusion within the biliary and pancreatic ductal systems. These catheters are long, thin polyethylene tubes that are placed endoscopically over a guidewire into the common bile duct or the pancreatic duct. In this procedure, the use of the terms "proximal" and "distal" are used opposite from other procedures. The distal end of the catheter is placed within the duct of choice. The proximal end of the tube is routed from the duct, through the duodenal bulb, stomach, and esophagus, exiting the patient's mouth. It is then rerouted from the patient's mouth, through the patient's nose, and connected to a drainage bag (see section on nasocatheter placement technique).

The tips of these catheters vary. NBCs come with either a pigtail or straight tip, whereas the NPCs only come in a straight tip. Both catheters have side ports that are placed within the duct to facilitate drainage and to prevent reflux from the duodenum.

Nasobiliary catheter

Indications for NBC placement include the following:
(a) Decompression of an obstructed bile duct in acute suppurative cholangitis.
(b) Temporary or short-term decompression of the common bile duct, similar to that which follows unsuccessful stone extraction after endoscopic sphincterotomy.
(c) Prevention of stone impaction after endoscopic sphincterotomy.
(d) Infusion of contrast medium for repeat cholangiography.
(e) Instillation of various therapeutic solutions, including monooctanoin (Moctanin, used for gallstone dissolution), antibiotics (for acute bacterial cholangitis), corticosteroids (for sclerosing cholangitis), or saline (to flush sludge or small stones after endoscopic sphincterotomy).
(f) Preoperative biliary decompression to decrease jaundice (thereby decreasing perioperative complications) in patients undergoing elective biliary tract surgery.
(g) Temporary biliary decompression in patients who are septic or who have severe coagulopathy. Once infection has been controlled or coagulopathy corrected, sphincterotomy can be performed, and a large stent can be inserted for long-term therapy.
(h) Access for intraluminal irradiation therapy.
(i) Aspiration of bile for chemical and bacteriological studies (e.g., to identify causative agents in bacterial cholangitis or to determine the lithogenicity of bile in patients with cholestasis).
(j) Facilitating the healing process in traumatic or surgical biliary fistulas.
(k) Management of common bile duct stones. NBC is used to outline the common bile duct for targeting the stones.

Nasobiliary catheter placement is contraindicated in patients with coagulopathy, sepsis, active pancreatitis or other infection, recent food ingestion, or any other contraindication to EGD. Some physicians will insert an NBC in the presence of the first three contraindications, if leaving the patient untreated would cause further harm.

Nasopancreatic catheter

Indications for NPC placement include the following:
(a) repeated or traumatic cannulation of the pancreatic duct;
(b) decompression and drainage of a pancreatic pseudocyst;
(c) postendoscopic balloon or catheter dilatation, or endoscopic sphincterotomy of the pancreatic duct;
(d) treatment of pancreatic duct stone during extracorporeal shock-wave lithotripsy; and
(e) infusion of contrast medium for repeated pancreatogram without scope insertion;

Nasobiliary/nasopancreatic catheter placement

The procedure endoscopic retrograde cholangiopancreatography (ERCP) is performed with the side viewing scope. A cholangiogram and/or pancreatogram is obtained. Once a diagnosis is confirmed and a decision to place an NBC or NPC is made, the procedure is conducted as follows.

Endoscopic sphincterotomy is optional. The duct of choice is cannulated, and a guidewire is inserted through the existing cannula. Once the guidewire is properly positioned, the cannula is withdrawn by the physician using fluoroscopic guidance while the nurse or associate continues to feed/advance the guidewire to maintain wire position within the duct. The gastroenterologist and the assistant must be diligent in matching movements to ensure the wire does not perforate the liver capsule, perforate the substance of the pancreas, or loop in the duodenum (which could cause the guidewire to whip out of the duct).

The portion of the guidewire that now protrudes from the duodenoscope is wiped with a moistened gauze pad. The nasocatheter of choice is selected and flushed with sterile saline or sterile water before passage so that it slides more easily over the guidewire. The physician advances the catheter over the guidewire, through the scope, and into position within the duct as the nurse or associate applies gentle back pressure to the guidewire. Fluoroscopy is utilized to check guidewire and catheter position throughout placement.

Once the NBC or NPC is in proper position within the desired duct, the guidewire is removed. The physician begins to feed/advance the catheter through the biopsy/accessory channel as the nurse or associate withdraws the endoscope in 1- to 2-cm increments. The NBC or NPC should remain stationary throughout the scope removal. When the end of the endoscope is visible in the patient's mouth, the endoscope and mouth guard are removed. At this point the NBC or NPC proximal tip is within the duct of choice, and the distal portion exits the patient's mouth.

The NBC or NPC is then rerouted through the patient's nose to allow normal ingestions of foods and liquids while the nasocatheter is in place. A specially designed 25- to 30-cm 14 Fr nasopharyngeal tube is advanced through the nose and brought out through the patient's mouth. The end of the NBC or NPC is threaded inside the oral end of the nasopharyngeal tube and advanced until it exits through the nasal end of the larger tube. The tube in the oropharynx is held firmly by the endoscopist or assistant to maintain its position during withdrawal through the nose, thereby preventing dislodgement of the drainage tube from the bile or pancreatic duct. The nasopharyngeal tube is then withdrawn slowly through the nostril until the tip of the NBC or NPC emerges from the nose. The nasopharyngeal tube is discarded. The excess portion of the NBC or NPC at the nose is transected and a Luer-lok valve is attached, creating an adapter for an appropriate biliary tract drainage system. The end of the NBC or NPC is taped to the cheek and connected to a drainage bag.

An NBC or NPC can remain in place indefinitely and will provide continuous access to the biliary tree or pancreatic duct. Two to four hours after the procedure, the patient may be permitted a diet as ordered.

Following insertion of the NBC or NPC, it is important to monitor and record the patient's vital signs; observe the patient for abdominal pain or distention; administer antibiotics as ordered; tape the NBC or NPC to the patient's cheek, avoiding sharp angles and kinks; and place adapters and a drainage bag on the catheter and secure the apparatus to the patient's gown, allowing enough tubing to prevent traction when the patient turns his or her head. The patient may experience some minor throat discomfort, and green or yellow fluid may appear in the tube. Some movement of the tube is to be expected during eating and drinking.

To check tube patency, strict tube output is monitored every shift. The physician should be notified if no output is recorded, because this could indicate tube position shift (or resolution of a leak if used for bile duct decompression in common bile duct injuries). On occasion, the bile collected from this tube will be fed back to the patient to prevent bile salt depletion.

In addition to the complications that are associated with ERCP, endoscopic sphincterotomy, or insertion of biliary stents, potential complications of inserting an NBC or NPC include blockage of the catheter, nasal irritation, and sore throat. Minor complications can be managed by proper care of the nostril and use of throat lozenges and mild analgesics. To prevent mucus from plugging the side holes of the NBC or NPC, it may be helpful to irrigate the NBC or NPC with 10 ml sterile saline every 3 to 4 hours. To straighten out a kink, a guidewire may be passed through the entire NBC or NPC under fluoroscopic control, followed by irrigation. If this fails, the NBC or NPC must be replaced.

If irrigations are ordered to maintain patency, they should be performed with slow, gentle pressure to avoid driving stone fragments or infected bile into the intrahepatics (in the case of a nasobiliary tube); when the tube is in the pancreatic ducts, excessive injection pressure could force pancreatic secretions into the ascini of the pancreas, leading to pancreatitis.

BILIARY STENTS

To provide palliative biliary drainage, a thin, hollow Teflon or polyethylene tube can be placed endoscopically during ERCP (Fig. 29-1). The objective of a biliary stent or endoprosthesis is to create a bridge between two normal anatomical sites that bypasses the diseased or obstructed portion of the duct.

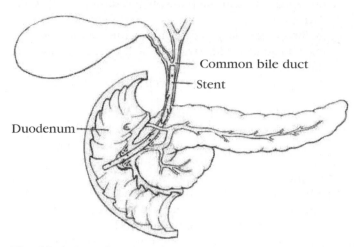

Fig. 29-1. Straight stent placement in common bile duct, draining to duodenum.

Two basic types of **biliary stents** are currently in use; the pigtail stent and the barbed stent. The length of the stent between the barbs may be 5 to 15 cm (2 to 6 inches), and the outside circumference ranges from 5 to 12 Fr. The scope channel size must accommodate the diameter of the stent. Each stent is provided with a number of side holes to facilitate drainage.

1. In the 5- or 7-Fr **pigtail stent,** one or both ends of the tube are coiled. This coiled shape disappears when the stent is pulled taut but quickly returns when allowed to relax. Pigtail stents can be introduced through a lateral-viewing endoscope. Because of a small diameter, these stents provide inadequate drainage in many cases and are used primarily to facilitate drainage when unremovable intraductal stones are present.

2. **Barbed stents** have projections, or "barbs," at each end that result from a diagonal cut of the stent wall. They range in size from 7 to 12 Fr and can be inserted by using lateral-viewing endoscopes. Barbed stents are used primarily for strictures of the common and/or pancreatic duct. Barbed stents have been shown to decrease morbidity; maintain their position with infrequent dislodgement; provide maximal flow; and decrease the risk for occlusion by sludge, stones, or tumor.

Regardless of the type of stent used, one end of the tube is seated above the ductal obstruction, and the other end protrudes into the duodenum. The configuration of the stent itself serves to secure it. The purpose of the stent is to allow free drainage or transhepatic **decompression.**

Placement of a biliary stent is indicated for the following:
  (a) relief of obstructive jaundice in patients with benign or malignant strictures of the bile duct;
  (b) palliative treatment of inoperable or metastatic pancreatic or periampullary neoplasms;
  (c) preoperative decompression to decrease complications associated with high bilirubin levels;
  (d) prevention of stone impaction in the ampulla in patients who are at high risk for surgery and have had

unsuccessful endoscopic sphincterotomy and stone extraction;

(e) maintaining biliary decompression in cases of sclerosing cholangitis with stricture of the extrahepatic bile ducts;

(f) protecting the area into which a biliary fistula drains; and

(g) postcholecystectomy Biliary leak (CBD).

Insertion of a biliary stent is associated with few major complications, a decreased incidence of procedure-related mortality, and a reduced number of hospital days.

Before the procedure it is important to determine whether the patient has had biliary surgery in the past. At least two gastroenterology nurses/associates will assist with the procedure; a nurse monitors the patient, and a nurse or associate assists the endoscopist. Endoscopy staff must be knowledgeable of labeling on stent packaging which reflects circumference first, and length second.

ERCP is performed first, to define the level and extent of the obstruction. A 5-mm sphincterotomy may be performed to allow easier passage of the stent (especially larger stents) and/or to facilitate drainage.

When placing a 5- or 7-Fr stent, a cannula is passed through a side-viewing duodenoscope with at least a 2.8-mm instrument channel and into the diseased duct. A 480-cm guidewire is passed through the cannula. The cannula is removed over the guidewire, which remains in place. The portion of the guidewire that protrudes from the duodenoscope is wiped with a gauze pad dampened with sterile saline or sterile water to remove residual contrast medium.

The stent is advanced over the guidewire, followed by a pusher tube that is the same diameter as the stent but of a different color. Once the stent has bypassed the obstructed area, the pusher tube and the guidewire are slowly removed. These maneuvers are all performed under fluoroscopic guidance. At this point, the distal end of the stent anchors itself in the duct, the midportion of the stent traverses the obstruction, and the proximal end lies free in the duodenum. Once the continuity of the duct is reestablished, the patient's condition should improve.

When placing a stent that is 10, 11.5, or 12 Fr, a guide catheter is used. A guide catheter is a long, polyethylene tube with a tapered tip. Most guide catheters measure 350 cm in length and 6 to 8 Fr. Guide catheters with increasing diameters are available to progressively dilate strictures to pass larger stents.

The guide catheter is passed over the guidewire through the channel of a 4.2-mm channel duodenoscope. The endoscopist guides the catheter through the stricture. A stent of predetermined size is passed over the guide catheter, followed by a pusher tube of the same size. The pusher tube should slide freely over the guide catheter but not over the stent. The stent is advanced over the guide catheter, into the common bile duct, and through the stricture. The properly positioned stent should protrude 1 cm into the duodenum. The gastroenterolgy nurse or assistant must assist the

endoscopist with coordinated movements and constant tension on the guidewire and guide catheter. After proper placement is determined, the pusher tube, guide catheter, and guidewire are slowly removed. Bile mixed with contrast medium should immediately escape through the stent. The guide catheter has radiopague markers on one end, which must be passed over the guidewire first. If not, the physician cannot utilize the markers for proper stent placement. Special attention to this item applies if repeated attempts are made to place the stent.

Because endoscopic placement of biliary stents can be a lengthy process, it is important to use as little fluoroscopy as possible during the procedure. To simplify stent placement, decrease fluoroscopy time, and therefore shorten overall procedure time, manufacturers have developed one-step stent kits. These stent-placement devices are preassembled guiding catheters and pusher tubes that feed directly over the guidewire. Some are preloaded with a stent as well. Those without a stent must have a stent backloaded onto the distal tip of the delivery device (the end that will be put through the scope) before passage over the guidewire and into the duct. Once the guiding catheter is advanced into the duct, the pusher tube is freed from the locked position with a twisting motion so that the physician can "push" the stent up the duct into position. The nurse or associate facilitates the stent delivery by pulling back on the guiding catheter as the stent is advanced into position. Once the stent is in place, the endoscopist holds the stent with the pusher tube as the guiding catheter and guidewire are removed.

During and after the procedure, the nurse should monitor and record the patient's vital signs and observe the patient for abdominal pain or distention. The nurse should document any existing pain before procedure. Before and during the procedure, monitoring should include continous ECG. Prophylactic antibiotics may be considered prior to placement. Serial blood studies are usually performed after placement of large stents to follow the patient's progress and to monitor the effectiveness of decompression. The serum bilirubin level usually declines progressively until it is nearly normal. The patient may be observed in the hospital or on an outpatient basis following the procedure. If a sphincterotomy has been performed, overnight hospital observation is recommended. The patient usually remains NPO for 2 to 4 hours after ERCP. The diet is then increased slowly as tolerated, preferably with a clear liquid diet for the first 24 hours post-ERCP. Some physicians recommend changing stents every 3 to 6 months to avoid plugging or breakage of stent material. Because the proximal portion of the stent protrudes into the duodenum, it can be withdrawn endoscopically by using a snare or stent-retrieving device, and it can be replaced fairly easily.

Potential early complications of stent placement include bleeding from the sphincterotomy or the tumor, cholangitis, pancreatitis, trauma to the biliary tract or duodenum, and obstruction of the pancreatic duct. Failure to place a stent properly is most commonly caused by either tumors involving the papilla of Vater, in which case the bile duct orifice cannot be identified, or hepatic neoplasms that cause a tight stricture of the intrahepatic ducts.

Recurrent jaundice is the most common delayed complication of biliary stent placement and is usually caused by clogging of the stent. Rarely, it may be a result of tumor growth along the prosthesis or metastatic spread of a malignant tumor to the liver. If occlusion of the prosthesis by cell detritus and viscous bile causes recurrent cholestasis and cholangitis, the endoprosthesis can be extracted with the aid of a polypectomy snare and replaced by a new prosthesis during the same session. Migration of the stent and erosion of the duodenal wall by the stent with ulcer formation or duodenal perforation are also potential delayed complications.

After biliary stent placement and before discharge, patients should be instructed to notify their physician when any symptoms of stent occlusion occur, such as pruritis, pain, or jaundice.

PANCREATIC STENTS

New endoscopic procedures have been developed in recent years to diagnose and treat pancreatic disorders. These techniques have been adapted from procedures initially used within the biliary system. Pancreatic stenting is one option.

Indications for pancreatic stenting include the following:

(a) unresolved pancreatitis;

(b) idiopathic acute pancreatitis;

(c) pancreas divisum with symptomatology;

(d) pancreatic duct disruption; traumatic, carcinoma, and idiopathic;

(e) prevention of post-ERCP pancreatitis;

(f) chronic pancreatitis;

(g) pancreatic strictures and/or stones; and

(h) sphincter of Oddi dysfunction.

Pancreatic stents are made from radiopaque polyethylene and come in 5, 7, and 10 Fr. The length is available from 1 to 12 cm. The stent is measured from the distal barb, which is positioned within the duodenum, to the proximal tip of the stent, which is positioned within the duct.

Placement of a pancreatic stent is similar in technique to the insertion of a biliary stent. Because of anatomical variations between the pancreatic duct and the biliary system, equipment has been modified for pancreatic therapeutics. More than one stent can be placed in the same procedure to facilitate difficult drainage.

Pancreatic stent placement

Placement of a pancreatic stent is similar to biliary stenting. The pancreatic duct is cannulated with the physician's preferred catheter. A pancreatogram is obtained, and a diagnosis is confirmed. The endoscopist then approves gentle flushing of the cannulating catheter with sterile saline or sterile water to clear the catheter of contrast medium and allow easier advancement of guidewires. Clarify amount of sterile saline or water with physician. It is important to note that when flushing the catheter, direct visualization with fluoroscopy is performed to decrease the chance of duct over-

fill. A guidewire of choice is advanced within the pancreatic duct. Choices in guidewires need to be explored to accommodate proper advancement of the catheter. For example, if a long tapered or dilating catheter has been used, a guidewire with a smaller diameter may be necessary.

Once the guidewire position is confirmed, the catheter is withdrawn as the nurse or associate advances the guidewire to maintain duct position. This is a synchronized effort in which communication between physician and nurse or associate plays a key role. The protruding guidewire is wiped with moist gauze to remove any remaining contrast medium, thus providing ease of insertion. The 5- or 7-Fr predetermined stent of choice is passed over the guidewire. A pusher tube follows the stent, pushing the stent along the guidewire and up into the pancreatic duct. As the endoscopist inserts the stent, the nurse or associate applies gentle back pressure on the guidewire. Fluoroscopy is utilized intermittently throughout. With the stent position verified, the guidewire is removed as the pusher tube holds the stent in place; then the pusher tube is removed. If a 10-Fr stent is the stent of choice, the addition of a guiding catheter is necessary, just as with biliary stents. The procedure order then becomes guidewire placement, guiding catheter over the guidewire, stent over the guiding catheter, and pusher tube to push the stent along the guiding catheter.

Postprocedure care is consistent with that of biliary stenting. Complications associated with pancreatic stenting include abdominal pain and mild pancreatitis. Sepsis is rarely noted. Clogging of the stents occurs in time frames extending from 6 weeks to 4 months. Migration of the pancreatic stent into the pancreatic duct or out of the pancreatic duct into the duodenum occurs in approximately 5% to 10% of the patients stented. There are some data to suggest that prolonged stent placement causes ductal changes similar to chronic pancreatitis, but these changes appear to be temporary and resolve once the stent is removed.

In addition, medical treatment of postoperative ileus or abdominal distention may include administration of IV Neostigmine (2mg dose over 5 minutes). Nursing should be alert to adverse effects such as respiratory depression/arrest, bronchospasm, or bradycardia. Keep Atropine at bedside.

METAL STENTS

Self-expanding metal stents (SEMS) are currently available endoscopically for esophageal, tracheobronchial, biliary, and colonic placement. These stents have also been used in vascular and urethral works, as well as in transjugular intrahepatic portosystemic shunt (TIPS) procedures.

In every case, metal stents are permanent and are not considered removable without surgery (although some covered and coiled stents have been successfully removed soon after placement). Therefore, SEMS are only inserted endoscopically for palliation of the patient who has been diagnosed with an obstructing neoplasm. Most symptoms from GI cancers come from the obstructive nature of the tumor preventing natural passage of oral intake through the GI tract or blocking bile flow. Placed within a malignant stricture, metal stents, with their wire memory, expend a greater radial force against an encroaching tumor. Maintaining luminal patency decreases symptoms, allows continued oral intake, and therefore improves the patient's quality of life.

Currently, metal stents are available in a spiral coil configuration, a tubular wire-mesh design, and a zigzag pattern (esophageal only).

SEMS continually benefit from technological advancements. At present, metal stents are available in open mesh and covered versions, each with their own set of problems. Uncovered SEMS are prone to tumor ingrowth. Covered stents have a greater potential for migration. Tumor ingrowth may be treated by placing additional stents (metal or polyethylene) within the existing stent or by thermal coagulation (heater probes or bipolar probes) used to melt away the obstruction. Uncovered SEMS enmesh with the GI wall and therefore are less likely to be displaced from the stricture by food bolus, peristalsis, and other complications. Manufacturers of covered stents compensate by flaring either end of the stent to anchor it in place and/or by only covering the center column of the stent, leaving the ends uncovered so they will bond with the GI tract. These changes are important, because covered stents are more effective in the treatment of tracheoesophageal fistulas.

SEMS are loaded, compressed, and stretched on their own delivery devices. As a result, some shorten 25% to 50% on deployment. Before stent placement, the stricture must be located, measured, and marked—either internally with contrast injection/instillation, or externally with radiopaque markers. Dilatation of the area to be stented may be done just before placement to ensure the stent delivery device can pass through the stricture, deploy the stent, and be removed successfully. The one absolute exception to this is colonic stent placement. Preplacement dilatation of colonic neoplasm is contraindicated because of the potential for perforation or rupture.

Each manufacturer's stent design and delivery device is slightly different. Until physician and endoscopy staff are experienced and comfortable with a metal stent and its delivery device, it is advisable to have a manufacturer's representative present during placement. Stent deployment should be slow, with diligent attention to the fluoroscopic image (and endoscopic image where applicable). When placing a SEMS across the gastroesophageal junction, in a distal biliary or ampullary stricture with a markedly dilated biliary tree above, or a colonic stricture with significant colonic dilatation proximal to the malignant obstruction, the tendency will be for the stent to shoot above the stricture into the dilated area. Depending on the SEMS and the device used, the metal stent may be recaptured and/or repositioned if 50% or less has been deployed.

Special considerations

1. Esophageal stents should be placed at least 2 to 3 cm below the cricopharynx to avoid interfering with the patient's airway. Placing the stent too high in the esophagus will cause coughing and gagging. It may also result in poor patient tolerance because of odynophagia or a constant sensation of an esophageal foreign body.
2. If the stent bridges the gastroesophageal junction, the patient should be instructed to follow antireflux measures and should be started on antireflux medications.
3. Following placement of an esophageal metal stent, patients should be instructed to notify their gastroenterologist for recurrent dysphagia, significant dyspnea, or persistent cough, which might indicate a fistula, tumor ingrowth, stent migration, or aspiration pneumonia.
4. Following biliary SEMS placement, as with other biliary stents, patients should be instructed to notify their gastroenterologist if symptoms of recurrent obstruction occur, such as pruritis, pain, or jaundice.
5. Following colonic SEMS placement, bowel control measures and dietary modifications are recommended based on stent location.
6. Reassure the patient that the metal stent will not set off a metal detector at the airport.
7. Manufacturers of these stents now provide endoprosthesis registration forms to track devices after stent implantation.

For stents in the sigmoid or left colon, the following postprocedure measures are recommended:

(a) daily stool softener;
(b) increased oral fluid intake;
(c) regular diet minimizing fresh vegetables and tough meats; and
(d) for each day the patient does not have a bowel movement, he or she should take Milk of Magnesia or a tablespoon of mineral oil.

For stents placed in the rectum, the following postprocedure measures are recommended:

(a) a daily stool softener *and* 1 tablespoon of mineral oil;
(b) soft diet without any fresh vegetables; and
(c) Fleet enema if no bowel movement for 2 days or a pressure sensation in the rectum.

INTESTINAL (NASOENTERIC) INTUBATION

Nasoenteric tubes are longer than nasogastric tubes. In the past, many were used to aspirate intestinal contents, lavage the intestinal tract, or to dislodge bowel obstructions. The Cantor tube, Kaslow tube, Harris tube and the Miller-Abbott tube were used with the injection of mercury as a weight but are not used today because of the danger of mercury.

Nasoenteric intubation is used for the following reasons:

(a) to aspirate intestinal contents for examination;
(b) to treat intestinal obstruction by providing intestinal decompression, relieving dilitation proximal to the obstruction, decreasing and diverting intestinal secretions and gas formation, and providing intestinal stenting;
(c) to prepare the intestinal tract for surgery by removing intestinal contents;
(d) to prevent postoperative nausea, vomiting, and abdominal distention;

(e) to provide enteral alimentation postoperatively until edema at the operative site has subsided or until peristalsis returns; and

(f) to provide enteral alimentation when the patient's condition prohibits gastric feeding.

There are many tubes from which to choose, depending on patient need and physician preference. They range from 8 Fr to 12 Fr in size. Some can be placed through an endoscope and then be transferred from oral to nasal by using an oral transfer tube. They have a luer loc adapter, attached so that they can be connected to a feeding pump. Others can be placed over a wire that has been passed through an endoscope and positioned either with or without fluoroscopy. The wire is kept in position as the endoscope is removed. The nasal transfer tube is passed through the chosen nostril and the tip brought out of the patient's mouth. The wire is then fed into the tip of the transfer tube until it exits the transfer tube through the nostril and into the GI tract. These tubes are usually 12 Fr or 60 inches long and can be placed well into the small bowel.

When the tube is in place, the patency must be checked frequently. Accurate intake and output records must be kept and frequent mouth and nostril care should be provided.

If used for suctioning, the amount, color, consistency, and odor of the drainage should be noted.

After removal of the tube, the patient is usually given food gradually, progressing from fluids to a regular diet. Initial feedings are small and frequent, and the amount of liquid given at any one time is limited.

Potential complications of intestinal intubation include otitis media resulting from eustachian tube irritation, although this is rare with small-bore tubes; intussusception; knotting of the tube; pressure necrosis with perforation; and rupture of esophageal varices. Indwelling nasoenteric decompression tubes may cause reflux esophagitis, inflammation of the nose or mouth, and ulceration of the nose and larynx.

COLON DECOMPRESSION

Colon decompression involves placement of a tube in the rectum or colon to relieve colonic distention. It is indicated in patients with colonic pseudo-obstruction (nontoxic megacolon or Ogilvie's syndrome), postoperative ileus, or colon distention secondary to flexible sigmoidoscopy or colonoscopy. Ogilvie's syndrome occurs in elderly patients who have a preexisting disease that necessitates bed rest. Without decompression, cecal perforation may result. Insertion of a rectal tube may be ordered every 2 to 3 hours in these patients.

Colon decompression is contraindicated in patients with recent rectal surgery, organic colon obstruction, recent surgical anastomosis, recent myocardial infarction, or diseases of the rectal mucosa.

Colon decompression can be accomplished by using a 22- to 32-Fr rectal tube of soft rubber or plastic, a small-lumen decompression tube, a large-lumen decompression tube, or an over-the-guidewire decompression tube. Tubes can be purchased in kits from different manufacturers.

1. If a **rectal tube** is to be used, the patient is placed in Sims' position and draped appropriately. The tube is lubricated with a water-soluble lubricant. The patient breathes slowly and deeply, and then bears down as for a bowel movement to relax the anal sphincter and facilitate insertion. The tube is inserted into the rectum and then advanced 15 cm. The proximal end of the tube should be taped to the lower buttock, and the end of the tube should be covered with a waterproof absorbent pad or connected to a drainage bag. Rectal tubes should be left in place for a maximum of 30 minutes. If no gas has been expelled, the procedure may be repeated in 2 to 3 hours.

   Rectal tubes attached to some type of drainage system may also be used to minimize excoriation and skin breakdown in incontinent patients who have watery diarrhea or in incontinent patients who have significant lower GI bleeding.

2. A **small-lumen decompression tube** can be passed through the biopsy channel of a colonoscope to the cecum. The colonoscope is removed while the tube is continually advanced through the channel. Tube placement is confirmed fluoroscopically, and the proximal end is secured to the buttock and attached to a drainage bag.

3. If a **large-lumen decompression tube** is to be used, biopsy forceps are passed through the channel of the colonoscope, and a suture is tied around the distal end of the decompression tube. The suture is grasped with the biopsy forceps, and the colonoscope and tube are passed side-by-side. Once the desired area is reached, the tube is released and the forceps are withdrawn from the colonoscope. The colonoscope is then withdrawn with care to avoid dislodging the tube, and confirmation is made of its placement fluoroscopically. The proximal end of the tube is secured to the buttock and attached to a drainage bag.

4. If an **over-the-guidewire decompression tube** is to be used, the colonoscope is inserted, and a 480-cm guidewire is passed through the channel. The colonoscope is removed while advancement of the guidewire is continued. The position of the guidewire is confirmed, the decompression tube is advanced over the guidewire, and placement is confirmed fluoroscopically. The guidewire is removed, and the proximal end of the tube is secured to the buttock and attached to a drainage bag.

Massive colonic distention may also be relieved by colonoscopic suction.

After placement of a rectal or decompression tube, it is important to ensure the patency of the tube and to assess the patient for relief of symptoms. The color, consistency, and amount of drainage and the character of the patient's abdomen should be noted. The patient should be told to expect drainage from the tube. The physician may order a rectal tube to be removed once the abdomen is flat and soft or if the tube is ineffective after 30 minutes.

Potential complications of decompression include perforation and clogging of the tube with stool.

ABDOMINAL PARACENTESIS

Abdominal **paracentesis** involves withdrawal of fluid from the peritoneal space for diagnostic and therapeutic purposes, using a large-bore needle or a trocar and cannula inserted in the abdominal wall. It may be performed at bedside or in a treatment room. Studies show therapeutic taps drain more fluid than midline taps especially in obese, cirrhotic patients. Ultrasound guided paracentesis is being used more frequently in patients with previous abdominal surgeries.

Paracentesis is indicated for the following:

(a) evaluation of ascites;

(b) determination of a perforated viscus following blunt trauma or symptoms of acute abdomen; and

(c) relief of dyspnea or abdominal pain secondary to tense ascites.

It is contraindicated in uncooperative patients and for patients with the following:

(a) severe coagulopathy;

(b) thrombocytopenia;

(c) intestinal obstruction;

(d) abdominal wall infection;

(e) previous multiple abdominal surgeries; and

(f) Portal hypertension with abdominal collateral circulation.

Paracentesis may be performed in patients with coagulopathy if small-gauge needles in the vascular midline are used. It must be performed cautiously in pregnant patients and in patients with unstable vital signs. Patients should also be on BP monitor to alert RN to developing hypotension.

Before paracentesis, it is important to have the patient void to reduce the risk of accidental injury to the bladder when the needle or trocar and cannula are inserted. Baseline vital signs, weight, and abdominal girth at the umbilical level should be recorded.

Depending on the physician's preference, the patient may be positioned in Fowler's position, the knee-hand position, or sitting on the side of the bed with the feet supported. The preferred position is usually recumbent, with a 30-degree elevation of the head. In this position, gravity causes fluid to accumulate in the lower abdominal cavity, and the pressure created by the abdominal organs facilitates fluid flow. The patient should be draped with a sheet exposing the abdomen. He or she should be cautioned to remain as still as possible to avoid injury from the needle or trocar and cannula.

With sterile technique and with the patient under local anesthesia, the needle or catheter is introduced in the midline between the umbilicus and pubis (Fig. 29-2). The risk of hemorrhage is reduced by entering through the avascular linea alba, but the catheter may be introduced laterally if necessary. The rectus muscles, upper abdomen, collateral venous channels, and areas of surgical scars should be avoided.

During the procedure the gastroenterology nurse should disinfect the skin, assist the physician in establishing and maintaining a sterile field, and draw up the local anesthetic. Specimen containers should be ready to receive fluid. The first 10 ml of fluid should be collected separately, followed by 50-ml aliquots. Ascitic fluid should be cultured using blood culture media bottles. Pulse and respiratory status should be monitored throughout the procedure.

Only a small amount of fluid is needed for diagnosis. Vacuum collection bottles, 500 to 1000 ml, and appropriate tubing often facilitate ease of fluid collection. If greater vol-

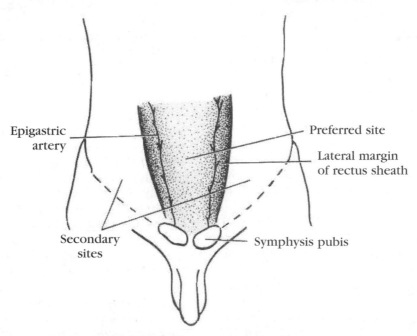

Fig. 29-2. Sites for paracentesis.

umes are to be withdrawn, a larger-gauge needle or catheter/needle assembly should be used. The physician may make a small incision with the scalpel before inserting the needle or trocar and cannula, usually 1 to 2 inches below the umbilicus.

After paracentesis is completed, an elasticized, adhesive dressing should be applied to the site. The patient should be helped to a comfortable position, and vital signs should be monitored and documented every 15 minutes. The patient should be observed closely for vertigo, faintness, diaphoresis, pallor, heightened anxiety, tachycardia, dyspnea, and hypotension. The physician should be notified if the patient's pulse rate increases and systolic blood pressure decreases, respiratory status changes, temperature is elevated, peritoneal fluid leaks from the site, or scrotal edema develops.

The color, amount, viscosity, and odor of any drainage should be noted. Specimens should be labeled and sent to the laboratory with the appropriate requisition slip. The patient's weight and abdominal girth should be compared with baseline figures.

Complications are rare in abdominal paracentesis but may include hemorrhage, perforation of the abdominal organs by the needle or the trocar and cannula, peritonitis, hepatic coma from decreased systemic circulation, reduced tissue perfusion, and wound infection. Aspiration of more than 1500 ml of peritoneal fluid may induce hypovolemic shock because of the sudden shift of fluid from the circulatory system to replace aspirated fluid.

If the patient shows signs of hypovolemic shock, the drainage rate should be slowed by reducing the vertical distance between the needle or trocar and cannula and the collection container. If necessary, the drainage may be stopped altogether. Colloid replacement with albumin is recommended with large-volume paracentesis.

CASE SITUATION

Mr. Jason Ruggles comes to his internist complaining of vague abdominal pain that is causing him some distress. He is willing to undergo whatever tests are necessary to find the cause of the problem.

Points to think about

1. Mr. Ruggles has abdominal pain; what might his internist do first?
2. If the internist refers Mr. Ruggles to a gastroenterologist, what type of diagnostic test might the gastroenterologist perform?
3. If the gastroenterologist believes that Mr. Ruggles has inflammation caused by overproduction of gastric acid, what tests could he perform to confirm his suspicions?
4. If Mr. Ruggles is not treated properly, what consequences can he expect?
5. If Mr. Ruggles must go through a lengthy series of tests and therapeutic procedures, he may become disheartened and

discouraged. Periodically, the nurse must reevaluate and, if necessary, intervene in Mr. Ruggles' struggle to cope during this stressful time. What are some behaviors that might indicate that intervention is needed?

Suggested responses

1. The internist sends Mr. Ruggles for an upper GI radiographic series, which outlines his esophagus, stomach, and duodenum. Although the films reviewed by the radiologist are normal, the internist knows that this normal x-ray examination does not necessarily mean there is nothing wrong with Mr. Ruggles, so he refers the patient to a gastroenterologist.
2. The gastroenterologist conducts a full history and physical examination and decides that an EGD is in order. The EGD is done, uneventfully, and the diagnosis is moderate duodenitis, gastritis, and esophagitis.
3. To confirm his suspicion that Mr. Ruggles is producing too much gastric acid, the gastroenterologist might order the following:
   (a) A gastric analysis, which measures the amount of acid produced. The nurse must know how to place a nasogastric tube appropriately for best drainage of the stomach (along the greater curvature with the tip in the antrum) and must collect specimens of gastric juice before and after stimulation with pentagastrin. Some gastroenterology nurses and associates also know how to titrate and calculate the acid content of these specimens; others have these measurements done by the chemistry laboratory.
   (b) An intraesophageal acid drip test (Bernstein test), which determines if the esophagitis is symptomatic. This also requires a nasogastric intubation with precise placement of the tube in the esophagus.
   (c) An intragastric instillation of acid, which can determine if acid is causing the abdominal pain. This test also requires placement of a nasogastric tube.
   (d) Serial blood tests, conducted over an hour after the administration of a pancreatic stimulant (secretin), which can determine if the excess acid production is caused by a tumor in the pancreas (Zollinger-Ellison syndrome).
   (e) An esophageal motility study, which will show whether the esophagus contracts properly to clear acid from the esophagus.
   (f) Twenty-four-hour pH monitoring, which will document the number of reflux episodes that occur. The motility study and the pH monitoring require two more nasogastric intubations.
4. If Mr. Ruggles is not treated properly, the following events could occur:
   (a) Mr. Ruggles could develop scarring and strictures from reflux of acid in the esophagus; this could require dilatation of the esophagus, perhaps on an ongoing basis.
   (b) Overacidity in the stomach can lead to peptic ulcerations, particularly in the prepyloric and pyloric chan-

nel area. This can lead to scarring and deformity or stenosis of the pyloric channel, causing gastric outlet obstruction, which would need to be dilated. Because dilatation of the pylorus is not usually as effective as dilatation of the esophagus, this may lead to gastric surgery to correct the problem.

(c) If medications do not control Mr. Ruggles' acid production, he may progress from inflammation to ulcerations with bleeding and attendant complications. This may require surgical intervention to control acid production (vagotomy and pyloroplasty, vagotomy and antrectomy, or highly selective vagotomy).

5. These are all difficult tests for the patient, requiring that the nurse is patient and caring and establishes a supportive, trusting relationship with the patient. Nasogastric intubation can be uncomfortable, but a skilled person can make the procedure much more tolerable. Some signs that may indicate Mr. Ruggles is not effectively coping with the stress involved include the following:

(a) nonperformance of activities of daily living;
(b) purposelessness;
(c) self-absorption;
(d) inflexibility;
(e) hopelessness;
(f) unconcern and detachment from usual social supports;
(g) nonproductive lifestyle; and
(h) excessive use of denial.

Indifference to social supports and demoralization are two negative manifestations of coping with the stress caused by illness. The nursing diagnosis "ineffective individual coping" is defined as impairment of adaptive behaviors and problem-solving abilities of a person in meeting life's demands and roles. Coping is a continual process, and numerous factors influence it, so the assessment of a person's coping mechanisms becomes an ongoing nursing responsibility.

REVIEW TERMS

barbed stents, biliary stents, decompression, french (in reference to circumference), lavage, nasobiliary catheters (NBCs), nasoenteric intubation, nasogastric tube, nasopancreatic catheters (NPCs), pancreatic stents, paracentesis, pigtail stent, proximal and distal (correct orientation), self-expanding metal stents (SEMS), "tense" acities

REVIEW QUESTIONS

1. If the patient belches after air is injected into a nasogastric tube, what is the most likely cause?
(a) The tube is curled in the patient's mouth or throat.
(b) The tube is in the patient's esophagus.
(c) Stomach contents are blocking the tube.
(d) The tube is blocking the patient's airway.

2. After insertion of an esophageal prosthesis, the patient should be able to feel the presence of the prosthesis:
(a) For a few hours.
(b) For a few days.
(c) Indefinitely.
(d) The patient should not be aware of the presence of the prosthesis.

3. The main advantage of using a double-lumen orogastric tube for gastric lavage is that:
(a) It permits continuous instillation of an irrigant.
(b) It permits rapid aspiration of large amounts of gastric contents.
(c) It can be inserted nasally if necessary.
(d) It is easier to insert.

4. After the patient's tolerance of gastric lavage has been established, what volume of irrigation solution is used for each subsequent instillation?
(a) 50 ml.
(b) 250 ml.
(c) 500 ml.
(d) 1000 ml.

5. Monooctanoin (Moctanin) is sometimes instilled through a nasobiliary catheter. Why?
(a) To treat bacterial cholangitis.
(b) To flush out small stones after endoscopic sphincterotomy.
(c) For gallstone dissolution.
(d) To treat sclerosing cholangitis.

6. For biliary decompression, a polyethylene tube (inserted via a duodenoscope) exits and drains to the outside through the patient's:
(a) Mouth.
(b) Nose.
(c) Abdominal wall.
(d) Gastrostomy tube.

7. The most common delayed complication of biliary stent placement is:
(a) Recurrent jaundice.
(b) Duodenal perforation.
(c) Hemorrhage.
(d) Pancreatitis.

8. A rectal tube should be left in place:
(a) Until decompression is achieved.
(b) For a maximum of 3 minutes.
(c) For a maximum of 30 minutes.
(d) For 2 to 3 hours.

9. Before abdominal paracentesis, it is important for the patient to void. Why?
(a) To keep the patient comfortable during the procedure.
(b) To reduce intraabdominal pressure.
(c) To give a more accurate measure of abdominal girth.
(d) To avoid injury to the bladder when the needle is inserted.

10. Biliary stenting is performed for all of the following except:
(a) Pancreatitis.
(b) Choledocholithiasis.
(c) Strictures.
(d) Cholangitis.

11. Metal stents currently available are:
    (a) Changed every 4 to 6 months.
    (b) Used only for benign tumors.
    (c) Permanent stents.
    (d) Removed easily with a snare.
12. One complication that is unique to pancreatic stenting is:
    (a) Stent migration.
    (b) Stent occlusion.
    (c) Stent-induced pancreatic ductal change.
    (d) They always require an endoscopic sphincterotomy before insertion.
13. Indications for pancreatic stent insertion include all *except*:
    (a) Pancreatic duct disruption.
    (b) Sphincter of Oddi dysfunction.
    (c) Pseudocyst.
    (d) Choledochocele.

BIBLIOGRAPHY

Axelrad, A.M., Fleischer, D.E. & Gomes, M. (1996). Nitinol coil esophageal prosthesis: advantages of removable self-expanding \p\pmetallic stents. *Gastrointest Endosc 43*(2), 155-60. Gastrointestinal Endoscopy.

Bernard, M. & Forlaw, L. (1984). Complications and their prevention. In Rombeau, J. & Caldwell, M. (Eds.), *Clinical nutrition: enteral and tube feeding vol 1*. Philadelphia: W.B. Saunders.

Carr-Locke, D.L. (1996, September). *Stent therapy of malignant biliary obstruction*. Presented at Therapeutic ERCP Course for GI Nurses and Associates, Milwaukee, WI.

Clausen, D. (1996). Drug forum: Moctanin. *Gastroenterol Nurs 19*(5), 183-5. Gastroenterology Nursing.

Cotton, P. & Williams, C. (1996). *Practical gastrointestinal endoscopy* (4th ed.). London: Blackwell Scientific.

Given, B. & Simmons, S. (1984). *Gastroenterology in clinical nursing* (4th ed.). St. Louis, MO: 1984, Mosby.

Hamilton, H. (Ed.) (1983). *Procedures, Nurse's Reference Library*. Springhouse, PA: Intermed Communications.

Krueger, J. & Ostrowski, P. (1986, September). *Pre- and postprocedural care of the ERCP patient*. Presented at Therapeutic ERCP Course for GI Nurses and Associates, Milwaukee, WI.

McFarland, G. & McFarlane, E. (1989). *Nursing diagnosis and intervention*. St. Louis, MO: Mosby.

McNally, P. R. (2001). *GI/Liver Secrets*. Philadelphia, Pennsylvania: Hanley & Belfus, Inc.

Miller, L. (1988). Endoscopic stent placement: a nursing perspective. In Trivits, S. (Ed.), *SGA Journal Reprints*, Rochester, NY: Society of Gastrointestinal Assistants.

Nelson, D.B., Silvis, S.E. & Ansel, H.J. (1994). Management of a tracheo-esophageal fistula with a silicone-covered self-expanding metal stent. *Gastrointest Endosc 40*(4), 497-99. Gastrointestinal Endoscopy.

Neuhaus, H. (1991). Metal esophageal stents. *Semin Interven Radiol 8*(4), 305-10. Seminars in Interventional Radiology.

Ravenscroft, M. & Swan, C. (1984). *Gastrointestinal endoscopy and related procedures: a handbook for nurses and assistants*. Baltimore, MD: Williams & Wilkins.

Smits, M.E. (1995). *New developments in endoscopic and pancreatic drainage*. Amsterdam.

Tytgat, G. & Classen, M. (Eds.) (2000). *Practice of therapeutic endoscopy*. Philadelphia: W.B. Saunders.

Waye, J., Geenen, J.E., Fleischer, D. (1992). *Techniques in therapeutic endoscopy* (2nd ed.). Philadelphia: W.B. Saunders.

All techniques in this chapter, except intestinal intubation and metal stents, are also discussed in:

Society of Gastroenterological Nurses & Associates, Inc. (2003). *Manual of gastroenterological procedures* (5th ed.). Baltimore, MD: Williams & Wilkins.

Chapter 30

EXCISION AND EXTRACTION

This chapter will acquaint the gastroenterology nurse with endoscopic procedures that are used for the removal of foreign bodies, polyps, and retained stones from the common bile duct and pancreatic duct. The use of lithotripsy for the disruption of gallstones is also discussed.

Learning objectives

After reviewing the content of this chapter, the gastroenterology nurse should be able to:

1. Describe techniques used for removal of foreign bodies and bezoars from the GI tract.
2. Explain the indications, contraindications, procedures, and potential complications of endoscopic polypectomy.
3. Describe the indications, contraindications, procedures, and risks of endoscopic sphincterotomy.
4. Discuss the use of biliary lithotripsy for the disruption of gallstones, and the use of pulsed-dye laser lithotripsy.

FOREIGN BODY REMOVAL

Endoscopic techniques may be used for extraction of foreign bodies from the esophagus, stomach, duodenum, or colon. Foreign bodies may be deliberately or accidentally swallowed or may be introduced into the lower GI tract from the rectum. Most foreign objects lodge at areas of anatomical or physiological narrowing, such as the cricopharyngeal or lower esophageal sphincter (LES). If a foreign body passes the esophagus, it will usually pass through the remainder of the GI tract without incident. Other sites of potential hang-up are the pylorus, the duodenal C-loop, the ligament of Treitz, the ileocecal valve, and the anus.

The most frequent victims of foreign body ingestion are young children who are between the ages of 6 months and 4 years, persons with dentures, and inebriated or mentally impaired individuals. Children most often ingest coins, toys, crayons, and ballpoint pen caps. Adults present with bones and meat impacted in the esophagus. Prisoners and psychiatric patients may ingest a variety of objects. In the lower GI tract, foreign objects are found predominantly in males who are between the ages of 24 and 65 years and who are either homosexuals or the victims of criminal assault. Foreign bodies may also be iatrogenic in origin, such as dental instruments, parts of nebulizers, tubes, prosthetic devices, or biopsy instruments, including small-bowel biopsy capsules that have been lost in the GI tract. A Given Imaging capsule can also act as a foreign body if it does not pass through the GI tract secondary to a small bowel obstruction or adhesions.

Of the foreign bodies that enter the GI tract, 80% to 90% pass through without incident, often within 48 hours; 10% to 20% need to be removed endoscopically, and 1% require surgery. Most foreign-body obstructions involve the esophagus, especially above a benign or malignant stricture, web, or ring.

Foreign bodies in the stomach cause few, if any, symptoms. Conservative management is in order for most foreign objects that have reached the stomach. Endoscopic or surgical removal of foreign bodies should not be attempted unless a week has passed without progress. Exceptions to this rule are objects containing lead or mercury or objects with sharp points, because of the risk of bleeding, obstruction, or perforation. Most ingested objects that have passed into the stomach will pass uneventfully through the pylorus and the rest of the GI tract. In children, pennies, nickels, and dimes will pass, but quarters may not.

Objects that have passed beyond the second portion of the duodenum cannot be retrieved endoscopically. Their progress may be followed radiologically, with surgical exploration as a last resort.

Swallowed objects that hang up in the cecum or sigmoid colon may be retrieved with a colonoscope. Biopsy forceps, pronged polyp-retrieval forceps, special foreign-body forceps and polyp retrieval nets may be useful in removing foreign bodies from the colon, but the polypectomy snare is the most versatile instrument.

Objects that have been inserted into the rectum and the sigmoid colon may be retrieved by using a flexible or rigid sigmoidoscope. In the case of large objects, the patient may require general anesthesia for cooperation and for relaxation of the anal sphincter. No cathartics or enemas should be given. Objects lying below the peritoneal reflection of the rectum can usually be grasped and removed by using a rigid anoscope or proctoscope. Early surgical consultation is advised for high colorectal foreign bodies.

Endoscopic or surgical removal of foreign bodies is indicated for the following:

(a) most foreign bodies lodged in the esophagus, with the possible exception of round objects or food boluses in the distal esophagus, which may pass spontaneously;

(b) sharp or pointed objects that could result in obstruction or perforation, such as pins, toothpicks, and bones, even if they have entered the stomach;

(c) long, narrow objects, such as wires (more than 6 cm in length for children and more than 13 cm in adults) that may not be able to negotiate the fixed duodenal angles;

(d) gastric foreign bodies greater than 2 cm in diameter, or any gastric foreign bodies that do not pass after a 2-week observation period;

(e) toxic foreign bodies, such as alkaline button batteries; and

(f) duodenal foreign bodies that do not pass within 6 days of ingestion.

Foreign body removal is contraindicated when the risk associated with removing the object is greater than the risk posed by the object itself. It is also contraindicated in uncooperative patients or in patients with a known or suspected perforated viscus.

Patients with foreign bodies may present with pain, sepsis, mediastinitis, peritonitis, hemorrhage, abscess, or an abdominal mass. It is important to obtain a history and description of the foreign body, including its location, length of time lodged, type and location of pain, previous x-ray examinations, any history of dysphagia, previous foreign body removal, or other pertinent history, information, or symptoms.

The physician should confirm the location of the foreign body with x-ray films of the neck, chest, and abdomen. Serial films may be helpful to monitor the progression of the object. It is also important to establish the time of last food or fluid ingestion. Barium swallows should be avoided if there is any evidence that the object is located at or just below the cricopharynx, but a thin suspension of barium may be given in small sips to help locate radiolucent foreign bodies in the lower esophagus.

A wide assortment of endoscopic snares and retrieval devices are available, including the following:

(a) laryngoscopes and curved forceps such as Kelly clamps for removal of objects that are lodged in the hypopharynx or are accidentally dropped into the hypopharynx during extraction;

(b) rat-tooth, alligator, or shark-tooth forceps to grasp and secure flat, metallic objects or objects that may be difficult to remove;

(c) tripod-type forceps to remove food boluses;

(d) w-shaped forceps or polypectomy snares/nets to remove coins;

(e) polypectomy snares to remove long, narrow objects, such as opened paper clips, stiff pieces of wire, or injector razor blades, or to remove oddly shaped objects, such as jacks or jewelry;

(f) pelican-type forceps, which are available in graduated sizes, for breaking up and removing food obstructions;

(g) stainless steel wire basket-type forceps for a variety of round objects, such as marbles or stones, or for meat boluses that can be removed in one piece;

(h) snares, grasping forceps, and baskets for removal of gastric foreign bodies;

(i) rubber-tip forceps for grasping needles and nails;

(j) magnetic extraction devices for removal of metallic objects (although caution is advised when withdrawing the object through the cricopharynx); and

(k) standard biopsy forceps for objects with a small central opening, through which closed biopsy forceps will pass but opened forceps will not.

It is important to confirm that the retrieval device will fit the channel size of the endoscope. It may also be helpful to obtain a similar object and practice grabbing it with various forceps, snares, and baskets to simulate the endoscopic situation and to determine which instrument is best suited in a particular case.

Use of a foreign body hood or **overtube** can sometimes be indicated. Endoscopic overtubes are polyvinyl sleeves that are used to facilitate various upper endoscopic procedures, including extraction of foreign bodies. The overtube protects the esophageal mucosa and the airway as the object is pulled out with the endoscope. An overtube should be used when sharp or pointed foreign bodies must be removed or when the endoscope must be passed several times, as for piecemeal removal of a soft bolus of meat. Overtubes cannot be used in the duodenum.

If an overtube is needed, one with an inner diameter approximately 2 mm larger than the outside diameter of the endoscope should be chosen. This size prevents mucosa catching between the overtube and the endoscope as the scope is advance or withdrawn. After it has been lubricated both inside and outside, it is slipped over the endoscope insertion tube. The patient is intubated in the usual manner with the overtube covering the endoscope as it is passed into the patient's esophagus. A mouth guard or bite block prevents the overtube from slipping into the patient's mouth.

In situations where a large or dangerous foreign body cannot be pulled far enough into the overtube, it is safer to use a latex hood. The hood is placed on the distal tip of the scope and folded back toward the controls for insertion. When the endoscope is withdrawn into the esophagus, the hood catches on the LES and is forced distally, thereby covering the object.

For removal of foreign bodies from the upper GI tract, the patient is placed in the left lateral position and antibiotic prophylaxis is administered if ordered. To reduce anxiety and promote cooperation, the patient may be premedicated and/or receive IV moderate sedation drugs during the procedure. Infants, children, or uncooperative patients may require general anesthesia with endotracheal intubation to protect their airway and provide patient safety.

During the procedure the nurse should monitor the patient's vital signs; the color, warmth, and dryness of the skin; the level of consciousness and pain tolerance. It is also important to observe the patient for symptoms of perforation (increase restlessness, pain, or tachycardia). Oral secretions should be suctioned. The airway must be protected and maintained, and steps should be taken to prevent aspiration.

Extraction of a foreign body from the esophagus requires good visibility, a firm grasp of the object, and removal without force. Pointed objects should be withdrawn with the point trailing. If the object is pointed on both ends, the proximal sharp end must be completely covered by the grasping forceps. If the object has a single pointed end that is directed cephalad, it can be carried into the stomach and turned so the pointed end trails before it is removed. Objects with sharp edges should be extracted with the aid of an overtube or hood.

Great care must be taken to avoid dropping the foreign body into the laryngopharynx on withdrawal. A laryngoscope with appropriate size blade and McGill forceps should be readily available in the event the foreign body is dropped into the patient's airway. The object should be grasped quickly from the patient's mouth to prevent it from falling into the trachea. Institutional policies should be followed for disposal of the retrieved foreign body.

After the object has been removed, it is important to monitor the patient's vital signs and to observe for bleeding, vomiting, abdominal or chest pain, continued abdominal distention, subcutaneous emphysema, or aspiration. When it is determined that the object has been removed without complications, the patient should be reevaluated to rule out any underlying disease that may have caused the obstruction, especially in the esophagus.

Although rare, potential complications of endoscopic foreign body removal include perforation, impaction of the foreign object, hemorrhage, localized inflammation or pressure necrosis, and aspiration of the object.

For patients with food impacted above an esophageal stricture, hydrostatic balloon dilatation of the stricture is an alternative method of treatment, providing the food bolus does not totally occlude the lumen. Once the stricture is dilated, the bolus can be pushed into the stomach. Medications such as glucagon should be available to promote relaxation of the esophagus, thereby facilitating passage of the foreign object into the stomach.

It is important to act quickly if a patient has swallowed a small, button-type battery. The alkaline substance from the battery acts rapidly on the mucosa, causing direct corrosive action, burns, and pressure necrosis. Direct corrosive activity frequently leads to perforation. Potentially catastrophic complications, such as esophagotracheal or esophago-aortic fistula, can ensue.

Occasionally, packets of cocaine are swallowed or placed in the rectum, often encased in condoms, in an attempt at concealment. The ingestion of 1 to 3 g of powdered cocaine can be fatal. Because rupture of even one packet carries the risk of death, the use of ipecac, lavage, enema, or cathartics should be avoided. Surgical removal is the treatment of choice in such cases.

BEZOAR REMOVAL

Bezoars are concretions of food or foreign matter that have undergone digestive change(s) in the GI tract. They include trichobezoars, which consist of matted hair, and phytobezoars, which consist of plant material. Symptoms associated with the presence of a bezoar range from a feeling of fullness in the upper quadrants to epigastric pain and periodic attacks of nausea and vomiting. Gastric outlet and intestinal obstruction are common complications.

The best way to diagnose and differentiate between bezoars is by gastroscopy. The standard treatment methods for phytobezoars include the following:

(a) physical disruption methods, including manual attempts at external disruption, a liquid diet, suction and lavage, and endoscopic internal fragmentation by using biopsy forceps and polypectomy snares;

(b) chemical attack with papain, acetylcysteine, or cellulase; and

(c) gastrotomy, if medical treatment fails.

Trichobezoars cannot be dissolved in vivo. Treatment of these large intragastric masses is always surgical.

POLYPECTOMY

GI polyps are lesions that may project from the mucosal surface into any part of the GI lumen. Some polyps are **pedunculated** (i.e., they are attached to the mucosa by a stemlike pedicle or stalk). **Sessile polyps** are attached to the mucosa by a broad base. Because of their protrusion into the lumen and the stresses of the fecal stream to which colonic polyps are subject, polyps occasionally bleed or cause abdominal pain or obstruction. However, symptomatic polyps are uncommon. The greatest concern is with their potential to become malignant.

Most polyps are removed by wire snares or with hot biopsy forceps, which are opened and closed by a gastroenterology nurse or associate. Commercial **polypectomy snares** come in various sizes and shapes.

Polyps are usually transected by use of a high-frequency current, which is produced by a generator attached to the sheathed snare. The current is applied for brief pulses until the polyp is transected. Electrical currents that have a pure cutting effect are never used in colonoscopic polypectomy. Electrocoagulation current alone may be used if the polyp is attached by a thin pedicle, but a blend of cutting and coagulation current is usually applied to thick-based polyps.

It is important to remember that different electrosurgical units (ESUs) may not provide the same current output. In addition, the characteristics of the snare used may alter the power setting on a given ESU. For example, a thin wire cuts through tissue more quickly than a thick wire. The operator must be familiar with the units that are available, and guidelines must be developed for each unit.

To guard against electrical hazards, a ground system must be established. The electrocautery equipment, including the connections and grounding pad, should be checked before each use. The snare should be checked to ensure that it is in working order and is conducting current. One way of testing the circuitry is to set the ESU at half power and then check for sparking between the side of the snare loop and the patient plate. ESU cutting and coagulation controls should be set in accordance with the physician's instructions.

Colonic polyps

Colonoscopic **polypectomy** is indicated for all polyps with a diameter of 1 cm or larger. Smaller polyps can usually be handled with cold or hot biopsy forceps, particularly if the polyp is sessile.

Contraindications to colonic polypectomy include the following:

(a) use of aspirin, nonsteroidal antiinflammatory drugs (NSAIDs), or anticoagulants;

(b) coagulopathy;

(c) polyps that appear malignant and are probably invasive;

(d) inadequate bowel preparation; and

(e) uncooperative patients.

Coagulation screening, blood count, and appropriate blood chemistry studies may be needed, in addition to a history and physical examination. The patient should be told how to obtain the results of pathological studies. Compliance with instructions for thorough bowel preparation is critical and must be confirmed.

The patient should be placed in the left lateral recumbent position, and a grounding pad should be applied to the patient, usually on the upper thigh or lower trunk, whichever is the largest tissue mass. All leads on the ESU should be checked for secure attachment. Cords and attachments should be inspected for fraying and wear. Cut and coagulation dials should be set according to the endoscopist's instructions, and verbal orders should be repeated back to the operator.

A colonoscope should be advanced as it would be for diagnostic colonoscopy. If diagnostic colonoscopy to the cecum has not been performed previously, it may be carried out before polypectomy. At a minimum, the scope should be advanced 20 to 25 cm beyond the polyp to remove fecal fluid.

When the polyp is in view, its shape, its size, and the length of its stalk must be evaluated. Based on these factors, the appropriate technique for polypectomy can be determined.

1. Small, sessile polyps less than 8 mm in diameter may be completely removed, recovered for biopsy examination, and ablated with hot biopsy forceps. The polyp is grasped between the jaws of the insulated forceps and lifted away from the intestinal wall by manipulating the angulation controls. This maneuver pulls the mucosa away from the submucosa and muscularis propria so the application of current causes only slight heating of the deeper tissues. With the grasped polyp pointed toward the lumen, coagulation current is applied, destroying the polyp. When the whitish area encircling the polyp base is 1 to 2 mm wide, the current is discontinued, and the polyp is pulled off its base.

2. Sessile polyps less than 1 cm in diameter can be removed in one piece by using the snare-cautery technique if their bases are not wide, and if a reasonable "pseudo-stalk" can be created at the base.

3. For most pedunculated polyps, a polypectomy snare is advanced so a wire loop is created, and the polyp is "lassoed" with the snare wire. The tip of the catheter is advanced to the base of the polyp, and the loop is gently tightened. The polyp is tented slightly into the center of the lumen to be certain that no adjacent normal mucosa is caught in the loop. If the polyp has a long stalk, it is best to leave at least 1 cm of the stalk. Polyps with short stalks are ensnared as close to their necks as possible. Pedunculated polyps are usually transected within 2 to 4 seconds; mucosal blanching is noted adjacent to the snare wire during transection. Following closure of the snare, the polyp will fall into the lumen and the coagulated stalk will be visible. A suction specimen trap may be placed between the endoscope suction port and the suction tubing to prevent accidental loss of the specimen.

4. For pedunculated polyps with large or lobulated heads, segmental resection of the head may be necessary before complete polypectomy can be done.

5. Broad-based pedunculated polyps may be bunched to acceptable resection size to permit single transection, or they may be managed by segmental resection.

6. Large sessile polyps more than 2 cm in diameter are also removed in a piecemeal fashion, beginning with two oblique cuts made at right angles to each other across one quarter to one third of the polyp. The remaining base of the polyp may be transected during the initial polypectomy or 4 to 8 weeks later, after the area of mucosal ulceration has healed. Injecting 1-2ccs of normal saline using an injection (sclerotherapy) needle close to the base of the polyp prior to the polypectomy can help to raise the base.

7. If a polyp is awkwardly located for snaring, it may be helpful to bypass it and advance the colonoscope through the rest of the colon. As the instrument is removed, the colon is straightened, thereby providing a better view of the polyp for removal. The patient may also be repositioned to improve the orientation of the polyp.

8. Snaring and retrieving multiple polyps may require passing the colonoscope several times.

When the physician is ready to use the ESU, the nurse should turn on the power and turn it off immediately after use. The nurse must also open and close the snare or biopsy forceps at the request of the physician. It is important to close the snare slowly while maintaining continual communication with the physician. Visualization of this procedure using a lecture scope or video monitor is an absolute necessity.

After polypectomy is complete, the next important step involves retrieval of the polyp. The polyp may be retrieved by taking the following measures:

(a) removing it in the cup of the forceps, if cold/ hot biopsy forceps were used for polypectomy;

(b) placing the tip of the colonoscope flush against the head of the polyp and applying suction;

(c) resnaring the cut polyp and withdrawing it by use of the colonoscope. If the resnared polyp is kept 3 to 5 cm from the instrument tip, the colon can be visualized during withdrawal;

(d) entrapment of the polyp with a basket, by a three-pronged polyp retriever or net or

(e) suction aspiration of the polyp through the suction line and into a suction specimen trap or one of the newer filtered polyp retrieval traps.

To locate a lost polyp, a bolus of water may be squirted through the biopsy channel to identify the path of gravity in the colon and thus determine the probable location of the resected polyp or to dislodge a small polyp that entered the scope's suction channel. A suction specimen trap must be in place prior to retrieving the small polyp lodged in the suction channel.

It may not be possible to pull large polyps through the anus with the colonoscope, but if the patient bears down, the polyp can be expelled. Sometimes, the polyp must be removed from the rectum by digital exam or by passing a rigid sigmoidoscope and grasping it with forceps.

Once the polyp has been retrieved, the colonoscope may be reinserted to inspect the polypectomy site and to determine that there is no serious complication at the polypectomy site.

A thorough histological examination of the entire polyp is essential to determine whether there is a possibility of malignant change. The specimen should be prepared and labeled in accordance with institutional policy. The polyp itself should be fixed in formalin solution and examined by serial section to determine the presence of epithelial atypia or frank cancer within the polyp or invading the stalk. A final determination must be made by the pathologist.

The most common types of polyps encountered in the distal portion of the colorectum are hyperplastic or metaplastic polyps. Hyperplastic polyps are characterized by an abnormal multiplication or increase in the number of normal cells in a tissue, whereas metaplasia refers to a change in the adult cells in a tissue to an abnormal form. Hamartomatous polyps, including juvenile polyps and Peutz-Jeghers polyps, are those in which the cells of a circumscribed area grow faster than those of surrounding areas.

There is no evidence that routine follow-up examination is necessary for patients with hyperplastic, inflammatory, or hamartomatous polyps. Carcinoma in situ does not recur or metastasize and requires no treatment other than polyp removal. Patients with sessile polyps that harbor invasive carcinoma and patients with pedunculated polyps with invasive carcinoma and no clear margin of resection should undergo surgery if feasible.

After the polypectomy procedure is completed, it is important to observe the patient for abdominal pain or distention. The nurse should monitor vital signs and instruct the patient regarding dietary and medication restrictions. For instance, intake of alcoholic beverages, aspirin, NSAIDs, or other medications that alter the clotting mechanism should be avoided for a period of time after the procedure to minimize the risk of delayed hemorrhage.

Polyps in the rectum and lower sigmoid colon can be resected more safely than those in the cecum and right side of the colon, where the wall is thinner. There are a number of potential complications of colonoscopic polypectomy.

1. Bleeding is the most common complication and may occur immediately or as long as 21 days after polypectomy.

2. Adverse reactions to sedation include hypotension, respiratory depression, bradycardia, nausea, vomiting, and sweating.

3. Vasovagal attack usually occurs when colonoscopy causes serious discomfort or pain or from excessive abdominal distention or pressure. Clinical manifestations include hypotension; bradycardia; and cold, clammy skin. Depending on the extent of the adverse response, intervention may include reducing the amount of air in the colon, scope withdrawal, IV Atropine, or termination of the procedure.

4. Transmural burns are manifested by abdominal pain, leukocytosis, and fever without evidence of free air or diffuse peritoneal signs. If any portion of the polyp head is permitted to come in contact with the intestinal wall, heat may be transferred through this point of contact, causing a burn of the wall adjacent to the polyp. To avoid this, the polyp may be jiggled to and fro, to move a small point of contact to various areas on the wall. Pedunculated polyps may be manipulated with the tip of the catheter or with suction, or the patient's position may be changed to provide better access and to bring the head of the polyp away from the bowel wall. If no perforation is present, the patient should be observed and treated with antibiotics if ordered, and solid food should be withheld. The syndrome usually resolves in 24 to 48 hours.

5. Perforation can occur if a portion of the wall of the colon is ensnared, if too much current is applied, or if there is substantial disruption of tissue by mechanical force during colonoscopy. Exploratory laparotomy with closure is the procedure of choice for the management of free perforation. Transmural burns and/or perforation from excessive coagulation is a more serious and more

common complication with sessile polyps, compared to pedunculated polyps.

6. The risk of explosion of flammable gases, such as hydrogen and methane, can be minimized by a good bowel preparation and by avoiding electrocautery in the presence of stool.

7. Current leakage from the ESU can cause thermal injury to the endoscopist, the patient, or the nurse.

Hemorrhage is a potential occurrence during any polypectomy but is most likely to occur when the polyp is large, in a difficult position, and/or has a thick stalk. Once the snare has been tightened around the polyp or its stalk, it should not be released or loosened, because if the tissue has been partially excised with the wire and it cannot be removed, bleeding may occur and vision may be impaired. Malfunctioning electrocoagulation equipment may also be a cause of post-polypectomy bleeding. If bleeding is suspected, IV fluids should be maintained. A large-bore needle should be used in case the patient needs blood.

If there is active pumping of blood from the stalk of a pedunculated polyp following polypectomy, the stalk may be regrasped with the snare, which should be tightened until the bleeding is stopped, and then coagulation current should be reapplied at successive intervals until hemostasis is achieved. If bleeding occurs following transection of a sessile polyp, an injection needle may be inserted through the instrument and diluted epinephrine given. A bipolar probe or heater probe or injection therapy may also be used to stop the bleeding.

During this emergency situation, it is best to have at least two nurses in attendance to control the situation. One nurse or associate should prepare equipment for coagulation, while another nurse attends to the patient and checks vital signs at frequent intervals. IV fluids will act to restore volume, transport oxygen, and remove waste products. Intake and output records should be established immediately. Blood loss should be assessed through the amount seen in the suction canister and rectal discharge. If not done before the procedure, laboratory work should be ordered, including hematocrit, hemoglobin, and coagulation studies. Blood should be typed and crossmatched. Oxygen should be administered via nasal cannula. The patient should be calmly reassured and should lie flat to encourage blood flow to the brain and other vital organs. The patient should be kept warm. Most of the time, bleeding can be controlled without surgery, but a surgeon should be notified in case surgery is needed. The patient should be prepared for admission to the hospital for observation.

Peutz-Jeghers syndrome

If the GI hamartomatous polyps typical of Peutz-Jeghers syndrome are fairly well localized to a short segment of intestine, segmental resection may be all that is required. Usually, however, polyposis is extensive and the patient requires multiple enterotomies throughout his or her life. The physician should target the larger polyps, which are most likely to be responsible for symptoms.

Gastric polyps

Gastric polyps are uncommon; most are solitary, small, hyperplastic polyps that may be either sessile or pedunculated. Gastric polyps are usually discovered in radiographic or endoscopic examinations in patients complaining of nausea, abdominal pain, and other GI symptoms, although it is unlikely that the polyps are responsible for these symptoms.

It is important to note that the gastric mucosa is more vascular than that of the colon, and slower closure of the snare handle is necessary during electrocautery to ensure hemostasis.

To enhance retrieval of resected polyps after polypectomy in the antrum and duodenum, IV glucagon may be given just before resection to inhibit peristalsis. Once located, the polyp should be grasped with a wire snare/net to provide additional traction as the polyp and instrument pass back through the cricopharynx. A foreign-body hood can be helpful during polyp removal to keep the polyp from falling into the trachea.

Gastroscopic polypectomy is indicated for most gastric polyps, but surgical excision is indicated for the following:

(a) sessile or broad-based polyps, in which no definitive diagnosis can be made by endoscopic biopsy examination;

(b) intramural polypoid lesions, such as leiomyomas; and

(c) any polypoid lesion that is believed to be responsible for symptoms and cannot be removed by endoscopic polypectomy.

Following removal of the gastric polyp, the denuded mucosa creates an iatrogenic ulcer. An antiulcer regimen with histamine$_2$ (H$_2$)-receptor antagonists and proton pump inhibitors for 4 weeks following gastric polypectomy may be recommended.

Patients with adenomatous gastric polyps should undergo repeat endoscopic surveillance every 1 to 2 years. Patients with hyperplastic gastric polyps do not require surveillance.

SPHINCTEROTOMY

Endoscopic retrograde sphincterotomy, also known as papillotomy, is an electrosurgical incision of the papilla of Vater and the fibers of the sphincter of Oddi during endoscopic retrograde cholangiopancreatography (ERCP). The terms **sphincterotomy** and **papillotomy** are often used interchangeably. The term papillotomy may be used by some to indicate only a mucosal cut rather than a submucosal cut, but this is difficult to determine endoscopically.

The objective of sphincterotomy is to sever the sphincter fibers and any soft tissue that impedes the passage of bile and/or common duct stones. It is the procedure of choice for management of recurrent common bile duct (CBD) stones after cholecystectomy. In fact, retained or recurrent CBD stones account for 83% of the sphincterotomies performed.

In addition to postcholecystectomy choledocholithiasis, indications for endoscopic sphincterotomy include the following:

(a) choledocholithiasis in patients with an intact gallbladder who are poor surgical risks or before laparoscopic cholecystectomy;

(b) papillary stenosis in patients with prolonged symptoms and severe disability who have been unresponsive to symptomatic treatment. Sphincterotomy in these patients serves to enlarge the papillary opening and decrease ductal pressure;

(c) obstruction of the CBD by ampullary tumors or distal CBD lesions (In this case, sphincterotomy is done to relieve ductal obstruction caused by tumor growth and to reduce the resultant jaundice. It may be performed in preparation for more extensive surgery or as palliation);

(d) gallstone pancreatitis;

(e) acute suppurative (purulent) cholangitis;

(f) sphincter of Oddi dysfunction;

(g) Choledochocele;

(h) Sump syndrome, a rare clinical entity involving the accumulation of gallstones or food debris in the defunctionalized segment of the distal CBD in patients who have had a side-to-side choledochoduodenostomy;

(i) in preparation for stent placement, Gruntzig balloon dilatation, or nasobiliary catheterization;

(j) HIV-related hepatobiliary disease (A sphincterotomy in these patients can relieve pain by reducing ductal pressure caused by AIDS cholangiopathy.); and

(k) to reduce pressure in the CBD with a bile duct leak after laparoscopic cholecystectomy injury.

Contraindications for sphincterotomy include the following:

(a) an uncooperative patient (The patient must be able to lie still, follow directions for posturing for radiographs, and follow other directions as needed.);

(b) significant coagulopathy;

(c) recent myocardial infarction or severe pulmonary disease;

(d) allergy to the contrast medium though some providers will use a lower ionized contrast medium with premedication of Benedryl or Solumedrol;

(e) the presence of an extremely large stone (greater than 20 or 25 mm in diameter), unless a lithotripter is available or stent placement is planned instead of surgery; and

(f) inability to properly position the **sphincterotome (papillotome).**

Periampullary diverticula do not necessarily constitute a contraindication to sphincterotomy, but patients with this condition are at additional risk.

In preparation for the procedure, a side-viewing duodenoscope with a nonmetal head should be checked for movement of the tip, good visibility, functioning of the forceps elevator, suction, and water channels. If the forceps elevator sticks, the tip of the scope should be soaked in tepid water until freed. Once it moves freely, silicone should be applied to maintain its motion.

The cannulating catheters used for dye injection should be filled with radiopaque contrast material and cleared of air bubbles. Sphincterotomes should be flexed to confirm full range of motion and smoothness of function. The sphincterotome should also be filled with the contrast medium. Retrieval balloon catheters should be filled with contrast material, cleared of air bubbles, and tested for balloon inflation.

Although ERCP can be safely performed on an outpatient basis, patients may be hospitalized post sphincterotomy because of the additional risks involved. Patients should be NPO for at least 6 hours before the procedure. Dentures or bridges should be removed, and a bite block should be used to protect the teeth and the scope. A topical anesthetic may be used to numb the throat. Prophylactic antibiotics usually are not necessary unless the patient has an underlying valvular heart disease, sepsis, biliary tract obstruction, or a pancreatic pseudocyst. It is recommended that two nurses/associates assist during sphincterotomy to help ensure patient safety: one nurse to monitor the patient, and the other to assist with the equipment.

Patients with underlying coagulation abnormalities should have necessary precautions taken, such as vitamin K injections, administration of fresh frozen plasma, or specific coagulation factors. Patients with abnormal coagulation studies should also be treated during the healing phase for 7 to 10 days following the procedure.

An IV line should be started, preferably in the patient's right hand or forearm, and run at a keep-open rate. The patient is usually placed in prone position on the x-ray table with their head turned towards the right to aid passage of the endoscope. They may be placed in the left lateral position to the far right side of the table, thereby making it relatively easy to roll them into the prone position once the scope is passed into the duodenum. The patient's left arm may be placed behind him or her to further facilitate prone positioning.

In preparation for sphincterotomy, the nurse applies the grounding pad and sets up the ESU as described in the section on polypectomy. The cutting currents used in sphincterotomy are composed of continuous sinusoidal waves or bursts that are active most of the time. These cutting currents produce intense heat at the point of contact, thus vaporizing and exploding cells.

The medications used for the procedure vary based on physician preference. Before intubation and during the procedure, the patient is sedated. Glucagon may be given to reduce duodenal motility before cannulation and sphincterotomy. Atropine may be needed to control the pulse rate if vagal response occurs. Pediatric patients may require general anesthesia. Opiates are generally avoided when Sphincter of Oddi manometric studies are anticipated because these agents may cause sphincter spasms, which alter the sphincter pressure and make cannulation difficult.

Narcotic and sedative antagonists should be on hand for reversal of drug effects. Emergency equipment should be available and functioning in the event of respiratory or cardiac arrest.

During the procedure the nurse should help the patient lie

as still as possible, give emotional support, and monitor the patient's vital signs including: skin color, warmth, and dryness; oral secretions; and position. Pillows may be needed to support the patient in the required position.

Once the ampulla of Vater is sighted, glucagon may be administered and a high-quality cholangiogram is obtained. The appropriate sphincterotome is selected, preflushed with contrast medium, inserted into the scope, and introduced into the CBD. The sphincterotome should be advanced only a short distance before contrast material is injected to confirm placement in the CBD. A wire-guided sphinctertome may be used to help direct the sphincterotome into the proper position.

Fluoroscopy demonstrates proper placement of the sphincterotome within the bile duct. The physician then directs the nurse to flex the sphincterotome slowly, and the cannula is withdrawn from the duct far enough so that approximately one half to two thirds of the wire is visible in the duodenum, outside the papillary orifice. The wire is oriented in a 12 o'clock position in relation to the papilla so the wire is held against the roof of the papilla during cutting.

Before starting the electrocautery incision, voice checks should be made between the endoscopist and the gastroenterology nurse concerning the following:

(a) application of the grounding pad on the patient and its connection (on most units an alarm warns personnel of these problems);
(b) attachment of the sphincterotome handle to the ESU;
(c) presetting of the ESU with the desired current setting;
(d) correct positioning of the foot pedal;
(e) control of duodenal motility using glucagon prn;
(f) degree of wire flexion required on the sphincterotome;
(g) switching on the power just before cutting; and
(h) removal of guidewire from sphinctertome if not a safety, non-conducting type.

Cutting is usually done with a partially flexed sphincterotome, with very short bursts of current (less than 1 second) to carry the incision through the sphincter 1 to 2 mm at a time.

The length of the sphincterotomy should be tailored to the size of the common duct stones. The apparent length of the intraduodenal segment of the CBD and the length of the narrow portion of the duct until the point where the duct becomes dilated are of great importance. The sphincterotomy must be extended to the dilated portion of the duct, but it must also remain within the intraduodenal segment of the duct. The usual length of the incision is 10 to 12 mm. As the current is being applied, the endoscopist may order changes in the flexion of the sphincterotome. The entire procedure should be done under direct visual guidance.

The completion of a sphincterotomy is usually signaled by a gush of bile that contains some blood, thus indicating that the sphincter fibers have been severed and usually that the sphincterotomy is adequate. After sphincterotomy is completed, the operator determines the size of the opening and patency to the bile duct by using a flexed sphincterotome or an inflated balloon catheter.

The ESU should be turned off as soon as the sphincterotomy is complete. If stones are present and do not pass spontaneously, a retrieval device should be passed into the duct to retrieve the stones. Alternative retrieval devices include occlusion balloons (the preferred method), baskets, or mechanical lithotripters.

1. Stones up to 12 mm in diameter can be extracted by using a balloon catheter. Balloons are passed up beyond the stone and then inflated to pull the stone down and drag it through the sphincterotomy incision. Balloons may also be used for determining the size of the incision, for determining the presence of and removing gravel, and for performing cholangiography after sphincterotomy or choledochoduodenostomy. Considerable traction is often required for pulling a stone through a sphincterotomy incision.

2. A basket can trap stones up to 15 mm in size (Fig. 30-1). Baskets are more difficult to introduce into the CBD than is a balloon or sphincterotome. Occasionally, the operator has difficulty entrapping stones in a basket, and there have been reports of impaction of baskets with entrapped stones in the distal portion of the CBD. Some patients have required surgical intervention for removal of impacted baskets with entrapped stones. Most baskets today have breakable wires that aid release of the basket if it becomes impacted. A mechanical lithotripter with a pair of wire cutters should always be readily available when baskets are used in the duct to remove stones.

3. A modified sphincterotome, similar to a polypectomy snare, can be used to hook the stone in a wire loop and extract it.

4. A mechanical lithotripter functions on the same principle as the basket, capturing the stone and then applying pressure against the trapped stone, causing fragmentation. The device is composed of a basket with high tensile strength wires with a Teflon sheath that can be removed and replaced by a coil spring sheath to allow application of traction on the stone. Mechanical cutting through the stone is accomplished by using wires for mechanical cutting and a coil spring sheath for firm traction on the stone.

5. Electric spark pulsing lithotripsy, which has been useful for removing stones from the urinary tract, can sometimes be effective in the removal of gallstones.

Gallstones have also been destroyed with lasers, but this method is not widely used at this time. Occasionally, large stones that cause ductal obstruction and cannot be removed endoscopically may be bypassed with a biliary stent.

If stones cannot be removed immediately after sphincterotomy, it is usually advisable to allow them to remain until the edema and reaction to the sphincterotomy have subsided. A nasobiliary catheter or plastic stent may be placed as a prophylactic measure to avoid obstruction. (Care of patients with nasobiliary tubes is discussed in Chapter 29.) The patient is reexamined in 5 to 14 days to determine whether the stones have passed. During this second examination, the operator may again consider extending the sphincterotomy

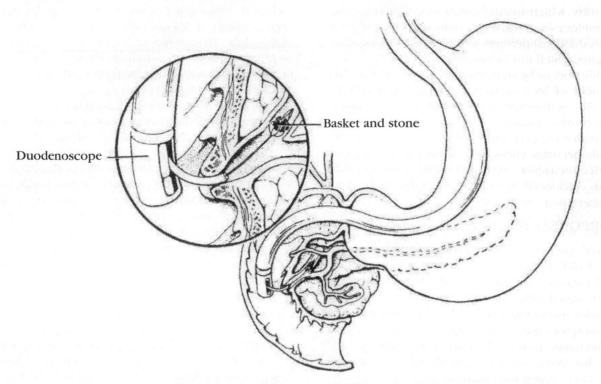

Fig. 30-1. Stone retrieval while basket is in the CBD.

and attempting extraction of the stones.

If these methods are unsuccessful, cholesterol stones may be dissolved by using oral **ursodeoxycholic acid**. This method dissolves the stones in approximately in 20% to 70% of cases or may soften large calculi so they can be extracted later as "mud." The time required for complete stone dissolution shows wide varation. Treatment should be withdrawn if patients show no radiologic evidence of gallstone dissolution after 6 months.

Methods for direct contact dissolution of gallstones using solvents have been used for many years in a few centers in the USA and Europe. Methyl tert-butyl ether (MTBE) is used for cholesterol dissolution, EDTA to enhance calcium solubility and N-acetylcysterine to promote mucin solubility. These solvents can be delivered during an ERCP using a nasobiliary tube or through a transhepatic approach.

If all attempts to remove stones fail, as outlined in Chapter 29, a stent can be inserted to facilitate biliary drainage and to keep the stone from impacting and causing biliary obstruction.

In patients with Billroth II gastrectomies, endoscopic access to the papilla and its subsequent cannulation and sphincterotomy can be difficult. Specially designed sphincterotomes are needed in this case that cut in a downward direction instead of the usual 12 o'clock position.

Following endoscopic sphincterotomy, antibiotics may be administered according to the physician's order. The patient's blood pressure, pulse, respirations, and oxygen saturation should be monitored for 1 hour, or per institution protocol. Any abdominal discomfort, nausea, or vomiting should be noted and treated as per physician order. Clear fluids are usually given on the same evening, and on the following day, if there are no adverse reactions, the diet is advanced to solid food.

PANCREATIC SPHINCTEROTOMY

Pancreatic sphincterotomy is done with small, specially shaped pancreatic stents and specially designed wire-guided sphincterotomes that are able to provide the endoscopist accurate positioning into the pancreatic duct. Pancreatic sphincterotomy may be indicated for the following diagnoses:

(a) symptomatic pancreatic obstruction;

(b) pancreatic calculi;

(c) pancreatic duct strictures, leaks, or pseudocysts;

(d) pancreas divisum; and

(e) pain relief for chronic pancreatitis.

Nursing care for endoscopic pancreatic sphincterotomy or stent placement is the same as for biliary duct interventions. Voice checks and teamwork between the endoscopist and gastroenterology nurse are essential. Experience with endoscopic therapeutic interventions in the pancreatic duct is limited; these procedures should be undertaken only by highly skilled endoscopists with experienced biliary GI nurses as their assistants.

The mortality rate for endoscopic sphincterotomy is considerably lower than for surgical removal of retained common duct stones. Reported complications include the following:

(a) bleeding, which is the most common complication and is responsible for half of the deaths. Bleeding can usually be managed by observation and/or transfusion;

(b) pancreatitis, which usually can be adequately treated with antibiotics and conservative follow-up;

(c) free retroduodenal perforation;

(d) cholangitis, which can be prevented by placing a stent in the bile duct or by adding a nasobiliary catheter; and

(e) entrapment of baskets, which can be eliminated by using balloons to extract stones or by ensuring that the sphincterotomy is adequate to allow the passage of a basket with a trapped stone.

If the papilla becomes edematous as a result of excessive probing or electrocoagulation, the retroduodenal artery may be displaced. Accidental severing of the artery caused by anatomical aberration may occur.

EXTRACORPOREAL SHOCK-WAVE LITHOTRIPSY

For selected patients, **extracorporeal shock-wave lithotripsy** (ESWL) is a noninvasive alternative to cholecystectomy. ESWL involves the use of shock waves generated in a specially designed table to fragment larger stones into smaller particles, most of which can then be passed spontaneously. Lithotriptors use either ultrasound or fluoroscopy to identify the target stones.

Candidates for ESWL are patients who have fewer than three stones. Other favorable predictors for success are low body mass and a good gallbladder function. ESWL is usually done on an outpatient basis under local anesthesia and moderate sedation.

Lithotripsy is generally applied in combination with dissolution therapy. Success of stone fragmentation is dependent on the size, composition, and number of stones. Stone clearance depends on the ability of the gallbladder to contract and expel the stone fragments. ESWL has been most successful with solitary stones that are less than 2 cm in size.

There have been no serious complications from ESWL, and no significant damage to surrounding organs has been reported. Petechiae on the abdominal wall is common and about 2% of patients can have microscopic hematuria. If large stone fragments remain following ESWL, CBD obstruction is a potential complication. Endoscopic sphincterotomy may be required in these patients. Compared with patients treated with cholecystectomy, patients who are treated with ESWL generally appear to have less pain, a shorter recovery period, and less chance of infection.

PULSED-DYE LASER LITHOTRIPSY

Stones in the gallbladder and CBD can also be destroyed with a pulsed-dye laser beam. Pulsed laser systems reduce the risk of thermal injury since power peaks are reached within fractions of a second. It permits precise targeting, thereby reducing the risk of bile duct injury. A quartz fiber is pushed up against the stone, and the laser fires. The beam creates a high-energy shock wave (a photo-acoustic effect) at the point of contact, and the stone is fragmented. Newer devices permit adjustment of the laser fiber by providing an acoustic signal that indicates the fiber is in contact with the stone or tissue. It is highly effective and safe for the fragmentation and extraction of difficult to treat gallstones. Due to the costs of laser lithotriptors, only a few centers will specialize in this modality.

A number of successful options have been developed for reaching the stones with the laser fiber.

1. **Laser lithotripsy** can be used during ERCP to treat ductal stones, either by threading the laser catheter through a smaller, flexible "baby" scope that is passed through the duodenoscope or by introducing a flexible radiopaque laser catheter through the duodenoscope.

2. In a percutaneous approach to fragmentation of ductal stones, the procedural cannula that leads the laser fiber to the stones can be inserted through either the tract formed by a T-tube left in place after cholecystectomy or the skin under fluoroscopic guidance.

Stones in the gallbladder can be fragmented by catheterizing the gallbladder through its free wall (cholecystolithotomy), and 2 weeks later, replacing this drainage catheter with a procedural catheter, through which an endoscope and a laser fiber are inserted.

Compared to ESWL, laser lithotripsy is less time consuming, eliminates the need for "long-term" dissolution therapy, and can be used for patients with a greater number of stones.

CASE SITUATION

Mr. Thomas Freeman is a 69-year-old man with a history of insulin-dependent diabetes. During his last visit to his internist, he complained of abdominal discomfort with early satiety and a general feeling of fullness in his stomach. The internist ordered an upper GI series. The x-ray film showed a gastric mass in the antrum, so the internist referred Mr. Freeman to a gastroenterologist, who will perform an esophagogastroduodenoscopy (EGD).

Points to think about

1. The gastroenterology nurse has done an assessment of Mr. Freeman before his EGD. Based on the knowledge of his symptoms and history, the most likely causes of the patient's symptoms are either a tumor or a bezoar. What equipment will the nurse set up for the procedure?

2. The nurse knows that this is a potentially time-consuming and resource-intensive procedure. What can be done to plan ahead?

3. The EGD confirms that Mr. Freeman has a phytobezoar. The gastroenterologist breaks up the bezoar, allows it to pass, and withdraws the scope. What might happen next?

4. Why would the gastroenterologist schedule Mr. Freeman for a repeat endoscopy?

5. What patient education would be helpful for Mr. Freeman?

Suggested responses

1. In setting up for Mr. Freeman's EGD, the gastroenterology nurse should consider the following:

   (a) The upper GI series shows a mass in the antrum. This could be a malignant lesion, so the nurse will set up to collect specimens for biopsy and cytology.

(b) Because Mr. Freeman is a diabetic, he may have decreased gastric motility caused by diabetic autonomic neuropathy and gastroparesis. This condition can allow food to remain in the stomach and collect into a phytobezoar. The nurse will set up equipment to be used to break up this concretion and allow it to pass through the stomach (e.g., rat-tooth forceps, snare, grasper).

(c) Some bezoars form because pyloric strictures prevent passage of food into the duodenum. It is possible that the nurse will need balloons to dilate the pyloric sphincter.

2. To plan for a potentially time-consuming and resource-intensive procedure, the nurse should complete the following steps:

(a) Place the procedure at the end of the schedule, rather than in the busiest part, to avoid feeling rushed. Allow at least an hour.

(b) Have all equipment readily available and checked with regard to proper working order.

(c) The procedure is much easier if the patient is comfortable and cooperative. The nurse should assess medication needs appropriately throughout the procedure and give additional doses as needed. The nurse should also monitor vital signs carefully and vigilantly, maintain the airway, and suction secretions.

3. After the bezoar has been broken up, and the endoscope has been removed, the nurse might expect the following:

(a) If the endoscopist has been able to ascertain that the pyloric sphincter is not stenosed, the particles should pass through. If not, the pyloric sphincter may need to be dilated.

(b) The physician may place Mr. Freeman on a full liquid diet for several days to help passage.

(c) Metoclopramide (Reglan) may be ordered to increase peristalsis.

(d) A repeat endoscopy may be ordered.

4. A repeat endoscopy might be ordered for the following reasons:

(a) It is often difficult to properly visualize the mucosa because of the bezoar, and it may be difficult to get past it to view the antrum and pylorus.

(b) Pyloric stenosis may require further evaluation and dilatation.

(c) Gastric carcinomas may be found distal to the bezoar, thereby causing obstruction. These should be examined by biopsy.

(d) Ulcerations may have been missed because of the presence of the bezoar.

(e) It is a good idea to check to be sure that the material has passed successfully through the pyloric sphincter.

5. Patient education considerations for Mr. Freeman could include the following:

(a) Poor dentition is often a problem in phytobezoars. The nurse might question Mr. Freeman about teeth and gum problems. He may have ill-fitting dentures or teeth in poor repair. The nurse might suggest a trip to the dentist.

(b) Poor eating habits may contribute to the formation of bezoars. Question Mr. Freeman about his diet and caution him to chew his food very well before swallowing. Consultation with a dietitian may be in order.

REVIEW TERMS

extracorporeal shock-wave lithotripsy, laser lithotripsy, overtube, papillotome, papillotomy, pedunculated polyps, polypectomy, polypectomy snares, sessile polyps, sphincterotome, sphincterotomy, ursodeoxycholic acid.

REVIEW QUESTIONS

1. Objects that are accidentally dropped into the hypopharynx during extraction should be removed using:
   (a) A polypectomy snare.
   (b) A wire basket.
   (c) A laryngoscope and curved forceps.
   (d) Biopsy forceps.

2. A polyvinyl overtube is useful for endoscopic removal of:
   (a) Foreign bodies from the duodenum.
   (b) Pointed objects.
   (c) Extremely large objects.
   (d) Small, round objects.

3. Individuals who have swallowed packets of cocaine in an attempt at concealment should be treated:
   (a) Endoscopically.
   (b) Surgically.
   (c) With observation only, permitting the packets to pass unimpeded.
   (d) With syrup of ipecac.

4. Polyps that are attached by a thin pedicle are usually transected by use of:
   (a) Cutting current alone.
   (b) Coagulation current alone.
   (c) Blended current.
   (d) Hot biopsy forceps.

5. Endoscopic polypectomy is contraindicated in patients with:
   (a) Gastric polyps.
   (b) Hyperplastic polyps.
   (c) Sessile polyps more than 2 cm in diameter.
   (d) Coagulopathy.

6. A polyp that entered the scope's suction channel may be retrieved by the following measure:
   (a) Depressing the suction button several times on the endoscope
   (b) Placing a specimen trap between the endoscope suction port and the suction tubing
   (c) Flushing water down the biopsy channel of the scope.

7. For endoscopic retrograde sphincterotomy, the ESU is turned on:
   (a) Only when the endoscopist indicates that he or she is ready to begin cutting.

(b) As soon as the grounding pad is securely attached.

(c) Once the patient is in position.

(d) As soon as fluoroscopy demonstrates proper placement of the sphincterotome within the bile duct.

8. The preferred method of retrieving stones that do not pass spontaneously after endoscopic retrograde sphincterotomy is:

(a) A mechanical lithotripter.

(b) A retrieval basket.

(c) A balloon catheter.

(d) Nasobiliary drainage.

9. Extracorporeal biliary lithotripsy disrupts gallstones using what mechanism?

(a) Ultrasonography.

(b) Chemical agents.

(c) Shock waves.

(d) Endoscopic removal.

10. Compared to ESWL, lasertripsy has the following advantages:

(a) It is faster.

(b) It does not require dissolution therapy.

(c) It can be used in patients with a greater number of stones.

(d) All of the above.

BIBLIOGRAPHY

Albert, M.B.. (1990). Successful outpatient treatment of gallstones with piezoelectric lithotripsy. *Ann Intern Med* 113, 164.

Bisson, B. (1997, July/August). Methane Gas Explosion during Colonoscopy. *Gastroenterology Nursing* 20, 136-7.

Brennan, K. & Johns, P. (1995, March/April). Esophageal Bezoar Formation in a tube-fed patient receiving sucralfate and antacid therapy: A case report. *Gastroenterology Nursing* 18, 46-8.

Carr-Locke, D.L. (1998, November/December). Technology Assessment Status Evaluation: Overtube use in Gastrointestinal Endoscopy. *Gastroenterology Nursing* 21, 265-67.

Cotton, P. & Williams, C. (1990). *Practical gastrointestinal endoscopy* (3rd ed.). Oxford: Blackwell Scientific.

Ferretis, C.B. & Malas, E.G.(1992). Endoscopic transpapillary catherization of the gallbladder followed by external shock-wave lithotripsy and solvent infusion for the treatment of gallstone disease. *Gastrointestinal Endoscopy* 38, 19.

Harz, C. (1991). Extracorporeal shockwave lithotripsy and endoscopy: combined therapy for problematic bile duct stones. *Surg Endosc* 5, 196.

Kozark, R.A. & Ball, T.J. (1994). Endoscopic pancreatic duct sphincterotomy: Indications, technique, and analysis of results. *Gastrointestinal Endoscopy* 40, 592.

Neuhaus, H. & Zillinger, C. (1998). Randomized Study of intracorporeal laser lithotripsy versus extracorporeal shock-wave lithotripsy for difficult bile duct stones. *Gastrointestinal Endoscopy* 47, 327.

Shields, N. (1990). Endoscopic retrograde sphincterotomy: special challenge for the GIA. In Trivits, S.(Ed.), Journal Reprints II, Rochester, NY: Society of Gastroenterology Nurses and Associates, Inc.

Sleisenger, M. & Fordtran, J. (1998). *Gastrointestinal disease: pathophysiology, diagnosis, management* (6th ed.). Philadelphia: W.B. Saunders.

Stone, J. & Schluterman, S. (1996, March/April). GI Nurses' Retrospective Look at Foreign Body Ingestions in Children. *Gastroenterology Nursing* 19, 70-1.

Tint, G.S. & Salen, G. (1982). Ursodeoxycholic acid: A safe and effective agent for dissolving gallstones. *Ann Internal Medical* 97, 351.

Wilkinson, M.L. (1998). Does laser lithotripsy hit the target? *GUT* 43, 740.

Yamada, T. Laine, L., Alpers, D.H. (1999). *Textbook of Gastroenterology* (3rd ed.). Philadelphia, Pennsylvania: Lippincott Williams.

Chapter 31

COMPLICATIONS AND EMERGENCIES

This chapter will acquaint the gastroenterology nurse with some of the complications and emergency situations that can occur in gastroenterology settings and will describe appropriate interventions for each situation. The topics covered include endoscopic and spontaneous perforations, hemorrhage, shock, adverse drug reactions, cardiac complications/arrest, respiratory depression, vasovagal reactions, aspiration, and pediatric complications.

Learning objectives

After reviewing the content of this chapter, the gastroenterology nurse should be able to:

1. Discuss the causes and risk factors for eight of the most important emergency situations and complications that are encountered in the gastroenterology laboratory.
2. Recognize the symptoms of these complications.
3. Explain the steps that must be taken to avoid or treat complications and emergencies associated with endoscopic procedures for adult and pediatric populations.

PERFORATION OF THE UPPER GASTROINTESTINAL TRACT

Perforation of the upper GI tract can be a result of blunt trauma, increased intraesophageal pressure, underlying pathology, ingestion of a foreign body, or mechanical trauma during upper endoscopy. It can occur in the esophagus, stomach, or duodenum. Perforation during diagnostic endoscopy is extremely rare. Predisposing factors include anterior cervical osteophytes, Zenker's diverticulum, stricture, malignancy, or an uncooperative patient. Therapeutic endoscopy carries a much greater risk of perforation.

Esophageal perforation during therapeutic endoscopy is most frequently seen with dilatation of strictures that are a result of radiation therapy, caustic ingestion, or malignancy. It can also be a result of instrument trauma (e.g., dilators, biopsy forceps, the endoscope, overtubes). Rates vary not only by the nature of the esophageal disorder but also with the aggressiveness of the management approach. There is an overall mortality rate of 25% with this complication.

Gastric perforation is less common than esophageal perforation and may be related to ulcer disease, biopsies of ulcerated lesions, and impaction of the endoscope in the hiatal hernia sac. With the advent of push enteroscopy and the use of an overtube, cases of gastric mucosal stripping and duodenal perforations have been reported. Perforations can also result from electrocautery of a bleeding ulcer in the duodenal bulb. Retroduodenal perforations can occur with sphincterotomy during endoscopic retrograde cholangiopancreatography (ERCP).

The most consistent clinical sign of upper GI perforation is pain. The type of pain and other signs and symptoms are determined by the site of the perforation.

1. If perforation has occurred in the cervical esophagus, the patient will have dysphagia, crepitus or stiffness of the neck, and neck and throat pain that is aggravated by swallowing or moving the cervical spine. The patient may also experience fever, tenderness in the affected area, or neck swelling.
2. Perforation of the thoracic esophagus typically results in substernal or epigastric pain that increases with respirations and movement of the trunk. Shortness of breath, cyanosis, pleural effusion, and back pain may also be present.
3. Perforation at the distal area of the esophagus, near the diaphragm, may lead to shoulder pain, dyspnea, severe back and abdominal pain, tachycardia, cyanosis, diaphoresis, and hypotension.
4. Boerhaave's syndrome is a spontaneous (nontraumatic) rupture of the esophagus that is commonly associated with dyspnea after a vomiting episode. It may cause severe chest and/or abdominal pain. The patient appears acutely ill and has hypotension, fever, subcutaneous

emphysema, unilateral absence of breath sounds, or evidence of pleural effusion.

5. Gastric perforation causes severe back and abdominal pain, tachycardia, cyanosis, diaphoresis, and hypotension with a drop in temperature, followed by a high fever. Patients may also experience prolonged distention of the abdomen following gastroscopy or disappearance of liver dullness on percussion.

6. After duodenal perforation, vital signs may remain stable initially. The patient then experiences sudden local or generalized abdominal pain. Although a brief period of improvement follows, peritonitis develops. The patient's abdomen becomes rigid. He or she has a high fever, hypotension, tachycardia, and severe pain that inhibits abdominal movement and the ability to breathe deeply. Both gastric and duodenal perforation can produce indications of leaking gastric or duodenal contents, such as acute upper abdominal pain and subsequent signs of guarding, rebound tenderness, or absent bowel sounds.

Contrast esophagography is the mainstay of diagnosis of esophageal perforation, although the false negative rate may be in excess of 10%. Gastrografin is used initially and followed by barium if no perforation is seen on the initial study.

Close observation and symptomatic treatment are important if perforation is suspected. Surgical advice should be sought immediately, even though perforations that are recognized early are sometimes treated conservatively with nasogastric or pharyngeal suction, parenteral nutrition, and broad-spectrum antibiotics. Conservative management is contraindicated if a major leak is apparent on contrast radiology, or if perforation occurs through an ulcer or tumor. Delay in diagnosis or inappropriate selection of a conservative management approach is likely to result in a negative patient outcome.

If necessary, cervical perforations may be sutured, and the patient may be treated with IV antibiotics. Surgery is more often recommended for intrathoracic perforations, which have a poorer prognosis. Contained thoracic perforations may be treated conservatively. If an intrathoracic perforation is not contained, urgent thoracotomy with chest and mediastinal drainage and esophageal suturing is indicated.

Small gastric perforations into the lesser sac of the peritoneal cavity can be managed conservatively. Anterior free gastric perforations with peritoneal signs and abdominal free air shown on x-ray film require surgical management. Retroduodenal perforations can be managed conservatively with bowel rest and duodenal suction. Perforations resulting from ERCP with sphincterotomy may require placement of a nasobiliary tube or stent.

PERFORATION OF THE LOWER GASTROINTESTINAL TRACT

Lower GI perforations can be spontaneous or mechanical. Certain factors are believed to put patients at higher risk. These include ischemic colitis, adhesions, strictures, radiation, diverticular disease, obstruction, inflammatory bowel

disease, malignancy, preexisting partial tears or necrosis, an uncooperative patient, or a poorly prepped bowel. They occur most often from mechanical trauma related to manipulation of the instrument during colonoscopy. It is worth noting that these perforations have been shown to be inversely related to the experience of the endoscopist.

Pneumatic perforation may result from overdistention with insufflated air. Initially, a linear tear of the serosa forms in the overdistended segment of bowel. The mucosa may then either herniate through the opening and burst or become progressively thinner until it is permeable to air.

The risk of perforation with polypectomy is almost twice as high as with diagnostic colonoscopy and is usually related to electrical injury of the bowel wall. Types of electrical injury include the following:

(a) excessive current applied to the base of the polyp before cutting;

(b) incidental injury to the opposite wall; and

(c) entrapment of normal mucosa in snare polypectomy.

Several predisposing factors can increase the risk of post-polypectomy perforation. These include large polyps, sessile polyps, and removal of lipomas. Perforations secondary to polypectomy may occasionally be delayed and have been reported to occur up to 2 weeks after the procedure. In addition to polypectomy thermal injuries, perforation has also occurred with laser therapy and a variety of thermal devices for treatment of arteriovenous malformations.

Initially, these patients may experience little or no pain secondary to the effects of the sedation utilized for the procedure. As the effects subside, the pain will progressively worsen. Signs of lower GI perforation include sudden, severe abdominal pain that becomes generalized, possibly accompanied by signs of peritonitis, abdominal distention, pneumoperitoneum, increased tympany, loss of hepatic dullness, malaise, fever, a change in vital signs, and bloody or mucopurulent rectal drainage. Increasing abdominal pain following an examination of the colon may also indicate a perforation. A hole in the colon may be seen by the examiner, or omentum may be visualized. On occasion, a colonic perforation is diagnosed radiographically, using plain abdominal radiographs in the supine position.

Most free colonoscopic perforations need to be treated promptly with surgical exploration. Patients with retroperitoneal perforations, which are usually pneumatic perforations, should receive symptomatic treatment and close observation. Surgical intervention is indicated only if signs progress.

GASTROINTESTINAL BLEEDING

GI **hemorrhage** may be associated with an underlying disease state, trauma or may arise as a rare complication of diagnostic endoscopy (Fig. 31-1). Therapeutic endoscopic procedures, including sclerotherapy, polypectomy, laser therapy, tumor ablation, and dilatation are more likely to cause bleeding. Hemorrhage is the most common complication of polypectomy. Inexperience or lack of expertise on the part of the electrosurgical unit (ESU) operator and/or malfunc-

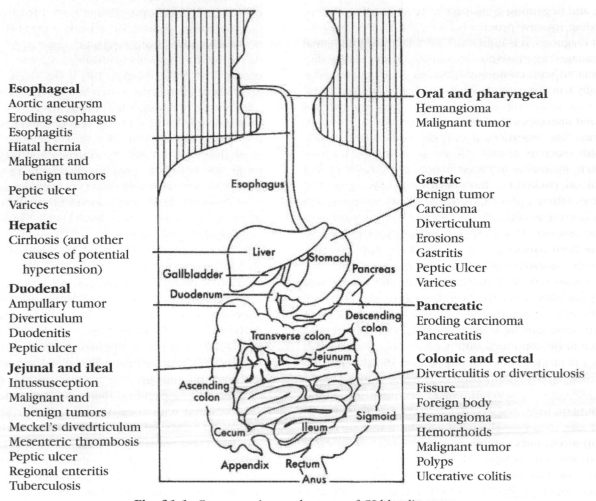

Esophageal
Aortic aneurysm
Eroding esophagus
Esophagitis
Hiatal hernia
Malignant and
  benign tumors
Peptic ulcer
Varices

Hepatic
Cirrhosis (and other
  causes of potential
  hypertension)

Duodenal
Ampullary tumor
Diverticulum
Duodenitis
Peptic ulcer

Jejunal and ileal
Intussusception
Malignant and
  benign tumors
Meckel's divedrticulum
Mesenteric thrombosis
Peptic ulcer
Regional enteritis
Tuberculosis

Oral and pharyngeal
Hemangioma
Malignant tumor

Gastric
Benign tumor
Carcinoma
Diverticulum
Erosions
Gastritis
Peptic Ulcer
Varices

Pancreatic
Eroding carcinoma
Pancreatitis

Colonic and rectal
Diverticulitis or diverticulosis
Fissure
Foreign body
Hemangioma
Hemorrhoids
Malignant tumor
Polyps
Ulcerative colitis

Fig. 31-1. Common sites and causes of GI bleeding.

tion can contribute to the risk of polypectomy-related hemorrhage.

Precipitating factors for upper GI bleeds include traumatization of recently bleeding esophageal varices; esophagitis, gastritis, or duodenitis; mucosal tears in patients with strictures; cardio-esophageal (Mallory-Weiss) tears; and a biopsy performed on a recently bleeding lesion or at the base of ulcers where larger vessels may be exposed. Peptic ulcer disease is the leading cause of upper GI hemorrhages, accounting for approximately 50% of cases. Esophageal variceal hemmorhage accounts for an estimated 10% of upper GI bleeding. Less common causes include Boerhaave's syndrome and Osler-Weber-Rendu disease.

Common causes of lower GI bleeding include diverticulosis, inflammatory bowel disease, colonic angiodysplasia, and hemorrhoids. Less-common causes include intussusception, rectal trauma, and anal disorders.

Upper GI bleeding is indicated by hematemesis, hypotension, tachycardia, or melena (liquid, tarry, foul-smelling black stools). Lower GI bleeding is associated with tachycardia, hypotension, weakness, pallor, bright red rectal bleeding (hematochezia), maroon or black stools, and possibly abdominal pain and distention. Bleeding as a complication

of polypectomy is most often intracolonic, resulting in obvious hematochezia.

The American Society for Gastrointestinal Endoscopy (ASGE) has advised that routine screening via laboratory testing is not recommended for all GI endoscopy. In patients with known or suspected liver disease, with bleeding disorders, or taking anticoagulants, some laboratory tests may be useful to minimize the risk of bleeding.

Evaluating a patient with suspected GI bleeding involves taking a thorough history, including any history of hematemesis or hematochezia, pain and abdominal tenderness, or severe retching. Routine medication usage, including over-the-counter drugs should be discussed. Any concomitant heart, lung, renal, liver, or central nervous system (CNS) disease should be considered. Vital signs should be monitored, including postural signs. A physical examination should be performed, including a rectal examination. Pallor of the lips, gums, ear lobes, and nail beds should be noted.

Initial management of upper GI bleeding should focus on maintaining the airway, providing oxygenation, monitoring of serum HCT levels every 6 hours during the acute phase, establishing a large-bore IV catheter, maintaining adequate fluid volume, stabilizing the patient's condition, stopping the bleeding, and beginning appropriate therapy to prevent further bleeding. Invasive procedures may be indicated to make a prompt diagnosis. It is imperative that patients with bleeding be managed aggressively because of the high mortality rate associated with continued bleeding or rebleeding. This is especially true for patients with esophageal and/or gastric varices.

Continued management of these patients may include central venous line insertion, and serial laboratory studies. Crystalloids (such as normal saline or Ringer's lactate solution, which maintains intravascular volume) and colloids (whole blood, packed red blood cells, and blood products such as fresh-frozen plasma, platelets, and albumin) should be administered as ordered by the physician. The patient should be assessed frequently for signs and symptoms of electrolyte disturbances, continued or recurrent bleeding.

Nasogastric aspiration and gastric lavage may be required, using an Ewald tube to remove clots from the stomach, if necessary for better visualization. If the return fluid from the nasogastric tube is clear initially, or if it clears promptly with lavage, the tube can be removed; if the return is bloody, lavage should be continued until clear. Nasal oxygen, pulse oximetry, and an electrocardiogram (ECG) may be needed in patients with hypovolemia to continually assess and combat ischemic effects.

Depending on the cause and site of upper GI bleeding, the physician may treat it with gastric lavage, drug therapy, balloon tamponade, injection sclerotherapy, thermal coagulation methods, endoscopic variceal ligation (banding), Hemoclip™ or EndoLoop™ application or surgery. Endoscopic techniques for the management of upper GI bleeding are discussed in detail in Chapter 28, including thermal coagulation methods, injection sclerotherapy, banding, and esophagogastric tamponade. Gastric lavage is discussed in Chapter 29.

In patients with acute upper GI bleeding, upper endoscopy may reveal stigmata of recent hemorrhage, such as a visible vessel, fresh blood clot, black eschar, or active bleeding. If an obvious bleeding source is identified, the endoscopist may choose to treat prophylactically (to prevent a rebleed); "tease" the bleeding site to determine the potential for rebleeding and treat if bleeding occurs; or treat medically/conservatively and monitor the patient for signs of recurrent bleeding. If no signs of recent hemorrhage are visible, medical treatment may be sufficient. In patients with continuing bleeding or stigmata of recent hemorrhage, therapeutic endoscopy or surgery may be indicated, in addition to further diagnostic tests.

The following steps should be taken to determine the source of lower GI bleeding:

1. Obtain a thorough history to determine symptoms that may pinpoint the cause of the bleeding. Painless bleed may indicate diverticular bleed, AVM, hemorrhoids, or neoplasm. Pain preceding the bleed may indicate ischemic bowel disease, inflammatory bowel disease, or infection. Information collected should include the color of the stool (i.e. black, maroon, or bright red) and the consistency characteristics of the stool (i.e. sticky, tarry, mucousy, or watery). This description can help identify the possible cause and location of the bleed.

2. Perform a physical examination, which should include a rectal examination and may also include anoscopy and sigmoidoscopy.

3. If no obvious bleeding site is found and the patient continues to bleed, perform esophagogastroduodenoscopy (EGD) to exclude an upper GI lesion (~ 5% of severe hematochezia is due to an upper GI source).

4. Perform technetium-99 tagged red blood cell scan, which can detect bleeding rates as low as 0.1 ml/min. Limitations with technetium-99 scans are encountered with patients experiencing intermittent bleeding, as seen in AVMs

5. Perform a colonoscopy. If the patient is hemodynamically stable, prepare the colon for examination using a standard prep.

6. If bleeding remains brisk, perform mesenteric arteriography.

7. If extravasation of contrast is seen, infuse vasopressin (Pitressin) or consider embolization therapy; if bleeding persists despite vasopressin or embolization, proceed with or continue replacement transfusion, and perform surgery.

8. If no extravasation is noted, but significant bleeding persists, consider exploratory laparotomy.

In patients with postpolypectomy hemorrhage, management involves stabilizing the patient; monitoring blood pressure, urine output, and central venous pressure in unstable patients; and transfusion (in 25% to 50% of patients). Endoscopic techniques for management of a lower GI bleed are also discussed in Chapter 28.

If emergency endoscopy is indicated to control GI bleeding, the nurse should verify signed informed consent; obtain the patient's medical history, including current medications and allergies and a history of the present bleeding episode; remove dentures; monitor vital signs at least every 15 minutes; monitor the patient's cardiac status using a heart monitor; monitor oxygen saturation with a pulse oximeter; establish large-bore IV line(s); obtain blood samples for complete blood count (CBC) and type and crossmatch as ordered; and start oxygen via nasal cannula as ordered. Staff should be prepared to perform gastric lavage using a large-bore orogastric or nasogastric tube.

After an emergency endoscopy, it is important for the nurse to monitor vital signs and observe the patient for bleeding; vomiting; or change in vital signs, pain, and abdominal distention. The type, amount, and times of replacement of IV fluids given should be documented.

Complications of GI bleeding may include the following:

(a) anemia from blood loss;

(b) cypovolemic shock from severe volume depletion;

(c) exsanguination from rapid massive intravascular blood loss;

(d) myocardial or cerebral infarction from acute hemoglobin depletion;

(e) disseminated intravascular coagulation from shock and clotting factor loss;

(f) peritonitis and sepsis from bowel rupture; and

(g) aspiration from massive upper GI bleeding.

SHOCK

Shock is a condition of acute peripheral circulatory failure caused by derangement of circulatory control or loss of circulating fluid. It may be endocrine, neurogenic, bacterial, cardiogenic, or hypovolemic in origin but is always characterized by decreased tissue perfusion and increased peripheral vasoconstriction. The two most common forms of shock in gastroenterology patients are hypovolemic shock and bacterial (septic) shock.

Hypovolemic shock

In hypovolemic shock, the loss of circulating volume may result from loss of blood or plasma, intestinal obstruction, nephrotic syndrome, dehydration, or trauma. In patients undergoing paracentesis, hypovolemic shock may result from the rapid shift of fluid from the circulatory system to the peritoneum as the body attempts to replace the aspirated fluid.

Hypovolemia causes the body to respond to the perceived volume loss by decreasing urinary output and constricting the caliber of peripheral blood vessels. At the same time, blood flow to the cerebral and cardiovascular systems increases.

Glycogen breakdown increases, insulin is suppressed, and hyperglycemia occurs. If cerebral blood flow is decreased and a subsequent loss of consciousness takes place, the central regulating centers may shut down.

Signs of shock include: altered mental status; restlessness; increased anxiety; pale, cool, clammy skin; collapse of peripheral neck veins; and tachycardia. Decreased capillary refill time may be present which is noted by pressing the fingernail. In the early stages, hypertension may occur. Hypotension is an advanced sign. The patient may also show diaphoresis, piloerection (goose bumps), muscle weakness, decreased urinary output, hyperventilation, abdominal distention, and electrolyte imbalance.

Treatment should focus on restoring tissue perfusion and reducing peripheral vasoconstriction. The patient should be positioned in a way that facilitates the blood supply to the brain and promotes venous return from the rest of the body. To promote respiration, the patient should lie flat with the legs elevated 20 degrees at the hips or with the head elevated slightly. To decrease oxygen use, activity should be minimized.

IV fluids should be administered to maintain the patency of the vascular system, to restore volume and an oxygen transport system, and to remove wastes. Depending on the patient's hematocrit, the fluid given may be blood, plasma, plasma expanders, or a balanced salt solution (Ringer's).

Vasoactive agents or steroids may be given. Steroids decrease peripheral resistance, increase tissue perfusion, increase venous return, and have a positive effect on the heart muscle. Metabolic acidosis is generally corrected by the administration of fluids. It may be necessary to use endotracheal intubation or a volume respirator to deliver oxygen.

Internal or external bleeding should be stopped. Depending on the bleeding site and the severity of the bleed, a gastroenterologist, interventional radiologist, and a surgeon may all be involved in the care of the patient with a GI bleed. Methods of controlling external bleeding are direct pressure, ligation, cautery, or application of topical medication. Central venous pressure readings may be ordered to monitor the course and effectiveness of treatment.

Septic shock

Septic shock or bacteremia is produced by direct invasion of the bloodstream by microorganisms or their toxins. Septic shock may be associated with peritonitis, infections such as cholecystitis or pancreatitis, bowel surgery or trauma, reduction of volvulus, or hemorrhage. Patients undergoing biliary stent replacements may experience bacteremia (or even sepsis) as a result of the "bacterial shower" into the blood stream that occurs as the obstructed stent is removed.

Initial symptoms of shock can be chills; fever; warm, flushed skin; a lesser degree of hypotension; and an increase of cardiac output. This is sometimes referred to as *warm shock*. Without treatment it can rapidly progress to the symptoms exhibited in hypovolemic shock. Treatment focuses on removing the cause, antibiotic therapy, and prevention of system failure, including the use of vasopressors such as Dopamine or Dobutamine during the initial phase before the antibiotics have had a chance to reach effective serum levels.

Although GI endoscopy, dilatation, and sclerotherapy are associated with transient episodes of bacteremia, antibiotic prophylaxis for prevention of endocarditis is controversial. However, most experts agree that prophylaxis for high-risk patients (those with prosthetic valves, a history of endocarditis, or a surgically constructed systemic pulmonary shunt) undergoing high-risk procedures (dilatation, sclerotherapy, or ERCP with bile duct obstruction) may help avoid the complication of bacteremia, which can lead to septic shock.

ADVERSE DRUG REACTIONS

In the gastroenterology laboratory, whenever a drug is administered it is important to be aware of potential side effects, toxic reactions, and allergic responses.

A side effect is any drug effect that is not intended. Some side effects are transient and subside as the patient develops a tolerance to the drug. In some patients, adjusting the drug dosage may control undesirable side effects, but in others, side effects contraindicate the use of a drug altogether.

Toxic reactions can be acute, resulting from excessive doses, or chronic, resulting from progressive accumulation of the drug in the body. Toxic reactions can also result from impaired metabolism or excretion that can cause elevated blood levels.

Chapter 31   Complications and emergencies   **347**

Table 31-1. Adverse drug reactions in the gastroenterology laboratory

Generic name	Trade name	Adverse effects
Narcotics and antagonists		
Meperidine HCl	Demerol, Pethadol, Pethidine	Respiratory depression, nausea and vomiting, hypotension, tachycardia
Fentanyl citrate	Sublimaze, Duragesic	Respiratory depression or apnea, hypotension, bradycardia, laryn-gospasm, muscular rigidity after rapid IV infusion, hypertensive crisis in patients taking MAO-inhibitors
Morphine sulfate	Duramorph, MS Contin, Roxanol	Respiratory depression, nausea and vomiting, bradycardia, ortho-static hypotension
Butorphanol tartrate	Stadol	Respiratory depression, nausea, bradycardia, palpitations, clammy skin, may cause withdrawal in patients addicted to narcotics
Naloxone HCl	Narcan	Hypertension, tremors, nausea and vomiting, sweating, tachycardia, withdrawal symptoms in patients addicted to narcotics
Sedatives and antagonists		
Diazepam	Valium	Respiratory depression, hypotension, tachycardia, laryngospasm
Midazolam HCl	Versed	Respiratory arrest, hypotension
Flumazenil	Romazicon	Dizziness, agitation, seizures, nausea and vomiting
Topical anesthetics		
Benzocaine	Hurricaine, Anbesol, Orajel, Cetacaine	Allergic reactions, anaphylaxis, methemoglobinemia in infants
Lidocaine HCl	Xylocaine	Respiratory depression and arrest, convulsions, bradycardia, cardiac arrest, anaphylaxis, excitatory and/or depressant CNS effects
Anticholinergics		
Atropine sulfate	Atropine	Hypertension or hypotension, ventricular tachycardia, paradoxical bradycardia, atrial or ventricular fibrillation, nausea and vomiting
Glycopyrrolate	Robinul	Palpitations, tachycardia, neuromuscular blockade (curare-like action) leading to muscle weakness and possible paralysis with overdosage
Antiemetics		
Droperidol	Inapsine	Hypotension, tachycardia, respiratory depression when used in combination with narcotics, laryngospasm, bronchospasm, restlessness/anxiety
Hormones		
Glucagon	Glucagon	Nausea and vomiting, hyperglycemia, hypokalemia

Drug allergy or hypersensitivity results from an antigen-antibody immune reaction in susceptible patients. Skin lesions (urticaria) and respiratory distress are the most common symptoms of drug allergies, but cardiovascular dysfunction and potentially fatal **anaphylaxis** may also be seen. It is vitally important to check for drug allergies before administering medications.

Table 31-1 lists several drugs used in the gastroenterology laboratory, with potential adverse reactions. Most adverse drug reactions in the GI laboratory are related to the drugs used for conscious sedation and analgesia. Sedatives can cause excessive depression of the central nervous system, particularly in elderly patients and in those with hypoalbuminemia.

Patients who have a known or suspected benzodiazepine dependence should be monitored carefully for seizure activity when receiving flumazenil as a reversal agent for benzodiazepines. All patients receiving this drug should be monitored for resedation, because sedation may outlast

reversal effects.

Narcotic analgesics such as meperidine (Demerol) are used to achieve analgesia, sedation, and euphoria. Side effects of meperidine include nausea and vomiting, respiratory depression, hypotension, and spasm of intestinal smooth muscle. Narcotic antagonists such as naloxone reverse the side effects of meperidine, but as with flumazenil, patients should be closely observed for resedation.

Anticholinergics and hormones

Anticholinergic agents and hormones, such as atropine, Robinul, and glucagon, all have side effects. These agents have been associated with reports of ileus, urinary retention, arrhythmias (bradycardia, tachycardia, and atrioventricular block), vomiting, and hyperglycemia. Atropine can increase intraocular pressure in patients with narrow-angle glaucoma.

To avoid adverse medication effects, it is important to administer medications cautiously. Titration should be performed slowly to the level of sedation required. The patient should be observed for signs of laryngospasm, bradycardia, excessive diaphoresis, hypotension, respiratory depression, or apnea. Resuscitation equipment and reversal agents should always be readily available. The staff should be alert to the danger of drug withdrawal when narcotic antagonists are given to drug users or patients who are being treated with narcotics.

A cart with equipment for cardiopulmonary resuscitation, including airway, bag-valve-mask resuscitation setup, oxygen supply tubing, suction, laryngoscope, IV infusion setup, drugs, and a defibrillator should be readily available on every endoscopy unit. This cart should be checked daily or in accordance with institutional policy and should be restocked if drugs are outdated. A supply of oxygen must be available whenever resuscitation is attempted.

Early diagnosis and treatment of anaphylactic reactions are necessary to avert death, which can occur within 15 minutes. There must be constant attention to an adequate airway and perfusion. Epinephrine and an antihistamine are usually used for treatment.

In addition to drug-induced anaphylaxis, allergies to latex have been identified as a cause of this type of adverse reaction. For patients with a documented history of latex allergy, every effort must be made to minimize exposure to products that contain latex. Common items in the GI lab include bite blocks, syringe plungers, adhesive tape, and tourniquets. Other patients at risk for developing this allergy are those who have had many surgical procedures, especially bowel surgeries, cesarean sections, or other procedures exposing them to equipment sterilized with ethylene oxide.

Additional emergency treatment for this type of anaphylactic reaction includes removal of the suspected antigens and changing IV catheters and tubing. All other treatment is aimed at correcting respiratory compromise, hypotension, and cardiovascular collapse.

CARDIAC COMPLICATIONS/ARREST

The most common complication of upper endoscopy, aside from miscellaneous medication reactions, is cardiopulmonary in nature. There is a mild to moderate amount of cardiovascular stress associated with upper GI endoscopy. Minor ECG changes during the procedure are common and can occur in up to 35% of patients. These are primarily sinus tachycardia, S-T-T segment changes, and premature atrial or ventricular contractions. These changes are more likely to occur in the elderly and in patients with ischemic heart disease or chronic lung disease. Serious ventricular arrhythmias and myocardial infarction are uncommon in the endoscopy setting. Some of the changes are related to anxiety and premedication rather than to the procedure itself. Patients with known heart disease should be monitored by ECG during upper GI endoscopy. ECG changes also occur during lower endoscopy, but these changes are usually transient. During colonoscopy, the procedure nurse must be mindful of grounding pad placement and the use of electric cautery for patients with a pacemaker and/or automatic internal defibrillator device (AIDD). To avoid the device firing inappropriately, the AIDD should be deactivated prior to using cautery. The AIDD must be reactivated postprocedure.

Some of the major causes of **cardiac arrest** in the gastroenterology unit are too-rapid administration or overdosage of medications; obstruction of the respiratory tract; and preexisting conditions, such as acute anxiety states, anemia, cardiac disease, dehydration, pulmonary edema, and shock.

Signs of impending cardiac arrest include the following:
  (a) signs of respiratory obstruction (cyanosis, gasping respiration, increased rate and shallowness of respiration);
  (b) pulse irregularities and rate changes;
  (c) muscle twitching; and
  (d) cold and clammy skin.

Initial signs of collapse of cardiopulmonary function are absent pulse and/or respiration and lifeless appearance. If these conditions are present, cardiopulmonary resuscitation (CPR) must begin immediately. In any situation, the most important principles of CPR include establishment of a patent airway, provision of ventilation, and restoration of cardiac pumping action.

When a patient experiences cardiac arrest, the nurse must act quickly. Brain damage or death can result if circulation is not restored within 3 to 6 minutes after cardiac and respiratory arrest. First, the resuscitation team or another source of assistance should be alerted. The patient should be placed on a flat, firm surface, and CPR should be initiated. The patient should be attached to an electrocardiograph or a defibrillator, and defibrillation should be performed by a qualified person. An IV line should be started by using a large-bore catheter, the oxygen apparatus should be set up, and oxygen should be administered. Tracheal suction apparatus and catheters should be prepared, and the patient should be suctioned as needed. The nurse may assist with intubation as needed. Events immediately preceding the crisis should be documented, and the necessary data should be provided to the resuscitation team. Vital signs should be monitored. The necessary equipment should be provided.

Any excess equipment and personnel should be removed from the area. Family members and visitors should be escorted to a waiting area and provided with emotional support. Other patients should be screened from activities. The attending physician should be notified if he or she is not in attendance.

If the resuscitation effort is successful, the patient should be transferred to a monitored area, and the physician should speak with the family. If it is unsuccessful, the physician should notify the family and provide emotional support. The physician may request consent for autopsy. If the family agrees, consent forms need to be completed and documented. Resuscitation equipment should be checked and restocked. The established protocol for a death in the gastroenterology unit should be followed.

RESPIRATORY DEPRESSION

In patients receiving anesthesia, sedatives, or narcotics, **res-**

piratory depression can occur, potentially leading to cardiovascular collapse. Symptoms of respiratory depression include a decrease in respiratory rate and/or tidal volume, oxygen desaturation as measured by pulse oximetry, Cheyne-Stokes respiration (rhythmic waxing and waning of respirations), periods of apnea, and cyanosis. These symptoms may be accompanied by extreme somnolence; skeletal muscle flaccidity; cold, clammy skin; and sometimes bradycardia and hypotension. When medications that have been associated with respiratory depression are used, such as narcotics and benzodiazepines, the drugs should be titrated to achieve maximum effect with minimum dose. Particular diligence should be paid to decreasing oxygen saturation. Inform the endoscopist of the decreasing saturation. Increasing the oxygen flow rate and the head tilt/chin lift maneuver may be all that is necessary to increase the oxygen saturation level to within acceptable limits and avoid serious complications.

Respiratory depression may be reversed with naloxone (Narcan) and/or flumazenil (Romazicon). Elderly patients and patients with underlying pulmonary disease may require smaller doses. Additional caution should be used sedating the elderly. Due to a slower metabolism, the sedation may require twice as long to take effect for these patients. If their metabolism is not taken into account, the elderly have greater potential for over-sedation. Patients who have hepatic and/or renal dysfunction may take twice as long to clear the drugs from their system. For this reason, patients with these coexisting conditions should be monitored more closely following their procedures when they are no longer being stimulated by the scope.

If the patient stops breathing, the physician should be notified at once. The most important factors are the establishment and maintenance of the patient's airway. These goals are accomplished by placing the patient in a supine position and tilting the head back, taking care to avoid hyperextension and subsequent closing of the airway. An oropharyngeal airway should be inserted quickly, and oxygen should be administered by a bag-valve-mask apparatus. The gastroenterology nurse should be prepared to assist with the intubation of the patient and to control respirations if necessary.

An appropriate IV dose of naloxone (Narcan) and/or flumazenil (Romazicon) should be administered simultaneously with efforts at respiratory resuscitation. The pulse should be checked. If the carotid pulse cannot be palpated, external cardiocompression should be started. Usually, once a reversal agent takes effect, the patient begins to awaken and breathe independently.

VASOVAGAL SYNCOPE

A **vasovagal episode** is a transient vascular and neurogenic reaction marked by pallor; nausea; diaphoresis; bradycardia; a rapid fall in blood pressure, which when below a critical level results in loss of consciousness (**vasovagal syncope**/fainting); and characteristic electroencephalographic changes. It is most often evoked by emotional stress associated with fear or pain. This response can also be seen prior to the procedure, with intravenous insertion. Vasovagal episodes have been reported during colonoscopy. There is no clear agreement as to cause, but several theories have been postulated, such as stretching of the mesentery and the presence of diverticular disease.

To treat a vasovagal reaction, the patient should be positioned with the head at a level with or lower than the rest of the body. Consciousness usually returns quickly once the patient is recumbent. Additional treatment may include IV fluids at an increased rate, supplemental oxygen, and IV atropine. If the vasovagal syncope is a response to patient discomfort, i.e., bearing down and holding his/her breath, the patient should be encouraged to breathe. Once the heart rate and blood pressure are adequate, additional sedation/analgesia may be necessary to increase patient tolerance.

POSTURAL HYPOTENSION

Postural hypotension may occur when the patient suddenly assumes an upright position. There is a fall in systolic and diastolic blood pressure, sometimes accompanied by weakness, dizziness, or syncope. Great care should be taken when discharging a patient who has undergone a bowel prep for their procedure. Postural hypotension is commonly associated with prolonged bed rest, volume depletion, neurological disease, and the use of narcotics in ambulatory patients. Dehydration can occur quickly in children and the elderly due to the fragile nature of their fluid and electrolyte balance.

ASPIRATION

Aspiration occurs when liquids or solids mistakenly enter the pulmonary system. The incidence of aspiration is only 0.8% but the mortality rate of this complication may reach 10%. Patients can aspirate saliva, gastric secretions, blood, or retained gastric contents/food residual.

Topical pharyngeal anesthesia, sedation, and supine positioning may all be contributing factors in aspiration and its sequelae. A full stomach, active bleeding, and retained gastric secretions, blood, or retained gastric contents/food residue. The elderly and any other patients who have depressed cough and gag reflexes are also at risk.

Aspiration is also a problem in patients who are receiving enteral nutrition. Aspiration of gastric secretions may be minimized by placing a feeding tube well beyond the pylorus into the duodenum, by controlling gastric volumes, and by elevating the patient's head and shoulders.

The question of whether percutaneous endoscopic gastrostomy tubes prevent or cause aspiration is debatable. Most of the literature agrees that the method of enteral formula administration (continuous versus intermittent infusion) does not affect the incidence of aspiration. It is difficult to determine in cases of aspiration pneumonia whether the source is oropharyngeal secretions or gastric secretions. Dyes, such as methylene blue, can be mixed in the enteral formula to determine if the tube feeding is the aspiration source.

During upper endoscopy, the nurse suctions the patient if

necessary to avoid aspiration. The risk of aspiration is also reduced by performing the procedure with the patient on the left side, with the head tilted to the side to allow secretions to run out.

PEDIATRIC COMPLICATIONS AND EMERGENCIES

Upper GI endoscopy and colonoscopy in pediatric patients are useful tools for diagnosis and management. Diagnostic endoscopic procedures generally are safe, with a rate of less than 1% for serious complications. As with the adult population, therapeutic procedures carry higher rates of complications but usually are also accomplished without significant problems.

Complications of upper endoscopy in children are the same as in the adult population, with the following exceptions:

(a) Oral trauma caused by the presence of loose baby teeth (assess the child or orthodonic appliances which could be dislodged and potentially aspirated);

(b) Upper airway obstruction caused by incorrect selection of scope size (observe for inspiratory stridor which could be caused by trachea compression by the endoscope);

(c) Oxygen desaturation caused by crying and struggling;

(d) Hypoxemia as a result of methemoglobinemia, which can develop after exposure to benzocaine or related medications;

(e) Over-distension of the abdomen can lead to respiratory compromise; and

(f) Arrhythmias are rare during endoscopy in the pediatric population.

In the event of a significant decreased oxygen saturation in a pediatric patient undergoing endoscopy, reposition the head, assess for abdominal distension, and consider aborting the procedure until the cause of respiratory compromise is identified and treated.

Complications during lower endoscopy have been reported infrequently, and data used have been extrapolated from the adult population.

Most problems during endoscopic procedures center around sedation and analgesia. Reports in the literature indicate that ineffective sedation in children is more common than oversedation and hypoxemia. In upper endoscopy, patients age 3 to 9 years prove to be the most difficult to sedate, and patients age 6 to 9 years require the highest doses of midazolam and meperidine. During lower endoscopy, doses follow more closely the recommendations utilizing body weight; age itself is not a factor. Procedures are contraindicated when patients cannot be adequately sedated. General anesthesia should be considered for these patients.

Depending on the procedure and condition of the patient, the gastroenterologist may decide that the child requires sedation in the operating room and be safely monitored by the anesthesiologist.

CASE SITUATION

It is midnight on a Friday night. The gastroenterology nurse on call is awakened by her beeper. She checks the number and calls the hospital. The intensive care unit (ICU) informs the nurse that they have just admitted a John Doe who is vomiting bright red blood. The gastroenterologist on call, is on his way in and has requested that the nurse on call meet him as soon as possible in the ICU. She rushes to get dressed. While driving to the hospital, she goes over what she will need to do.

Points to think about

1. Because this is a new patient, the gastroenterology nurse has no history on which to rely and must think of all possible causes of upper GI bleeding that she may be able to treat endoscopically. What will she take to the bedside?

2. Because this patient is a John Doe, he is either too disoriented to provide his name or is unconscious and has no identification. If the patient is conscious, some quick questions might help the nurse assess possible problems. What would she ask?

3. The gastroenterologist arrives, and together he and the nurse plan the course of action. He decides the nasogastric aspirate is clear enough to proceed, and the nurse prepares the patient for endoscopy. During the procedure the patient will be at risk for the serious complication of aspiration. How should the nurse address this issue?

4. Assessing the amount of blood lost is important when judging the amount of fluid needed to reverse volume depletion. What can the nurse learn from laboratory data about this?

5. What should the nurse know about how each body system responds to massive GI bleeding?

6. John Doe's inability to provide his name and address leads the nurse to the nursing diagnosis "altered thought processes caused either by loss of consciousness or disorientation to time, place, and person." (Data have not been provided to determine whether this patient is unconscious or disoriented.) What are the seven areas of cognitive assessment in which a nurse ordinarily endeavors to obtain data for this diagnosis?

Suggested responses

1. The gastroenterology nurse might take the following equipment to the bedside:

(a) Banding equipment and at least 2 injector needles, if the physician uses that technique. The vomiting of bright red blood may indicate variceal bleeding. Alternative medications for therapeutic injection should the sclerosant fail to control the bleeding.

(b) Gastric lavage equipment (Ewald tube and large irrigating syringes). Large amounts of blood in the stomach make it difficult to visualize bleeding sites, and it is often difficult to get supply items from central service in the middle of the night.

(c) The electrocautery device that the gastroenterology department uses (bipolar probe, heater probe, or cautery unit) and an extra probe. If the probe comes in more than one diameter (i.e., 7Fr +10Fr) be sure to take the size appropriate for the scope channel diameter. The laser can be used for GI bleeding, but it usually cannot be transported to the ICU because of its specific electrical and plumbing needs. Late at night is not an optimal time to do emergency endoscopy in the gastroenterology unit, because there are usually not enough personnel present to handle any complications that occur.

(d) The usual sedatives and emergency drugs. The ICU may stock most things, but it is better to plan ahead because the pharmacy may not be open.

(e) Cover gowns; protective eyewear; masks; and enough gloves for the gastroenterology nurse, the physician, and the ICU nurse, who may have to help the gastroenterology nurse.

(f) The largest channel gastroscope available or a double-channel gastroscope. The nurse should ensure that equipment is checked and working properly before going to the bedside.

(g) A second scope compatible with banding equipment and/or capable of better flexibility to visualize and treat bleeding in the duodenal bulb.

(h) Tubes for esophagastric tamponade should all measures fail to control the bleeding i.e. Sengstaken-Blakemore three-lumen tube or the four lumen Minnesota Sump tube (along with a manometer, clamps, etc., as necessary for use with tubes).

2. If the nurse was able to ask John Doe some questions, she might ask the following:

(a) Whether he has had a bleeding episode such as this before or has been previously diagnosed or treated for ulcer disease. Recurrent ulcerations are common; however, in 40% of patients, the new bleeding will stem from a different lesion.

(b) If he is allergic to any medication, and what medications he has been taking at home. Many patients forget about over-the-counter medications, and the nurse should specifically ask about aspirin, cold remedies, or ibuprofen (Advil, Nuprin, Motrin). Also, she should ask about specific anticoagulants, which may prolong bleeding time.

(c) If he had vomiting of gastric contents before the onset of vomiting of blood. Forceful vomiting can cause a tear in the lower esophagus or gastric cardia, which can bleed profusely (Mallory-Weiss tear).

(d) If he consumes much alcohol. Sometimes it helps to ask about specific quantities; that is, "Do you drink beer? If so, one or two six-packs a day?" "Do you drink vodka, whiskey, or rum? If so, one or two pints a day?" If a family member is present, he or she may give more accurate information than the patient. Excessive alcohol consumption can cause gastritis or ulcers that bleed excessively. Alcoholic liver damage may be evi-

dent on physical examination (ascites, spider angiomata, enlarged liver, or gynecomastia). If liver damage is probable, the nurse may suspect esophageal varices as a cause of bleeding. Clotting mechanisms would also be affected. In this patient an INR and platelet count should be assessed prior to endoscopy, as time and urgency permit.

(e) What the state of his general health is, with particular attention to cardiac, respiratory, or renal problems. Patients with concomitant health problems are at higher risk for complications.

3. To address the issue of the possibility of aspiration during endoscopy, the gastroenterology nurse can take the following precautions:

(a) Recognize that all patients undergoing upper endoscopy are at risk of aspirating saliva, gastric secretions, and blood. Patients most at risk are those who have recently eaten a meal, those who have active upper GI bleeding, those with recent stroke, and those with pyloric obstruction and gastric retention.

(b) An overtube may be employed to help protect the airway and minimize gagging, especially if the scope and/or gastric lavage may be passed more than once.

(c) Use a topical throat anesthetic sparingly, if at all. Local pharyngeal anesthesia interferes with swallowing and gag reflex and alters coordination of the pharynx and upper esophageal sphincter.

(d) Minimize the use of sedative medications in patients at high risk for aspiration. IV sedation and analgesia causes depression of the respiratory system and CNS and can also suppress the laryngeal closure reflex for 5 to 10 minutes.

(e) Keep the patient in the left lateral position until sedation wears off. Have adequate, working oral suction available with Yankauer suction tips. Monitor the patient carefully throughout the procedure and during recovery, with special attention to color, blood pressure, secretions, and sensorium.

4. Loss of 10% to 25% of blood volume is considered a moderate bleed; over 25% is considered a massive bleed. The normal adult has a circulating blood volume of 75 ml/kg body weight. A man who weighs 154 lb (70 kg) will have about 5250 ml of circulating blood volume; 20% of that is about 1 L. Therefore, if he loses a single liter, he will experience a moderate bleed, with a corresponding drop in blood pressure, rapid pulse, labored breathing, loss of sensorium, anxiety, or a feeling of impending doom.

(a) Blood pressure. Lying and standing blood pressures can help determine the extent of depleted circulating blood, shock and hypotension. If, on standing, the blood pressure falls 30 mm Hg or more from baseline or the apical pulse rate increases 20 to 30 beats per minute, there is significant postural hypotension. If the patient is "shocky" in the recumbent position, he may already have lost more than 50% of his circulating volume. This will be a more accurate indication of the significance of the bleed.

(b) Hemoglobin and hematocrit. Hemoglobin and hematocrit levels are always done and may give an indication of the duration of hemorrhage, rather than provide information about the amount of acute blood loss. The patient can exsanguinate with a normal hemoglobin and hematocrit. It can take from 12 to 36 hours for hemoglobin and hematocrit values to drop in acute bleeding.

(c) Blood urea nitrogen (BUN). A BUN level above 40 mg (in patients without previous renal disease) indicates a significant bleed. Blood in the gut is partially digested and proteins are absorbed, which elevate BUN, and volume depletion produces a prerenal azotemia with consequent elevation of BUN.

(d) Coagulation studies. Coagulation studies are important because clotting factors will be used up quickly, and patients with underlying liver disease will have difficulty keeping up with the demand.

(e) Arterial blood gases (ABGs). ABGs should be drawn to check for lactic acidemia, which can occur as a result of severe tissue hypoxia because there is less blood carrying less oxygen to cells. Hypoperfusion causes potential complications to each body system as a result of hemorrhage.

5. The different body systems respond to massive GI bleeding in the following ways:

(a) Cardiovascular system. The heart's workload increases during periods of hypovolemia and reduced tissue oxygenation. A diseased heart may not be able to provide the increased output needed to maintain adequate tissue perfusion. The heart itself needs a lot of blood and oxygen and can suffer from myocardial ischemia during GI bleeding.

(b) Respiratory system. Hemorrhage can worsen preexisting pulmonary disease. Ventilation and perfusion may be impaired by white blood cells clumping in the lung's tiny blood vessels, and adult respiratory distress syndrome may result. This may occur 12 to 28 hours after hemorrhage; the ABGs should be monitored.

(c) Hematological system. Coagulation problems frequently occur following hemorrhage, because the clotting factors are used more rapidly than they are produced.

(d) Renal system. Prolonged low renal blood flow causing hypoxia leads to renal failure. Acute tubular necrosis can occur when large myoglobin molecules in the bloodstream (released from other cells being destroyed) become lodged in tiny tubules. Watch for decreased urine output. The serum creatinine is a more reliable indication of kidney function than the BUN.

(e) Metabolic system. When the compensatory hormone regulation fails to maintain fluid and electrolyte concentrations, metabolic derangement can follow, including decreased serum pH (acidosis), decreased potassium (hypokalemia), increased sodium (hypernatremia), and serum hyperosmolality, which causes movement of fluid into the vascular space from the extravascular space to maintain circulating volume. This must be corrected.

6. The seven areas of cognitive assessment are as follows:
(a) level of consciousness;
(b) orientation;
(c) memory;
(d) judgment/intellectual functioning;
(e) thought flow;
(f) thought content; and
(g) perception.

REVIEW TERMS

anaphylaxis, aspiration, cardiac arrest, hemorrhage, hypovolemia, perforation, respiratory depression, shock, vasovagal syncope

---

REVIEW QUESTIONS

1. Substernal or epigastric pain that increases with respirations and movement of the trunk is associated with perforation of what portion of the GI tract?
(a) Cervical esophagus.
(b) Thoracic esophagus.
(c) Distal esophagus, near the diaphragm.
(d) Stomach.

2. Conservative management of upper GI perforations may include:
(a) Suction.
(b) IV nutrition.
(c) Administration of antibiotics.
(d) All of the above.

3. Hematochezia is generally a symptom of:
(a) Bleeding esophageal varices.
(b) Bleeding ulcers.
(c) Gastritis.
(d) Lower GI bleeding.

4. In a patient with upper GI bleeding, if the return fluid from gastric lavage promptly becomes clear, the next step is to:
(a) Continue lavage.
(b) Remove the nasogastric tube.
(c) Use an Ewald tube to remove clots from the stomach.
(d) Begin balloon tamponade.

5. In patients suffering from hypovolemic shock, circulation to the heart and the brain initially:
(a) Increases.
(b) Decreases.
(c) Remains the same.
(d) Stops.

6. An important side effect of topical pharyngeal anesthesia is:
(a) Vomiting.
(b) Increased intraocular pressure.
(c) Allergic reactions.
(d) Superficial phlebitis.

7. When a patient experiences cardiac arrest, what is the first

action the gastroenterology nurse should take?

(a) Call for help.

(b) Initiate CPR.

(c) Attach the patient to a monitoring device.

(d) Remove family members and visitors from the room.

8. What drug is used to reverse narcotic-induced respiratory depression?

(a) Physostigmine (Antilirium).

(b) Naloxone (Narcan).

(c) Flumazenil (Romazicon).

(d) Epinephrine.

9. To treat a vasovagal attack, it is important to:

(a) Offer fluids.

(b) Begin CPR.

(c) Position the patient with the head at the level of or below the rest of the body.

(d) Keep the patient warm.

10. To avoid aspiration during upper endoscopy, the nurse usually:

(a) Maintains the patient in the supine position.

(b) Encourages the patient to breathe deeply.

(c) Provides suction as necessary.

(d) Intubates the patient.

BIBLIOGRAPHY

Aliperti, G. (1996). Complications related to diagnostic and therapeutic endoscopic retrograde cholangiopancreatography. *Gastrointest Endosc Clin North Am 6*, 397-407 1996. Gastrointestinal Endoscopy Clinics of North America.

Bloomfield, R.S. & Rockey, D.C. (2000, January). Diagnosis and Management of Lower Gastrointestinal Bleeding. *Current Opinion in Gastroenterology 16*(1), 89-97.

Cappell, M.S. & Iacovone, F.M. (1999, January). Safety and Efficacy of Esophagogastroduodenoscopy after Myocardial Infarction. *American Journal of Medicine, 106* (1), 29-35.

Chan, M. (1996). Complications of upper endoscopy. *Gastrointest Endosc Clin North Am 6*, 287-303. Gastrointestinal Endoscopy Clinics of North America.

Chung, J.K. (2002, June). Evaluation of Endoscopic Hemostatis in Upper Gastrointestinal bleeding related to Mallory-Weiss Syndrome. *Endoscopy 34*(6), 474-9.

Chung, J.K. (2001, November). Endoscopic Factors Predisposing to rebleeding following Endoscopic Hemostasis in bleeding peptic ulcers. *Endoscopy 11*(33), 969-75.

Clouse, R. (1996). Complications of endoscopic gastrointestinal dilation techniques. *Gastrointest Endosc Clin North Am 6*, Danmore, L. (1996). Colonoscopic perforations: etiology, diagnosis and management. *Dis Colon Rectum 39*, 1308-14. Diseases of the Colon and Rectum.

Dorland's Illustrated Medical Dictionary (29th ed.) (2000). Philadelphia: W.B. Saunders.

Eastwood, G. & Avunduk, C. (1994). *Manual of gastroenterology: diagnosis and therapy* (2nd ed.). Boston: Little, Brown.

Engstrom, P. & Goosenberg, E. (1999). *Diagnosis and Management of Bowel Diseases*. Philadelphia: Professional Communications, Inc.

Feldman, M., Friedman, L.S. & Sleisenger, M.H. (2002). *Sleisenger & Fordtran's Gastrointestinal and Liver Disease: Pathophysiology, Diagnosis, Management*. Philadelphia: Elsevier Science Health Science.

Fox, V. (1997). Complications following percutaneous endoscopic gastrostomy and subsequent catheter replacement in children and young adults. *Gastrointest Endosc 45*, 64-71. Gastrointestinal Endoscopy.

Gedebou, T. (1996). Clinical presentation and management of iatrogenic colon perforations, *Am J Nurs 172*, 454-8. American Journal of Nursing.

Gitnick, G. & Hollander, D. (Eds.) (1994). *Principles and practice of gastroenterology and hepatology* (2nd ed.). New York: Elsevier.

Huang, S.P. & Wang, H.P. (2002, June). Endoscopic Hemoclip Placement and Epinephine Injection for Mallory Weiss Syndrome with Active Bleeding. *Gastrointestinal Endoscopy 55*(7), 842-6.

Kavic, S. & Basson, M. (2001, April). Complications of endoscopy. *American Journal of Surgery 181*(4), 319-32.

Laine, L. & Estrada, R. (2002, January). Randomized trial of normal saline solution injections versus bipolar electrocoagulation for treatment of patients with high-risk bleeding ulcers: is local tamponade enough? *Gastrointestinal Endoscopy 55*(1), 6-10.

Landi, B. (1996). Duodenal perforation occurring during push-enteroscopy. *Gastrointestinal Endoscopy 43*, 631 (letter).

Medical Economics (Ed.) (2001). *Physicians' desk reference* (56th ed.) Oradell: Author.

Minocha, A. (2000). *2001 Minocha's Guide to Digestive Diseases.* McLean, Virginia.: International Medical Publishing, Inc.

Morse, T. (2000, May). *Presenting the core complications and emergencies*. Presented at the 27th Annual Meeting of the Society of Gastroenterology Nurses and Associates.

Nettina, S.M. (2000). (Ed.). *The Lippincott manual of nursing practice* (7th ed.). Philadelphia: J.B. Lippincott.

Odom, J. (2000, May). *Wink, Blink, and a Nod: A tale of Conscious Sedation*. Presented at the 27th Annual Meeting of the Society of Gastroenterology Nurses and Associates, Chicago, Illinois.

Redmond, M. (1996). Latex allergy: recognition and perioperative management. *Post Anesth Nurs 2*, 6-12. Post Anesthesia Nursing.

Rothbaum, R. (1996). Complications of pediatric endoscopy. *Gastroendosc Clin North Am 6*, 445-9. Gastrointestinal Endoscopy Clinics of North America.

Schapiro, G. & Edmundowicz, S. (1996). Complications of percutaneous endoscopic gastrostomy. *Gastrointest Endosc Clin North Am 6*, 409-22. Gastrointestinal Endoscopy Clinics of North America.

Society of Gastroenterological Nurses and Associates, Inc. (2003). *Manual of Gastrointestinal Procedures* (5th ed.). Chicago, IL.

Shannon, M.T., Stang, C.L. & Wilson, B.A. (2001). *Nurses' drug guide 2002*, Stanford, CT: Prentice Hall.

Sivak, M. (1997). *Gastroenterology endoscopy* (2nd ed.). Philadelphia: W.B. Saunders.

Taylor, M. (Ed.) (1996). *Gastrointestinal emergencies*. Baltimore, MD: Williams & Wilkins.

Waye, J., Kahn, O. & Auerbach, M. (1996). Complications of colonoscopy and flexible sigmoidoscopy. *Gastrointest Endosc Clin North Am 6*, 343-77. Gastrointestinal Endoscopy Clinics of North America

Yang, R. & Laine, L. (1995). Mucosal stripping: a complication of push enteroscopy. *Gastrointestinal Endoscopy 41*, 156-8.

Chapter 32

SURGICAL INTERVENTIONS

This chapter will acquaint the gastroenterology nurse with surgical interventions in the GI tract. An overview of indications, procedures, and possible associated complications will be discussed. Understanding these surgical interventions will help the GI nurse to anticipate client needs when providing outpatient follow-up and assisting with endoscopy and other related procedures.

The gastroenterology nurse is an integral part of the team responsible for management of the GI surgical patient. In the outpatient clinic setting, the GI nurse is often the first person the surgical patient encounters before any diagnostic workup. From that point, the patient continues to interact with GI professional nurses throughout the preoperative period and during diagnostic testing, medical intervention, and therapeutic endoscopy procedures. In the postoperative period, the surgical patient encounters GI nurses in the outpatient clinic, as well as during any endoscopic procedures performed to evaluate the effectiveness of surgery or to provide treatment for postoperative complications. The GI surgery patient has a tremendous need for education and emotional support, both of which are provided by the GI nurse during all phases of care.

Learning objectives

After reviewing the content of this chapter, the gastroenterology nurse should be able to:

1. Identify common GI disorders that require surgical intervention.
2. Describe common surgical procedures performed for GI disorders.
3. Identify complications associated with surgical interventions of the GI tract.
4. Discuss nursing interventions related to treating patients who have undergone surgery for GI disorders.

SURGICAL INTERVENTIONS FOR ESOPHAGEAL DISORDERS

Many esophageal disorders are endoscopically diagnosed and initially treated by medical management. When medical management fails or when the disorder is chronic, the patient and physician may choose surgical correction of the disorder. After surgical intervention, the patient may undergo endoscopy to allow for evaluation of the surgical repair and recurrence of disease. Common problems requiring surgical intervention include gastroesophageal reflux disease (GERD), achalasia, esophageal cancer, and perforation of the esophagus.

Gastroesophageal reflux disease

Surgery for **GERD** is indicated when medical management fails to adequately treat symptoms, leading to such complications as Barrett's esophagus or bleeding, and when symptoms are potentially harmful or life threatening, such as aspiration pneumonia, exacerbation of pulmonary disease, or bradycardia. Infants are especially prone to GERD due to transient lower esophageal sphincter relaxations (TLESRS) as lower esophageal sphincter tone is not well developed, even in the premature infant. Reflux resolves in the majority of infants by age 18 months. Therefore, surgical correction in infants is usually reserved for those with harmful or life-threatening symptoms.

The most common surgical procedure used to treat gastroesophageal reflux is the **Nissen fundoplication** or one of its variants. The Nissen procedure can be performed through laparotomy or laparoscopy. In either procedure, the gastric fundus is wrapped 360 degrees around the distal esophagus and sutured into place, creating a tightened lower esophageal sphincter (Fig. 32-1). In pediatric patients, a gastrostomy tube is frequently placed to allow for gastric decompression. Interestingly, results of a pediatric series of

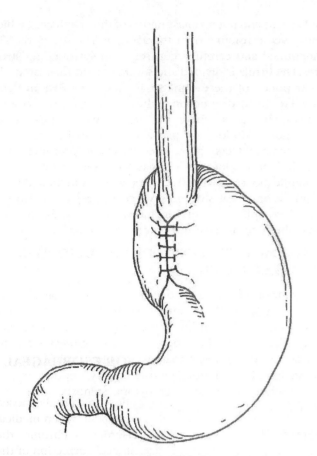

Fig. 32-1. Nissen fundoplication to treat GERD. (Redrawn from Ellett M: Pediatric esophageal reflux: a nursing perspective, *SGA J* 2(1) 1988.)

laparoscopic fundoplications suggest that the results and complication rates are similar to those of the open procedure, but the hospitalization is shortened.

Complications include inability to belch or vomit, "gas bloat syndrome" (distention, inability to vomit, abdominal pain, and severe irritability), and recurrence of symptoms with a need to repeat the surgical procedure after a period of time (a "failed" or "slipped" fundoplication). The rate of pediatric failed or slipped fundoplications is 0.9-13%.

Other surgical procedures used to correct gastroesophageal reflux include the Belsey Mark IV repair and the Hill posterior gastropexy. When surgical correction such as Nissen fundoplication is not feasible, a jejunal feeding tube may be placed endoscopically or surgically to allow feedings to bypass the stomach, decreasing the risk of reflux. Hiatal hernia carries a high risk for reflux symptoms and is discussed later in this chapter.

Until recently, treatment options for GERD included ongoing drug therapy, lifestyle changes, or invasive surgery. New endoscopic treatment options are becoming available but at this printing are still investigational.

The concept of intraluminal gastroplication was first introduced by Swarn in 2001. A plication is a type of "pleat" in the tissue secured by an intraluminal suturing device. Plications are placed in the stomach, at or just below the squamocolumnar junction, to enhance the competency of the LES (lower esophageal sphincter) and prevent reflux of gastric contents into the esophagus.

Endoscopic valvuloplasty has been investigated in the animal model. This involves intussusception of the gastroesophageal junction into the stomach to create a nipple-type valve. This augments function of the cardia and improves competency of the LES.

Achalasia

Surgical intervention for treatment of **achalasia** is generally reserved for patients who have not responded adequately to the medical or endoscopic measures discussed in Chapter 13. The traditional surgical procedure for achalasia is **Heller's myotomy** or one of its variants.

Heller's myotomy requires an abdominal incision or left thoracotomy to approach the esophagus. Surgical incisions are made in the anterior and posterior portions of the distal esophageal musculature that extends into the gastric cardia. The muscle tissue is then divided longitudinally to the mucosal layer, allowing for relaxation of the lower esophagus. A modified Heller's myotomy may be performed, incising only the anterior wall of the esophagus. Gastroesophageal reflux is common following Heller's myotomy; therefore, an antireflux procedure is usually also performed.

Esophageal cancer

Successful surgical intervention for esophageal cancer requires accurate diagnosis and careful staging, which are frequently performed in the endoscopy suite. Surgical resection is the treatment of choice for tumors of the distal two thirds of the esophagus, if preoperative staging suggests that there is no metastatic disease and the patient is otherwise in good health and able to withstand the rigors of major surgery.

Several techniques may be used to remove the diseased esophagus and to restore continuity to the alimentary canal. Typically, an abdominal incision is made and the stomach and duodenum are mobilized. The thoracic esophagus is then identified and the diseased area excised. An esophageal replacement procedure may be indicated. There is usually a gastric pull-through that attaches the stomach to the proximal esophagus. A gastrostomy tube is placed at the time of surgery to allow for enteral nutrition.

Complications of this procedure include recurrence of cancer at anastomotic sites, esophageal strictures, gastroesophageal reflux, and dysphagia. Postoperative esophageal strictures may require multiple dilatation sessions and may be extremely tight, because they are fibrous.

Preoperative staging of esophageal cancer using EUS (endoscopic ultrasound) has been shown to be a well-tolerated and cost-effective tool for patients and physicians. Stage I and IV tumors may be treated with combined modality therapies, including surgery, which spares patients discomfort and risk and saves considerable health cost expenditure.

Early stage esophageal cancers, involving the epithelium or mucosa without lymph node involvement, may also be treated endoscopically with EMR (endoscopic mucosal resection). This technique involves using submucosal saline injection with a specialized cautery loop technique, using a two-channel therapeutic endoscope. In some instances, EMR is combined with PDT (photodynamic therapy) for treatment of Barrett's esophagus with neoplasia.

Perforation of the esophagus

Perforation of the esophagus may be associated with esophageal instrumentation (including endoscopes, esophageal dilators, guidewires, and biopsy forceps), surgery, swallowed foreign bodies, penetrating trauma, peptic ulceration, and Boerhaave's syndrome. **Boerhaave's syndrome** is an uncommon but catastrophic event in which the lower thoracic esophagus is completely torn away from the gastric cardia.

Esophageal perforation is a potentially life-threatening condition that requires prompt recognition and may require immediate surgical intervention. Although the physician and endoscopy nurse may actually see the esophageal tear during the course of the procedure, many perforations are not detected until after the procedure is complete. As a result, patients who undergo endoscopy on an outpatient basis must receive detailed instructions regarding reporting of symptoms of possible perforation. Symptoms such as fever, abdominal or chest pain, dyspnea, abdominal distention, abdominal rigidity, increased heart rate, and increased respiratory rate should receive immediate attention. Hypotension is a late and ominous sign of impending shock and circulatory collapse. Perforation is confirmed by x-ray examination, demonstrating free air within the chest or abdominal cavities.

Early treatment of esophageal perforation includes stabilization of respiratory status, antibiotic therapy, volume replacement, and chest-tube drainage. When surgery becomes necessary, the site of perforation dictates the surgical approach. Generally, the esophageal tear is closed with sutures and the sutured area is reinforced with pleural or intercostal flaps in a thoracic esophageal injury and with a diaphragmatic flap in the event of a distal injury.

Complications associated with repair of esophageal perforation depend on the site of the repair. Dysphagia and airway difficulties may be associated with repair of the upper esophagus, whereas gastroesophageal reflux may be associated with repair of the lower esophagus. Stricture is a potential complication of repair to any area of the esophagus.

Esophageal atresia

Esophageal atresia (EA) is a congenital malformation, affecting between 1 in 2000 and 1 in 5000 live births, that necessitates surgical correction in the neonatal period. In EA, the esophagus ends in a blind pouch instead of attaching to the stomach. It is associated with **tracheoesophageal fistula** (TEF) in 85% of cases. TEF is an open communicating channel between the trachea and esophagus. EA and TEF are frequently associated with other congenital anomalies.

The mainstay of surgical management is surgical ligation of the TEF and end-to-end anastomosis of the esophagus, which is achieved through a right thoracotomy. The site of the TEF is identified and carefully cut free from surrounding structures. The fistula is divided and sutured or suture-ligated. The upper pouch of the esophagus is then identified and connected to the lower portion of the esophagus (primary anastomosis). In cases where the gap between ends of the esophagus is too long for primary anastomosis, delayed primary repair may take place after the infant has gained sufficient weight to allow for the anastomosis to succeed.

Complications associated with repair of EA include dysphagia and esophageal strictures. When TEF repair is also performed, complications may include respiratory compromise and inability to manage respiratory secretions.

SURGICAL INTERVENTIONS FOR DISORDERS OF THE STOMACH

Many disorders of the stomach are endoscopically diagnosed and initially treated by medical management. Depending on the nature of the surgical correction, many patients require further endoscopy after surgery. Common disorders of the stomach that may require surgical intervention include hiatal hernia, morbid obesity, peptic ulcer disease, perforated peptic ulcer, pyloric stenosis, and gastric cancer.

Hiatal hernia

Hiatal hernia is a common disorder, frequently associated with gastroesophageal reflux symptoms. The most common

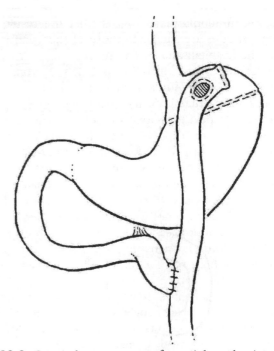

Fig. 32-2. Gastric bypass surgery for weight reduction in the morbidly obese. Note staple line across the gastric fundus, which excludes the body and the Roux-en-Y reconstruction with gasrojejunostomy and duodenojejunostomy.

type of hiatal hernia is the **sliding hiatal hernia,** in which a portion of the stomach slides up through the opening in the diaphragm. Medical measures used to treat reflux symptoms may not be effective or practical for use on a chronic basis in some patients.

Repair of hiatal hernia includes reduction of the herniated portion of the stomach through an abdominal incision. Following reduction of the hernia, the hiatus is repaired using sutures, and the gastroesophageal junction is fixed beneath the diaphragm. A Nissen fundoplication may be indicated to prevent reflux postoperatively.

Morbid obesity

Several therapeutic treatments have been developed for the treatment of morbid obesity because of its close association with serious health problems. Unfortunately, surgical intervention may be the only effective long-term treatment for obesity in some patients.

Two surgical procedures are commonly performed to treat morbid obesity: **vertical banded gastroplasty** and **Roux-en-Y gastric bypass** (Fig. 32-2). In either procedure, the stomach is approached via midline incision, and incidental cholecystectomy may be performed. Banded gastroplasty is achieved by placing a double row of staples from the fundus to the proximal lesser curve to exclude the remainder of the stomach and to create a 15- to 30-ml gastric reservoir. A constricting band is placed around the distal portion of the reservoir to form an outlet with a maximum diameter of

approximately 12 mm. Food is able to pass to the unaltered area of the stomach and then to the small bowel in the usual fashion. Similarly, gastric bypass surgery involves placing a double row of staples across the gastric fundus to form a 15- to 30-ml reservoir. The jejunum is divided, attaching the distal limb to the gastric pouch in a side-to-side anastomosis and the proximal limb to the small bowel by end-to-end anastomosis.

Complications associated with surgery for morbid obesity include excessive weight loss, iron-deficiency anemia, macrocytic anemia, reflux gastritis (reflux of intestinal contents into the stomach), and diarrhea. Complications of vertical banded gastroplasty are usually caused by the constricting band at the exit of the gastric pouch. The band may ulcerate into the lumen of the stomach or outward into the liver. Stomal stenosis is common with both vertical banded gastroplasty and Roux-en-Y gastric bypass and may require endoscopic dilatation.

Peptic ulcer disease

Although antral and duodenal ulcers may have different clinical presentations, they are usually discussed together because they share common pathophysiology and surgical intervention. Surgery was once the definitive treatment for peptic ulcer disease. The introduction of effective medical therapy, as well as recognition of the role of *Helicobacter pylori (H pylori)* in peptic ulcer disease, has made these procedures less common.

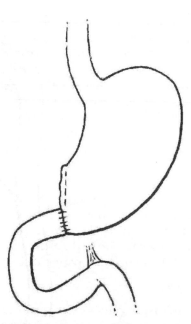

Fig. 32-3. Billroth I (gastroduodenostomy) surgery for gastric ulcers. The antrum has been resected and the duodenum reanastomosed to the gastric remnant.

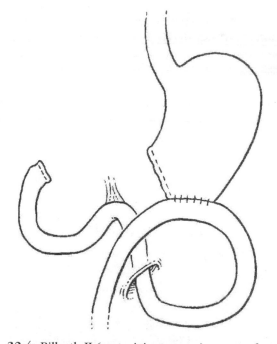

Fig. 32-4. Billroth II (gastrojejunostomy) surgery for gastric and duodenal ulcers. The distal portion of the stomach and proximal duodenum have been resected, with the jejunum reanastomosed to the gastric remnant.

Indications for surgical treatment of peptic ulcer disease include patient noncompliance with medical therapy and peptic ulcers that are refractive to medical therapy or remain active despite eradication of *H. pylori* infection. Several surgical procedures have been developed for the treatment of peptic ulcer disease: partial gastrectomy to reduce the number of parietal cells in the stomach, antrectomy to abolish the gastric phase of secretion and to promote gastric emptying, and selective vagotomy to negate the cephalic phase of secretion and to reduce parietal cell sensitivity to secretory stimulus. In practice, the surgeon often selects a combination of these interventions. Three surgical procedures are indicated for the treatment of peptic ulcer disease: partial gastrectomy with gastroduodenostomy (Billroth I procedure), partial gastrectomy with gastrojejunostomy (Billroth II procedure), and highly selective vagotomy.

1. The **Billroth I procedure** (Fig. 32-3) sacrifices the distal portion of the stomach, pylorus, and duodenal bulb. The duodenum is then reattached by anastomosis with the remaining portion of the stomach.
2. The **Billroth II procedure** (Fig. 32-4) also sacrifices a distal portion of the stomach and a portion of the proximal duodenum. The proximal duodenum is closed, and a segment of proximal jejunum is attached to the gastric remnant with an end-to-end or side-to-side anastomosis.
3. Vagotomy (Fig. 32-5) is frequently included with the Billroth I and Billroth II procedure. Vagotomy alone can be used to treat ulcer disease, but it must be performed with caution. Truncal vagotomy causes complete denervation of the stomach by severing the anterior and posterior vagal trunks. Innervation of the gallbladder is also lost, and cholelithiasis is a recognized complication. Selective vagotomy spares gallbladder innervation. **Highly selective vagotomy** interrupts the nerve fibers to the antrum but preserves the innervation to the

pyloric region (acid production is diminished, but pyloric motility is maintained).

Surgical treatment of bleeding secondary to peptic ulcer disease may involve simple ligation of the bleeding vessel and closure of the ulcer. Complications associated with surgery for peptic ulcer disease include weight loss, iron-deficiency anemia, macrocytic anemia, reflux gastritis, and diarrhea.

Perforated peptic ulcer

Perforation of an ulcer through the wall of the stomach or duodenum into the peritoneum is a catastrophic event, requiring emergent treatment. There is a high incidence of malignancy associated with perforated gastric ulcers.

Signs and symptoms of perforation from a peptic ulcer include generalized epigastric pain, pain referred to the shoulder, abdominal tenderness with guarding, abdominal rigidity, absent bowel sounds, and progressive abdominal distention. Signs of related shock and impending circulatory collapse include tachycardia; tachypnea; decreased blood pressure; and shallow, grunting respirations. X-ray diagnosis is by acute series with an anteroposterior (AP) chest x-ray and upright and supine kidney, ureter, and bladder (KUB) x-rays. Acute series is used to confirm perforation by demonstrating air-fluid levels in loops of small bowel and free air under the diaphragm.

Surgical management involves closure of the perforation with sutures. Identification and resection of malignancy is an essential part of surgical management. Definitive surgery for peptic ulcer disease (discussed in the previous section) may be performed at the time the perforation is repaired or may be reserved for a later date.

Pyloric stenosis

Hypertrophic **pyloric stenosis** is a common disorder of infancy, with an occurrence of approximately 1 in 500 live births. The treatment of choice is pyloromyotomy. Pyloromyotomy involves incision of the muscle surrounding the pylorus, accessing this region via an abdominal incision.

In adults, chronic ulceration with subsequent scarring in the pyloric channel and duodenum can result in pyloric stenosis and gastric outlet obstruction. Pyloric stenosis can also be caused by inflammatory edema surrounding an acute channel ulcer.

Pyloric stenosis in adults may be treated by dilatation. Surgical intervention is indicated when pyloric stenosis is secondary to peptic ulcer disease. A truncal vagotomy and gastric outlet drainage procedure (Billroth I) may be indicated to treat the underlying peptic ulcer disease.

Gastric cancer

Resection of gastric carcinoma remains the only treatment to offer a chance of cure or long-term survival. The extent of gastric resection is dictated by the location and extent of the lesion.

Total gastrectomy is indicated when the length of the neoplasm is less than that required to obtain good margins,

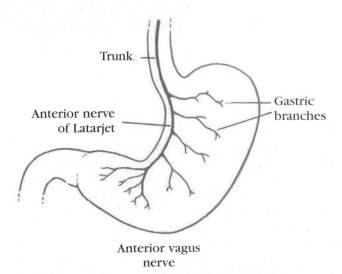

Fig. 32-5. Anterior vagal nerve distribution. Note trunk, gastric branches, and anterior nerve of Latarjet. Truncal vagotomy disrupts the entire vagal network, whereas highly selective vagotomy interrupts only the antral innervation.

when the cancer involves two or all three sections of the stomach, and when the carcinoma is diffuse. A Billroth I procedure is usually performed for cancers in the distal portion of the stomach. If total gastrectomy is performed, a Roux-en-Y or Hunt-Lawrence pouch procedure may be indicated. In either procedure, the esophagus is connected to a segment of the jejunum. Inoperable cancers of the stomach or of the pancreatobiliary system may cause duodenal obstruction and may be palliated by formation of an antecolic gastroenterostomy at the greater curvature of the stomach. Complications associated with gastrectomy for gastric cancer include weight loss, iron-deficiency anemia, macrocytic anemia, reflux gastritis, and diarrhea.

EUS (endoscopic ultrasound) has been shown to be an accurate and cost-effective tool in preoperative staging of gastric cancer. Accurate staging prior to surgical intervention enables the physician to plan the most appropriate treatment.

Early-stage cancers, confined to the mucosal layer without lymph node involvement, may possibly be removed by EMR (endoscopic mucosal resection), as described in the section on esophageal cancer. Successfully performed, this would eliminate the need for surgical intervention.

SURGICAL INTERVENTIONS FOR PANCREATIC DISORDERS

Two general conditions require pancreatic surgery: chronic pancreatitis and pancreatic cancer.

Chronic pancreatitis

Surgery is considered the last resort for chronic pancreatitis and should be reserved for patients with unbearable pain and life-threatening episodes of acute pancreatitis. Resection is based on the belief that removal of diseased tissue diminishes or eliminates pain associated with pancreatitis, as well as the risk of further complications. Total pancreatectomy is unacceptable to most patients and is reserved for patients in whom other surgical procedures have failed. Pancreaticoduodenectomy (see the following section) provides pain relief and may cause fewer metabolic deficits than distal pancreatectomy. Resection of the pancreatic head provides drainage for the duct of Wirsung, the duct of Santorini, and the tributary ducts associated with the head of the pancreas.

Pancreatic cancer

The majority of patients with pancreatic cancer have disease in the head, neck, or uncinate process of the gland. The only potentially curative treatment for patients with cancer of the pancreas is **pancreaticoduodenectomy,** also called **Whipple's procedure** (Fig. 32-6).

Whipple's procedure involves removal of approximately 50% of the stomach and all of the duodenum, along with the proximal jejunum. The pancreatic head, neck, and uncinate process are resected, along with the gallbladder and distal biliary tree. The **modified Whipple's procedure** leaves the entire stomach and 2 to 4 cm of the proximal duodenum, preserving peptic acid-inhibiting hormones, prevent-

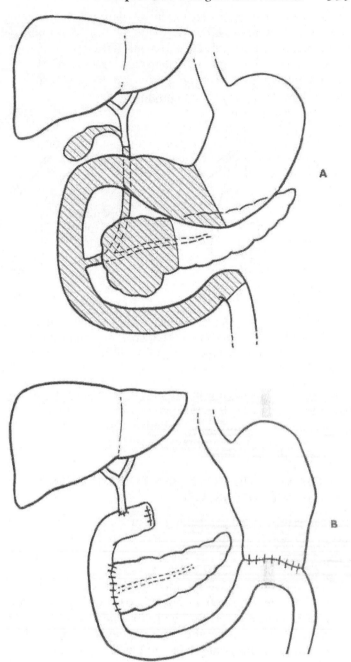

Fig. 32-6. Whipple's procedure (pancreaticoduodenectomy.) **A,** Shaded areas indicate gallbladder and segments of common bile duct, stomach, pancreas, and duodenum that are resected. **B,** Typical postprocedure anatomy with choledochojejunostomyh, pancreaticojejunostomy, and gastrojejunostomy.

ing postoperative peptic ulceration. In the pylorus-preserving pancreaticoduodenectomy, the second, third, and fourth portions of the duodenum; the neck, head, and uncinate process of the pancreas; and the gallbladder and distal biliary tree are removed. Three anastomoses are necessary for reconstruction: an end-to-end pancreaticojejunostomy, an end-to-end hepaticojejunostomy, and an end-to-end duodenojejunostomy.

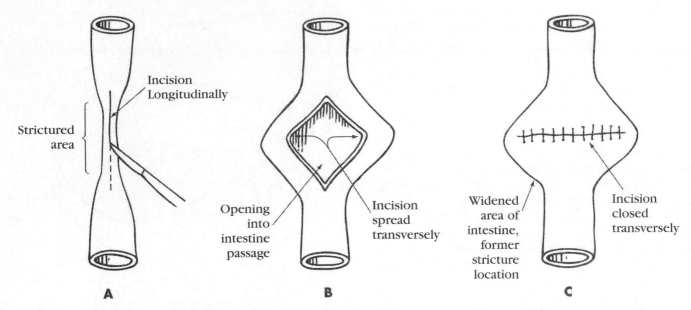

Fig. 32-7. Surgical treatment for small intestine strictures. **A,** The strictured area is identified, and the bowel is opened longitudinally. **B,** The incision is spread transversely. **C,** The incision is closed transversely.

Outcomes in managing pancreatic cancer have improved over the past decade. If performed before nodal spread, pancreaticoduodenectomy is an effective approach. Survival is increased if adjunctive therapy consisting of radiotherapy and chemotherapy is given.

SURGICAL INTERVENTIONS FOR DISORDERS OF THE BILIARY TRACT

Cholecystitis, usually resulting from cholelithiasis, is the most common indication for surgery of the biliary tract.

Cholecystitis

The traditional surgical intervention is open cholecystectomy, performed through a right subcostal incision dividing the rectus muscle to expose the gallbladder. Calot's triangle (cystic duct, cystic artery, and common hepatic duct) is identified, and both the cystic duct and cystic artery are ligated before removal of the gallbladder. Intraoperative cholangiography is often performed by inserting a catheter through the cystic duct into the common bile duct. Radiopaque contrast is injected into the common bile duct, and x-rays are taken to detect gallstones or other obstructions in the common bile duct. In the presence of stones or obstruction, a choledochostomy is performed to explore the common bile duct. Sphincteroplasty may also be performed if intractable obstruction or dense strictures are found in the ampulla. When the gallbladder has been previously removed and recurrent obstruction of the common bile duct occurs, choledochoenterostomy is indicated. This procedure involves a side-to-side anastomosis of the common bile duct to the first part of the duodenum. Laparoscopic cholecystectomy allows for surgical resection of the gallbladder without a large abdominal incision. The gallbladder is approached by laparoscope through a small incision just below the umbilicus. Additional small puncture wounds are made in the upper abdomen to allow for insufflation of carbon dioxide and insertion of surgical instruments. Dissection of the gallbladder is performed with either laser or diathermy, and the gallbladder is removed through the abdominal incision. Gallstones remaining in the common bile duct may be removed endoscopically at a later time. Complications of cholecystectomy include injury to the common bile duct and anastomotic strictures of the common bile duct.

SURGICAL INTERVENTIONS FOR DISORDERS OF THE SMALL INTESTINE

Common surgical interventions involving the small intestine include resection because of a variety of diseases and disorders, as well as Crohn's disease.

Disorders necessitating small intestine resection

Removal of portions of the small intestine may be necessary for a variety of reasons. At birth, congenital anomalies such as duodenal atresia, jejunal atresia, ileal atresia, gastroschisis, or omphalocele may dictate removal of affected parts of the small intestine. In infancy, necrotizing enterocolitis may lead to resection. In children and adults, problems that may cause a need for small intestine resection include trauma, obstruction, infection, and Crohn's disease.

In general, resection of the small intestine involves removal of the affected portion of bowel and end-to-end anastomosis of the remaining healthy segments. The ability to create a primary anastomosis (performed at the time of initial surgery) depends on the length of resection and the integrity of the remaining tissue. Creation of a temporary or permanent ostomy may be necessary with massive resection or dictated by poor tissue integrity.

Complications associated with small intestine resection include stricture, adhesions and scarring, diarrhea, and malnutrition. The degree of malnutrition associated with small intestine resection depends on the location and the length of the resection. Massive small intestine resection may result in the need to maintain nutrition by total parenteral nutrition on a long-term or permanent basis.

Crohn's disease

Surgical resection of lengths of small bowel in Crohn's disease is reserved for patients who have not responded to aggressive medical treatment. Although prolonged remission may occur after resection, a majority of patients receiving surgery for Crohn's disease require additional surgery within a few years.

Indications for small intestine surgery in Crohn's disease include intestinal obstruction, fistula, abscess, uncontrolled hemorrhage, perforation, and growth failure in children who have localized disease. Resection or strictureplasty may be performed when stricture occurs in the small intestine. Strictureplasty involves a longitudinal incision made across the area of stricture; the incision is then sutured in a horizontal direction, creating a wider lumen (Fig. 32-7). Complications associated with surgery for Crohn's disease include diarrhea, weight loss, and recurrence of disease.

SURGICAL INTERVENTIONS FOR DISORDERS OF THE COLON AND RECTUM

Indications for surgical intervention in the colon and rectum are numerous and fall into several broad categories. These categories include but are not limited to congenital anomalies, trauma, inflammatory diseases, and neoplastic disease. Common disorders include Hirschsprung's disease, inflammatory bowel disease (Crohn's disease and ulcerative colitis), colorectal cancer, and perforation.

Hirschsprung's disease

The incidence of Hirschsprung's disease is uncertain but may range from 1 in 5000 to 1 in 10,000 live births. Hirschsprung's disease is the congenital absence of intramural ganglia in the intestinal tract, most frequently of the anorectum and variable lengths of the distal colon. Treatment is surgical and involves removal of the affected portion of the colon.

The most commonly used surgical procedures include the rectosigmoidectomy (Swenson's procedure), retrorectal transanal pull-through (Duhamel's procedure), and endorectal pull-through (Soave's procedure) (Fig. 32-8). Swenson's procedure involves removal of the rectum and anastomosis of the normal ganglionic bowel to a 1- to 2-cm rectal cuff. In Duhamel's procedure, the aganglionic rectum is left in place, and the normal ganglionic bowel is pulled down behind the rectum and through an incision in the posterior rectal wall at the level of the internal sphincter. The original Duhamel's procedure was an anastomosis of the ganglionated proximal bowel to the closed native rectum at the anal

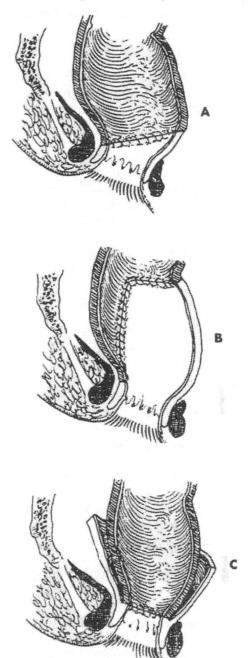

Fig. 32-8. The three major operative procedures for Hirschsprung's disease. **A,** Swensen's procedure (rectosigmoidoscopy). **B,** Duhamel's procedure (retrorectal transanal pull-through). **C,** Soave's procedure (endorectal pull-through). The unshaded native rectum is aganglionic, and the shaded pull-through bowel contains ganglion cells. (From Walker WA et at: *Pediatric gastrointestinal disease,* vol 2, ed 2, St . Louis, 1996, Mosby. Modified from philippart AL: Hirschsprung's disease. In Ashcraft KW, Holder TM, eds: *Pediatric surgery,* ed.2, Philadelphia, 2993, WB Saunders.)

verge. Dilatation of the rectum by fecal retention led to Martin's modification, which added a proximal suture anastomosis of the anterior native rectum to the pulled-through colon. Complications associated with surgical intervention for Hirschsprung's disease include anal stenosis, obstructive symptoms, fecal incontinence, constipation, and enterocolitis.

Inflammatory bowel disease

Although Crohn's disease may affect any part of the GI tract, ulcerative colitis affects only the large intestine. As a result, the colon may be the site of disease activity for both of these chronic illnesses. In ulcerative colitis, surgery is a definitive cure for the disease.

Surgery is indicated when medical therapy fails to prevent significant physical and emotional morbidity. Indications for colectomy in acute ulcerative colitis include uncontrolled hemorrhage, severe colitis that is refractory to aggressive medical therapy, toxic megacolon, stricture, or perforation. Elective colectomy is indicated in patients with prolonged dependence on steroids to maintain disease control, patients who develop complications secondary to steroid use, retardation of growth or sexual maturation despite nutritional support, and epithelial dysplasia (indicating an increased risk for carcinoma).

The current standard of care is to perform an abdominal colectomy, rectal mucosectomy, and endorectal ileoanal pull-through and anastomosis. Usually this procedure is performed in the following stages: colectomy; ileoanal anastomosis with creation of a rectal "pouch" and diverting ileostomy; and (after 2 to 6 months) closure of the ileostomy. If the colitis is severe at the time of surgery, a subtotal colectomy is performed, leaving a rectal stump and creating a terminal ileostomy. Rectal mucosectomy and ileoanal pull-through and anastomosis are performed after the patient recovers. Complications associated with these procedures include diarrhea, perianal irritation, incontinence, anastomotic strictures, and inflammation of the rectal pouch ("pouchitis"). Unlike ulcerative colitis, in which disease is limited to the colon and surgery is curative, no definitive surgical procedure exists for treatment of Crohn's disease.

Intractable colitis is managed by proctocolectomy or colectomy with ileorectal anastomosis if the rectum is free of disease. Ileostomy is necessary when the rectum is diseased. The endorectal pull-through procedure used for ulcerative colitis is contraindicated in patients with Crohn's disease because of the high risk of postoperative perianal disease, including fistulas and abscesses. Complications of this procedure include fistulas, abscess formation, diarrhea, pouchitis, and recurrence of disease.

Colorectal cancer

Surgical treatment of colorectal cancer typically involves removal of the affected segment of colon as an attempt to cure or palliate. A right hemicolectomy is indicated for cancers found in the cecum and ascending colon. In this procedure, the mesocolic vessels are isolated and divided, and the ileum is divided above the ileocecal valve. The transverse colon is divided at a point beyond the hepatic flexure. An end-to-end ileocolonic anastomosis is usually made. An extended right hemicolectomy is similar, but it sacrifices the terminal ileum and the portion of the colon that lies distal to the sigmoid. An ileosigmoidal anastomosis is then formed. In a similar fashion, a left hemicolectomy is performed when indicated by a lesion in the area of the splenic flexure; end-to-end anastomosis of the transverse colon and rectosigmoid is usually made to retain bowel continence. Lesions in the sigmoid or rectosigmoid colon are usually treated with an anterior resection. In this setting, the sigmoid and a segment of the rectum are resected, with the descending colon anastomosed to the rectal remnant.

Perforation of the colon

Perforation of the colon may occur secondary to acute inflammatory bowel disease, inserted foreign bodies, and penetrating trauma, as well as during surgical and endoscopic procedures. Perforation during an endoscopic procedure usually occurs secondary to instrumentation, including the endoscope or biopsy forceps. The risk of perforation is increased when polypectomy is performed and in patients with diminished mucosal integrity, such as those with inflammatory bowel disease.

Perforation of the colon is a potentially life-threatening condition that requires prompt recognition and may require immediate surgical intervention. Endoscopic visualization of an open defect in the bowel wall, visible fatty tissue (such as the omentum), or actual abdominal organs is clear indication of a perforation. Unfortunately, not all perforations of the colon are easily detected. As a result, patients should be closely monitored for signs and symptoms of perforation after the procedure is completed. Patients who take immunosuppressive medications (e.g., cyclosporine, azathioprine, mercaptopurine, prednisone) may not demonstrate all the classic signs and symptoms of perforation, because these symptoms are dictated by immune response. As a result, these patients should be vigilantly monitored for complications.

Those who undergo colonoscopy on an outpatient basis must receive detailed instructions regarding reporting of symptoms of possible perforation, as well as other possible complications related to the procedure. Symptoms such as fever, abdominal or rectal pain, abdominal distention, abdominal rigidity, increased heart rate, or increased respiratory rate should receive immediate attention. Hypotension is a late and ominous sign of impending shock and circulatory collapse. Perforation is confirmed by x-ray, demonstrating free air under the diaphragm.

Early treatment of colon perforation includes stabilization of respiratory status, antibiotic therapy, and resuscitative measures such as volume replacement. The degree of fecal contamination of the abdominal cavity and resultant peritonitis may depend on the adequacy of the bowel preparation done before the procedure. When surgery becomes necessary, the tear is generally closed with sutures and the abdominal cavity thoroughly rinsed with an antibiotic solution. In cases of severe injury to the colon and surrounding structures, partial or total colectomy with creation of an ostomy may be indicated. Ability to create an anastomosis to the rectum after the patient has stabilized will depend on the degree of injury to the rectum.

Complications associated with repair of perforation of the colon depend on the site and degree of the repair. Anastomotic strictures may form at the repair site. Repair in the rectal area may result in bowel incontinence and rectal strictures.

REVIEW TERMS

achalasia, Billroth I procedure, Billroth II procedure, Boerhaave's syndrome, EMR, EUS, esophageal atresia, gastroplication, GERD, Heller's myotomy, highly selective vagotomy, modified Whipple's procedure, Nissen fundoplication, PDT, pancreaticoduodenectomy, pyloric stenosis, Roux-en-Y gastric bypass, sliding hiatal hernia, tracheoesophageal fistula, vagotomy, vertical banded gastroplasty, Whipple's procedure

BIBLIOGRAPHY

Behar, J. (1990). Normal Anatomy, histology and physiology of the upper gastrointestinal tract. In Molinoff, P. (Ed.), *Peptic Ulcer Disease: Mechanisms and Management*. Rutherford, NJ: The Healthpress Publishing Group Inc.

Bevan, P.G. & Donovan, I.A. (1992). *Handbook of general surgery*. Oxford: Blackwell Scientific.

Buttar, N., Wang, K., Lutzke, L., Krishnadath, K. & Anderson M. (2001, December). Combined endoscopic mucosal resection and photodynamic therapy for esophageal neoplasia within Barretts' esophagus. *Gastrointestinal Endoscopy 54*(6),.

Cameron, J.L. (1997). Current management of pancreatic cancer. *Pract Gastroenterol 21*(3), 28-37. Practical Gastroenterology.

Cucchiara, S., Bartolotti, M., Minella, R. (1993). Fasting and postprandial mechanisms of gastroesphageal reflux in children with esophageal reflux disease. *Dig Dis Sci 38*(1), 86-92, 1993. Digestive Disease Science.

Cuschieri, A., Giles, G.R. & Moossa, A.R. (Eds.)(1995), *Essential surgical practice* (3rd ed.). Oxford: Butterworth-Heinemann.

Deebas, H.T. & Orloff, S.L. (1995). Surgery for peptic ulcer disease and postgastrectomy syndromes. In Yamada, T. (Ed.), *Textbook of gastroenterology* (2nd ed.). Philadelphia: J.B. Lippincott.

Dent, J., Halloway, R.H., Touvli, Jr., & Dodds, W.J. (1998). Mechanisms of lower esophageal sphincter incompetence in patients with symptomatic gastroesophageal reflux. *Gut 29*, 1020-8.

DeVault, K. & Castell, D. (1995). Guidelines for the diagnosis and treatment of gastroesophageal reflux disease. *Archives of Internal Medicine 155*(21), 2165-73.

Filipi, D. (2001). Transoral flexible endoscopic suturing for treatment of GERD: A multicenter trial. *Gastrointestinal Endoscopy, 53*(4), 416-22.

Ho, S.H. & Frey, C.F. (1997). Surgery for acute and chronic pancreatitis. *Pract Gastroenterol 21*, 30. Practical Gastroenterology.

Johnston, D. & Sue-Ling, H. (1995). Surgical management of morbid obesity. In Cuschieri, A., Giles, G.R. & Moossa, A.R. (Eds.), *Essential surgical practice* (3rd ed.). Oxford: Butterworth-Heinemann.

Lloyd-Jones, W. & Giles, G.R. (1995). The colon, rectum and anal canal. In Cuschieri, A., Giles, G.R. & Moossa, A.R. (Eds.), *Essential surgical practice* (3rd ed.). Oxford: Butterworth-Heinemann.

Mason, R. (1997, March). A new intoluminal esophageal reflux procedure in baboons. *Gastrointestinal Endoscopy 45*(3) .

Mulholland, M.W., Moossa, A.R. & Liddle, R.A. (1995). Pancreas: anatomy and structural anomalies. In Yamada, T. (Ed.), *Textbook of gastroenterology* (2nd ed.). Philadelphia: J.B. Lippincott.

Nahara, H. (2000, December). Effectiveness of endoscopic mucosal resection with submucosal saline injection technique for superficial squamous carcinomas of the esophagus. *Gastrointestinal Endoscopy 52*(6).

NASPGHAN GER (North American Society for Pediatric Gastroenterology, Heptalogy and Nutrition). (2001). Pediatric gastroesophageal reflux clinical practice guidelines. *Journal of Pediatric Gastroenterology Nursing 32* (Suppl 2), S1-31.

Omari, T., Miki, K. & Fraser, R. (1995). Esophageal body and lower esophageal sphincter function in healthy premature infants. *Gastroenterology 109*, 1757-64.

Rothenberg, S.S. (1998). Experience with 220 consecutive laparoscopic Nissen fundoplications in infants and children. *J Pediatric Surgery 33*, 274-8. Journal of Pediatric Surgery.

Shumaker, D., deGarmo, P. & Faigel, D. (2002, September). Potential impact of preoperative EUS on esophageal cancer management and cost. *Gastrointestinal Endoscopy 56*(3)

Tovar, J.A., Olivares, P., Diaz, M., Pace, R.A., Prieto, G. & Molina M. (1998). Functional results of laparoscopic fundoplication I children. *Journal of Pediatric Gastroenterology Nursing 26*, 429-31.

Walker, W. Durie, P.R., Hamilton, J.R., Watkins, J.B., Walker-Smith. (1996). *Pediatric gastrointestinal disease* (2nd ed.). St. Louis, MO: Mosby.

Yamada, T. Laine, L., Alpers, D.H. (1999). *Textbook of Gastroenterology Vol. 2* (3rd ed.). Philadelphia: Lippincott.

Answers to Review Questions

Chapter 1
1. c
2. a
3. b
4. a
5. d
6. b
7. b
8. c
9. a
10. a

Chapter 2
1. b
2. c
3. a
4. b
5. d
6. b
7. c
8. b
9. c
10. d

Chapter 3
1. b
2. b
3. a
4. c
5. d
6. a
7. c
8. b
9. b
10. c

Chapter 4
1. a
2. b
3. d
4. d
5. b
6. d
7. b
8. a
9. d
10. d

Chapter 5
1. d
2. c
3. c
4. c
5. c
6. a
7. b
8. b
9. d
10. b

Chapter 6
1. b
2. d
3. a
4. d
5. a
6. d
7. d
8. d
9. b
10. a
11. c

Chapter 7
1. a
2. b
3. b
4. d
5. c
6. c
7. b
8. a
9. c
10. c

Chapter 8
1. a
2. d
3. d
4. b
5. d
6. c
7. a
8. c
9. c
10. c

Chapter 9
1. c
2. b
3. c
4. d
5. a
6. b
7. c
8. b
9. a

Chapter 10
1. a
2. d
3. d
4. a
5. d
6. c
7. c
8. c
9. a
10. c

Chapter 11
1. a
2. c
3. d
4. d
5. c
6. b
7. d
8. a
9. d
10. b

Chapter 12
1. a
2. d
3. c
4. c
5. b
6. b
7. d
8. c
9. a

Chapter 13
1. b
2. c
3. d
4. a
5. a
6. c
7. d
8. c
9. a
10. c

Chapter 14
1. a
2. c
3. b
4. c
5. b
6. a
7. a
8. d
9. c
10. c

Chapter 15
1. c
2. b
3. c
4. c
5. d
6. b
7. a
8. b
9. d
10. c

Chapter 16
1. b
2. a
3. d
4. b
5. d
6. b
7. c
8. c
9. b
10. d
11. b

Chapter 17
1. b
2. b
3. c
4. d
5. c
6. b
7. a
8. c
9. c
10. a
11. e

Chapter 18

1. a
2. b
3. d
4. b
5. b
6. d
7. a
8. a
9. d
10. a
11. d
12. a
13. c

Chapter 19

1. b
2. c
3. a
4. d
5. d
6. a
7. a
8. b
9. c
10. d

Chapter 20

1. c
2. a
3. a
4. c
5. c
6. c
7. a
8. a
9. d
10. a

Chapter 21

1. c
2. b
3. a
4. b
5. b
6. d
7. c
8. a
9. b
10. b

Chapter 22

1. b
2. d
3. a
4. a
5. a
6. b
7. d
8. c
9. d
10. b

Chapter 23

1. c
2. b
3. d
4. c
5. a
6. b
7. d
8. b
9. a
10. c

Chapter 24

1. b
2. b
3. c
4. d
5. a
6. c
7. a
8. b
9. d
10. c

Chapter 25

1. b
2. c
3. a
4. c
5. d
6. b
7. b
8. a
9. a
10. c

Chapter 26

1. d
2. a
3. c
4. a
5. c
6. d
7. c
8. a
9. b
10. c

Chapter 27
1. b
2. c
3. a
4. b
5. c
6. c
7. a
8. b
9. a

Chapter 28
1. d
2. d
3. b
4. b
5. c
6. a
7. b
8. a
9. d
10. b

Chapter 29
1. b
2. a
3. a
4. c
5. c
6. b
7. a
8. c
9. c
10. d
11. a
12. c
13. c
14. d

Chapter 30
1. c
2. b
3. b
4. b
5. d
6. b
7. a
8. c
9. c
10. d

Chapter 31
1. b
2. d
3. d
4. b
5. a
6. c
7. a
8. b
9. c
10. c

Glosssary

abetalipoproteinemia. A hereditary syndrome characterized by a lack of beta-lipoproteins in the blood, acanthocytosis, hypocholesterolemia, progressive ataxic neuropathy, atypical retinitis pigmentosa, and malabsorption.

achalasia. A combined defect of absent peristalsis of the esophageal body and elevated lower esophageal sphincter pressure.

achlorhydria. Absence of free hydrochloric acid in the stomach. May be caused by gastric cancer, ulcer, pernicious anemia, adrenal insufficiency, or chronic gastritis.

acinus. A small saclike dilatation, especially a functional unit of the liver, which is supplied by terminal branches of the portal vein and the hepatic artery, and drained by a terminal branch of the bile duct.

activated partial thromboplastin time. A measure of the rapidity of blood clotting, which examines factors I, II, V, VIII, IX, X, XI, and XII.

actual health problem. A health condition that is identified as presently causing some difficulty for the patient.

adenomatous polyp. A benign polypoid adenoma.

advocacy. The act of speaking or writing in support of another or in protection of another's rights.

Alagille's syndrome. See

a1-antitrypsin deficiency. Lack of a plasma protein that is produced in the liver.

ambulatory pH monitoring. A 24-hour test that records fluctuations in esophageal pH and correlates them with symptoms of esophageal reflux.

amebiasis. The state of being infected with

American dilator. One of a series of radiopaque, tapered, polyvinyl dilators that are passed over a guidewire for the purpose of widening a gastrointestinal lumen.

American Nurses Association (ANA). A professional society for nursing in the United States.

amino acid. A class of organic compounds containing an amino group and a carboxyl group. Amino acids form the chief structural components of proteins, and several are essential in human nutrition.

ampulla of Vater. The dilatation formed by the junction of the common bile duct and the pancreatic duct proximal to their opening into the duodenum.

anabolism. Any constructive process by which simple substances are converted by living cells into more complex compounds, especially into living matter.

anaphylaxis. An unusual or exaggerated allergic reaction to a foreign protein or other substance.

anemia. A reduction below normal in the number of erythrocytes. See also

anesthetic. A drug or agent used to abolish the sensation of pain, particularly before surgery or other painful procedures.

angiography. The roentgenographic visualization of blood vessels following introduction of contrast material.

annular pancreas. A developmental anomaly in which the pancreas forms a ring entirely surrounding the duodenum.

anorexia. Lack or loss of appetite for food.

anoscopy. Examination of the anus and lower rectum using a specially designed speculum.

antacid. A substance that counteracts or neutralizes acidity, usually gastric acidity.

antibiotic. An agent that inhibits the growth of or kills microorganisms, used in the treatment of infectious diseases.

anticholinergic. An agent that blocks the parasympathetic nerves.

antidiarrheal. An agent that combats abnormally frequent and liquid fecal discharges.

antiemetic. An agent that prevents or alleviates nausea and vomiting.

antiflatulent. An agent that disperses or prevents the formation of air or gas pockets in the gastrointestinal tract.

antifungal. An agent that is destructive to fungi, suppresses their growth or reproduction, or is effective against fungal infections.

antrum. The constricted, elongated, lower portion of the stomach.

anus. The terminal orifice of the gastrointestinal tract.

argon. An inert gas that is used in lasers.

Argon Enhanced Coagulation. Radio frequency coagulation from an electrosurgical generator that is capable of delivering monopolar current through a flow of ionized argon gas.

arteriography. Roentgenography of an artery after injection of a contrast medium.

ascending colon. The portion of the large intestine between the cecum and the hepatic flexure.

ascites. The effusion and accumulation of serous fluid in the abdominal cavity.

aspiration. (1) The act of inhaling, including the accidental inhalation of solids or liquids; (2) the removal of fluids or gases from a cavity by the application of suction. See also *aspiration biopsy.* A biopsy in which the tissue is obtained by the application of suction through a needle attached to a syringe.

assessment. Continuous, systematic collection, validation, and communication of patient data for the purpose of planning, implementing, and evaluating nursing care directed toward the attainment of specific patient outcomes.

atresia. Congenital absence or closure of a normal body orifice or tubular organ.

audit. A review of documentation for the purpose of determining whether or not specific objectives were met (i.e., patient goals were achieved, nursing standards of care were met, or structural or environmental criteria were attained) during the period of time outlined in a goal or standard. See also and

Auerbach's plexus. The part of the enteric plexus that is within the muscularis. Also called the myenteric plexus.

authority. The legal or rightful power to command or act.

balloon tamponade. Esophageal-gastric tamponade, involving exertion of pressure against bleeding esophageal varices by inflation of esophageal and usually gastric balloons.

barbed stent. A stent with projections or "barbs" at each end that result from a diagonal cut in the stent wall and serve to hold the stent in place.

barium enema. A suspension of barium that is injected into the rectum and retained in the intestines during roentgenological examination. Also called a contrast enema.

barium sulfate. A bulky, fine, white powder without odor or taste, and free from grittiness, that is used as a contrast medium in roentgenography of the digestive tract.

barium swallow. Ingestion of a thick barium solution for the purpose of radiographic examination of the esophagus.

Barrett's esophagus. Replacement of the normal squamous epithelium of the esophagus by columnar epithelium.

beaking/bird's beak. Tapering of the esophagus at the gastric cardia seen on barium esophagram, characteristic of patients with achalasia.

Bernstein test. Attempted simulation of noncardiac chest pain by instillation of hydrochloric acid through one of the ports of a manometry catheter or a nasogastric tube that is positioned in the esophagus.

bezoar. A concretion of foreign material that builds up in the stomach.

bile. An alkaline golden brown to greenish-yellow fluid that is secreted by the liver and poured into the small intestine via the bile ducts. Important constituents include conjugated bile salts, cholesterol, phospholipid, bilirubin diglucuronide, and electrolytes.

biliary colic. Paroxysms of pain and other severe symptoms resulting from the passage of gallstones along the bile duct.

biliary stent. A stent inserted into the common bile duct or pancreatic duct.

Billroth I procedure. Surgical procedure sacrificing the distal portion of the stomach, pylorus, and duodenal bulb.

The duodenum is then reattached by anastomosis with the gastric remnant.

Billroth II procedure. Surgical procedure sacrificing the distal portion of the stomach and a portion of the proximal duodenum. The proximal duodenum is closed, and a segment of proximal jejunum is attached to the gastric remnant with end-to-end or side-to-end anastomosis.

biopsy. The removal and examination, usually microscopic, of tissue from the living body, performed to establish a precise diagnosis. See also and

biopsy forceps. An instrument that can be passed through the biopsy channel of an endoscope for the purpose of excising pieces of living tissue from a suspected pathological site. See also

bipolar electrocoagulation. An electrocoagulation method in which the electrical current flows between two small electrodes on the tip of the probe, both of which are in contact with the target tissue.

bipolar probe. A specialized bipolar hemostatic probe that is inserted through the instrument channel of an endoscope.

body. The largest and most important part of the stomach, lying between the fundus and the antrum.

Boerhaave's syndrome. Catastrophic event in which the lower thoracic esophagus is completely torn away from the gastric cardia.

borborygmi. Rumbling noises caused by the propulsion of gas through the intestines.

bougie. A slender, flexible, cylindrical instrument for introduction into a tubular organ, usually for the purpose of dilating a constricted area. See also and

bougienage. The passage of a slender, flexible cylindrical instrument into a tubular organ to dilate a stricture.

Brunner's gland. A tubulo-alveolar gland in the submucosa of the duodenum, which opens into a crypt of Lieberkühn.

candidiasis. Infection with a fungus of the genus cannula. A tube for insertion into a duct or cavity; sometimes passed over a guidewire.

capital budget. Planning document used to anticipate costs for durable equipment with purchase price greater than $500 and expected life of greater than 5 years.

carbohydrate. An aldehyde or ketone derivative of a polyhydric alcohol; the hydrogen and oxygen are usually in the proportion to form water. The most important carbohydrates are the starches, sugars, celluloses, and gums.

cardia. The portion of the stomach surrounding the esophagogastric junction, which contains cardiac glands but lacks parietal and chief cells.

cardiac arrest. Sudden cessation of cardiac function, with disappearance of arterial blood pressure, connoting either ventricular fibrillation or ventricular standstill.

cardiac gland. A gland located distal to the esophagogastric junction that secretes mucus and pepsinogens.

cardiac sphincter. See

care conference. A collaborative meeting of nurses and possibly other health and allied health professionals for the purposes of planning and evaluating nursing management of a patient's health problem or set of problems. It represents a brainstorming effort to generate creative, comprehensive, or more aggressive approaches to care, usually for long-term patients with complicated problems whose previous management has failed to bring about desired outcomes.

catabolism. Any destructive process by which complex substances are converted by living cells into more simple compounds.

cathartic. An agent that causes evacuation of the bowels by increasing bulk (bulk cathartic), stimulating peristaltic action (stimulant cathartic), softening the feces and reducing friction between them and the intestinal wall (lubricant cathartic), or increasing fluidity of the intestinal contents by retention of water by osmotic forces and indirectly increasing motor activity (saline cathartic).

catheter. A tubular, flexible surgical instrument for withdrawing fluids from, or introducing fluids into, a cavity of the body. See also and

cecum. The first part of the large intestine, forming a dilated pouch into which open the ileum, the colon, and the vermiform appendix.

celiac sprue. A malabsorption syndrome affecting both children and adults, precipitated by the ingestion of gluten-containing foods. Pathologically, the proximal intestinal mucosa loses its villous structure, surface epithelial cells exhibit degenerative changes, and their absorptive function is severely impaired.

cell. Any one of the minute protoplasmic masses that make up organized tissue, consisting of a nucleus surrounded by cytoplasm that contains the various organelles and is enclosed in the cell or plasma membrane. A cell is the fundamental structural and functional unit of living organisms. See also **G cell, goblet cell, Kupffer cell, oxyntic cell, Paneth's cell, parietal cell, red blood cell, white blood cell,** and

Centers for Disease Control and Prevention (CDC). The federal public health agency within the Public Health Service that investigates specific disease outbreaks and formulates general guidelines for disease control.

central tendency. The grouping or score that occurs with the greatest frequency, used in describing a mass of data.

certification. The process by which a nongovernmental agency or association grants recognition to an individual who has met certain qualifications that have been predetermined by that agency or association.

Certifying Board of Gastroenterology Nurses and Associates, Inc. A volunteer, nonprofit organization of gastrointestinal clinicians and physicians formed for the purpose of testing the knowledge, understanding, and skill of practitioners engaged in the field of gastroenterology and endoscopy.

chief cell. A cell located in the parietal glands of the stomach; chief cells secrete pepsinogens.

cholangiogram. A roentgenogram of the gallbladder and bile ducts, following intravenous injection of contrast medium. See also

cholangitis. An inflammation of a bile duct. See also

cholecystitis. Inflammation of the gallbladder.

cholecystokinin. A polypeptide hormone secreted by the mucosa of the upper small bowel, which stimulates contraction of the gallbladder (with release of bile) and secretion of pancreatic enzymes.

choledocholithiasis. The presence of gallstones in the common bile duct.

cholelithiasis. The presence or formation of gallstones.

cholestasis. Stoppage or suppression of the flow of bile, having either intrahepatic or extrahepatic causes.

cholinergic. Stimulated, activated, or transmitted by choline (acetylcholine); a term applied to nerve fibers that liberate acetylcholine at a synapse when a nerve impulse passes; an agent that produces such effects.

chyme. A relatively homogeneous semiliquid combination of food and digestive juices found in the stomach and small bowel.

cirrhosis. A liver disease characterized pathologically by loss of the normal microscopic lobular architecture, with fibrosis and nodular regeneration.

coagulating current. An electric current that is applied for the purpose of coagulating tissue.

coagulation. The process of clot formation; in surgery, the disruption of tissue by physical means to form an amorphous residuum, as in electrocoagulation and photocoagulation.

colitis. Inflammation of the colon. See also and

collaborative diagnosis. Statements of actual or potential health problems that occur from complications of disease, diagnostic studies, or therapeutic procedures, for which the nurse identifies a need to work with other members of the healthcare team toward resolution. See also and

colloid. A state of matter made up of very small, insoluble, nondiffusible particles that remain in suspension in a dispersion medium. The particles in a colloid are larger than ordinary crystalloid molecules, but they are not large enough to settle out under the influence of gravity. See also

colon. The part of the large intestine that extends from the cecum to the rectum. See also and

colonoscopy. Endoscopic examination of the colon.

common bile duct. The duct formed by the union of the cystic duct and the hepatic duct.

comparison group. A group of subjects whose scores on a dependent variable are used as the basis for evaluating the scores of an experimental group or the group of primary interest. "Comparison group" is used rather than "control group" when the investigation does not use a true experimental design. See also

computed tomography. The process of moving an x-ray source in one direction as the film is moved in the opposite direction, thus showing in detail a predetermined plane of tissue while blurring or eliminating detail in other planes. The emergent x-ray beam is measured by a scintillation counter and the electronic impulses are recorded on a magnetic disk, then processed by a minicomputer for reconstruction display of the body in cross-section on a cathode-ray tube. Also called a CT scan.

concurrent audit. An evaluation of nursing care and patient outcomes performed while the patient is receiving care. It is performed by using direct observation of nursing care, patient interview, and/or chart review.

constipation. Infrequent or difficult evacuation of feces; passage of unduly hard or dry fecal material.

consultation. A meeting of two or more professionals to exchange ideas concerning patient care or to seek advice, instruction, or information.

contrast roentgenography. Roentgenography performed after the administration of a contrast medium, often barium sulfate, which facilitates interpretation of the film by accentuating differences in the densities of different regions and structures.

control group. The subjects not receiving an experimental treatment or intervention, whose performance provides a baseline against which the effects of the treatment can be measured. See also

corticosteroid. Any of the steroids elaborated by the adrenal cortex (excluding sex hormones of adrenal origin) in response to the release of corticotropin by the pituitary gland, or any of the synthetic equivalents of these steroids.

counseling. The act of rendering short-term, long-term, or motivational guidance to a patient/significant other, an act that may involve the patient in problem solving.

criterion. A measurable quality, attribute, behavior, or characteristic that specifies a skill, knowledge, or health state that is met at the point a health goal is achieved. Plural: criteria.

critical item. An instrument or object that is introduced directly into the bloodstream or into other normally sterile areas of the body.

Crohn's colitis. Crohn's disease, confined to the colon.

Crohn's disease. A chronic granulomatous inflammatory disease involving any part of the GI tract, but commonly involving the terminal ileum, with scarring and thickening of the bowel wall. It frequently leads to intestinal obstruction and fistula and abscess formation and has a high rate of recurrence after treatment. Also known as regional enteritis.

cryoprecipitate. Any one of a group of serum proteins, including factors VIII, XIII, and fibrinogen, that settle out of solution at temperatures below 20° C.

crypt of Lieberkühn. A simple tubular gland in the mucous membrane of the intestine, opening between the bases of the villi and containing argentaffin cells.

crystalloid. A substance that, in solution, passes readily through animal membranes, lowers the freezing point of the solvent containing it, and is generally capable of being crystallized. See also

culture. The propagation of microorganisms or of living tissue cells in special media conducive to their growth.

Curling's ulcer. A stress ulcer that appears in patients with serious burn injuries.

Cushing's ulcer. A stress ulcer that appears in patients with intracranial trauma.

cutting current. An electrical current applied for the purpose of dissection or fulguration.

cystic duct. The passage connecting the neck of the gallbladder and the common bile duct.

cystic fibrosis. A hereditary disorder of infants, children, and young adults, in which there is widespread dysfunction of the exocrine glands. It is characterized by signs of chronic pulmonary disease caused by excess mucus production in the respiratory tract, pancreatic deficiency, abnormally high levels of electrolytes in the sweat, and occasionally by biliary cirrhosis.

cytology. The study of cells, their origins, structure, function, and pathology. See also

cytology brush. A sheathed, disposable brush that can be passed through the biopsy channel of an endoscope for the purpose of obtaining specimens for microscopic examination.

data. The material or collection of facts upon which a discussion or an inference is based. See also and

database. A foundation of subjective and objective patient information that enables the design and implementation of a comprehensive and effective plan of care.

decompression. The removal of pressure, as in the removal of excess gas from the intestinal tract.

decontamination. The removal of gross soils and the reduction of the number of microorganisms to the point where an item may be considered safe for handling.

dependent intervention. Nursing action performed under the supervision or direction of a physician.

dependent variable. A concept capable of taking on different values whose value is affected by, or determined by, other variables.

descending colon. The portion of the colon between the splenic flexure and the sigmoid colon at the pelvic brim.

desiccation. The act of drying up, especially the treatment of a tumor or other disease by drying up the part by the application of laser or electrical energy.

dextrose. D-Glucose monohydrate. A monosaccharide that occurs as colorless crystals or as a white, crystalline or granular powder; used chiefly as a fluid and nutrient replenisher, usually administered by IV infusion. Also used as a diuretic and alone or in combination with other agents for other clinical purposes.

diaphragmatic hiatus. An opening in the diaphragm where the esophagus enters the abdominal cavity.

diarrhea. Abnormally frequent and liquid fecal discharges.

diffuse esophageal spasm. Repetitive, prolonged simultaneous contractions along the length of the esophagus, with intermittent normal peristalsis.

dilator. An instrument that is used to enlarge an orifice or canal by stretching. See also and

disaccharide. Any of a class of sugars that yield two monosaccharides on hydrolysis and have the general formula $C_n(H_2O)_{n-1}$

disinfection. A physical or chemical process that kills or destroys most pathogenic microorganisms, but rarely kills all spores.

dispersive electrode. Grounding pad.

diverticulitis. Inflammation of a diverticulum, especially inflammation related to colonic diverticula, which may undergo perforation with abscess formation.

diverticulosis. The presence of diverticula, particularly colonic diverticula, in the absence of inflammation.

diverticulum. An outpouching of one or more layers of the wall of a tubular organ. See also

documentation. The act of collecting, abstracting, and coding of patient data and therapeutic processes for the purposes of communicating patient care, supplying a supporting reference concerning the status or progress of a patient, and archiving evidence of care rendered.

double-blind. An experiment in which neither subjects nor investigators are aware of which subjects are in the experimental group and which subjects are in the control group.

double-contrast roentgenography. Mucosal relief roentgenography; involves injection and evacuation of a barium enema, followed by inflation of the intestine with air under light pressure. The light coating of barium on the walls of the inflated intestine in the roentgenogram clearly reveals even small abnormalities.

dry swallow. Performing the action of swallowing during esophageal manometry without ingesting liquid. See also

duct. A passage with well-defined walls, especially a tube for the passage of excretions or secretions. See also and

duct of Santorini. The minor pancreatic duct, draining a part of the head of the pancreas into the minor duodenal papilla.

duct of Wirsung. Pancreatic duct; the main excretory duct of the pancreas, which usually unites with the common bile duct before entering the duodenum at the major duodenal papilla (papilla of Vater).

dumping syndrome. A group of disabling symptoms associated with rapid gastric emptying that mimic the symptoms of hypoglycemia.

duodenum. The first, or proximal, portion of the small bowel, extending from the pylorus to the jejunum.

dyspepsia. Impairment of the power or function of digestion, usually applied to epigastric discomfort following meals.

dysphagia. A sensation of difficulty in swallowing.

D5W. Five percent dextrose in water; given as an intravenous solution.

edrophonium chloride. Tensilon; a cholinesterase inhibitor that is administered by IV bolus in a provocative test designed to reproduce noncardiac chest pain caused by esophageal dysmotility.

electrocautery. An instrument used to destroy tissue, using an electrical current.

electrocoagulation. Coagulation of tissue, using either a monopolar or a bipolar electrical current. See also and

electrolyte. A substance that dissociates into ions when fused or in solution and thus becomes capable of conducting electricity.

electrosurgical unit (ESU). An apparatus for cutting or coagulating tissue, using a high-frequency electrical current.

endogenous. Produced or arising from within a cell or organism.

endoscopic retrograde cholangiopancreatography (ERCP). An endoscopic technique for radiological visualization of the biliary and/or pancreatic ducts.

endoscopic variceal ligation (EVL). The endoscopic introduction of rubber bands or O-rings for the treatment of bleeding varices.

endoscopy. Visual inspection of any cavity of the body by means of an endoscope.

enema. A liquid injected into the rectum. See also

enteral nutrition. Administration of a prescribed diet by means of a flexible tube inserted into the stomach or small bowel transnasally, surgically, or endoscopically.

enteric plexus. A plexus of autonomic nerve fibers within the wall of the digestive tube, and made up of the submucosal, myenteric, and subserosal plexuses.

enteritis. Inflammation of the intestine, especially of the small bowel. See also and

enterochromaffin cell. A basal granular cell whose granules stain readily with silver and chromium salts and which is a site of synthesis and storage of serotonin; includes argentaffin cells and agyrophilic cells.

enteroclysis. The injection of a nutrient or a medicinal liquid into the bowel.

enterocolitis. Inflammation involving both the small bowel and the colon.

erythrocyte. A red blood cell; one of the elements found in peripheral blood; normally, in humans, the mature form is a nonnucleated, yellowish, biconcave disk, adapted, by virtue of its configuration and its hemoglobin content, to transport oxygen.

esophageal atresia. Birth defect characterized by a markedly dilated blind upper esophageal pouch, a variable esophageal defect, and a lower pouch terminating as a fistula communicating with the posterior trachea.

esophageal reflux. Reflux of gastric or duodenal contents back into the esophagus.

esophageal rings and webs. Thin, circumferential mucosal shelves appearing in the esophagus. See also

esophagitis. An inflammation of the esophageal mucosa.

esophagogastroduodenoscopy (EGD). Endoscopic examination of the esophagus, stomach, and duodenum.

esophagus. The musculomembranous tubular portion of the GI tract that extends from the pharynx to the stomach.

ethylene oxide. A colorless, flammable gas used to sterilize instruments.

evaluative statement. A statement defining an actual outcome; for example, skills developed, knowledge obtained, or change in health status.

exfoliative cytology. Microscopic examination of cells desquamated from the body surface or a lesion as a means of detecting malignancy and microbiological changes, to measure hormonal levels, etc. Cells may be obtained by such procedures as aspiration, washing, smears, and scraping, and the technique may be applied to vaginal secretions, sputum, urine, abdominal fluid, prostatic secretions, etc.

exogenous. Originating outside an organ or part.

experimental group. The subjects receiving an experimental treatment or intervention.

familial polyposis. Multiple adenomatous polyps with high malignant potential lining the mucous membrane of the intestine, particularly the colon, beginning about puberty.

fatty acid. Any monobasic aliphatic acid containing only carbon, hydrogen, and oxygen and made up of an alkyl radical attached to the carboxyl group. Saturated fatty acids have the general formula $C_nH_{2n}O_2$. There are also several series of unsaturated fatty acids having one or more double bonds, and a few cyclic acids.

fiber optics. The transmission of an image along flexible bundles of coated parallel fibers that propagate light by internal reflections.

fine-needle aspiration. Sampling of pancreatic tissue for the purpose of cytological examination. Used in the diagnosis of pancreatic cancer.

fistula. An abnormal passage between two internal organs. See also

fluoroscopy. Examination of deep structures by means of roentgen rays; uses a screen covered with crystals of calcium tungstate, on which are projected the shadows of x-ray beams passing through the body from the source of irradiation.

Food and Drug Administration (FDA). The federal regulatory agency responsible for controlling the safety and effectiveness of drugs, devices, and instrumentation and approving products for disinfectant registration by review of labeling and supporting data submitted by the registrants.

French unit. A unit for denoting the size of catheters or other tubular instruments, each unit being roughly equivalent to 0.3 mm in diameter. (i.e., 18 French [Fr] indicates a diameter of 6 mm).

frozen section. A tissue biopsy obtained during endoscopy that is sent for immediate microscopic examination by a pathologist to determine the type of abnormal tissue present.

fulguration. Destruction of living tissue by electric sparks generated by a high-frequency current.

fulminant hepatic failure. Massive liver cell death that occurs within 2 months of the development of acute hepatitis.

functional organization. A form of organizational structure that is designed to allow specialists in given areas to give and enforce recommendations within a clearly defined scope.

fundus. The proximal portion of the stomach, which lies above and to the left of the lower esophageal sphincter.

G cell. A cell type located in the pyloric glands of the stomach; G cells secrete gastrin.

gallbladder. The pear-shaped reservoir for bile on the posteroinferior surface of the liver, between the right and the quadrate lobe; from its neck, the cystic duct projects to join the common bile duct.

Gardner syndrome. Familial polyposis of the colon (with malignant potential), supernumerary teeth, fibrous dysplasia of the skull, osteomas, fibromas, and epithelial cysts.

gastric baseline. Manometric tracing showing a relatively flat, smooth tracing with a small pressure increase on inspiration or abdominal pressure. Indicates all catheter recording ports are in the patient's stomach.

gastric ulcer. Ulcer of the gastric mucosa.

gastritis. An inflammation of the gastric mucosa.

gastroenterology associate. A non-RN healthcare professional with varied educational background who is engaged in the field of gastroenterology.

gastroenterology nurse. A registered nurse who specializes in the field of gastroenterology.

gastroesophageal reflux disease (GERD). Backward flow of gastric contents into the esophagus when the pressure in the stomach is greater than in the esophagus. Associated with pregnancy, obesity, or incompetence of the lower esophageal sphincter.

gastroesophageal sphincter. See

giardiasis. Infection with the flagellate protozoan characterized by protracted, intermittent diarrhea with symptoms suggesting malabsorption, and by abdominal pain, distention, and flatulence; light infections are usually asymptomatic.

gland. An aggregation of cells, specialized to secrete or excrete materials not related to their ordinary metabolic needs. See also and

glucose. A monosaccharide, $C_6H_{12}O_6$, found in certain foodstuffs, especially fruits, and in the normal blood of all animals. It is the chief energy source for living organisms, its utilization being controlled by insulin.

glutaraldehyde. A high-level disinfectant that is effective against vegetative gram-positive, gram-negative, and acid-fast bacteria, some bacterial spores, some fungi, and viruses.

glycerol. A trihydric sugar alcohol that is the alcoholic component of the fats; it is soluble in water and alcohol and is an intermediate in the metabolism of fatty acids.

glycogen. A polysaccharide that is the chief carbohydrate storage material in animals. It is a long-chain polymer of glucose, formed in and largely stored in the liver and to a lesser extent in muscles, being depolymerized to glucose and liberated as needed.

goal. (1) A desired outcome that should reflect the mission statement of an organization. (2) A desired patient outcome, which must be realistic, usable, observable, and specific.

goblet cell. A unicellular mucous gland found in the epithelium of various mucous membranes, especially in the respiratory passages and the intestines. Droplets of mucigen collect in the upper part of the cell and distend it, while the basal end remains slender and the cell assumes the shape of a goblet.

greater curvature. The lower lateral border of the stomach.

greater omentum. A layer of visceral peritoneum that hangs from the greater curvature of the stomach over the anterior side of the abdominal viscera.

grounding pad. A dispersive electrode that is securely attached to the patient's skin and serves to complete the current flow from a monopolar electrosurgery probe, through the patient's body, and back to the generator. Also known as a grounding plate.

halon. Bromotrafluoromethane. A commercial product used in fire extinguishers that are safe for use in areas containing sensitive electrical equipment.

haustrum. Sacculation in the wall of the colon produced by adaptation of its length to that of the tenia coli, or by the arrangement of the circular muscle fibers. Plural: haustra.

health problem. A condition related to health that requires intervention if disease or illness is to be prevented or resolved and if coping and wellness are to be promoted. See also and

heartburn. A retrosternal sensation of warmth or burning that occurs in waves and tends to rise toward the neck. Also known as pyrosis.

heater probe. A hollow aluminum cylinder with an inner heat coil and an outer coating of Teflon that is applied directly to a bleeding vessel to produce hemostasis using bipolar electrocoagulation.

Helicobacter pylori. A gram-negative curved or special rod that is microaerophilic. Formerly

Heller's myotomy. Surgical procedure performed to treat achalasia.

hematochezia. The passage of bloody stools.

hematocrit. The volume percentage of red blood cells in whole blood.

Hemoccult. The trademark for a modification of the guaiac test for occult blood, in which guaiac-impregnated filter paper is used; the test is positive if the specimen turns blue.

hemochromatosis. A disorder of iron metabolism characterized by excess deposition of iron in the tissues, especially in the liver and pancreas, and by bronze pigmentation of the skin, cirrhosis, diabetes mellitus, and associated bone and joint changes.

hemoglobin. The oxygen-carrying pigment of the red blood cells.

hemolysis. The liberation of hemoglobin from the red blood cells and its appearance in the plasma.

hemorrhage. Bleeding; the escape of blood from the blood vessels.

hepatic duct. The duct that is formed by the union of the right and left hepatic ducts and in turn joins the cystic duct to form the common bile duct.

hepatic encephalopathy. A condition usually occurring secondary to advanced liver disease but also seen in the course of any severe disease or in patients with portacaval shunts. Marked by disturbances of consciousness that may progress to deep coma (hepatic coma), psychiatric changes, flapping tremor, and fetor hepaticus. Also called portal-systemic encephalopathy.

hepatic flexure. The right flexure of the colon; the bend in the large intestine at which the ascending colon becomes the transverse colon.

hepatitis. Inflammation of the liver.

hepatocyte. A parenchymal liver cell.

hepatorenal syndrome. A syndrome characterized by functional renal failure, oliguria, and low urinary sodium concentration, without pathological renal changes, associated with cirrhosis and ascites or with obstructive jaundice.

hiatal hernia. Occurs when a portion of the stomach protrudes through the diaphragmatic hiatus into the thoracic cavity.

high-level disinfection. Process of cleaning instruments that destroys all vegetative microorganisms but not necessarily all bacterial spores.

highly selective vagotomy. Surgical procedure interrupting the nerve fibers to the antrum but preserving the innervation of the pyloric region.

Hirschsprung's disease. Megacolon caused by congenital absence of myenteric ganglion cells in a distal segment of the colon. The resultant loss of motor function causes massive hypertrophic dilatation of the normal proximal colon; the aganglionic segment usually remains narrowed but may dilate passively. The condition appears soon after birth, is more common in males, and causes extreme constipation, abdominal distention, sometimes vomiting, and when severe, growth retardation. Also known as congenital megacolon or aganglionic megacolon.

histamine. A decarboxylation product of histidine found in all body tissues. Cellular receptors of histamine include H_1 receptors, which mediate the effects of histamine on smooth muscle and capillaries; and H_2 receptors, which mediate the acceleration of heart rate and the promotion of gastric acid secretion.

histamine2 (H2) blocker. An agent that blocks the cellular receptor site for histamine that is responsible for stimulating the heart rate and gastric secretion.

histology. The study of the minute structure, composition, and function of the tissues; also called microscopical anatomy.

hot biopsy forceps. A type of biopsy forceps that is insulated by a nonconducting sheath and attached to an electrocoagulation snare handle.

Hurst bougie. One of a series of blunt-tipped, mercury-filled tubes of graded diameter used for dilating esophageal strictures.

hydrogen breath test. A measure of the amount of hydrogen expelled in the breath after ingestion of a carbohydrate drink; used to detect carbohydrate malabsorption, abnormal gastrointestinal transit time, or bacterial overgrowth in the small bowel.

hydrostatic balloon. A polyethylene balloon that can be inserted into the GI tract and inflated with fluid to a specified pressure; used primarily for the dilatation of strictures.

hypertonic. A term denoting a solution that, when bathing body cells, causes a net flow of water across the semipermeable cell membrane out of the cell. Also denotes a solution having a greater tonicity than another solution (e.g., the blood), to which it is being compared.

hypoalbuminemia. An abnormally low albumin content in the blood.

hypoglycemia. An abnormally low glucose content in the blood, which may lead to tremulousness, cold sweat, pilo-erection, hypothermia, and headache, accompanied by confusion, hallucinations, bizarre behavior, and ultimately, convulsions and coma.

hypopharyngeal sphincter. See

hypothesis. A declarative conjectured statement posing a relationship between two or more variables; hypotheses lead to empirical studies that seek to confirm or disconfirm the relationships. See also

hypotonic. A term denoting a solution that, when bathing body cells, causes a net flow of water across the semipermeable cell membrane into the cell; also denotes a solution having less tonicity than another solution (e.g., the blood), to which it is being compared.

hypovolemia. Abnormally decreased volume of circulating fluid in the body.

ileocecal valve. A functional valve at the junction of the ileum and cecum, consisting of circular muscle of the terminal ileum.

ileum. The distal portion of the small intestine, extending from the jejunum to the cecum.

independent intervention. Nursing action initiated without direction or supervision of other healthcare professionals. Independent nursing intervention is instituted as the result of a nursing assessment.

independent variable. A concept capable of taking on different values whose value is unaffected by other variables in a given study.

indicator. A measurable variable that is used to measure the degree to which standards are met.

infantile hypertrophic pyloric stenosis. Congenital obstruction of the pyloric lumen caused by pyloric muscular hypertrophy.

infectious waste. Waste capable of producing an infectious disease; includes human, animal, or biological wastes and any items that may be contaminated with pathogens.

infiltration. The diffusion or accumulation in a tissue or cells of substances not normal to it or in amounts in excess of the normal.

inflammatory bowel disease. A general term for inflammatory diseases of the bowel of unknown etiology, including Crohn's disease and ulcerative colitis.

informed consent. An interaction between physician and patient in which a meaningful exchange of information concerning an impending healthcare ministration occurs. Consent is not valid without fulfillment of these four requirements: full disclosure, competent judgment and decision-making ability, comprehension of the procedure and its associated risks and aftereffects, and free will.

insufflation. The act of blowing a vapor, gas, or air into a body cavity.

interdependent intervention. Nursing action performed in concert with the efforts of other healthcare professionals.

intervention. All those activities the nurse identifies that directly relate to the nursing diagnosis and are directed toward improving the patient's problem. See also and

interview. A meeting of patient and nurse to gather data concerning a patient's health status, health problems, risks, weaknesses, strengths, and need for nursing care.

intestinal pseudoobstruction. A condition characterized by constipation, colicky pain, and vomiting, but without evidence of organic obstruction.

intrahepatic biliary dysplasia. A rare autosomal-dominant liver disease that incorporates a combination of anomalies in conjunction with chronic cholestasis.

intussusception. The prolapse of one part of the intestine into the lumen of an immediately adjoining part.

ionizing radiation. High-energy radiation that interacts with matter to produce ion pairs.

irritable bowel syndrome. A chronic noninflammatory disease characterized by excessive secretion of mucus and disordered colonic motility with consequent colic, constipation, and/or diarrhea with the passage of mucus. It is a common disorder with a psychophysiological basis.

ischemic colitis. Acute vascular insufficiency of the colon usually involving the portion supplied by the inferior mesenteric artery. The classic radiological sign is thumbprinting caused by localized elevation of the mucosa by submucosal hemorrhage or edema. Ulceration may follow.

islet of Langerhans. One of the irregular microscopic structures scattered throughout the pancreas and comprising the endocrine portion of the pancreas.

isotonic. A term denoting a solution in which body cells can be bathed without a net flow of water across the semipermeable cell membrane. Also denotes a solution having the same tonicity as another solution (e.g., the blood), to which it is being compared.

jaundice. A syndrome characterized by hyperbilirubinemia and deposition of bile pigment in the skin, mucous membranes, and sclera with resulting yellow appearance of the patient.

jejunum. The portion of the small bowel that extends from the duodenum to the ileum.

Joint Commission on Accreditation of Healthcare Organizations (JCAHO). An independent credentialing agency that grants approval to healthcare facilities that voluntarily comply with the agency's standards for public and patient health and safety.

Kupffer cell. A large, star-shaped or pyramidal cell with a large oval nucleus and a small prominent nucleolus. These intensely phagocytic cells line the walls of the sinusoids of the liver and form part of the reticuloendothelial system.

lactase deficiency. A deficiency in the brush-border enzyme lactase, which causes malabsorption of the disaccharide lactose; patients typically experience distention, flatulence, cramping, and diarrhea within minutes of ingesting milk or milk products.

lamina propria. The connective tissue coat of a mucous membrane.

laparoscope. A fiberoptic instrument that permits inspection of the peritoneal cavity.

laparoscopy. Examination of the interior of the abdomen using a laparoscope.

laparotomy. A surgical incision made through the abdomen.

laser. Light Amplification by Stimulated Emission of Radiation. A device that transforms light of various frequencies into an extremely intense, small, and nearly nondivergent beam of monochromatic radiation in the visible region with all the waves in phase. Capable of mobilizing immense heat and power when focused at close range, it is used as a tool in surgical procedures, in diagnosis, and in physiological studies.

Latex Allergy. Certain proteins in latex may cause sensitization or symptoms. Reactions may be mild with skin redness, hives, or itching. More serious reactions may involve respiratory such as runny nose and scratchy throat, Rarely, shock may occur.

lavage. The irrigation or washing out of an organ, such as the stomach or bowel.

laxative. An agent that acts to promote evacuation of the bowel.

lesser curvature. The upper lateral border of the stomach.

lesser omentum. A layer of visceral peritoneum that attaches the lesser curvature of the stomach to the underside of the liver.

leukocyte. A white blood cell.

liability. Legal responsibility for one's acts (or failure to act), including the responsibility for financial restitution in the event of demonstrable damages resulting from negligent acts.

ligament of Treitz. Suspensory muscle of the duodenum; a flat band of smooth muscle originating from the diaphragm and continuous with the muscular coat of the duodenum at its junction with the jejunum.

line organization. A traditional form of organizational structure, in which each position has authority over a lower one in the organization.

Linton tube. A three-lumen tube used for esophageal-gastric tamponade; it has a gastric balloon but no esophageal balloon, and ports for both gastric and esophageal aspiration.

lipid. A fat or fatlike substance that is easily stored in the body and serves as a source of fuel. They include the fatty acids, neutral fats, waxes, and steroids; compound lipids include glycolipids, lipoproteins, and phospholipids.

lithotripsy. The crushing of gallstones or bladder calculi, either by using a mechanical lithotripter or by focusing shock waves on the stone.

lower esophageal sphincter (LES). A group of thickened circular muscles at the distal end of the esophagus, which regulate the entry of food into the stomach. Also known as the cardiac sphincter or gastroesophageal sphincter.

malabsorption. Impaired intestinal absorption of nutrients.

maldigestion. Impaired digestion.

Mallory-Weiss tear. A mucosal rent at the gastroesophageal junction that is associated with prolonged forceful vomiting.

malnutrition. Any disorder of nutrition, whether caused by unbalanced or insufficient diet or by defective assimilation or utilization of foods.

Maloney bougie. One of a series of mercury-filled bougies similar to the Hurst bougie but with a conical tip.

malrotation. Failure of normal rotation of an organ, as of the gut, during embryonic development.

manometry. Measurement of pressure or contraction, especially within the GI tract.

matrix organization. A type of organizational structure that looks at individual subsystems within a complex structure. These subsystems can be viewed anywhere on the continuum from totally dependent to totally autonomous.

mean. The index of central tendency usually referred to as the average; it is the sum of the values in a set, divided by the total number of elements in the set.

Meckel's diverticulum. An occasional sacculation or appendage of the ileum, derived from an unobliterated yolk stalk.

median. That point in a set of values above which and below which 50% of the values lie.

medical diagnosis. Classification of a patient's medical condition, based on interpretation of data related to pathology and etiology; usually implies a course of treatment.

megacolon. Abnormally large or dilated colon; the condition may be congenital or acquired, acute or chronic. See also

Meissner's plexus. The part of the enteric plexus that is situated in the submucosa. Also called the submucosal plexus.

microorganism. A minute living organism, usually microscopic, including bacteria, viruses, fungi, and protozoa.

microvillus. A minute cylindrical process on the free surface of a cell, especially in the intestinal epithelium.

mineral. A nonorganic, homogeneous solid substance, usually a constituent of the earth's crust.

minimum effective concentration. Threshold strength below which a disinfecting solution should not be used.

Minnesota tube. A four-lumen tube used for esophageal-gastric tamponade; it has both gastric and esophageal balloons and ports for gastric and esophageal aspiration.

mission statement. A statement that describes the intent of a specific organization. The statement should include the unit's overall goals, objectives, services, and the intent of the quality to be delivered.

mode. The numerical value in a set of values that occurs most frequently.

modified Whipple's procedure. Pylorus-preserving pancreaticoduodenectomy.

monitoring. The measurement of physiological parameters, including the use of mechanical devices and clinical observations.

monoglyceride. A compound consisting of one molecule of fatty acid esterified to glycerol.

monopolar electrocoagulation. An electrocoagulation method in which the electrical current flows between a small, active electrode that is in contact with the target tissue and a larger grounding pad that is attached to the patient's skin.

monosaccharide. A simple sugar; a carbohydrate that cannot be decomposed by hydrolysis. The monosaccharides are colorless crystalline substances, with a sweet taste, and which have the general formula CH_2O.

narcotic. An agent that depresses the central nervous system, reduces pain, and sometimes produces sleep.

narcotic antagonist. An agent that opposes the action of narcotics on the nervous system.

nasobiliary catheter (NBC). A catheter that is inserted endoscopically into the common bile duct during ERCP, with the opposite end brought out through the patient's nostril. Its purpose is to provide drainage or to allow the instillation of therapeutic solutions.

nasoenteric intubation. Insertion of a tube that is passed through the naris, into the stomach, and then into the intestinal tract; used primarily to remove intestinal contents or to provide for tube feeding (enteral nutrition).

nasogastric tube. A soft rubber or plastic tube that is inserted through a nostril and into the stomach, for instilling liquid foods or other substances, or for withdrawing gastric contents.

nasopancreatic catheter. Long, thin, polyethylene tube placed endoscopically into the pancreatic duct and routed through the nose for short-term decompression or perfusion.

Nd:YAG (neodymium:yttrium-aluminum-garnet). A mineral crystal that is used as a laser medium to produce 1060-nm light.

needle. A sharp instrument used for suturing or puncturing. See also

Nissen fundoplication. Open abdominal surgical antiesophageal reflux procedure.

nitrogen balance. A state of the body in regard to ingestion and excretion of nitrogen. In negative nitrogen balance the amount of nitrogen excreted is greater than the quantity ingested; in positive nitrogen balance the amount excreted is smaller than the amount ingested.

noncritical item. An item that either does not ordinarily touch the patient or touches only intact skin. Washing with a detergent is often sufficient cleaning for these items.

normal saline. An isotonic solution of sodium chloride for temporarily maintaining living cells. Also known as physiological saline.

null hypothesis. The hypothesis that states that there is no relationship between the variables under study. It is used primarily in connection with tests of statistical significance as the hypothesis to be rejected.

nursing audit. The method of evaluating care, the outcomes of care, or the process by which these outcomes are achieved by using a review of patient records.

nursing diagnosis. A statement of an actual or potential health problem that can be alleviated or prevented by independent nursing intervention.

nursing examination. A physical assessment focused on functional abilities, usually performed in head-to-toe format, during which objective data about a patient's health status is gathered; steps in the examination include inspection, auscultation, percussion, and palpation.

nursing history. An interview-style assessment that is performed to evaluate a patient's health status, health problems, risks, weaknesses, strengths, and need for nursing care.

nursing order. A prescription for the nursing care that is to be given to achieve patient health goals.

nursing process. A systematic approach to nursing care using problem-solving techniques. It encompasses assessment, diagnosis, outcome identification, planning, implementation, and evaluation.

nutcracker esophagus. Esophageal peristalsis with a contractile amplitude two to three times the normal volume.

nutrition. The processes involved in taking nutriments and assimilating and using them. See also and

objective. An observable activity that is developed to help achieve the established goals of an organization.

objective data. Facts perceptible by the senses of one observer that can be verified by another person observing the same data.

observation. Systematic, deliberate use of the five senses to gather data.

obstipation. Intractable constipation.

occult blood. Blood present in such small quantities that it can be detected only by chemical tests of suspected material, or by microscopic or spectroscopic examination.

Occupational Safety and Health Administration (OSHA). The federal regulatory agency responsible for enforcing safety and health regulations in the workplace.

odynophagia. Painful swallowing.

oral. Pertaining to the mouth; taken through or applied in the mouth.

organizational structure. A structure that determines the process by which a group of people distribute responsibilities, establish lines of communication, identify relationships, and establish accountability. See also and

osmosis. The passage of a solvent from a solution of lesser to one of greater solute concentration when the two solutions are separated by a membrane that selectively prevents the passage of solute molecules but is permeable to the solvent.

outcome. The end product of nursing care; measurable changes in a patient's health or behavior.

outcome identification. An actual or potential health problem exhibited by an individual through the process of clinical reasoning and judgement functions that nurses by virtue of their education and experience are capable and licensed to treat independently.

outcome standard. A patient-focused standard that addresses changes in the patient's health status or the results of nursing care.

overtube. A polyvinyl sleeve that fits over an endoscope and serves to protect the esophageal mucosa and the airway during various upper GI procedures, including extraction of foreign bodies.

oxyntic cell. See

pancreas. A large, elongated gland situated transversely behind the stomach, between the spleen and the duodenum. See also and

pancreas divisum. A developmental anomaly in which the pancreas is present as two separate structures, each with its own duct.

pancreatic enzyme insufficiency. A deficiency in pancreatic exocrine function, leading to malabsorption of fats and other nutrients.

pancreatic fistula. An abnormal passage between the pancreas and another organ or, more often, between the pancreas and the exterior, often following pancreatic trauma, external drainage of a pseudocyst, or pancreatic surgery.

pancreaticoduodenectomy. Surgical procedure indicated as therapy for chronic pancreatitis and its inherent complications and as a therapy for pancreatic cancer.

pancreatitis. Acute or chronic inflammation of the pancreas.

Paneth's cell. A narrow, pyramidal, or columnar epithelial cell with a round or oval nucleus close to the base of the cell, occurring in the fundus of the crypts of Lieberkühn; Paneth's cells contain large secretory granules that may contain peptidase.

papillotome. A cutting instrument for incising the papilla of Vater.

papillotomy. Incision of a papilla.

paracentesis. Surgical puncture of a cavity for the aspiration of fluid, especially the abdominal cavity.

paralytic ileus. Obstruction of the intestines resulting from inhibition of bowel motility, which may be produced by numerous causes, most frequently by peritonitis.

parenteral. Administration of medications or nutrition by an injection route, such as subcutaneous, intramuscular, or intravenous.

parietal cell. A cell type located in the parietal glands of the stomach and that secretes hydrochloric acid and intrinsic factor. Also known as oxyntic cells.

pathology. The structural or functional manifestations of disease.

pedunculated polyp. A polyp that is attached to the mucosa by a stemlike pedicle or stalk.

peptic ulcer. An ulceration of the mucous membrane of the esophagus, stomach, or duodenum, caused by the action of the acid gastric juice.

peracetic acid. A chemical solution used for high-level disinfection.

percutaneous endoscopic gastrostomy (PEG). A technique for the endoscopic insertion of a gastrostomy feeding tube, for the purpose of providing enteral feeding.

percutaneous endoscopic jejunostomy (PEJ). A technique for the endoscopic insertion of a feeding tube through a PEG tube and into the jejunum, for the purpose of providing enteral feeding.

percutaneous liver biopsy. Aspiration biopsy of the liver by using a needle that has been inserted through a small incision in the skin.

percutaneous transhepatic cholangiogram. A roentgenogram of the hepatic and biliary ductal systems following injection of contrast directly into an intrahepatic bile duct, using a needle that is introduced percutaneously into the liver, through the eighth or ninth intercostal space.

perforation. A hole made through a body part.

performance improvement. See .

peripheral parenteral nutrition (PPN). Intravenous administration of a prescribed diet by means of a catheter inserted into a peripheral vein.

peristalsis. A distally progressive band of circular muscle contraction that causes the gradual progression of digestive contents through the GI tract.

peritoneoscopy. Examination of the peritoneal cavity by an instrument (laparoscope) that is inserted through the abdominal wall.

peritoneum. The serous membrane that lines the abdominopelvic walls and holds the viscera in place.

pernicious anemia. A megaloblastic anemia occurring in children or more commonly in later life, characterized by histamine-fast achlorhydria; laboratory and clinical manifestations are based on malabsorption of vitamin B_{12} because of a failure of the gastric mucosa to secrete adequate and potent intrinsic factor.

Peutz-Jeghers syndrome. A hereditary syndrome characterized by gastrointestinal polyposis associated with excessive melanin pigmentation of the skin and mucous membranes; gastrointestinal bleeding and intussusception are common complications.

Peyer's patch. An oval elongated area of lymphoid tissue on the mucosa of the small intestine, composed of many lymphoid nodules closely packed together.

philosophy. Major beliefs held by an individual or the members of a group.

phlebitis. Inflammation of a vein.

photocoagulation. Condensation of protein material by the controlled use of an intense beam of light.

physiograph. Device that produces a graphic display of test results.

pigtail stent. A stent that is coiled at one or both ends. The coiled shape straightens out when the stent is pulled taut but returns when it is allowed to relax.

placebo effect. An assumed psychological response to administration of a treatment suggested by the process of taking a medicine; usually encountered in drug testing, these effects are discounted from the real effects of the drug under study.

planning. The development of patient goals based on nursing diagnoses for the purpose of preventing, reducing, or resolving health problems through nursing intervention.

plasma. The fluid portion of the blood, in which the particulate components are suspended.

plasmolysis. Contraction or shrinking of a cell caused by the loss of water by osmotic action.

platelet. A disk-shaped structure found in the blood of all mammals and chiefly known for its role in blood coagulation.

plexus. A general term for a network of lymphatic vessels, nerves, or veins. See also and

pneumatic balloon. A balloon that is inserted over a guidewire into the lower esophageal sphincter and then inflated to a preset pressure and left in place for a period of time; used in the treatment of patients with achalasia.

pneumoperitoneum. The presence of gas or air in the peritoneal cavity; it may occur spontaneously, as in a subphrenic abscess, or be deliberately introduced as an aid to radiological examination and diagnosis.

polyp. A protruding growth from any mucous membrane; includes gastric polyps. See also and

polypectomy. Surgical or endoscopic removal of a polyp.

polypectomy snare. A sheathed wire loop that can be passed through the instrument channel of an endoscope; it may be attached to an electrosurgical unit and used to apply coagulation current for removal of gastrointestinal polyps, or it may be used to remove foreign bodies.

polyposis. The development of multiple polyps on a part. See also

population. All of the members of a group in which a survey researcher is interested; the entire set of people, objects, etc., with characteristics in common.

porphyria. Any of a group of disturbances of porphyrin metabolism, characterized by marked increase in formation and excretion of porphyrins or their precursors.

portal hypertension. Abnormally increased blood pressure in the portal venous system, a frequent complication of cirrhosis of the liver.

portal triad. The grouping of the tributaries of the hepatic artery, hepatic vein, and bile duct at the angles of the lobules of the liver.

position description. A delineation of the responsibilities of an individual in an organization, including the title of the position, the department, the person to whom the individual is responsible, a job summary, job qualifications, and specific duties and functions.

possible health problem. A health condition that has a high probability of developing because of an existing condition or disease.

potential health problem. A health condition that does not presently exist, but because of the presence of identified risk factors, requires that the nurse take preventive measures.

pressure transducer. A transducer is a device that translates one form of energy to another; in the case of manometric pressure transducers, changes in pressure are translated into electrical signals.

primary sclerosing cholangitis. A rare and serious condition in which inflammation involves the entire biliary tract; often related to GI or biliary tract infection.

priority setting. The activity concerned with ranking nursing diagnoses in order of actual or potential threat to the patient's well-being.

process improvement. A systematic approach to the way work is designed and performance is measured, assessed, and improved.

process standard. A standard that focuses on the nature and sequence of activities carried out by nurses implementing the nursing process; describes an acceptable level of performance of nursing actions.

proctoscopy. Inspection of the rectum with a speculum or tubular instrument with appropriate illumination.

proctosigmoidoscopy. Examination of the rectum and sigmoid colon with an instrument designed for illuminating and viewing those areas.

project organization. An organizational structure that is designed to complete a specific task.

prostaglandin. A group of naturally occurring, chemically related, long-chain hydroxy fatty acids that stimulate contractility of smooth muscle and have the ability to lower blood pressure, regulate acid secretion of the stomach, regulate body temperature and platelet aggregation, and control inflammation and vascular permeability; they also affect the action of certain hormones. There are six types: A, B, C, D, E, and F, with the degree of saturation of the side chain of each being designated by subscripts 1, 2, and 3.

protein. Any of a group of complex organic compounds, which contain carbon, hydrogen, oxygen, nitrogen, and usually sulfur, the characteristic element being nitrogen. Proteins are of high molecular weight and consist essentially of combinations of α-amino acids in peptide linkages.

prothrombin. Coagulation factor II, a protein present in the plasma that is converted to thrombin. See also

prothrombin time. A measure of the rapidity of blood clotting that examines coagulation factors I, II, V, VII, and X.

pseudocyst. An abnormal or dilated space resembling a cyst but not lined by epithelium as is a true cyst. A pancreatic pseudocyst is an encapsulated collection of pancreatic juice and cellular debris that has escaped from the pancreas, the wall being formed by inflammatory fibrosis of serosal surfaces of adjacent organs; pseudocysts most commonly occur in the lesser sac of the peritoneum.

pseudomembranous colitis. An acute inflammation of the bowel mucosa with the formation of pseudomembranous plaques overlying an area of superficial ulceration and the passage of the pseudomembranous material in the feces; may result from shock and ischemia or be associated with antibiotic therapy. Also called necrotizing enterocolitis.

pyloric gland. A gland located in the antrum or pylorus of the stomach; contains mucous cells and G cells.

pyloric sphincter. The thickened muscular sphincter that controls the passage of food from the stomach into the duodenum.

pyloric stenosis. Obstruction of the pyloric sphincter at the outlet of the stomach.

pylorus. The most distal portion of the stomach, lying between the antrum and the duodenum.

pyrosis. See

qualitative. Pertains to describing or analyzing qualities, attributes, or characteristics.

quality. In healthcare, the degree to which actions taken or not taken maximize the probability of beneficial outcomes.

quantitative. Pertaining to or measuring quantity.

radiation enteritis. Radiation injury to the intestines, usually occurring as a result of radiotherapy for pelvic, intraabdominal, or retroperitoneal malignancies.

radiography. The making of film records (radiographs) of internal structures of the body by passage of x-rays or gamma rays through the body to act on specially sensitized film. See also

random sample. Selection from the population (or a subpopulation) at large performed in such a way that each member of the population has an equal probability of being included in the sample.

range. The highest score (or value) minus the lowest score in a given set of values.

rapid pull-through. A technique whereby a manometry catheter is withdrawn steadily through the esophagus while the patient is not breathing or swallowing.

rectosigmoidoscopy. Endoscopic visualization of the lower portion of the sigmoid colon and the upper portion of the rectum.

rectum. The distal portion of the colon, beginning anterior to the third sacral vertebra as a continuation of the sigmoid and ending at the anal canal.

red blood cell. See

referral. The process of sending a patient to another source for aid or to another professional for appropriate action; also, a patient received from another source.

regional enteritis. See

regurgitation. A backward flowing of undigested food.

respiratory depression. A decrease in the rapidity and depth of respirations.

respiratory inversion point. During station pull-through, manometry of the lower esophageal sphincter, the point at which the tracing goes down (rather than up) with an inspiration. Indicates the point at which the recording port moves from the abdominal cavity into the thoracic cavity.

retrospective audit. An evaluation of nursing care and patient outcomes performed after discharge of the patient. Postdischarge questionnaires, interviews (over the telephone or face-to-face), or chart review are retrospective auditing techniques.

Ringer's solution. A sterile solution containing sodium chloride, potassium chloride, and calcium chloride in water for injection; used as a topical physiological salt solution.

roentgenography. The making of a record (roentgenogram) of internal body structures by passing x-rays through the body to act on specially sensitized film. See also and

role delineation. A statement of the behaviors that are expected of an individual in a certain position, as of a gastroenterology nurse or associate.

Roux-en-Y gastric bypass. Surgical procedure performed to treat morbid obesity.

ruga. A wrinkled ridge in the interior wall of the stomach. Plural: rugae.

sample. The portion of a group or population that is targeted for a survey. See also

sanitation. A process capable of destroying or reducing the number of microbial contaminants to a relatively safe level, as judged by public health requirements.

Savary-Gilliard dilator. One of a series of semiflexible, tapered polyvinyl chloride bougies that are passed over a guidewire for the purpose of widening a gastrointestinal lumen.

Schatzki's ring. One of a series of thin, concentric membranes located at the esophagogastric junction.

Schilling test. A test for gastrointestinal absorption of vitamin B_{12}, in which a measured amount of radioactive vitamin B_{12} is given orally and the percentage of radioactivity in the urine excreted over a 24-hour period is determined.

Schindler, Gabriele. The wife of pioneer gastroscopist Dr. Rudolph Schindler. She assisted her husband with gastroscopic procedures and is considered a role model for today's professional gastroenterology nurses and associates.

Schwachman-Diamond syndrome. Pancreatic insufficiency, cyclic neutropenia, metaphyseal dysostosis, and growth retardation. Second most common cause of pancreatic insufficiency in children.

scintigraphy. The production of two-dimensional images of the distribution of radioactivity in tissues after the internal administration of radionuclide, with the images obtained by a scintillation camera.

sclerotherapy. The injection of sclerosing solutions in the treatment of hemorrhoids, varicose veins, or esophageal varices.

scope of practice. A statement of the dimensions of a professional practice that outlines the functions of individuals in that profession.

secretin. A strongly basic polypeptide hormone secreted by the mucosa of the duodenum and jejunum when acid chyme enters the intestine. Carried by the blood, it stimulates the secretion of a watery pancreatic juice high in salt content but low in enzymes. It has a lesser stimulatory effect on bile and intestinal secretion.

sedation and analgesia. Describes a state that allows patients to tolerate unpleasant procedures while maintaining protective reflexes.

sedative. An agent that allays excitement.

self-expanding metal stents. Compressed and stretched metal devices that increase in diameter and decrease in length automatically on deployment to relieve strictures in lumens of various body structures.

semicritical item. An item or instrument (including endoscopes) that may come in contact with intact mucous membranes but does not ordinarily penetrate body surfaces. Meticulous physical cleaning followed by high-level disinfection is required for these items.

Sengstaken-Blakemore tube. A three-lumen tube used for esophageal-gastric tamponade; it has both gastric and esophageal balloons and a port for gastric aspiration.

serum. The cell-free portion of the blood from which the fibrinogen has been separated in the process of clotting.

sessile polyp. A polyp that is attached to the mucosa by a broad base.

shock. (1) A condition of acute peripheral circulatory failure caused by derangement of circulatory control or loss of circulating fluid; marked by hypotension, coldness of the skin, usually tachycardia, and often anxiety. (2) An extreme stimulation of the nerves, muscles, etc., accompanying the passage of electrical current through the body.

short bowel syndrome. Any of the malabsorption syndromes resulting from massive resection of the small bowel, the degree and kind of malabsorption depending on the site and extent of the resection; characterized by diarrhea, steatorrhea, and malnutrition.

sigmoid colon. The S-shaped part of the colon, lying in the pelvis, extending from the pelvic brim to the third segment of the sacrum, and continuous above with the descending (iliac) colon and below with the rectum.

sigmoidoscopy. Inspection of the sigmoid colon through the use of an endoscope.

sinusoid. A form of terminal blood channel consisting of a large, irregular anastomosing vessel; found in the liver, suprarenals, heart, parathyroid, carotid gland, spleen, hemolymph glands, and pancreas.

sliding hiatal hernia. Common type of hiatal hernia in which the gastroesophageal junction and a portion of the stomach slide upward into the mediastinum.

small bowel. The proximal portion of the intestine.

small bowel enteroscopy. Visualization of the small bowel with a long, thin, extremely flexible endoscope.

Society of Gastroenterology Nurses and Associates, Inc. (SGNA). The professional society for registered nurses and other healthcare personnel involved in the practice of gastroenterology.

solid-state catheter. A long, flexible manometry catheter that contains a series of miniature pressure transducers that directly record gastrointestinal contractions.

sphincter. A ring-like band of muscle fibers that constricts a passage or closes a natural orifice. See also and

Sphincter of Oddi. The sheath of muscle fibers surrounding bile and pancreatic ducts as they pass through the wall of the duodenum.

sphincterotome. An electrosurgical instrument for cutting through a sphincter, specifically the sphincter of Oddi.

sphincterotomy. Division of a sphincter, especially division of the sphincter of Oddi during ERCP.

splenic flexure. The left flexure of the colon; the bend at which the transverse colon becomes the descending colon.

sprue. A chronic form of malabsorption syndrome that occurs in both tropical and celiac forms. See also and

staff organization. A type of organizational structure that requires staff to assist management but allows them no authority.

standard. An acceptable, expected level of performance established by authority, custom, or consent. Standards in nursing define optimum levels of actual and expected performance. See also and

standard deviation. An average-size spread among values in a set around the average value in the set; how far away the numbers in a list are from their average.

standard for practice. An authoritative statement of the expected outcomes of professional practice, established through research and/or professional consensus.

standard of care. A measurable statement that defines the means to accomplish a practice outcome.

standard precautions. A system of infection-control guidelines developed by the Centers for Disease Control and Prevention that advises healthcare workers to take specific steps to minimize exposure to blood and body fluids of all patients, regardless of their infective status.

station pull-through. A technique whereby a manometry catheter is withdrawn through the esophagus in a stepwise fashion while the patient breathes slowly and evenly.

steatorrhea. Excessive amounts of fat in the feces, as in malabsorption syndromes.

stent. A hollow tube or endoprosthesis that is inserted for the purpose of bypassing diseased or obstructed parts of a duct or tubular organ. See also

sterilization. The destruction of all microbial life, including spores.

stoma. An opening established in the abdominal wall by colostomy, ileostomy, etc.

stress ulcer. A form of acute gastritis that is related to a severe trauma, illness, or chronic ingestion of certain drugs.

stricture. A narrowing of a canal, duct, or other passage as a result of scarring or deposition of abnormal tissue.

structural standard. A standard concerned with the environment in which care is provided.

subjective data. Perceptions by an affected person that cannot be perceived or verified experimentally.

suction biopsy. A method of obtaining tissue specimens from the rectum or small bowel, by creating a vacuum in a specially designed capsule or tube.

syncope. A temporary suspension of consciousness caused by generalized cerebral ischemia; faint.

syndrome. A set of symptoms that occur together; the sum of signs of any morbid state; a symptom complex.

tamponade. Compression of a part. See also

tenesmus. Straining, especially ineffectual and painful straining at stool or in urination.

tenia coli. Three thickened flat bands, about one-sixth shorter than the colon, formed by the longitudinal fibers in the muscular tunic of the colon and extending from the root of the vermiform appendix to the rectum, where they spread out and form a continuous layer encircling the tube.

threshold. Acceptable rates of activity that determine when to evaluate care.

tonicity. The effective osmotic pressure equivalent.

topical. Pertaining to a particular surface.

total parenteral nutrition (TPN). The intravenous administration of the total nutrient requirements of a patient with gastrointestinal dysfunction, accomplished via a central venous catheter, usually inserted in the superior vena cava.

toxic megacolon. Acute dilatation of the colon associated with amebic or ulcerative colitis; it may precede perforation of the colon.

tracheoesophageal fistula. Abnormal passage between the trachea and esophagus.

transverse colon. The portion of the colon that runs transversely across the upper part of the abdomen, from the right to the left colic flexure.

triglyceride. A compound consisting of three molecules of fatty acid esterified to glycerol; it is a neutral fat synthesized from carbohydrates for storage in animal adipose cells. On enzymatic hydrolysis, it releases free fatty acids in the blood.

trocar. A sharp-pointed instrument contained in a cannula, used to puncture the wall of a body cavity; usually used for insertion of the cannula.

tropical sprue. A malabsorption syndrome occurring in the tropics and subtropics. Protein malnutrition is usually precipitated by malabsorption, and anemia caused by folic acid insufficiency is particularly common.

ulcer. A local defect, or excavation, of the surface of an organ or tissue, which is produced by the sloughing of inflammatory necrotic tissue. See also and

ulcerative colitis. Chronic, recurrent ulceration in the colon, chiefly of the mucosa and submucosa, of unknown cause; manifested clinically by cramping, abdominal pain, rectal bleeding, and loose discharges of blood, pus, and mucus with scanty fecal particles.

ultrasonography. Mechanical radiant energy with a frequency greater than 20,000 hertz (cycles per second); ultrasonography is the visualization of deep structures of the body by recording the reflections (echoes) of ultrasonic waves directed into the tissues. Diagnostic ultrasonography uses a frequency range of 1 million to 10 million Hz, or 1 to 10 MHz.

upper gastrointestinal (UGI) series. A series of radiographs taken to visualize the esophagus, stomach, and sometimes the small bowel, following the ingestion of a barium solution.

upper esophageal sphincter (UES). The sphincter located at the upper end of the esophagus. Also known as the hypopharyngeal sphincter.

vagotomy. Surgical deenervation of vagus nerve.

validation. Verification; confirmation.

Valsalva maneuver. Forcible exhalation against a closed glottis, resulting in an increase in intrathoracic pressure.

variability. A concept concerned with how spread out or dispersed the data values are about the mean; the degree to which subjects in a sample vary from one another with respect to some critical attribute.

variable. A measured concept or construct; a characteristic or attribute of a person or object that takes on different values within the population under study. See also and

varix. An enlarged and tortuous vein or artery. Plural: varices.

vasovagal reaction. A transient vascular and neurogenic reaction marked by pallor, nausea, sweating, bradycardia, and rapid fall in arterial blood pressure which, when below a critical level, results in loss of consciousness and characteristic EEG changes. It is most often evoked by emotional stress associated with fear or pain.

vermiform appendix. A worm-like diverticulum of the cecum, ranging from 3 to 6 inches in length.

verres needle. A disposable or reusable needle that is used in laparoscopic procedures for the creation of pneumoperitoneum.

vertical banded gastroplasty. Surgical procedure performed to treat morbid obesity.

videoendoscopy. Visualization of gastrointestinal structures through an endoscope that has a distal sensing device in the tip, which electronically transmits an image to a video processor for display on a television monitor; the procedure is then performed by reference to the monitor.

villus. A small vascular process or protrusion, especially such a protrusion from the free surface of a membrane; the intestinal villi are the numerous threadlike projections that cover the surface of the mucosa of the small bowel and serve as the sites of absorption of fluids and nutrients.

vision. A statement that sets direction for a unit, department, or institution.

vitamin. An organic substance that occurs in foods in small amounts and that is necessary in trace amounts for the normal metabolic functioning of the body.

volvulus. Intestinal obstruction caused by a knotting and twisting of the bowel.

washing. Collection of a specimen for culture or cytology by injecting and then aspirating 20 to 30 ml of nonbacteriostatic saline.

water perfusion catheter. A long, multilumen manometry catheter that is continuously perfused with water. Each lumen has a separate recording port that is attached to a separate external pressure transducer; when a port is occluded by gastrointestinal contractions, the resulting pressure change is recorded on a physiograph.

webs. See

wet swallow. Swallowing 3 to 5 ml of water during esophageal manometry. See also

Whipple's disease. A malabsorption syndrome characterized by diarrhea, steatorrhea, skin pigmentation, arthralgia and arthritis, lymphadenopathy, and central nervous system lesions.

Whipple's procedure. Pancreaticoduodenectomy.

white blood cell. See

whole blood. Blood from which none of the elements have been removed.

Wilson's disease. Hepatolenticular degeneration. A rare progressive disease, inherited as an autosomal-recessive trait, and caused by a defect in the metabolism of copper; a pigmented ring at the outer margin of the cornea is pathognomonic.

x-ray. Electromagnetic vibrations of short wavelengths that are produced when high-velocity electrons impinge on various substances. X-rays are able to penetrate some substances much more readily than others and to affect a photographic plate, thus making them useful for taking roentgenograms of various parts of the body. They also cause certain substances to fluoresce, allowing fluoroscopic observation of the size, shape, and movements of various organs.

Zollinger-Ellison syndrome. A triad comprising intractable, sometimes fulminating and in many ways atypical peptic ulcers; extreme gastric hyperacidity; and gastrin-secreting, nonbeta islet cell tumors of the pancreas.

zymogen cell. See chief cell.

Resources

BOOKS AND GUIDELINES

For specific references, refer to the Bibliography at the end of each chapter.

Ackley, B. & Lodwig, G. (2001). *Nursing Diagnosis Handbook* (5th ed.). St. Louis, MO: Mosby.

Agency for Healthcare Research and Quality (1997). *Case Studies from the Quality Improvement Support System* (Publication No. 97-0022). Washington DC: U.S. Government Printing Office.

Albanese, J. (1982). *Nurses' drug reference* (2nd ed.). New York: McGraw-Hill.

Alfaro, R. (1999). *Applying Nursing Process: A Step-By-Step Guide* (4th ed.). Philadelphia: J. B. Lippincott.

Alfaro-LeFevre, R. (2002). *Applying nursing process: Promoting Collaborative Care* (5th ed.). Philadelphia: Lippincott, Williams and Wilkins.

Alvarado, C.J. & Reichelderfer, M. (2000). APIC Guideline for Infection Prevention and Control in Flexible Endoscopy. *American Journal of Infection Control 28*, 139.

American Academy of Pediatrics. (1997). *Recommended childhood immunization schedule: United States.* (Position Statement 99(1). pp.136-137). Elk Grove Village, Illinois: Author.

American Medical Association, Department of Drugs, Division of Drugs and Toxicology: *Drug evaluations annual 1991,* Chicago, 1991, AMA.

American Nurses Association: *Standards of clinical nursing practice.* Kansas City, Mo, 1991, ANA.

American Nurses Association. (1996). *Quality assurance workbook.* Kansas City, MO: Author.

American Society of Anesthesiologists (2002). *Practice guidelines for sedation and analgesia by nonanesthesiologists. Anesthesiology 96,* 1004-17.

Anderson, K., Keith, J. & Novak, P. (Eds.) (2001). *Mosby's Medical Nursing & Allied Health Dictionary* (6th ed.).

Association of periOperative Registered Nurses. (2002). *Recommended Practices for Safe Care Through Identification of Potential Hazards in the Surgical Environment.* Denver, CO: Author.

Association of periOperative Registered Nurses. (2002). *Recommended Practices for Environmental Responsibility.* Denver, CO: Author.

Association of periOperative Registered Nurses. (2002). *Latex Guidelines.* Denver, CO: Author.

Association of periOperative Registered Nurses. (2002). *Recommended Practices for Laser Safety in Practice Setting.* Denver, CO: Author.

Association of periOperative Registered Nurses. (2002). *Recommended Practices for Electrosurgery.* Denver, CO: Author.

ASHP. (1999). ASHP Therapeutic Guidelines for nonsurgical antimicrobial prophylaxis. *Ameri JourHealth Syst Pharma 56,* 1201-50. Philadelphia: W.B. Saunders.

Arky, R. (1996). *Physician's desk reference.* Montvale, NJ: Medical Economics.

Avilo, R. (1999). *Full leadership development: building the vital forces in organizations.* Thousand Oaks, CA; Sage.

Association of Operating Room Nurses. (1991). *AORN standards and recommended practices for perioperative nursing,* Denver: AORN.

Ballinger, P. (1995). *Merrill's Atlas of Radiographic Positions and Radiologic Procedures, Vol. 2&3* (8th ed.) St. Louis, MO: Mosby.

Barkin, J.S. (Ed.). (1994). *Advanced therapeutic endoscopy* (2nd ed.). Philadelphia: Lippincott-Raven.

Barnhart, E. (Ed.) (1997). *Physicians' desk reference* (51st ed.) Oradell, NJ: Medical Economics.

Beare, P. & Meyers, J. (1998). *Principles and practice of adult health nursing.* St. Louis, MO: Mosby.

Benitz, W.E. & Tatro, D.S. (1995) *The pediatric drug handbook* (3rd edition). St. Louis MO: Mosby.

Bevan, P.G. & Donovan, I.A. (1992). *Handbook of general surgery.* Oxford: Blackwell Scientific.

Beyea, S. (1996). *Critical pathways for collaborative nursing care.* Menlo Park, CA: Addison-Wesley

Birdsall, C. & Sperry, S. (1997). *Clinical pathways in medical surgical practice.* St. Louis MO: Mosby.

Blake R, Mouton J. (1964). *The managerial grid.* Houston: Gulf Publishing.

Blume, D. (1980). *Dosages and solutions* (3rd ed.). Philadelphia: F.A. Davis.

Bongiovanni, G. (Ed) (1988). *Essentials of clinical gastroenterology* (2nd ed.), New York: McGraw-Hill.

Bowlus, B. (Ed.). (1998). *Gastroenterology Nursing: a core curriculum* (2nd edition), St. Louis, MO: Mosby.

Boyce, J.M. & Pittet, D. (2002). Guideline for hand hygiene in health care settings, Atlanta, Georgia, Centers for Disease Control and Prevention.

Brent, N. (1997). *Nurses and the Law, A Guide to Principles and Applications.* Philadelphia, Pennsylvania: W.B. Saunders.

Broadwell, D.C. & Jackson, B.S. (1982). *Principles of ostomy care.* St. Louis, MO: Mosby.

Bums, N. & Grove, S.K. (1997). *The practice of nursing research: conduct, critique, and utilization* (3rd ed.). Philadelphia: W.B. Saunders.

Cardiner, G. (2001). *21st century manager.* Princeton, NJ: Peterson's Pacesetter Guides.

Carpenito, L. (1997). *Handbook of Nursing Diagnosis* (7th ed.). Philadelphia: J. B. Lippincott.

Carpenito, L. (1999). *Nursing Care Plans and Documentation* (3rd ed.). Philadelphia: J. B. Lippincott.

Carpenito, L. (2002). *Nursing diagnosis: application to clinical practice* (9th ed.). Philadelphia: Lippincott, Williams & Wilkins.

Castell, D. & Richter, J. (2002). *The Esophagus.* (2nd ed.). Philadelphia, Pennsylvania: Lippincott.

Castell, D. (Ed.). (1999). *Endoscopy in The Esophagus.* Philadelphia, PA: Lippincott Williams & Wilkens.

Castell, D., Richter, J. & Dalton, C., (Eds.) (1987). *Esophageal motility testing.* New York: Elsevier.

Cecil, R.L., Bennet, J.C., and Goldman, L. (2000). *Cecil Textbook of Medicine* (20th ed.). Philadelphia: W.B. Saunders.

Chobanian, S. & Van Ness, M. (Eds). (1994). *Manual of clinical problems in gastroenterology.* Boston: Little, Brown.

Chopra, S. & May, R. (Eds.) (1989). *Pathophysiology of gastrointestinal diseases.* Boston: Little, Brown.

Christopher, W.F. (1994). *Vision, mission, total quality.* Portland, OR: Productivity Press.

Cleary, P., Faven, E. & Intenzo, D. (Eds.). (1989). *Fundamentals of nursing, the art and science of nursing care.* Philadelphia: J.B. Lippincott.

Coco, C. (1980). *Intravenous therapy: a handbook for practice.* St. Louis, MO: Mosby.

Coleman, D. (1987). *Anatomy and physiology of the small bowel* (2nd ed.). *SGA J 10,* 44-5. Society of Gastrointestinal Assistants.

Cotton, P. & Williams, C. (1996). *Practical gastrointestinal endoscopy* (4th ed.). London: Blackwell Scientific.

Craven, R. & Hirnle, C. (2003). *Fundamentals of Nursing: Human Health and Function* (4th ed.). Philadelphia: Lippincott, Williams, and Wilkins.

Cuschieri, A., Giles, G.R. & Moossa, A.R. (Eds.).(1995), *Essential surgical practice* (3rd ed.). Oxford: Butterworth Heinemann.

Damsgard, C. (1985). *Gastrointestinal Assistant certification review manual.* Rochester, NY: Society of Gastrointestinal Assistants.

Doenges, M. & Moorhouse, M. (2000). *Nurses Pocket Guide, Diagnosis, Interventive, Rationale* (7th ed.). Philadelphia: F.A. Davis.

Dorland's Illustrated Medical Dictionary (29th ed.) (2000). Philadelphia: W.B. Saunders.

Dunitz, M. & Bloom, S. (Eds.) (2002). *Practical gastroenterology.* Florence, KY: Taylor & Francis.

Eastwood, G. & Avunduk, C. (2002). *Manual of gastroenterology: diagnosis and therapy* (3rd ed.). Boston: Lippincott, Williams & Wilkins.

Elkin, M., Perry, A. & Potter, P. (2000). *Nursing Interventions and Clinical Skills,* (2nd ed.). St. Louis, MO: Mosby.

Emmert P, Barker L: *Measurement of communication behavior,* New York, 1989, Longman Publishing.

Fielder, F. (1967). *A theory of leadership effectiveness* (1st ed.). New York; McGraw-Hill.

Finkler, S. & Kovner, C. (2000). *Financial management for nurse managers and executives* (2nd ed.). Philadelphia: W.B. Saunders.

Fisher, K. (1999). *Leading self-directed work teams: a guide to developing new team leadership skills* (2nd ed.). New York: McGraw-Hill.

Gardner, P. (2003). *Nursing Process in Action.* Independence, KY: Delmar Learning.

Gitnick, G. & Hollander, D. (Eds.) (1994). *Principles and practice of gastroenterology and hepatology* (2nd ed.). New York: Elsevier.

Given, B. & Simmons, S. (1984). *Gastroenterology in clinical nursing* (4th ed.). St. Louis, MO: Mosby.

Goldberg, K. (Ed.) (1986). *Gastrointestinal problems, Nurse Review Series.* Springhouse, PA: Springhouse.

Gordon, M. (1984). *Manual of nursing diagnosis 1984-1985.* New York: McGraw-Hill.

Hamilton, H. (Ed.) (1983). *Procedures, Nurse's Reference Library.* Springhouse, PA: Intermed Communications.

Hamilton, H. (Ed.) (1985). *Diseases, Nurse's Reference Library Series.* Springhouse, PA: Springhouse.

Haubrich, W.S., Schaffner, F. & Berk, J.E. (Eds). (1995). *Bockus gastroenterology, Vol. 1* (5th ed.). Philadelphia: W.B. Saunders.

Henry, J. (1996). *Clinical diagnosis and management by laboratory methods* (19th ed.). Philadelphia: W.B. Saunders.

Huber, D. (2000). *Leadership and nursing care management* (2nd ed.), Philadelphia: W.B. Saunders.

Ignatavicius, D. & Hausman, K. (1995). *Clinical pathways for collaborative practice.* Philadelphia: W.B. Saunders.

Iyer, P., Taptich. B. & Bernocchi-Losey, D. (1995). *Nursing process and nursing diagnosis* (3rd ed.). Philadelphia: W.B. Saunders.

Jarvis, C. (2000). *Physical Examination and Health Assessment* (3rd ed.). Philadelphia.: W.B. Saunders.

Johns Hopkins Medical Laboratories (2000). *Department of Pathology Alphabetical Test Listings.* Baltimore, MD: Author.

Johns Hopkins Pathology. (2003). *Pancreas cancer fine needle aspiration.* Baltimore, MD: Johns Hopkins Hospital.

Johnson & Johnson Medical, Inc. (1994). *Material Safety Data Sheet, Enzymatic Detergent.* New Brunswick, New Jersey: Author.

Johnson, L.R. (Ed.) (1994). *Physiology of the gastrointestinal tract* (3rd ed.). Philadelphia: Lippincott-Raven.

Johnson, M., Bulechek, G., McCloskey, J., Maas, M., and Morehead, S. (2001). *Nursing Diagnoses Outcomes & Interventions.* St. Louis, Missouri: Mosby.

Joint Commission on Accreditation of Healthcare Organizations (1994). *Framework for Improving Performance.*

Joint Commission on Accreditation of Healthcare Organizations (2002). *Primer on indicator development and application.* Oakbrook Terrace, IL: JCAHO.

Joint Commission on Accreditation of Healthcare Organizations (2000). *Comprehensive Accreditation Manual for Hospitals.* Chicago: JCAHO.

Kahrilas, P., Clouse, R. & Hogan, W. (1994). An American Gastroenterological Association medical position statement on the clinical use of esophageal manometry. *Gastroenterology 107,* 1865-84.

Keighley, M. & Williams, N. (1999). *Endoscopy, Surgery of the Anus, Rectum and Colon* (2nd ed.). London: W. B. Saunders.

Kelly-Heidenthal, P. (2003). *Nursing leadership and management.* Clifton Park, NY: Delmar Publishing.

Kiernan, M. (1996). *The 11 commandments of 21st century management.* Englewood Cliffs, NJ: Prentice Hall.

Kneedler, J. & Dodge, G. (Eds.) (1989). *Perioperative patient care* (2nd ed.). Palo Alto, CA: Blackwell Scientific.

Kouzes, J.M. & Posner, B.Z. (1995). *The leadership challenge: how to get extraordinary things done in organizations.* San Francisco: Jossey-Bass.

Kozier, B., Berman, A.J., & Erb, G.(1999). *Fundamentals of nursing: concepts, process, and practice* (6th ed.). Upper Saddle River, New Jersey: Prentice-Hall.

Langfitt, D. (1984). *Critical care: certification preparation and review.* Bowie, MD: Brady Communications.

Langmore, S. (2001). *Endoscopic Evaluation & treatment of Swallowing Disorders.* New York: Thieme Medical Publishers, Inc.

Lankisch, P.G., Banks, P.A. (1998). *Pancreatitis.* New York: Springer-Verlag.

Lewis, S., Heitkemper, M. & Dirksen, S. (2000). *Medical Surgical Nursing, Assessment and Management of Clinical Problems.* St. Louis, MO: Mosby.

Mammett, J. & Dougherty, L. (Eds.). (2000). *Royal Marsden Manuel of Clinical Nursing Procedures* (5th ed.). Oxford: Blackwell Science.

Marquis, B.L. & Huston, C.J. (2000). *Leadership roles and management functions in nursing* (3rd ed). Philadelphia: Lippincott.

Martin, D. (2002). *Practical gastroenterology.* Florence, KY: Taylor and Francis.

Mayo, F. (1949). *The social problems of an industrial civilization.* Boston: Routledge.

McFarland, P. & McFarlane, J. (1997). (Ed.), *Nursing diagnosis and intervention.* (3rd Edition) St. Louis, MO: Mosby.

McNally, P. R. (2001). *GI/Liver Secrets.* Philadelphia, Pennsylvania: Hanley & Belfus, Inc.

Medical Devices Agency (1996). *Latex Sensitization in the health care setting: use of latex gloves.* London: HMS.

Medical Devices Agency (1998). *Latex Medical Gloves (Surgeons) and Examination Powered Latex Medical Gloves.* London: HMS.

Medical Economics (Ed.). (2001). *Physicians' desk reference* (56th ed.) Oradell: Author.

Merriam-Webster's collegiate dictionary (10th ed.) (1998). Springfield, MA. Merriam-Webster

Microvasive Product Information. Natick: MA: Author.

Minocha, A. (2000). *2001 Minocha's Guide to Digestive Diseases.* McLean, Virginia.: International Medical Publishing, Inc.

Misiewicz, J. J., Bartram, C.I., Cotton, P.B. (1994). *Atlas of clinical gastroenterology* (2nd ed.). London: Gower Medical.

Molinoff, P. (Ed.) (1990). *Peptic Ulcer Disease: Mechanisms and Management.* Rutherford, NJ: The Healthpress Publishing Group Inc.

Moorehead, G., & Griffin, R.W. (2001). *Organizational behavior: managing people in organizations* (6th ed.). Boston: Houghton Mifflin.

Nettina, S.M. (Ed.). *The Lippincott manual of nursing practice* (7th ed.). Philadelphia: J.B. Lippincott.

Nightingale, F. (1859) *Notes on Nursing: What it is and what it is not.* Philadelphia: J.B. Lippincott.

North American Nursing Diagnosis Association (1989). *Taxonomy I with official diagnostic categories.* St Louis, MO: Author.

North American Nursing Diagnosis Association (2000). *Taxonomy of nursing diagnoses.* St. Louis MO: NANDA.

NASPGHAN GER (North American Society for Pediatric Gastroenterology, Heptalogy and Nutrition). (2001). Pediatric gastroesophageal reflux clinical practice guidelines. *Journal of Pediatric Gastroenterology Nursing 32* (Suppl 2), S1-31.

Ogilvie, J. Norwitz, L., Kalloo, A.N., Kallo, A.N. (2002). *Johns Hopkins Manual for Gastrointestinal Endoscopy Nursing.* Thorofare, NJ: Slack Inc.

Perry, A.G. & Potter, P.A. (1994). *Clinical nursing skills and techniques* (3rd ed.). St. Louis, MO: Mosby.

Physicians' Desk Reference (55th ed.) (2001). Montvale, NJ: Medical Economics.

Polit, D.F., Beck, C.T. & Hungler, B.P. (2001). *Essentials of nursing research: methods, appraisal, and utilization.* Philadelphia: J.B. Lippincott.

Price, S.A. & Wilson, L.M. (1992). *Pathophysiology: clinical concepts of disease processes* (4th ed.). St. Louis, MO: Mosby.

Ravenscroft, M. & Swan, C. (1984). *Gastrointestinal endoscopy and related procedures: a handbook for nurses and assistants.* Baltimore, MD: Williams & Wilkins.

Rayhorn, N. (Ed.) (1995). *Manual of gastrointestinal procedures: pediatric supplement.* Chicago: Society of Gastroenterology Nurses and Associates.

Remington's pharmaceutical sciences (1995). Easton, PA: Mark Publishing.

Rodwell-Williams, S. & Schlenker, E. (2002). *Essentials of nutrition and diet therapy* (8th ed.). St. Louis, MO: Mosby.

Rombeau, J. & Caldwell, M. (Eds.). (1984). *Clinical nutrition: enteral and tube feeding vol 1.* Philadelphia: W.B. Saunders.

Roy, C.C., Silverman, A. & Alagille, D. (Eds.) (1995). *Pediatric clinical gastroenterology* (4th ed.). St. Louis, MO: Mosby.

Rubenfeld, M.G. & Scheffer, B.K. (1999). *Critical Thinking in Nursing: An Interactive Approach* (2nd ed.). Philadelphia: J. B. Lippincott.

Rybacki, J.J. & Long, J.W. (1997). *The essential guide to prescription drugs.* New York: Harper Perennial-Harper Collins Publishers.

Sachar, D., Waye, J. & Lewis, B. (Eds.) (1989). *Gastroenterology for the house officer.* Baltimore, MD: Williams & Wilkins.

Schaffner, M. (Ed.) (1994). *Manual of gastrointestinal procedures* (3rd ed.). Baltimore, MD: Williams & Wilkins.

Schiff, E.R., Sorrett, M.R. & Maddrey, W.S. (Eds.) (1999). *Schiff's Diseases of the Liver* (8th ed.). Philadelphia: Lippincott-Raven.

Schroeder, S., Krupp, M. & Tierney, L. Jr. (Eds.) (1988). *Current medical diagnosis and treatment.* Norwalk, CN: Appleton and Lange.

Semour, S. & Block, S. S. (Eds.) (2000). *Disinfection, sterilization and preservation* (5th ed.). Philadelphia: Lippincott Williams & Wilkins.

Shannon, J.T., Wilson, B.A. & Stang, C.L. (1995). *Gouani and Hayes drugs and nursing implications* (8th ed.). Stamford, CN: Appleton and Lange.

Shannon, M.T., Stang, C.L. & Wilson, B.A. (2001). *Nurses' drug guide 2002,* Stanford, CT: Prentice Hall.

Shortell, S. & Kaluzyny, A. (2000). *Health care management: organizational design and behavior* (4th ed.). Clifton Park, NY: Delmar Publishing.

Silverman, A. & Roy, C. (1991). *Pediatric clinical gastroenterology* (4th ed..). St. Louis, MO: Mosby.

Silvis, S. (Ed.) (1985). *Therapeutic gastrointestinal endoscopy.* New York: Igaku-Shoin.

Sivak, M. (2000). *Gastrointestinal Endoscopy, Volume 1 and 2* (2nd ed.). Philadelphia, Pennsylvania: W.B. Saunders.

Sivak, M. Jr. & Petrini, J. (Eds.) (1986). *Gastrointestinal endoscopy: old problems, new techniques: Gastrointestinal Series Volume 4.* New York: Praeger.

Sleisenger, M. & Fordtran, J. (Eds.) (2002). *Gastrointestinal disease: pathophysiology, diagnosis, management* (7th ed.). Philadelphia: W.B. Saunders.

Smeltzer, S.C. & Bare, B.G. (2000). *Textbook of Medical Surgical Nursing* (9th ed.). Philadelphia, Pennsylvania: Lippincott.

Smits, M.E. (1995). *New developments in endoscopic and pancreatic drainage.* Amsterdam: Author.

Society of Gastroenterological Nurses and Associates, Inc. (2003). *Manual of Gastrointestinal Procedures* (5th ed.). Chicago: SGNA.

Society of Gastroenterology Nurses and Associates Inc. (1998). Standards of Clinical Nursing Practice and Role Delineation Statements. Chicago, IL: Author.

Society of Gastroenterology Nurses and Associates, Inc (2002). Statement on reprocessing of water bottles used during endoscopy. *Gastroenterol Nurs 25,* 5.

Society of Gastroenterology Nurses and Associates, Inc. (2000). Standards for infection control and reprocessing of flexible gastrointestinal endoscopes [Monograph]. *Gastroenterology Nursing : 23(4),* pp. 172-179.

Society of Gastroenterology Nurses and Associates, Inc. (2000). Guidelines for nursing care of the patient receiving sedation and analgesia in the gastrointestinal endoscopy setting [Monograph], *Gastroenterol Nurs 23(3),* 125-9. Lippincott, Williams & Wilkins.

Society of Gastroenterology Nurses and Associates, Inc. (2001). Role delineation of unlicensed assistive personnel in gastroenterology. *Gastroenterol Nurs 24(4),* 208-9. Lippincott, Williams & Wilkins

Society of Gastroenterology Nurses and Associates, Inc. (2001). Role delineation of the licensed practical/vocational nurse in gastroenterology. *Gastroenterol Nurs 24(4),* 204-5. Lippincott, Williams & Wilkins.

Society of Gastroenterology Nurses and Associates, Inc. (2001). Role delineation of the registered nurse in a staff position in gastroenterology. , *Gastroenterol Nurs 24(4),* 202-3. Lippincott, Williams & Wilkins.

Society of Gastroenterology Nurses and Associates, Inc. (2001). Standards for practice, *SGNA Monograph Series, Chicago, Illinois.*

Society of Gastroenterology Nurses and Associates, Inc. (2001, January). *Safe Operation of Radiographic Equipment during GI Endoscopic Procedures.* Chicago: Author.

Society of Gastroenterology Nurses and Associates, Inc. (2002). *Reprocessing of endoscopic accessories and valves* (position statement). Chicago: Author.

Society of Gastroenterology Nurses and Associates, Inc. (2002). *Reuse of single-use critical medical devices* (position statement). Chicago: Author.

Society of Gastroenterology Nurses and Associates, Inc. (January, 2001). Radiation Safety in the Endoscopic Setting. *Gastroenterology Nursing 24: 3,* 143-6.

Springhouse Corporation. (1999). *Handbook of Infusion Therapy.* Philadelphia: Springhouse.

Springhouse. (1990). *Nursing90 Books: Nursing90 drug handbook,* Springhouse, PA: Springhouse.

Suchy, F.J. (Ed.) (2001). *Liver disease in children* (2nd ed.). St. Louis, MO: Lippincott, Williams & Wilkins.

Sugawa, C. & Schuman, B. (1981). *Primer of gastrointestinal fiberoptic endoscopy.* Boston: Little, Brown.

Taketomo, C., Hodding, J. & Kraus, D. (1996). *Pediatric dosage handbook.* Washington, DC: American Association for Clinical Chemistry.

Tappen, R. N. (2001). *Nursing leadership and management concepts and practice* (4th ed.). Philadelphia: F.A. Davis.

Taylor, F. (1998). *Scientific management.* New York: Dover Publisher.

Taylor, M. (Ed.) (1996). *Gastrointestinal emergencies.* Baltimore, MD: Williams & Wilkins.

Thompson, J., McFarlane, G., Hirsh, J. & Tucker, S. (2002). *Diagnostic . Procedures and Tests: Mosby's Clinical Nursing* (5th ed.). St. Louis MO: Mosby.

Tytgat, G. & Classen, M. (Eds.) (2000). The *Practice of therapeutic endoscopy.* Philadelphia: W.B. Saunders.

Udall, S. & Hiltro, J. M. (1996). *The accidental manager.* New York: Prentice Hall.

Van Ness, M. & Gurney, M. (Eds.) (1989). *Handbook of gastrointestinal drug therapy.* Boston: Little, Brown.

Walker, W.A., Durie, P., Hamilton, J.R., Watkins, J.B. and Walker-Smith, J.A. (2000). *Pediatric gastrointestinal disease: Pathophysiology, diagnosis, management. (2nd ed.).* Ontario, Canada: Decker.

Waltz, C., Strickland, 0. & Lenz, E. (1991). *Measurement in nursing research* (2nd ed.). Philadelphia: I.A. Davis.

Watson, D. (1990). *Monitoring the patient receiving local anesthesia.* Denver, CO: Association of Operating Room Nurses.

Waye, J. Geenen, J.E., and Fleischer, D. (1987). *Techniques in therapeutic endoscopy.* (2nd ed.). Philadelphia: W.B. Saunders.

Weinstein, S. (2001). *Plumers Principles and Practice of Intravenous Therapy* (7th ed.). Philadelphia: Lippincott, Williams & Wilkins.

Weinstock, D., Andrews, M. & Cray, J. (Eds.) (1998). *Nurse's Reference Library Series: Diseases* (6th ed.). Springhouse, PA: Springhouse.

Worman, H. J. (1999). *The Liver Disorders Sourcebook*. Chicago: Lowell House.

Yamada, T. Laine, L., Alpers, D.H. (1995). *Textbook of Gastroenterology Vol. 2* (2nd ed.). Philadelphia: Lippincott.

JOURNAL ARTICLES AND UNPUBLISHED PAPERS

Current volumes of SGNA's official journal, *Gastroenterology Nursing*, published by Williams & Wilkins, provide an invaluable resource. Individual articles are cited in chapter reference lists but are not reproduced in this bibliography.

Abele, J.E. (1992). The physics of esophageal dilatation. *J-Iepalo Gastroenterol 39*, 486-9.

Albert, M.B.. (1990). Successful outpatient treatment of gallstones with piezoelectric lithotripsy. *Ann Intern Med 113*, 164.

Aliperti, G. (1996). Complications related to diagnostic and therapeutic endoscopic retrograde cholangiopancreatography. *Gastrointest Endosc Clin North Am 6*, 397-407 1996.

Alter, M.J. (1990). The hepatitis C virus and its relationship to the clinical spectrum of NANB hepatitis. *J Gastroenterol Hepatol 5(Suppl 1)*, 78-94.

Alter, M.J. (1990). Risk factors for acute non-A, non-B hepatitis in the United States and association with hepatitis C virus infection. *JAMA 264*, 2231-5.

Alter, M.J. (1991). Hepatitis C: a sleeping giant? *Am J Med 91*, 112S-115S.

Alter, M.J. (1992). The natural history of community-acquired hepatitis C in the United States: The sentinel counties chronic non-A, non-B hepatitis study team, *N Engl J Med 327*, 1899-1905.

Alter, M.J. (1993). Community acquired viral hepatitis B and C in the United States. *Gut 34 (Suppl. 1)*, S17-S19.

Alter, M.J. (1995). Epidemiology of hepatitis C in the West. *Semin Liver Dis 15*, 5-14.

American Cancer Society (2003). Can Colon Cancer be detected? [On-line]. Available: www.cancer.org.

American Society of Gastroenterological Endocopists (2000). Endoscopic therapy of chronic pancreatitis. *Gastrointestinal Endoscopy 52*, 843-8.

American Society of Gastrointestinal Endoscopy (1995). Antibiotic Prophyalaxis for Gastrointestinal Endoscopy, Clinical Guideline. *Gastrointestinal Endoscopy 42*, 630-5.

Andersen, G. (1998). Assessing the Older Patient. *RN .61:3*, 47-51.

Anderson, C. (Ed.) (2001). Defining the Severity of Workplace Violent Events among medical and nonmedical samples. *Gastroenterology Nursing 24:5*, 225-230.

Angelucci, P. (1995). TIPS for controlling bleeding. *Nursing 95 25*, 43.

Arndorfer, R. (1988). Techniques of esophageal manometry. In Trivits, S. (Ed.), *SGA Journal Reprints*, Rochester, NY: Society of Gastrointestinal Assistants.

Aronson, B. (1998). Update on peptic ulcer drugs. *American Journal of Nursing 98(1)*, 41-7.

Axelrad, A.M., Fleischer, D.E. & Gomes, M. (1996). Nitinol coil esophageal prosthesis: advantages of removable self-expanding metallic stents. *Gastrointest Endosc 43(2)*, 155-60. Gastrointestinal Endoscopy.

Bahr, A. (1988). The large intestine. In Trivits, S. (Ed.), *SGA Journal Reprints*. Rochester, NY: Society of Gastrointestinal Assistants.

Ballard, K.A., Arborgast, D., Boeckman, J., Conlon, P., Cox, J.A., Dayhoff, N.E., Fournier, J., Hozdic, L., Murcko, A., Peters, D.A., Staudt, G.A., Stordahl, N., Waszak, L.C. (2003) ANA Standards of Clinical Nursing Practice, Draft published for Public comment. American Nurses Publishing, Washington, D.C., http://www.nursingworld.org/

Bank, S. & Indaram, A. (1999). Causes of acute and recurrent pancreatitis: clinical considerations and clues to diagnosis. *Gastroenterology Clinics of North America 28*, 571-89.

Barnie, D. (1989). Evaluation of nursing specialties. *SGA J 11*, 214-216. Williams & Wilkins.

Barnie, D. (1990). Percutaneous endoscopic gastrostomy tubes: the nurse's role in a moral, ethical, and legal dilemma. *Gastroenterol Nurs 12*, 250-4.

Barnie, D. (1990a). Care planning in the endoscopy unit: master care plan for the intraprocedure patient. *Journal Reprints II*, Rochester, NY: Society of Gastroenterology Nurses and Associates.

Barnie, D. (1990b). Care planning in the endoscopy unit: master care plan for the postprocedure patient. *Journal Reprints II*, Rochester, NY: Society of Gastroenterology Nurses and Associates.

Barnie, D. (1990c). Care planning in the endoscopy unit: master care plan for the pre-endoscopy patient. *Journal Reprints II*, Rochester, NY: Society of Gastroenterology Nurses and Associates.

Baron, T.H. & Morgan, D.E. (1999). Acute necrotizing pancreatitis. *New England Journal of Medicine 340*, 1412-1417.

Barrish, J.O. & Gilger, M.A. (1993). Colon cleanout preparations in children and adolescents. *Gastroenterol Nurs 16*, 106.

Batalden, P.B. & Stoltz, P.K. (1993). A Framework for the Continual Improvement of Health Care: Building and Applying Professional and Improvement Knowledge to Test Changes in Daily Work. *Joint Commission Journal on Quality Improvement 19(10)*; 424-52.

Beck, M. (1986). Reflux esophagitis. *SGA J 9*, 77-8.

Beck, M. (1989). Percutaneous endoscopic gastrostomy. *Nursing 89 19*, 76 7.

Bender, A., Motley, R., Pierotti, R.J., Bischof, R.O. (1999). Quality and Outcomes Management in the Primary Care Practice. *Journal of Medical Practice Management 14(5)*, 236-40.

Berstein, D.I. (2002, August 1). Management of natural rubber latex allergy. *J Allergy Clin Immunol 100(2Suppl)*, S111-6. Journal of Allergy and Clinical Immunology.

Bertagnolli, M. (1990). Use of endoscopic ultrasound in patients with esophageal motility disorders. In Trivits, S. (Ed.), *Journal Reprints II*, Rochester, NY: Society of Gastroenterology Nurses and Associates.

Bharucha, A.E. (2001, March). Slow transit constipation. *Gastroenterol Clin North Am 30(1)*, 77-95.

Bisson, B. (1997, July/August). Methane Gas Explosion during Colonoscopy. *Gastroenterology Nursing 20*, 136-7.

Black, M. (1988). Documentation in the GI lab. In Trivits, S (Ed), *SGA Journal Reprints*. Rochester, NY: Society of Gastrointestinal Assistants.

Black, M. (1989). Crohn's disease: pathophysiology, diagnosis and management. *Gastroenterol Nurs 11*, 259-63.

Bloomfield, R.S. & Rockey, D.C. (2000, January). Diagnosis and Management of Lower Gastrointestinal Bleeding. *Current Opinion in Gastroenterology 16(1)*, 89-97.

Bodinsky, G. (1989). Documentation: charting to standardize. *SGNA Monograph Series*. Rochester, NY: Society of Gastroenterology Nurses and Associates.

Brady, P. (1994). Management of esophageal and gastric foreign bodies: Clinical Update. *ASGE 2(1)*, 1-4.

Branski, D., Faber, J. & Shiner, M. (1996). A comparison of small-intestinal mucosal biopsies in children obtained by blind suction capsule with those obtained by endoscopy. *J Pediatr Gastroenterol Nutr 22*, 194-6.

Brennan, K. & Johns, P. (1995, March/April). Esophageal Bezoar Formation in a tube-fed patient receiving sucralfate and antacid therapy: A case report. *Gastroenterology Nursing 18*, 46-8.

Brewer, J. (1988). The anatomy and physiology of the pancreas. In Trivits, S. (Ed.) *SGA Journal Reprints*. Rochester, NY: Society of Gastrointestinal Assistants.

Brugge, W.R., (Ed.). (2002). Cystic Diseases of the Pancreas. *Gastrointestinal Endoscopy Clinics of North America 12*, 1-828.

Buttar, N., Wang, K., Lutzke, L., Krishnadath, K. & Anderson M. (2001, December). Combined endoscopic mucosal resection and photodynamic therapy for esophageal neoplasia within Barretts' esophagus. *Gastrointestinal Endoscopy 54(6)*,.

Cameron, J.L. (1997). Current management of pancreatic cancer. *Pract Gastroenterol 21(3)*, 28-37.

Campbell, T. & Lunn, D. (1997). Intravenous therapy: current practice and nursing concerns. *Brit J Nurs 6,21*, 1218-1228.

Cappell, M.S. & Abdullah, M. (2000). High risk, underappreciated, obscure, or preventable causes of gastrointestinal bleeding. *Gastroentero Clinics 29(1)*, 125-67.

Cappell, M.S. & Iacovone, F.M. (1999, January). Safety and Efficacy of Esophagogastro-duodenoscopy after Myocardial Infarction. *American Journal of Medicine, 106* (1), 29-35.

Carlson, L. & Anderson, B. (1988). Sphincter of Oddi dysfunction: a cause of biliary obstruction. In Trivits, S. (Ed.), *SGA Journal Reprints*, Rochester, NY: Society of Gastrointestinal Assistants.

Carr-Locke, D.L. (1991). Pancreas divisum: the controversy goes on. *Endoscopy 23,* 105-10.

Carr-Locke, D.L. (1996, September). *Stent therapy of malignant biliary obstruction.* Presented at Therapeutic ERCP Course for GI Nurses and Associates. Milwaukee, WI.

Carr-Locke, D.L. (1998, November/December). Technology Assessment Status Evaluation: Overtube use in Gastrointestinal Endoscopy. *Gastroenterology Nursing 21,* 265-67.

Cassidy, C. (1999). Want to Know How You're Doing? *AJN 99:9,* 51-59.

Castilla, A. (1993). Lymphoblastoid alpha-interferon for chronic hepatitis C: a randomized controlled study. *Am J Gastroenterol 88,* 233-9.

Center for Disease Control. (2003, February 14). *Safety of blood supply in the United States.* [On-line.] Available: www.CDC.org.

Chan, M. (1996). Complications of upper endoscopy. *Gastrointest Endosc Clin North Am 6,* 287-303.

Chang, K.J. & Wiersema, M.J. (1997). Endoscopic ultrasound-guided fine-needle aspiration biopsy and interventional endoscopic ultrasonography. *Gastrointest Endosc Clin North Am 7*(2), 221-35.

Chen, P., Wu, C. & Liaw, Y. (1986). Hemostatic effect of endoscopic local injection with hypertonic saline-epinephrine solution and pure ethanol for digestive tract bleeding. *Gastrointest Endosc 32,* 319-23.

Choo, Q.L. (1989). Isolation of a cDNA clone derived from a blood-borne non-A, non-B viral hepatitis genome. *Science 244,* 359-62.

Christensen, R. (2000). What's Your Diagnosis? *Nursing 2000.* 32 hn 1 – 32 hn 4.

Chung, J.K. (2001, November). Endoscopic Factors Predisposing to rebleeding following Endoscopic Hemostasis in bleeding peptic ulcers. *Endoscopy 11*(33), 969-75.

Chung, J.K. (2002, June). Evaluation of Endoscopic Hemostatis in Upper Gastrointestinal bleeding related to Mallory-Weiss Syndrome. *Endoscopy 34*(6), 474-9.

Clancy, C.M. (1998). Continuous Quality Improvement and Primary Care. *Medical Care 36(5),* 619-20.

Clark, C.H. (1999). Hepatitis C: Role of the advanced practice nurse. *AACN Clinical Issues 10,* 455-63.

Clausen, D. (1996). Drug forum: Moctanin. *Gastroenterol Nurs 19*(5), 183-5. Gastroenterology Nursing.

Claussen, D.S. (1994). Versed administration for IV conscious sedation. *Gastroenterol Nurs 17*(2), 80-4.

Claussen, D.S. (1995). The newest proton pump inhibitor. *Gastroenterol Nurs 18*(6), 235-6.

Claussen, D.W. (1995). A clinical pathway for endoscopy. *Gastroenterol Nurs 18*(5), 182-5.

Clouse, R. (1996). Complications of endoscopic gastrointestinal dilation techniques. *Gastrointest Endosc Clin North Am 6,*

Danmore, L. (1996). Colonoscopic perforations: etiology, diagnosis and management. *Dis Colon Rectum 39,* 1308-14.

Cote, D. & Amedee, R. (1995). Zenker's diverticulum. *Otolaryngol Head Neck Surg Rep 144,* .

Crass, R. & Vanderveen, T. (1988). IV pumps and controllers: new technology stimulates increased sophistication. *J Healthcare Materials Management 6,* 51-61.

Craxi, A. (1994). Third-generation hepatitis C virus tests in asymptomatic anti-HCV-positive blood donors. *J Hepatol 21,* 730-4.

Cucchiara, S., Bartolotti, M., Minella, R. (1993). Fasting and postprandial mechanisms of gastroesphageal reflux in children with esophageal reflux disease. *Dig Dis Sci 38*(1), 86-92, 1993.

Dalton, C., Richter, J. & Castell, D. (1990). Esophageal manometry. In Trivits, S. (Ed.), *Journal Reprints II*, Rochester, NY: Society of Gastroenterology Nurses and Associates.

Dalzell, A.M. (1992). Esophageal stricture in children: fiber-optic endoscopy and dilatation under fluoroscopic control. *J Pediatr Gastroenterol Nutr 15,* 426-30.

Damsgard, C. (1988). Pancreatic disorders: an overview. *SGA J 11,* 117-19.

Davis, G. (1989). Treatment of chronic hepatitis C with recombinant Interferon alfa: a multicenter randomized controlled trial. *New Engl J Med 321,* 1501-6.

Davis, G.L. (1994). Interferon treatment of chronic hepatitis C. *Am J Med 96,* 41S-46S.

Davis, P., Drumm, M. & Konstan, M. (1996). Cystic fibrosis. *Am J Resp Crit Care Med 154(5),* 1229-56.

De Medina, M. & Schiff, E.R. (1995). Hepatitis C: diagnostic assays. *Semin Liver Dis 15,* 33-40.

De Vault, K. R. (1999, December). Overview of medical therapy for gastroesophageal reflux disease. *Gastroenterol Clinics 28,* 831-48.

Dennison, A. (1989). The management of hemorrhoids. *Am J Gastroenterol 84,* 475.

Dent, J., Halloway, R.H., Touvli, Jr., & Dodds, W.I. (1998). Mechanisms of lower esophageal sphincter incompetence in patients with symptomatic gastroesophageal reflux. *Gut 29,* 1020-8.

DeVault, K. & Castell, D. (1995). Guidelines for the diagnosis and treatment of gastroesophageal reflux disease. *Archives of Internal Medicine 155*(21), 2165-73.

DeVault, K. (1996). Current management of gastroesophageal reflux disease. *Gastroenterol 4(1),* 24-32.

Dewalt, S. (2002, April). *Interferons: what are the differences? Hepatitis,* 26-9.

Di Bisceglie, A.M. (1991). Long-term clinical and histopathological follow-up of chronic posttransfusion hepatitis. *Hepatology 14,* 969-74.

Dietitics.com. (2002, Fall). Dietary reference intakes released for carbohydrates, fats, protein, fiber, and physical activity. *Dietitics in Practice 2*(2).

DiMarino, A.J., Gage, T., Leung, J., Ravich, W., Wolf, D., Zuckerman, G. & Zuccaro, G. (1996). American Society of Gastrointestinal Endoscopy: Reprocessing of flexible gastrointestinal endoscopes. *Gastrointest Endosc 43,* 540-6.

Dunham-Taylor, J. (2000). Nurse executive transformational leadership found in participative organizations. *Journal of Nursing Administration, 30(5),* 241-250.

Durkin, S. (1999). Photodynamic therapy: a cancer treatment for the 21st century. *Gastroenterology Nursing 22(3),* 115-20.

Edel, E., Johnson, P. & Tiller, S. (1989). Perioperative documentation: incorporating nursing diagnoses into the intraoperative record. *AORN J 50,* 596-600.

Ellett, M. & Beausang, C. (2002). Introduction to qualitative research. *Gastroenterol Nurs 25,* 10.

Emslie, J. (1996). Technetium-99m-labeled red blood cell scans in the investigation of gastrointestinal bleeding. *Dis Colon Rectum 39*(7), 750-4.

Engstrom, P. & Goosenberg, E. (1999). *Diagnosis and Management of Bowel Diseases.* Philadelphia: Professional Communications, Inc.

Esteban, J.I., Genesca, J. & Alter, H.J. (1992). Hepatitis C: molecular biology, pathogenesis, epidemiology, clinical features, and prevention. *Prog Liver Dis 10,* 253-82.

Fennerty, M.B. & Peura, D.A. (1995, December). Helicobacter pylori: a primer for internal medicine physicians. *Intern Med,* 32-50.

Ferretis, C.B. & Malas, E.G. (1992). Endoscopic transpapillary catherization of the gallbladder followed by external shock-wave lithrotripsy and solvent infusion for the treatment of gallstone disease. *Gastrointestinal Endoscopy 38,* 19.

Filipi, D. (2001). Transoral flexible endoscopic suturing for treatment of GERD: A multicenter trial. *Gastrointestinal Endoscopy, 53*(4), 416-22.

Flaherty, G. & Fitzpatrick, J. (1978). Relaxation techniques to increase comfort of postoperative patients. *Nurs Res 27,* 3525.

Fleischer, D. (1988). BICAP tumor probe therapy for esophageal cancer: a practical guide. *Endosc Rev 5,* 2-13.

Fleischer, D. (1988). The therapeutic use of lasers in GI disease. In Trivits, S. (Ed.), *SGA Journal Reprints.* Rochester, NY: Society of Gastrointestinal Assistants.

Fleischer, D.E. (1989). A marked guidewire facilitates esophageal dilatation. *Am J Gastroenterol 84*, 359-61

Foglia, R. (1994). Esophageal disease in the pediatric age group. *Chest Surg Clin North Am 4(4)*, 785-809.

Food & Drug Administration [FDA] and Center for Disease Control [CDC], (1999). *Public Health Advisory: Infections from Endoscopes Inadequately Reprocessed by an Automated Endoscope Reprocessing System.* [On-line.] Available: http:// www.fda.gov/cdrh/safety/endoreprocess.html

Fowler, P. (2003). *Nursing Process: Implementation and Evaluation* (Fall 2002) [On-line.]. Available: http://www.rsu.edu/faculty/PFowler/Implementation%20and%20evaluation.ppt.

Fox, D. & Bignall, S. (1996). Management of gastro-oesophageal reflux. *Paediatr Nurs 8(1)*, 17-20.

Fox, V. (1997). Complications following percutaneous endoscopic gastrostomy and subsequent catheter replacement in children and young adults. *Gastrointest Endosc 45*, 64-71.

Franciscus, A. (2003). *How does interferon work?* [On-line.] Available: http://www.hcvadvocate.org/Oldsite/200205/interferon.htm.

Fried, M.W. & Hoofnagle, J.H. (1995). Therapy of hepatitis C. *Semin Liver Dis 15*, 82-91.

Friesen, C. (1995). Grasp biopsy, suction biopsy, and clinical history in the evaluation of esophagitis in infants 0-6 months of age. *J Pediatr Gastroenterol Nutr 20*, 300-4.

Fullenkamp, P. (1990). Gluten-sensitive enteropathy, Part II; Dietary treatment of celiac disease. In Trivits, S. (Ed.), *Journal Reprints II.* Rochester, NY: Society of Gastroenterology Nurses and Associates.

Fullhart, J.W. (1993). Generating ideas for research. *Gastroenterol Nurs 15*, 244.

Garcia-Samaniego, J. (1994). Hepatitis B and C virus infections among African immigrants in Spain. *Am J Gastroenterol 89*, 1918-9.

Gardner, S. (1988). Colorectal cancer. In Trivits, S. (Ed.), *SGA Journal Reprints.* Rochester, NY: Society of Gastrointestinal Assistants.

Gedebou, T. (1996). Clinical presentation and management of iatrogenic colon perforations, *Am J Nurs 172*, 454-8.

Geramizadeh, B. (2002). Brush cytology of gastric malignancies. *Acad Cytol 46(4)*, 693-6.

Gilger, M.A. (1993). Conscious sedation for endoscopy in the pediatric patient. *Gastroenterol Nurs 16*, 75.

Gregory, K. (2000, September). Nurse the Patient. *RN 63:9*, 52-4.

Griffith, H., Thomas, N. & Griffith, L. (1991). MDs bill for these routine nursing tasks. *American Journal of Nursing 91*, 22-27.

Grossweiner, L.J. (1995). Photodynamic therapy. *J Laser Appl 7*, 51-7.

Gruber, M. & Camara, D. (1988). Injection sclerotherapy: seven years' experience. In Trivits, S. (Ed.), *SGA Journal Reprints,* Rochester, NY: Society of Gastrointestinal Assistants.

Gruber, M. & Camara, D. (1988). Injection sclerotherapy: seven years' experience. In Trivits, S.(Ed.), *SGA Journal Reprints.* Rochester, NY: Society of Gastrointestinal Assistants

Gruber, M. (1995). Understanding published research reports, or how to "study" a study. *Gastroenterol Nurs 18*, 33.

Han, J.H. (1991). Characterization of the terminal regions of hepatitis C viral RNA: identification of conserved sequences in the 5` untranslated region and poly(A) tails at the 3` end. *Proc Natl Acad Sci USA 88*, 1711-5.

Harz, C. (1991). Extracorporeal shockwave lithotripsy and endoscopy: combined therapy for problematic bile duct stones. *Surg Endosc 5*, 196.

Haught, J. (1988). Zollinger-Ellison syndrome: an overview. In Trivits, S. (Ed.), *SGA Journal Reprints.* Rochester, NY: Society of Gastrointestinal Assistants.

Hayes, A. & Buffum, M. (2001). Educating patients after conscious sedation for gastrointestinal procedures. *Gastroenterol Nurs 24*, 54.

Hays, T.L., Saavedra, J.M., Mattis, L.E. (1995). The use of high-fat low-carbohydrate diets for advancement of enteral feedings in children with short bowel syndrome. *Top Clin Nutrition 10(4)*, 35-41.

Henderson, B.W. & Dougherty, T.J. (1992). How does photodynamic therapy work? *Photochem Photobiol 55(1)*, 145-57.

Hino, K. (1994). Genotypes and titers of hepatitis C virus for predicting response to interferon-alfa. *J Med Virol 42*, 299-305.

Hirschowitz, B. Curtiss, L. & Pollard, A. (1958). Demonstration of a new gastroscope, the "fiberscope." *Gastroenterology 35*, 50-53.

Ho, S.H. & Frey, C.F. (1997). Surgery for acute and chronic pancreatitis. *Pract Gastroenterol 21*, 30. Practical Gastroenterology.

Howden, C. & Hunt, R. (1998). Guidelines for the management of helicobacter pylori infection. *Amer J. Gastroent 93*(12), 2330-8.

Huang, S.P. & Wang, H.P. (2002, June). Endoscopic Hemoclip Placement and Epinephine Injection for Mallory Weiss Syndrome with Active Bleeding. *Gastrointestinal Endoscopy 55*(7), 842-6.

Huey, F. (1988). Working smart. *Am J Nurs 86*, 679-84.

Hunt, R.H. (1996). Eradication of Helicobacter pylori infection. *Am J Med 100*, 5A42S-5A50S.

Hyman, P. (1994). Gastroesophageal reflux: one reason why baby won't eat. *J Pediatr 125(6)*, S103-S109.

Intravenous Nurses Society (1990). Intravenous nursing standards of practice. *J Intraven Nurs Suppl,* S1-S98.

Jackson, B. (1989). Care of patients after percutaneous endoscopic gastrostomy (PEG) tube placement. *Gastroenterol Nurs 12*, 131.

Jagger, J. & Bentley, M. (DATE). Injuries from vascular access devices high risk preventable. *J Intrav Nurs 20, 65,* 533-37. Journal of Intravenous Nursing.

Jakobsen, E. (1990). Three new ways to deliver care. *Am J Nurs 90*, 24-6.

Joint Commission on Accreditation of Healthcare Organizations (2002, August). *The 2003 National Patient Safety Goals.* [On-line.] Available: www.JCAHO.org.

Jordan, S. (1996). Using glutaraldehyde-based instrument sterilants safely. *Infection Control Steriliz- Technology 2:11*, 30-5.

Kato, N. (1990). Molecular cloning of the human hepatitis C virus genome from Japanese patients with non-A, non-B hepatitis. *Proc Natl Acad Sci USA 87*, 9524-8.

Kavic, S. & Basson, M. (2001, April). Complications of endoscopy. *American Journal of Surgery 181(4)*, 319-32.

Kessler, D., Pape, S. & Sundwall, D. (1987). The federal regulation of medical devices. *New England Journal of Medicine 336*, 317-57.

Kirby, D. (1989). Management of esophageal varices: a review of treatment options and the role of the gastroenterology nurse and associate. *Gastroenterol Nurs 12*, 10-4.

Kirsch, M. (1991). Intralesional steroid injections for peptic esophageal strictures. *Gastrointest Endosc 37*, 180-2.

Kirschner, B.S. (1988). Inflammatory bowel disease in children. *Pediatr Clin North America 35*, 189-208.

Kleinbeck, S. (1989). Developing nursing diagnoses for a perioperative care plan: a classroom research project. *AORN J 49*, 1613-25.

Kneedler, J. (1976). A standard: what is it and how to use it. *AORN J 23:55*, 1-554. AORN

Kobayashi, Y. (1993). Quantitation and typing of serum hepatitis C virus RNA in patients with chronic hepatitis C treated with interferon-beta. *Hepatology 18*, 1319-25.

Kochhar, R. (1999, April). Intralesional steroids augment the effects of endoscopic dilation in corrosive esophageal strictures. *Gastrointest Endosc 49*,.

Konishi, M. (1994). Titration and genotyping of hepatitis C virus RNA in chronic hepatitis C patients treated with interferon. *Nippon Shokakibyo Gakkai Zasshi 91*, 147-53.

Kotton, C., (2002). *MEDLINE plus Medical Encyclopedia: Rectal Culture, VeriMed HealthCare Network.*: A.D.A.M., Inc.

Kozark, R.A. & Ball, T.J. (1994). Endoscopic pancreatic duct sphincterotomy: Indications, technique, and analysis of results. *Gastrointestinal Endoscopy 40*, 592.

Kraft, S. (1988). Ulcerative colitis. In Trivits, S. (Ed.), *SGA Journal Reprints.* Rochester, NY: Society of Gastrointestinal Assistants.

Krueger, J. & Ostrowski, P. (1986, September). *Pre- and postprocedural care of the ERCP patient.* Presented at Therapeutic ERCP Course for GI Nurses and Associates, Milwaukee, WI.

Kundtz, J. (1988). PEG/PEJ: implications for nursing care. In Trivits, S. (Ed.), *SGA Journal Reprints,* Rochester NY: Society of Gastrointestinal Assistants.

Kuo, G. (1989). An assay for circulating antibodies to a major etiologic virus of human non-A, non-B hepatitis. *Science 244,* 362-4.

Labar, C. (1986). Filling in the blanks on prescription writing. *American Journal of Nursing 86,* 31-3.

LaFontaine, P. (1989). Alleviating patients' apprehensions and anxieties. *Gastroenterol Nurs 11,* 256-7.

Laine, L. & Estrada, R. (2002, January). Randomized trial of normal saline solution injections versus bipolar electrocoagulation for treatment of patients with high-risk bleeding ulcers: is local tamponade enough? *Gastrointestinal Endoscopy 55*(1), 6-10.

Laine, L. & Peterson, W. (1994). Bleeding peptic ulcer. *Med Prog 331,* 717-27.

Landi, B. (1996) Duodenal perforation occurring during push-enteroscopy. *Gastrointestinal Endoscopy 43,* 631 (letter).

Lankisch, P. (2001). Natural course of chronic pancreatitis. *Pancreatology* 1, 3-14.

Larson, D. (1987). Advanced anatomy and physiology of the colon. *SGA J 10,* 92-97.

Lerner, A., Branski, D. & Lebenthal, E. (1996). Pancreatic diseases in children. *Pediatr Gastroenterol 3(1),* 125-37.

Levine, M. (1995). Role of the double-contrast upper gastrointestinal series in the 1990s. *Gastroenterol Clin North Am 24(2),* 289-308.

Levy, M. (2002, February). The hunt for microlithiasis in idiopathic pancreatitis: Should we abandon the search or intensify our efforts? *Gastrointest Endosc 55,.*

Lewis, B. & Czachor, K. (1990). Small bowel enteroscopy: the GIA's role. In Trivits, S. (Ed.), *Journal Reprints II,* Rochester, NY: Society of Gastroenterology Nurses and Associates.

Liese, A. (2003, January). *Ways to Choose the Right Answer on the NCLEX Exam* [On-line]. Available: http://www.angelfire.com/ga/anneliese/page2.htm.

Lightdale, C. (1995). Photodynamic therapy with porfirmer sodium versus thermal ablation therapy with Nd:YAG laser for palliation of esophageal cancer: a multicenter randomized trial. *Gastrointest Endosc 42*(6), 507-12. Gastrointestinal Endoscopy.

Liquid disinfecting and sterilizing reprocessors used for flexible endoscopes, Health Devices. 23:212-253,1994.

MacDonald, W.C., Trier, J.S. & Everett, N.B. (1964). Cell proliferation and migration in the stomach, duodenum and rectum of man: Radioautographic studies. *Gastroenterology 46,* 405-17.

MacKenzie, P.S. & Beresford, L. (1988). Planning and documentation: addressing patient needs in a day surgery setting. *AORN J 47,* 526-37.

Malen, A. (1986). Perioperative nursing diagnoses: what, why, and how. *AORN J 44,* 829-39.

Mansell, C.J. & Locarnini, S.A. (1995). Epidemiology of hepatitis C in the East. *Semin Liver Dis 15,* 15-32.

Maradieque, A. (1989). Quality assurance as reflected in documentation. *SGNA Journal 12,* 135-7.

Marcellin, P. (1991). Second generation (RIBA) test in diagnosis of chronic hepatitis C. *Lancet 337,* 551-2.

Marousky, R. (1991). The Material Safety Data Sheet (MSDS): A guide to chemical safety in the OR. *Today's OR Nurse 13,* 6-11.

Masci, E., Testoni, P.A., Passaretti, S. (1985). Compararison of ranitidine, domperidone maeleate and ranitidine and domperidone maleate in the short term treatment of reflux esophagitis. *Drugs EXP Clin Res 11,* 687-92.

Mason, R. (1997, March). A new intoluminal esophageal reflux procedure in baboons. *Gastrointestinal Endoscopy 45*(3) .

Mathews, J., Maher, K. & Cattau, E. Jr (1990). The role of endoscopic retrograde cholangiopancreatography injection training sessions for the gastroenterology nurse and associate. In Trivits, S. (Ed.), *Journal Reprints II,* Rochester, NY: Society of Gastroenterology Nurses and Associates.

Matsumoto, A (1994). Viral and host factors that contribute to efficacy of interferon-alpha 2a therapy in patients with chronic hepatitis C. *Dig Dis Sci 39,* 1273-80.

Matthews, J., Maher, K., & Cattau, E. Jr. (1990). The role of endoscopic retrograde cholangiopancreatography injection training sessions for the gastroenterology nurse and associate. In Trivits, S. (Ed.) *SGA Journal Reprints II,* Rochester, NY: Society of Gastroenterology Nurses and Associates.

Mattsson, L. (1991). Antibodies to recombinant and synthetic peptides derived from the hepatitis C virus genome in long-term-studied patients with posttransfusion hepatitis C. *Scandanavian Journal of Gastroenterol 26,* 1257-62.

Mattsson, L., Weiland, O. & Glaumann, H. (1988). Long-term follow-up of chronic post-transfusion non-A, non-B hepatitis: clinical and histological outcome. *Liver 8,* 184-8.

McAloose, B. & Gruber, M. (1990). SGNA standards of practice for gastroenterology nurses and associates. *Gastroenterol Nurs 12,* 229-31.

McDonald, D. (1986). Nurses on ethical teams—expanding their decision-making role. *AORN J 44,* 83-5. Association of Operating Room Nurses.

McGregor, P. (1987). Developing a patient questionnaire. *SGA J 10,* 50-1. Society of Gastrointestinal Assistants Journal.

McGregor, P. (1988). Your patient's escort: teaching the significant other. *SGA J 10,* 234-5.

Meenan, J., Rauws, E. & Huibretse, K. (1996). Benign biliary strictures and sclerosing cholangitis. *Gastrointest Endosc Clin North Am 6(1),* 127-38.

Messner, R. (1988). Infection control in total parenteral nutrition. In Trivits, S. (Ed.), *SGA Journal Reprints,* Rochester NY: Society of Gastrointestinal Assistants.

Mikels, C. (1988). Patient education guidelines. *SGA J 11,* 43-4. Society of Gastrointestinal Assistants Journal.

Mikels, C. (1989). Patient education for enhancement of compliance. *Gastroenterol Nurs 12,* 60-2.

Miller, L. (1988). Endoscopic stent placement: a nursing perspective. In Trivits, S. (Ed.), *SGA Journal Reprints,* Rochester, NY: Society of Gastrointestinal Assistants.

Mills, A. (1989). Pancreatitis: disruption in structure and function. *Gastroenterol Nurs 12,* 63-5.

Mita, E. (1994). Predicting interferon therapy efficacy from hepatitis C virus genotype and RNA titer. *Dig Dis Sci 39,* 977-82.

Monroe, D. (1990). Patient teaching for x-ray and other diagnostics. *RN 53,* 52-6.

Morse, T. (2000, May). *Presenting the core complications and emergencies.* Presented at the 27th Annual Meeting of the Society of Gastroenterology Nurses and Associates.

Nahara, H. (2000, December). Effectiveness of endoscopic mucosal resection with submucosal saline injection technique for superficial squamous carcinomas of the esophagus. *Gastrointestinal Endoscopy 52*(6)

National Digestive Diseases Information Clearinghouse (2002, May 11). *Chronic hepatitis C: current disease management.* [On-line.] Available: http://www.niddk.gov/health.digest/pubs/chrnhepc/chrnhepc.htm.

National Institutes of Health (1994). *NIH consensus statement: Helicobacter pylori in peptic ulcer disease* 1(12), 1-22. Washington, DC: Department of Health and Human Services.

Needlestick Safety and Prevention Act, HR5178, Law 106 430 (2000, November 6). Available: http://www.thomas.loc.gov.

Nelson, D.B., Silvis, S.E. & Ansel, H.J. (1994). Management of a tracheoesophageal fistula with a silicone-covered self-expanding metal stent. *Gastrointest Endosc 40(4),* 497-99.

Neuhaus, H. & Zillinger, C. (1998). Randomized Study of intracorporeal laser lithotripsy versus extracorporeal shock-wave lithotripsy for difficult bile duct stones. *Gastrointestinal Endoscopy 47,* 327.

Neuhaus, H. (1991). Metal esophageal stents. *Semin Interven Radiol 8(4),* 305-10.

Nostrant, T.T. (1995). Esophageal dilatation. *Digest Dis 13,* 337-55. Oakbrook Terrace, IL: Author.

Occupational Safety & Health Administration (2001). *Compliance Directive: Bloodborne Pathogens Standard* [On-line]. Available: http://www.needle-stick-syringe-injury.com/pgs/needle-stick-osha.html.

Odom, J. (2000, May). *Wink, Blink, and a Nod: A tale of Conscious Sedation*. Presented at the 27th Annual Meeting of the Society of Gastroenterology Nurses and Associates, Chicago, Illinois.

O'Donoghue, J. (1995). Adjunctive endoscopic brush cytology in the detection of upper gastrointestinal malignancy. *Int Acad Cytol 39*(1), 28-34.

Ogilvie, J. (1995). Botulinum toxin: a new therapeutic use. *Gastroenterol Nurs 18(3)*, 92-95.

Omari, T., Miki, K. & Fraser, R. (1995). Esophageal body and lower esophageal sphincter function in healthy premature infants. *Gastroenterology 109*, 1757-64.

Ord, B. (1990). Communication: care plan sharing. *Nurs Times 86,* 40-1.

Osmond, D.H. (1993). Risk factors for hepatitis C virus seropositivity in heterosexual couples, *JAMA 269,* 361-5.

Palmer, K.R. & Choudari, C.P. (1995). Endoscopic intervention in bleeding peptic ulcer. *Gut 37*, 161-4.

Palmieri, M. (1988). Pathophysiology of the pancreas. In Trivits, S. (Ed.) *SGA Journal Reprints,* Rochester, NY, Society of Gastrointestinal Assistants.

Pashankar, D.S. & Bishop, W.P. (2001, September). Efficacy and optimal dose of daily polyethylene glycol 3350 for treatment of constipation and encopresis in children. *JPediatrc 139*(3), 428-32.

Patterson, P. (1991). Advice for users on Compliances with Devices Act. *OR Manager 7*, 1.

Patterson, P., (Ed.) (1991). Advice for users on compliance with devices act. *OR Manager 7:1,*

Peck, S. & Altschuler, S. (1992). Pseudoobstruction in children. *Gastroenterol Nurs 14(4),* 184-8.

Pennazio, M. (1995). Clinical evaluation of push-type enteroscopy. *Endoscopy 27,* 164-70.

Peters, J. (1996). Laparoscopic surgery for the treatment of gastroesophageal reflux disease (article 2 in the series). *Pract Gastroenterol 20(3),* 8.

Peterson, W.L. (1991). Helicobacter pylori and peptic ulcer disease. *N Engl J Med 324,* 1043-8.

Pezzi, J.S. & Shiau, Y. (1995). Helicobacter pylori and gastrointestinal disease. *Am Fam Physician 52,* 1717-25.

Phaosawasdi, K. (1988). Cryptosporidiosis in the immunocompetent host: a case report and an examination of an increasingly important parasite. *SGA J 11,* 80-4.

Plumeri, P.A. (1990). Informed consent for endoscopy. In Trivits, S. (Ed.), *Journal Reprints II,* Rochester, NY: Society of Gastroenterology Nurses and Associates.

Poley, G. & Slater, J. (2000, September). Current reviews of allergy and clinical immunology. *J Allergy Clin Immunology 106(3),* 585-90.

Price, A. & Price, B. (2000). Problem-Based Learning In Clinical Practice Facilitating Critical Thinking. *Journal for Nursing in Staff Development 6:6,* 66-68.

Rayhorn, N. (1992). Colonoscopy and the pediatric patient. *Gastroenterol Nurs 15(1),* 18-22.

Redmond, M. (1996). Latex allergy: recognition and perioperative management. *Post Anesth Nurs 2,* 6-12.

Reeder, J. (1989). Secure the future: a model for an international nursing ethic. *AORN J 50,* 1298-1307.

Robinson, M. & Garnett, W. (1996). Marketing heartburn relief: evolution in the treatment of heartburn and gastroesophageal reflux disease and its impact on patients and physicians. *Pract Gastroenterol 20(8),* 36-42.

Rosch Endoscopy paper on 1001 cases of CP

Rothbaum, R. (1996). Complications of pediatric endoscopy. *Gastroendosc Clin North Am 6,* 445-9.

Rothenberg, S.S. (1998). Experience with 220 consecutive laparoscopic Nissen fundoplications in infants and children. *J Pediatric Surgery 33,* 274-8. Journal of Pediatric Surgery.

Rutala, W. A. (1996). APIC guideline for selection and use of disinfectants. *American Journal of Infection Control 24,* 45-7.

Rutala, W. A., Clontz, E.P., Weber, D.J. & Hoffman, K. K. (1991). Disinfection practice for endoscopes and other semi-critical items. *Infection Control Hosp Epidemiol 12,* 282-8.

Ryan, E.T. (1992). Hirschsprung's disease: associated abnormalities and demography. *J Pediatr Surg 27(1),* 76-81. Journal of Pediatric Surgery.

Saunderlin, G. (1996, May 20). *Small bowel enteroscopy*. Paper presented at the Twenty-Third Annual Course of the Society of Gastroenterology Nurses and Associates, Las Vegas, NV.

Schapiro, G. & Edmundowicz, S. (1996). Complications of percutaneous endoscopic gastrostomy. *Gastrointest Endosc Clin North Am 6,* 409-22.

Schapiro, M. (1989). The gastroenterologist and the treatment of hemorrhoids: is it about time? *Am J Gastroenterol 84,* 493-5.

Schmelzer, M. & Wright, K.B. (1996). Enema administration techniques used by experienced registered nurses. *Gastroenterol Nurs 19,* 171.

Schmelzer, M. (2001). Understanding the research methodology: should we trust the researchers' conclusions? *Gastroenterol Nurs 23,* 269.

Seeff, L.B. (1992). Long term mortality after transfusion-associated non-A, non-B hepatitis: The National Heart, Lung, and Blood Institute Study Group. *N Engl J Med 327,* 1906-11.

Shaffer, F. (1988). Nursing care plan for fiberoptic procedures. *SGA J 11,* 124-5.

Shah, J. (2002). *MEDLINEplus Medical Encyclopedia: Liver biopsy, VeriMEd Healthcare Network.*: A.D.A.A., Inc.

Shah, J. (DATE). *Updater MEDLINEplus Medical Encyclopedia: Small bowel biopsy, VeriMEd Healthcare Network.*: A.D.A.M., Inc.

Sharma, V.K. & Howden, C.W. (1999). Meta-analysis of randomized controlled trials of ERCP and endoscopic sphincterotomy for the treatment of acute biliary pancreatitis. *American Journal of Gastroenterology 94,* 3211-4.

Sheck, P. (1988). GI assistant's role in laser therapy. In Trivits, S.(Ed.), *SGA Journal Reprints.* Rochester, NY: Society of Gastrointestinal Assistants.

Shields, N. (1987). The role of professional organizations in the practice of GI nursing, *SGA J 10,* 112-113. Williams & Wilkins.

Shields, N. (1988). The role of the GIA in electrosurgery. In Trivits, S.(Ed.), *SGA Journal Reprints.* Rochester, NY: Society of Gastrointestinal Assistants.

Shields, N. (1990). Endoscopic retrograde sphincterotomy: special challenge for the GIA. In Trivits, S.(Ed.), *Journal Reprints II,* Rochester, NY: Society of Gastroenterology Nurses and Associates, Inc.

Short, N. (1989). Gastrointestinal intubations: nursing considerations. *Gastroenterol Nurs 12,* 43-9.

Shumaker, D., deGarmo, P. & Faigel, D. (2002, September). Potential impact of preoperative EUS on esophageal cancer management and cost. *Gastrointestinal Endoscopy 56(3)*

Sievert, W. (2002). Management issues in chronic viral hepatitis: hepatitis C. *J Gastroenterol Hepatol 17,* 415-22.

Smith, J.M. (2002). Alert! New revisions to HIPPA privacy rules. *Journal of the National Medical Association May: 94(5),* 285-6.

Sol, A.H. (1996). Medical treatment of peptic ulcer disease: practice guidelines. *JAMA 275,* 622-9.

Solberg, L.I., Brekke, M.L., Kottke, T.E. & Steel, R.P. (1998). Continuous Quality Improvement in Primary Care: What's Happening? *Medical Care 36(5):* 625-35.

Squires, R.H. & Colleti, R.B. (1996). Indications for pediatric gastrointestinal endoscopy: A medical position statement of the North American Society for Pediatric Gastroenterology and Nutrition. *Journal of Pediatric Gastroenterology Nursing. 23,* 107 -10.

Stachner, G., Kiss, A. & Wiesnagrotzki, S. (1986). Oesophageal and gastric motility disorders in patients categorized as having primary anorexia nervosa, *Gut 27,* 1120-6.

Stephens Scientific, a Division of Richard-Allen Scientific (1996). *Material Safety Data Sheet (MSDS): Formaldehyde 4% Solution.* Kalamazoo, Michigan.

Stone, J. & Schluterman, S. (1996, March/April). GI Nurses' Retrospective Look at Foreign Body Ingestions in Children. *Gastroenterology Nursing 19,* 70-1.

Surana, R., Quinn, F.M.J. & Puri, P. (1994). Short-gut syndrome: Intestinal adaptation in a patient with 12 cm of jejunum. *J Pediatr Gastroenterol Nutr. 19,* 246-9.

Swartz, M. (1989). Beyond the scope: a nursing view of the extraintestinal manifestations of inflammatory bowel disease. *Gastroenterol Nurs 12,* 172-8.

Swartz, M. (1990). Cytotec (misoprostol). *Gastroenterol Nurs 13,* 37-9.

Swartz, M. (1990). Losec (omeprazole/MSD). *Gastroenterol Nurs 12,* 274-6.

Swartz, M., Carey, K. & Danzi, J. (1989). Laser therapy of the gastric lesions of the Osler-Weber-Rendu syndrome, *SGA J 12,* 143-4.

Takahashi, M. (1993). Natural course of chronic hepatitis C. *Am J Gastroenterol 88,* 240-3.

Tanner, C. (2000, November). Critical Thinking: Beyond Nursing Process. *Nursing Education 39:8,* 33-

Tealey, A.R. (1994). Percutaneous endoscopic gastrostomy in the elderly. *Gastroenterol Nurs 16,* 151.

Telford, J., Farrell, J., Saltzman, J., Shields, S., Banks, P., Lichtenstein, D., Johannes, R., Kelsey, P. & Carr-Locke, D.L., (2002). Pancreatic stent placement for duct disruption. *Gastrointestinal Endoscopy 56,* 18-24.

Tham, T.C.K., Lichtenstein, D.R., Vandervoort, J., Wong, R.C.K., Slivka, A., Banks, P.A., Yim, H.B. & Carr-Locke, D.L. (2000, April). Pancreatic Duct Stents for "Obstructive Type" Pain in Pancreatic Malignancy. *The American Journal of Gastroenterology. 95,* 956-60.

Thampanitchawong, P. & Piratvisuth, T. (1995). *Liver biopsy: complications and risk factors.* World J. *Gastroenterology 5*(4), 301-4. World Journal of Gastroenterology.

Thome, S.E., Radford, M.J. & Armstrong, E. (1997). Long-term gastrostomy in children: caregiver coping. *Gastroenterol Nurs 20,* 46.

Thompson, G. (1997). Ways of avoiding latex allergy. *Community Nurse 3,* 2, 33-4.

Thurlow, J. (1989). Informed consent: every patient's right. *Gastroenterol Nurs 12,* 132-4.

Tinstman, C. (1995). Understanding the role of the Institutional Review Board. *Gastroenterol Nurs 18,* 153.

Tint, G.S. & Salen, G. (1982). Ursodeoxycholic acid: A safe and effective agent for dissolving gallstones. *Ann Internal Medical 97,* 351.

Toouli, J., Brooke-Smith, M., Bassi, C., Carr-Locke, D.L., Telford, Freeny, P., Imrie, C. & Tandon, R. (2002). Working Party Report from the 2002 World Congresses of Gastroenterology: Guidelines for the Management of Acute Pancreatitis. *Journal of Gastroenterology and Hepatology 17 (Suppl.),* 15-39.

Torbey, C. & Richter, J. (1995). Gastrointestinal motility disorders in pregnancy. *Semin Gastrointest Dis 6*(4), 203-16.

Tovar, J.A., Olivares, P., Diaz, M., Pace, R.A., Prieto, G. & Molina M. (1998). Functional results of laparoscopic fundoplication I children. *Journal of Pediatric Gastroenterology Nursing 26,* 429-31.

Tremolada, F. (1992). Long-term follow-up of non-A, non-B (type C) post-transfusion hepatitis. *J Hepatol 16,* 273-81.

Tsubota, A. (1993). Factors useful in predicting the response to interferon therapy in chronic hepatitis C. *J Gastroenterol Hepatol 8,* 535-9.

Tsubota, A. (1994). Factors predictive of response to interferon-alpha therapy in hepatitis C virus infection. *Hepatology 19,* 1088-94.

U.S. Veterans Affairs (2002, November 17). *Treatment Recommendations for Patients with Chronic Hepatitis C 2002* (version 1.0). [On-line.] Available: http://www.va.gov/hepatitisc.

Ulrich Chemical, Inc. (1997). *Material Safety Data Sheet (MSDS): Isopropyl Alcohol 70%.* Indianapolis, Indiana: Author.

Vilmann, P. (1994). Endoscopic ultrasonography-guided fine-needle aspiration biopsy of lesions in the upper gastrointestinal tract. *Gastrointest Endosc 41*(3), 230-5.

Wai, D.M. (Ed.) (2001). A Guide to Caring for your Latex Allergic Patient. *Gastroenterology Nursing 22:6,* 262-5.

Walina, C. (1988). Occupational Hazards in the Endoscopy Suite. *SGA Journal 11,* 100-5.

Wallace, M.R. & Oldfield, E.C (2001, September). The role of antibiotics in the treatment of infectious diarrhea. *Gastoenterol Clin North Am 30*(3), 817-36.

Walton, M. (1986). *The Deming management method.* New York: Pergee Books.

Waye, J. (1988). Light in the right lower quadrant during colonoscopy: a comparison of fiberoptic versus video colonoscopes. *SGA J 11,* 157-8.

Waye, J., Kahn, O. & Auerbach, M. (1996). Complications of colonoscopy and flexible sigmoidoscopy. *Gastrointest Endosc Clin North Am 6,* 343-77.

Weaver, L.T., Austin, S. & Cole, T.J. (1991). Small intestinal length: a factor essential for gut adaptation, *GUT 32,* 1321-1523.

Weiner, A.J. (1991). Variable and hypervariable domains are found in the regions of HCV corresponding to the flavivirus envelope and NS1 proteins and the pestivirus envelope glycoproteins. *Virology 180,* 842-8.

Wells, S. (1995). Gastroesophageal reflux: the use of pH monitoring. *Curr Probl Surg 30*(6), 431-558. Current Problems in Surgery.

Wheeler, B. (1988). Crisis intervention. *AORN J 47,* 1242-8.

Whitcomb, D.C. (2000). Genetic predispositions to acute and chronic pancreatitis. *Medical Clinics of North America 84,* 531-47.

Widell, A. (1991). Hepatitis C virus RNA in blood donor sera detected by the polymerase chain reaction: comparison with supplementary hepatitis C antibody assays. *J Med Virol 35,* 253-8.

Wiersema, M. Combined endosonography and fine-needle aspiration cytology in the evaluation of gastrointestinal lesions, *Gastrointest Endosc 40*(2), 199-206.

Wiersema, M.J. (Ed.). (1997). Emerging technologies in gastrointestinal endoscopy. *Gastrointestinal Clinical of North America 7,* 191.

Wiggins, M. & Sesin, P. (1990). Guidelines for administering IV drugs, *Nursing 90*(20), 145-52.

Wilkinson, M.L. (1998). Does laser lithotripsy hit the target? *GUT 43,* 740.

Williams, S. & DiPalma, J. (1990). Constipation in the long-term care facility. *Gastroenterol Nurs 12,* 179-82.

Williams, S. & Westaby, D. (1995). Recent advances in the management of variceal bleeding. *Gut 36,* 647-8.

Wilmore, D.W. (1972). Factors correlating with a successful outcome following extensive intestinal resection in newborn infants. *J Pediatr. 80,* 88-95.

Winchester, C. (1991). A new approach to esophageal varices: endoscopic variceal ligation. *Gastroenterol Nurs 14,* 5-8.

Wong, R.C.K., Carr-Locke, D.L. (1998). Endoscopic stents for palliation in patients with pancreatic cancer. In Reber, E.H. (Ed.), *Pancreatic Cancer.* Totowa, NJ: Humana Press.

Yang, R. & Laine, L. (1995). Mucosal stripping: a complication of push enteroscopy. *Gastrointestinal Endoscopy 41*

Yim, H.B., Jacobson, B.C., Saltzman, J.R., Johannes, R.S., Bounds, B.C., Lee, J.H., Shields, S.J., Ruymann, F.W., Van Dam, J. & Carr-Locke, D.L. (2001). Clinical outcome of the use of enteral stents for palliation of patients with malignant upper GI obstruction. *Gastrointestinal Endoscopy 53,* 329-32..

Young, R.J. (1996). Pediatric constipation: an overview of gastroenterology nursing. *Gastroenterol Nurs 19,* 88-95.

Yu, M. (2002). M2A TM Capsule Endoscopy: A breakthrough diagnostic tool for small intestine imaging. *Gastroenterology Nursing 25,* 1.

Yurko, L.C., Coffee, T. L., Fusilero, J., Yowler, C. J., Brandt, C. & Fratienne, R. B. (2001). Management of an inpatient outpatient clinic: an eight year review. *Journal of Burn Care and Rehabilitation (22),* 250-254.

Zfass, A. & Brennan, P. (1988). Endoscopy of the bowel. In Gitnick, G. & Hollander, D. (Eds.), *Principles and practice of gastroenterology and hepatology.* New York: Elsevier.

Zinberg, S. (1989). A personal experience in comparing three nonoperative techniques for treating internal hemorrhoids. *Am J Gastroenterol 84,* 488 92.

INTERNET

The World Wide Web (WWW), part of the Internet, is the quickest access to resources of all kinds. The Internet is a collection of information of all types stored in computers located throughout the world. After gaining access through a computer Internet browser, you can input a specific address or use a search engine to find the site address you require. Search engines allow you to type a word or words and run searches on those words (see listing of search engines below). The search engine then generates a list of hypertext links to specific addresses called Uniform Resource Locators (URLs). Hypertext links are easily identified because they are usually underlined or a different color than surrounding text. Clicking on a hypertext link allows you to view information presented in the link text.

In addition to online resources, there are a number of print resources available for locating information on the Internet. These include Internet Yellow Pages, Harley Hahn; New Riders' Official World Wide Web Yellow Pages; and World Wide Web Directory, Kris A. Jamsa.

Internet sites

Selected sites on the WWW. Each of these sites will have links to many other sites of interest.

ACG	http://www.acg.gi.org
ASGE	http://www.asge.org
CDC	http://www.cdc.gov
EPA	http://www.epa.gov
FDA	http://www.fda.gov
Gastroenterology Nursing	http://www.wwilkins.com/SGA
JCAHO	http://www.jcaho.org
National Council State Boards of Nursing	http://www.ncsbn.org
National Health Information Center	http://nhic-nt.health.org
National Institute of Nursing Research	http://www.nih.gov/ninr
Nurseweek	http://www.nurseweek.com
Nursing World	http://www.ana.org
Nursing Page	http://www.uwm.edu/people/brodg/ nurspage.htm
SGNA	http://www.sgna.org
Sigma Theta Tau	http://stti-web.iupui.edu
Virtual Hospital	http://vh.org
Yahoo Nursing	http://www.yahoo.com/health/nursing

Internet search engines

Alta Vista
Excite
Google
Hotbot
InfoSeek
Lycos
MSN
Open Text
Webcrawler
Yahoo

LIBRARIES

Hospital and university libraries offer access to nursing and medical literature, journals, computerized databases, and interlibrary loans. Each library will provide instruction on the use of computerized and hard copy databases such as the Cumulative Index to Nursing and Allied Health Literature (CINAHL) and the Medical Literature Analysis and Retrieval System (MEDLARS) (called MEDLINE) on the Internet.

PROFESSIONAL ORGANIZATIONS

Nursing and medical professional organizations offer literature, guidelines, position statements, and other information specific to their members' interests. Most organizations now have a home page on the WWW that provides access to their information, as well as links to other Internet sites of interest.

The following is a listing of some of the organizations; publishers of nursing and medical books, journals, audio/video tapes, computer diskettes/CD-ROMs; and Internet sites of specific interest to the gastroenterology nurse or associate. This is not an all-inclusive listing, and some telephone numbers and Internet sites will change. Many new sites are being generated daily. As you explore and find new interesting sites, contact the SGNA so these can be added to the links provided on the SGNA home page for all gastroenterology nurses and associates.

PUBLICATION CATALOGS

American Nurses Publishing	800-637-0323
Association of Operating Room Nurses	800-755-2676
Lippincott-Raven	800-777-2295
Mosby	800-325-4177
National League for Nursing	800-669-9656
Saunders	800-318-8596
Society of Gastroenterology Nurses and Associates	800-245-SGNA
Springer Publishing	212-431-4370
Springhouse	800-346-7844
Williams & Wilkins	800-882-8532

Journals

Nursing

Advances in Nursing Science
American Journal of Nursing
AORN Journal
Clinical Nurse Specialist
Clinical Nursing Research
Gastroenterology Nursing
Image: Journal of Nursing Scholarship
Journal of Advanced Nursing
Journal of Intravenous Nursing
Journal of PeriAnesthesia Nursing
Nursing 98
Nursing Clinics of North America
Nursing Economic$
Nursing Management
Nursing Outlook
Nursing Research
Nursing Science Quarterly
Nursing Times
OR Manager
Pediatric Nursing
RN
Today's OR Nurse

Medical

American Journal of Gastroenterology
Annals of Internal Medicine
Digestive Diseases and Sciences
Endoscopy Review
Gastroenterology
Gastroenterology Clinics of North America
Gastroenterology and Endoscopy News
Gastrointestinal Endoscopy
GUT
Hepatology
JAMA
Journal of Gastroenterology and Hepatology
Journal of Pediatric Gastroenterology and Nutrition
Lancet
New England Journal of Medicine
Seminars in Liver Disease
Transplantation

Healthcare

American Journal of Infection Control
Health Devices
Infection Control and Hospital Epidemiology
Infection Control and Sterilization Technology
Journal of Healthcare Material Management

INDEX